Radiology of Infectious and Inflammatory Diseases - Volume 5

Hongjun Li • Shinong Pan • Jun Zhou
Editors

Radiology of Infectious and Inflammatory Diseases - Volume 5

Musculoskeletal system

Science Press
Beijing

Springer

Editors
Hongjun Li
Beijing Youan Hospital
Beijing, China

Shinong Pan
Department of Radiology
Shengjing Hospital of China Medical University
Shenyang, Liaoning, China

Jun Zhou
Department of Radiology
The Fourth People's Hospital of Shenyang
Shenyang, Liaoning, China

ISBN 978-981-16-5002-4　　ISBN 978-981-16-5003-1　(eBook)
https://doi.org/10.1007/978-981-16-5003-1

Jointly published with Science Press
The print edition is not for sale in China (Mainland). Customers from China (Mainland) please order the print book from: Science Press.

This Springer imprint is published by the registered company Springer Nature Singapore Pte Ltd.
The registered company address is: 152 Beach Road, #21-01/04 Gateway East, Singapore 189721, Singapore

Preface I

Amidst the rapid development of society and economy, people's lifestyles and population mobility have changed, resulting in that the impact on the survival of mankind and social economic growth by infection and inflammatory diseases is ever-growing. The document issued by the National Health Commission stresses that all the hospitals at level II and above need to set up an infectious diseases department and an infection control office, to attach the greatest importance to the hazards of infectious diseases on human health. During the past 30 years, the development of medical imaging diagnosis and treatment technologies has greatly boosted the improvement on diagnosis and treatment modes in modern times. Since the modern medicine is highly dependent on medical imaging technologies, the medical imaging is granted an important mission in diagnosis and differential diagnosis of infection and inflammatory diseases.

During long-term clinical practices and scientific researches, my team and I realized that due to the neglect and lack of construction for key discipline system of infection and inflammatory diseases as well as researches on related theory system and specification guidance, the quality and effectiveness of the diagnosis and treatment provided for patients have been seriously affected, resulting in the abuse of clinical antibiotics, thus compromising patients' health and quality of life and increasing the economic burden on family and society. Based on the above considerations, the Book gathers a number of experts and scholars from the Infectious Diseases Group of the Chinese Association of Radiology, Infection Imaging Professional Committee of the Chinese Medical Doctor Association Radiological Branch, Professional Committee on Radiology of Infection and Inflammation of the Chinese Research Hospital Association, Working Committee on Infection (Infectious Disease) Imaging of Chinese Association of STD and AIDS Prevention and Control; Infectious Disease Imaging Group of Avocation of Infections Disease Hospital and Beijing Imaging Diagnosis and Treatment Technology Innovation Alliance. Clinical resources associated with infection and inflammatory diseases across the nation are integrated and the imaging characteristics and evolution rules of infection and inflammatory disease are summarized herein. Meanwhile, this book has revealed the pathological basis of infections and inflammatory diseases and put forward the essential points of imaging diagnosis and differential diagnosis of infectious and inflammatory diseases. It is believed that the publication of this series of monographs will boost the academic development of infections and inflammatory diseases in terms of prevention and control, rational drug use, and radiological diagnosis in China, and effectively serve the accurate clinical diagnosis and treatment.

This series of books systematically introduces the theory of the radiology of infection and inflammation for the first time. Divided into six volumes (Brain and Spinal Cord, Head and Neck, Heart and Chest, Abdomen and Pelvis, Skeletal Muscle, and Children), it covers four types of pathogens related to infectious diseases (bacteria, fungi, viruses, and parasites) and inflammatory diseases such as autoimmune diseases.

This series of books has three features: ① It is closely related to clinical practice, introduces almost all the types of diseases concerning, and encompasses clinically common, multiple, and rare infections and inflammatory diseases; ② In addition to sharing complete data, this series also focuses on providing an objective basis for diagnosis, especially the integrity, representativeness, continuity, and authenticity of cases and images involved; and ③ The editors, by virtue of their accumulated clinical experience and practice, contribute most of the data, and some materials adopted herein have been authorized by international peers. By absorbing and quoting the latest research results at home and abroad, this series of books brings readers a refreshing feel both in compilation form and contents.

An advisory committee and an expert committee are specially established to ensure the smooth publication of this series of books while upholding the principle of "scientific design and systematic demonstration." It took more than one year to accomplish the compilation from designing the outline to revising the final version. While the Chinese version is published at home, the English one will be simultaneously released by the publisher Springer. The editorial board put a high premium on the compilation of this series and organized several activities for the members of the domestic editorial board, such as training on standardized writing, and instruction in the professional review and finalization of drafts. In the meantime, the editorial board also assigned specific personnel to engage in the review, revision, and supplement. As the editor-in-chief, I would like to express my cordial thanks for their unremitting efforts. Unfeigned gratitude is also extended to the members of the National Infectious Disease Imaging Group who devoted themselves to the compilation of this book.

Facing the severe situation of prevention and treatment of infections and inflammatory diseases, this series of monographs will serve as another powerful tool fighting against infections and inflammatory diseases and play an essential role in raising the physicians' level of diagnosis and treatment, improving patients' quality of life and prolonging their lives.

During the process of scientific development, our knowledge and understanding are being perfected as well, where errors are also inevitable. We sincerely welcome your criticisms and suggestions and seek further improvement.

Beijing, China Hongjun Li
November 2019

The original version of this chapter was revised by modifying the affiliation of editors in the copy right page and by modifying the affiliation of associate editors and contributors under the section 'Editors and contributors' in front matter. Their affiliation is also modified accordingly in the chapters they have contributed. The correction to this book is available at https://doi.org/10.1007/978-981-16-5003-1_10

Preface II

The *Radiology of Infection and Inflammation* is a series of academic monographs led by Professor Hongjun Li and elaborately compiled by experts experienced in imaging diagnosis, teaching, and clinical diagnosis and treatment of infections and inflammatory diseases across the country. The series is divided into six volumes: Brain and Spinal Cord, Head and Neck, Heart and Chest, Abdomen and Pelvis, Skeletal Muscle, and Children. Informative and illustrated, it is a novel academic monograph, with rich content both in breadth and depth.

The *Radiology of Infection and Inflammation: Skeletal Muscle* is approximately 550,000 words in length and contains more than 600 illustrations. In addition to the clinically common infectious diseases of bones and joints, this book also gives a detailed introduction to the bone and joint infection in children, AIDS-related musculoskeletal infection, and other diseases. During the process of compilation, each editor has integrated relevant knowledge of the epidemic disease, microbiology, pathology, physiology, clinical medicine, imaging, and other disciplines in combination with their own clinical experience, in order to provide both the clinical and imaging practitioners with a systematic and comprehensive reference book on infections and inflammatory diseases. In terms of the imaging diagnosis of each disease, the book systematically summarizes the evolution of the disease and its imaging characteristics of different periods. The complete and consecutive images of each case are helpful for readers to sort out the essential points of diagnosis in the evolution of each disease. In terms of research status and progress, this book gives an additional introduction to the new imaging examination techniques in recent years and their application value and prospect. It is believed that this book will not only be a crucial reference book for practitioners in medical imaging, but also an intellectual mentor for clinicians. It will also be a worthy collection for medical students and graduates.

It is hereby expressed the appreciation for all the editors' hard work and dedication. Special gratitude is also extended to peers who provided the rare case images for this book. While we strive to provide comprehensive, detailed, and profound contents with an easy-to-understand approach, there remain some shortcomings and omissions in this book due to the editors' limited knowledge. Please do not hesitate to give your criticisms and suggestions, in order to produce a better second edition.

Shenyang, China — Shinong Pan
November 2019

Preface III

Infection is a clinically common local or systemic inflammatory response caused by the invasion of pathogens. It is mainly manifested as fever, pain, dysfunction, rash, vomiting, fatigue, etc. Severe cases may present sepsis. Some infections are contagious and some pathogen infections may be fatal. The infectious diseases of the musculoskeletal system, featured by complex and changeable nature, involve various organs and sites. In serious cases, they may be life-threatening. It is hard to make an early diagnosis and quantitive diagnosis for infectious diseases of the musculoskeletal system. Even for the musculoskeletal infection with a definite diagnosis, it is also tough to perform an imaging analysis and provide clear and efficient diagnosis and treatment information due to the difficulty in treating chronic diseases. With the development of new imaging techniques, imaging has been more widely used in diseases of the musculoskeletal system. At present, the number of patients with musculoskeletal infections is increasing, and great changes occur, which poses a substantial challenge to the multi-modal diagnosis and analysis of musculoskeletal imaging. Nonetheless, it also provides us with a new basis for diagnosis.

The *Radiology of Infection and Inflammation: Skeletal Muscle* is a specialist monograph on the imaging diagnosis of infection of skeletal muscles, approximately 550,000 words in length and containing more than 600 illustrations. Divided into nine chapters, it covers a general introduction to the infection of skeletal muscles, infectious lesions of bones and joints, spinal infection, bone and joint infection in children, AIDS-related musculoskeletal infection, soft tissue infection, and lesions of bones and joints associated with rheumatic disease. This book discusses and analyzes each disease from the aspects of overview, pathophysiology, imaging findings, essential points of diagnosis, differential diagnosis, research status, and progress. It is an optimal learning material for physicians working in the fields of imaging and clinical medicine.

This book is replete with the many years of the editors' clinical experience. Special gratitude is extended to peers who provided the case images for this book; some of these cases are very special, and their images are both valuable and rare. While the editors have all spared no effort in compiling this book, there remain shortcomings due to the variety of diseases involved, the short time of editing, and the limited capacity of the editors. We sincerely welcome your criticisms and suggestions.

Shenyang, China
December 2019

Jun Zhou

Introduction

The Book integrates multidisciplinary contents including pathology, physiology, microbiology, clinical work, and imaging of skeletal muscle systemic infection and inflammatory diseases. Divided into 9 chapters, the Book involves infectious lesions of bones and joints, spinal infection, bone and joint infection in children, AIDS-related musculoskeletal infection, soft tissue infection, and lesions of bones and joints associated with rheumatism. All the lesions are discussed and analyzed in terms of overview, pathophysiology, imaging findings, essential points of diagnosis, differential diagnosis, research status and progress, with up-to-date imaging examination techniques added.

The Book strives to be comprehensive and exhaustive, and explains profound theories in simple language. Besides an important reference book for medical imaging workers, it also provides clinicians who work on infection and inflammatory diseases, medical students, and graduate students with useful and valuable guidance.

Contents

About the Editors

Editor-in-Chief

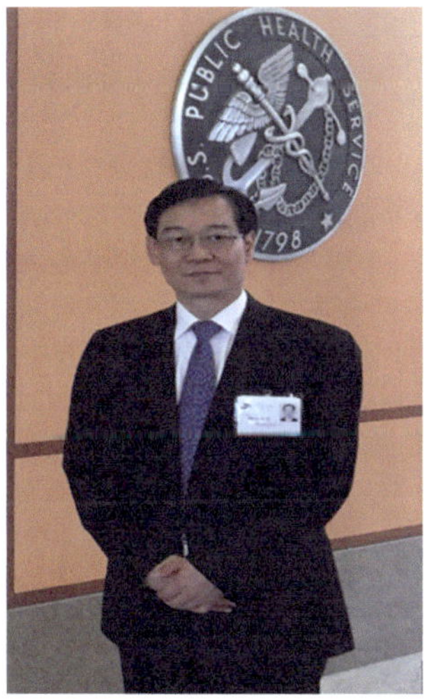

Hongjun Li is a M.D., a professor, a chief physician, and a doctoral supervisor. As one of the returned talents from overseas, he is the specialist in radiology of legal infectious diseases, the founder of the international standard system for the imaging innovation discipline of legal infectious disease, as well as the main pioneer of the theoretical system for medical imaging of legal infectious diseases. He is an expert who enjoys the special government allowance from the State Council and the outstanding contribution expert; He is listed in first batch of Beijing "Ten Hundred Thousand Excellent Health Professionals," and is included in the first batch of academic leader (backbone) of senior health talents in Beijing 215 talent training program (namely, selection of 20 leading talents, 100 academic leaders, and 500 academic backbones). His team has been awarded "Science & Technology Innovation Cultivation Team" by the Beijing Municipal Commission of Health and Family Planning, and awarded "Hongjun Li Science & Technology Innovation Studio" jointly by Beijing Municipal Science and Technology Commission and Beijing Federation of Trade Unions under the signature of science and technology leader. In 2019, Hongjun Li won the titles "Accomplished Teacher for Training an Apprentice" and "People's Doctor." In 2020, Beijing Municipal Science and Technology Commission and Beijing Federation of Trade Unions awarded "Hongjun Li Demonstration Science and Technology Innovation Studio."

Research field: Radiology of infectious diseases.

Present titles: The Director of the Medical Imaging Center of Beijing Youan Hospital, Capital Medical University; the Deputy Director of Medical Imaging Department of Capital Medical University; the Founding Editor-in-Chief of the International English Periodical *Radiology of Infectious Diseases* (under the supervision of the National Health Commission) and the Deputy Chief Editor of *BMC Neurology*.

Outstanding contributions: He has pioneered the creation of innovative disciplines and systematic innovative theoretical systems, technical norms, guidelines, standards, disciplinary systems and diagnostic, treatment, and testing platforms for the imaging of global infectious diseases, broken the academic and application gaps of modern imaging techniques in the field of infectious diseases at home and abroad, and promoted the development of infectious disease prevention, diagnosis, and treatment technologies in China and even in the world.

Concurrent academic posts: Head of Infectious Diseases Group of Radiology Branch under Chinese Medical Association; Chairman of the Infection Imaging Professional Committee of the Chinese Medical Doctor Association Radiological Branch; Chairman of the Professional Committee on Radiology of Infection and Inflammation of the Chinese Research Hospital Association; Chairman of the Working Committee on Infection (Infectious Disease) Imaging of Chinese Association of STD and AIDS Prevention and Control; Chairman of Radiology Professional Committee under the National Health Technology Promotion and Inheritance Application Project; Leader of Infectious Disease Imaging Management Group of Infectious Disease Management Branch under Chinese Hospital Association; Vice Chairman of Evidence-based Medicine Branch under China Association for the Promotion of International Exchanges in Healthcare; Head of Infectious Diseases Group of General Radiological Equipment Professional Committee under China Association of Medical Equipment; President of the Beijing Imaging Diagnosis and Treatment Technology Innovation Alliance; Standing Member of General Radiological Equipment Professional Committee under Chinese Medical Equipment Association; Standing Member of Radiology Branch of Beijing Medical Association; Committee of Chinese Society of Medical Imaging Technology; Deputy Chief Editor of the *New Medicine*; and Editorial Board Member of 12 professional academic journals including *Chinese Medical Journal.*

Hongjun Li has served as the evaluation expert of projects under the National Key Medical Research Center; the evaluation expert of the National Award for Science and Technology Progress; the evaluation expert of Chinese Medical Science and Technology Progress Award; the comprehensive evaluation expert in examination and verification of medical standards of the State Food and Drug Administration; the special review expert of the National Major Infectious Diseases; the special review expert in the major science and technology research and development of the Ministry of Science and Technology; the head of final review group of the China's Major AIDS Projects under the 12th Five-Year Plan; the evaluation expert of projects under the National Natural Science Foundation of China; the evaluation expert of projects under Beijing Municipal Natural Science Foundation; and the evaluation expert of projects supported by China Scholarship Council.

Academic performance: Hongjun Li has been serving as the person in charge of the national science and technology research and development projects of major infectious diseases and key projects of the National Natural Science Foundation of China. He has been a Chinese Most Cited Researcher in the field of infectious disease imaging published by Springer for consecutive years, with top 50% of international medical attention and academic influence (2019). In the past 5 years, he has been approved to preside over scientific research and development special projects for major infectious diseases under the Ministry of Science and Technology, key projects of the National Natural Science Foundation, many projects of national Natural Science Foundation of China, as well as more than 20 projects including those under Beijing Natural Science Foundation, Sail Plan (Radiology of Major Infectious Diseases), and Technology Research and Development Programme. He has published more than 200 core papers and English papers, 62 of which are written in English. He has won 9 provincial and ministerial awards such as the Chinese Medical Science and Technology Award, 2 national invention patents, and 20 intellectual property and software copyright registrations. He has created 1 product of artificial intelligence integrated machine for clinical transformation of infectious diseases with medico engineering cooperation and discipline integration; and he has edited 38 medical monographs, 3 textbooks, 2 guidelines, and 8 standards; The professional original works in English edited by him, including *Atlas of Differential Diagnosis in HIV/AIDS, Radiology of Infectious Diseases 1–2, Radiology of HIV/AIDS, Radiology of Influenza A/H1N1, Radiology of Parasitic Diseases, Radiology of Influenza,* and other 8 works in English, have been published in series by the internationally renowned Springer Nature and PMPH; his representative works of *Radiology of Infectious Diseases 1–2* and *Radiology of HIV/AIDS* had been awarded the annual "Export Excellent Book Award" in 2014 and 2015, respectively, and in 2017, both works were awarded the "Universal Rewards" in respect of copyright by the State Administration of Press and Publication. He has been supported by the National Natural Science Publishing Foundation of China for many times, and several works have been selected as the national key publications of textbooks and reference books and one of the western medicine reference books for "Going Out" Project. In light of the benevolence of the doctor and with no view to selfish gains, I will lead the team to make global contributions to the integrated precise prevention and control of infectious diseases.

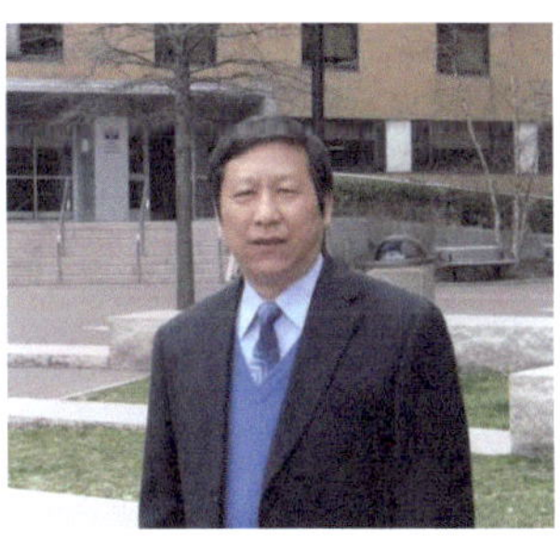

Shinong Pan is a professor and a chief physician of the radiology department of the Shengjing Hospital of China Medical University; a doctoral candidate/postdoctoral supervisor; a member of Radiological Society of North America; a vice leader of bone and joint professional team of the Chinese Society of Radiology; a standing committee member of sport anatomy branch of the Chinese Society for Anatomical Sciences; a standing committee member of the Liaoning Society of Osteoporosis and Bone Mineral Research; a vice chairman of the first sports medicine branch of Shenyang Medical Association; an editorial board member of the *Chinese Journal of Radiology* and *Chinese Journal of Magnetic Resonance Imaging*; and a reviewer of the *Chinese Medical Journal* and *Radiology of Infectious Diseases*.

He has engaged in the first-line imaging diagnosis and teaching for decades and is skilled in analyzing diseases by comprehensive imaging findings, in particular the imaging diagnosis for bones and joints system, facial features, and nervous system. In addition, he has rich experiences in the diagnosis of infectious lesions in bones and joints, tumor lesion, and lesions in bones and joints associated with rheumatism and has prominent attainments on diagnosis and differential diagnosis of complicated bones and joints diseases in children. He has trained more than 50 doctoral and master candidates. In recent years, Shinong Pan has undertaken 7 projects, participated in editing 4 textbooks as an associate editor, and published more than 90 papers.

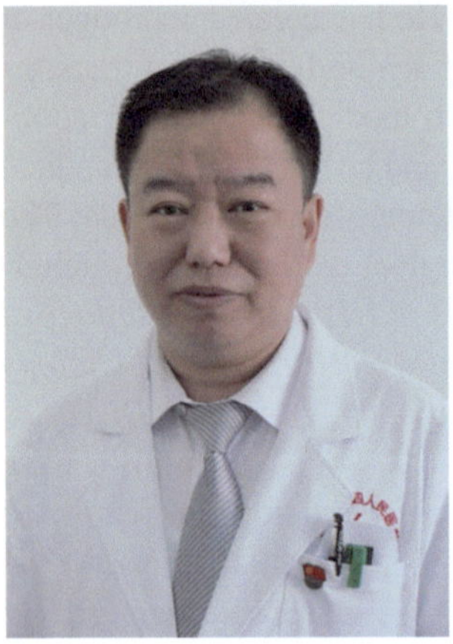

Jun Zhou is a chief physician; a Director of the Radiology Department of The Fourth People's Hospital of Shenyang; a Director of Shenyang Radiodiagnosis Quality Control Center; a Director of the Imaging Center of Remote Consultation Center; a member of infection (infectious diseases) imaging working committee of Chinese Association of STD and AIDS Prevention and Control; a member of Radiology Professional Committee of Osteoporosis Committee of China Gerontological Society; a member of Radiology Branch of Liaoning Medical Association; a member of Imaging Physician Branch of Liaoning Physician Association; a member of Liaoning Medical Image Quality Control Center; a Deputy Chairman of Shenyang Radiology Branch; a council member of Liaoning Medical Imaging Association; and a council member of Foot and Ankle Surgery Branch of Liaoning Society for Cell Biology.

Jun Zhou has engaged in the imaging diagnosis for more than 30 years and is skilled in diagnosing complicated lesions in bones and joints, facial features, and chest and abdomen, with special understanding in bones and joints diseases and orbital diseases. He is adept in diagnosing infectious lesions in bones and joints, and lesions in bones and joints associated with rheumatism, and has accumulated rich experiences in diagnosis and differential diagnosis of orbit diseases by CT and MRI. He edited *Writing Skills for X-ray Diagnosis Report, Writing Skills for CT Diagnosis Report,* and *Writing Skills for MRI Diagnosis Report,* which won the *2016 Excellent Book Award* issued by Shenyang Health and Family Planning Commission.

Editors and Contributors

Associate Editors

Junyan Yang Department of Radiology, The Sixth People's Hospital of Shenyang, Shenyang, Liaoning, China

Hongjun Fu Department of Radiology, The Tenth People's Hospital of Shenyang, Shenyang, Liaoning, China

Rongjie Bai Department of Radiology, Beijing Jishuitan Hospital, Beijing, China

Wei Li Department of Radiology, Shengjing Hospital of China Medical University, Shenyang, Liaoning, China

Dechun Li Department of Radiology, Xuzhou Central Hospital, Xuzhou, Jiangsu, China

Contributors (Ranked by Alphabetical Order of Family Name)

Hui Guo Department of Radiology, The First Affiliated Hospital of Xinjiang Medical University, Ürümqi, Xinjiang, China

Junlin Li Department of Radiology, People's Hospital of Inner Mongolia Autonomous Region, Hohhot, The Inner Mongolia, China

Li Li Department of Radiology, Beijing Youan Hospital, Capital Medical University, Beijing, China

Qi Li Department of Radiology, Liaoning Electric Power Central Hospital, Shenyang, Liaoning, China

Zhen Liu Department of Radiology, Shengjing Hospital of China Medical University, Shenyang, Liaoning, China

Xiaohong Lv Department of Radiology, The First Affiliated Hospital of Jinzhou Medical University, Jinzhou, Liaoning, China

Shi Qi Department of Radiology, Beijing Youan Hospital, Capital Medical University, Beijing, China

Zhanhua Qian Department of Radiology, Beijing Jishuitan Hospital, Beijing, China

Yuan Qu Department of Radiology, The Fourth People's Hospital of Shenyang, Shenyang, Liaoning, China

Jiye Song Department of Radiology, The Sixth People's Hospital of Shenyang, Shenyang, Liaoning, China

Na Su Department of Radiology, The Sixth People's Hospital of Shenyang, Shenyang, Liaoning, China

He Sun Department of Radiology, The Fourth Affiliated Hospital of China Medical University, Shenyang, Liaoning, China

Fengzhe Wang Department of Radiology, The Fourth People's Hospital of Shenyang, Shenyang, Liaoning, China

Ping Wang Department of Radiology, The Tenth People's Hospital of Shenyang, Shenyang, Liaoning, China

Su Wu Department of Radiology, Shengjing Hospital of China Medical University, Shenyang, Liaoning, China

Liwei Xie Department of Radiology, The Tenth People's Hospital of Shenyang, Shenyang, Liaoning, China

Huili Zhan Department of Radiology, Beijing Jishuitan Hospital, Beijing, China

Peng Zhang Department of Radiology, The Sixth People's Hospital of Shenyang, Shenyang, Liaoning, China

Heng Zhao Department of Radiology, The First Affiliated Hospital, Hengyang Medical School, University of South China, Hengyang, Hunan, China

Jing Zhao Department of Radiology, Beijing Youan Hospital, Capital Medical University, Beijing, China

Yuan Zhao Department of Radiology, The First Affiliated Hospital of Xinjiang Medical University, Ürümqi, Xinjiang, China

Wei Zhou Department of Radiology, The General Hospital of Northern Theater Command, Shenyang, Liaoning, China

Part I

General Introduction to Infection of Skeletal Muscles and Inflammatory Diseases

1 Imaging Examination Techniques

Shinong Pan, Yuan Zhao, and Su Wu

The infectious diseases of the musculoskeletal system, featured by complex and changeable nature, involve various organs and sites. In serious cases, they may be life-threatening. It is hard to make an early diagnosis and qualitative diagnosis for infectious diseases of the musculoskeletal system. Even for the musculoskeletal infection with a definite diagnosis, it is also tough to perform an imaging analysis and provide clear, targeted, and accurate diagnosis and treatment information due to the difficulty in treating chronic diseases. In 1895, the German physicist Röntgen discovered X-rays and took the first X-ray film of the human skeleton. The multimodal examination in medical imaging has played an essential role in the diagnosis, treatment, and follow-up of various orthopedic diseases over the last 100 years. Currently, various imaging examination techniques are applied in the musculoskeletal system, including conventional X-ray, CT, MRI, musculoskeletal ultrasound (MSKUS), PET/CT, and molecular imaging [1]. Different imaging methods having their own strengths and limitations. With the development of new imaging techniques, imaging examination has been more widely used in musculoskeletal diseases. Yet, the number of patients with musculoskeletal infection is increasing across the world, and great changes occur, which poses a substantial challenge to the multi-modal diagnosis and analysis of musculoskeletal imaging. This chapter briefly introduces various imaging examination techniques applied in the musculoskeletal system (including their characteristics and differences as well as the development of the new imaging techniques), describes the imaging characteristics of infectious diseases of the musculoskeletal system along with their clinical, bacteriological, and pathological characteristics and changes from the perspectives of bacteriology and pathology, and discusses the analysis strategy and the principle of diagnosis of the disease involved.

S. Pan (✉)
Department of Radiology, Shengjing Hospital of China Medical University, Shenyang, Liaoning, China
e-mail: cjr.panshinong@vip.163.com

Y. Zhao
Department of Radiology, The First Affiliated Hospital of Xinjiang Medical University, Ürümqi, Xinjiang, China

S. Wu
Department of Radiology, Shengjing Hospital of China Medical University, Shenyang, Liaoning, China

1.1 X-Ray Imaging Techniques

1.1.1 General Examination

As the preferred examination method for assessing the diseases of the musculoskeletal system, conventional X-ray plain film can generate a clear image with a high spatial resolution. With this technique, a good contrast of tissues among the fat, muscle, and skeleton can be obtained based on the principle that tissues vary in the absorption of X-ray. With the development of computer and network technology, radiography of most institutes has realized digital acquisition, browsing, and storage. Digital images may encompass various techniques such as image processing, stitching, and measurement. A picture archiving and communication system (PACS) can ensure the comparison and analysis of images obtained in different periods, and also allow for remote radiological diagnosis and real-time consultation. However, in the X-ray examination of the skeletal muscle, the in vitro artifacts and structural overlap may result in missed diagnosis and misdiagnosis. The resolution of the soft tissue structures is greatly limited by the conventional X-ray plain film as the X-ray attenuation of most soft tissue structures is within a very narrow range.

1.1.2 Special Examination

1.1.2.1 Fluoroscopy

The fluoroscopy technique, easy to operate, utilizes X-ray sources (similar to standard radiography) to provide real-time and dynamic video images. Yet, it generates a rela-

H. Li et al. (eds.), *Radiology of Infectious and Inflammatory Diseases - Volume 5*,
https://doi.org/10.1007/978-981-16-5003-1_1

tively high radiation dose. At present, fluoroscopy is often used for fracture reduction, orthopedic intervention, and other operations.

1.1.2.2 Examination of Stress Distribution

Standard radiography is a static evaluation of the structures of the musculoskeletal system. Ligament injury can be indirectly evaluated with the joint imaging under passive or active stress. For example, cervical hyperextension and hyperflexion can provide valuable information about the stability of the atlantoaxial joints [2].

1.1.2.3 Arthrography

Arthrography refers to an imaging technique that displays the normal anatomic structures and pathological changes in the joints by injecting a radiopaque contrast agent into the articular cavity under the guidance of fluoroscopy or ultrasound. A dynamic evaluation is performed with fluoroscopy. With the injection of local anesthetic drugs, arthrography provides diagnostic information to patients with suspicious joint lesions, which helps to make a definite diagnosis of the disease. With the advent of CT images that provide detailed and direct information about the joint structure, arthrography is now often used in combination with MRI.

1.1.2.4 Tomosynthesis

Tomosynthesis represents a conventional X-ray that has been modified. It is a multi-slice and low-dose imaging where the body position is projected by X-ray bulb tubes placed at different angles. At present, mammography is generally mature, and the application of digital tomography in the musculoskeletal system and other sectors is also expanding. According to the preliminary studies, the metal artifacts generated with tomography are smaller than those produced by CT. Moreover, it is well applied in the imaging of the orthopedic prosthesis, which lessens the diagnostic difficulties caused by superimposed images in traditional X-ray examination [2].

1.2 CT Imaging Techniques

1.2.1 Conventional CT

Thanks to the invention and application of computed tomography (CT), modern medical imaging has achieved leapfrog development. CT is featured by the acquisition of an image at the transverse plane and high spatial resolution. Among all the imaging techniques, CT shows the optimal performance in presenting the details of the skeletons. Compared with the traditional X-ray examination, CT can be used to detect inflammatory changes in the musculoskeletal system earlier and better evaluate the details of skeletons, which makes it a better imaging approach in diagnosing the inflammatory changes in the musculoskeletal system. Additionally, CT can be used to assess the soft tissues around the bone lesions. After decades of technical improvement and exploration, remarkable progress has been made in CT, from single axial scan to helical scan based on slip-ring technique, from single-row detector array to multi-row detector array, and from single axial image to volume data. Besides, isotropic and arbitrarily oriented imaging reconstruction has also been accomplished in CT. At present, CT has entered the era of three dimensions. By virtue of 3D reconstruction, an orthopedist can have a better understanding of the lesions and develop a more targeted surgical treatment plan, thus improving the diagnostic rate and operation success rate. However, due to limited ability in distinguishing soft tissues, CT is limited in some aspects. For example, it is less sensitive and specific than MRI in showing the lesions at the early stage of the musculoskeletal infection and medullary lesions.

1.2.2 Progress and Improvement of CT

Most progress of the modern CT is made by decreasing the radiation dose while ensuring image quality. For instance, many hospitals use low-dose CT to replace the X-ray plain film of the skeleton (a scan from head to knee) in patients with multiple myeloma. Various techniques such as multiplane image acquisition and iterative reconstruction have been widely used.

1. **Dual-energy CT.** Dual-energy CT allows for the synchronous acquisition of images at different energy levels by two X-ray bulb tubes placed at an angle of 90° and their respective detectors. It can show the bone contusion caused by bone marrow changes after trauma which the traditional CT cannot display.
2. **Energy spectrum CT metal artifacts reduction system (MARs).** An energy spectrum MARs can provide accurate projection data of the metal and its surrounding tissues and effectively suppress the common metal artifacts. Energy spectrum CT single energy image can be used to remove the common beam hardening artifacts. With this technique, a good imaging effect can be achieved in the re-examination of metal implants of bone and bone joints, especially in the evaluation of bone infection after the implantation of metal, which once being a tough problem. As a result, the energy spectrum CT can provide effective information for clinical diagnosis [2].

1.3 MR Imaging Techniques

Magnetic resonance imaging (MRI) is a revolution in medical imaging. It is different from the X-ray technique and is based on the principle that the attenuation of the released energy varies in different structure environments within the substance. MRI detects the electromagnetic wave emitted by the external gradient magnetic field and then obtains the images with diagnostic value via image post-processing. MRI, featured by high spatial resolution and tissue resolution, can not only clearly show muscles, cartilage, tendons, and ligaments but also reflect the pathophysiological changes of the disease at the molecular level. It fundamentally changes the imaging of skeletal muscle structures, with rapid changes in application in bone imaging and great potentials for further development.

As MRI can evaluate the condition of the skeleton and its surrounding soft tissues, it becomes the preferred examination method for most infections of skeleton muscles. If the bone marrow is normal on all pulse sequences, then osteomyelitis can be excluded by MRI with a 100% negative predictive value. It can be used to detect acute osteomyelitis at an early stage of the disease. Intravenous injection of the gadolinium contrast agents can be used to identify soft-tissue abscesses and sinus, distinguish the degree of synovial thickening, and evaluate spinal infections. At present, high-field-strength MRI has been applied in clinical practice, which further improves the resolution of MRI images and increases the accuracy of display in anatomical details and lesions. With the development of functional MRI and MRI spectrum, medical imaging has entered the field of functional imaging research.

1.3.1 Conventional Sequences

In the MRI examination of the musculoskeletal system, the conventional sequences include T_1 weighted image (T_1WI), T_2 weighted image (T_2WI), fat-suppressed sequence, and proton density-weighted image (PDWI). T_1WI reflects the difference of *T_1 value* among the tissues; T_2WI reflects the difference of *T_2 value* among the tissues; PDWI reflects the difference of proton density and relaxation time among the tissues. Normal adipose tissues appear hyperintense in both T_1WI and fast spin echo (FSE) T_2WI [3]. The use of a short time inversion recovery (STIR) or a fat-saturated T_2-weighted sequence (FS-T_2WI) can uniformly reduce the intensity of fat signals and highlight the focus of the musculoskeletal system. Since T_1 value, T_2 value, and proton density and relaxation time vary in different tissues or lesions, the signal intensity is different in T_1WI, T_2WI, and PDWI, showing different gray levels. MRI is used to diagnose diseases based on the changes of different gray levels.

1.3.2 Diffusion-Weighted Imaging

Diffusion-weighted imaging (DWI) reflects the characteristics of motion of water molecules in the tissues, which presents as the changes of diffusibility in the diseased tissues. The apparent diffusion coefficient (ADC) map mainly reflects the diffusion amplitude of water molecules, whose black-and-white degree is opposite to DWI. In terms of musculoskeletal disease, DWI can be used in the diagnosis and differential diagnosis of musculoskeletal infection and abscess. Especially in the case of atypical clinical manifestations, DWI sequences can provide valuable information for the diagnosis of osteomyelitis. Intravoxel incoherent motion diffusion weighted imaging (IVIM-DWI) is a new MR imaging sequence developed on the basis of DWI. It mainly obtains the diffusion and perfusion information of tissues with a double-exponential model [4]. In DWI imaging, water molecules in the blood vessels of single voxel have a fast diffusion rate (similar to free water), with the same probability of diffusing in all directions. This phenomenon is called IVIM. In a double-exponential model constructed based on IVIM and DWI with multiple b values, the ADC value of in vivo *tissues* contains the information of diffusion and microcirculatory blood perfusion of tissues and is highly sensitive to bone marrow perfusion, BMD, the relative content of bone marrow cells and water content. Therefore, it can obtain noninvasively more detailed information on the architecture of bone marrow cells and bone marrow neovascularization. *D* value (for assessment of the structure of tissue cells), *D** value, *f* value derived from IVIM-DWI are helpful to construct an accurate system for functional MRI evaluation of bone marrow microarchitecture and provide a new approach for noninvasive evaluation of bone marrow lesions [5].

1.3.3 Magnetic Resonance T_2 Mapping Technique

As a noninvasive MRI imaging technique using a multi-echo sequence, magnetic resonance (MR) T_2 mapping technique mainly reflects the specificity of tissues with attenuation of magnetization in the transverse plane. It can directly show the changes in the signal intensity of the lesions and reflect the microscopic changes of biological tissues at the molecular level by measuring the T_2 value. As a noninvasive quantitive examination technique for cartilage, T_2 relaxation time mapping is currently used to assess the damage and degeneration of articular cartilage. Application of the conventional MR sequence and T_2 mapping can significantly improve the diagnostic sensitivity of cartilage lesions since the changes of collagen, matrix structure and water content in cartilage correlate to the variation of T_2 value. There are few studies where this technique is applied in musculoskeletal infection. Some studies have shown that the T_2 relaxation time mapping can be used to quantitatively evaluate spinal infections (e.g., changes in the composition of tissues in tuberculosis lesions) and is of considerable value in the diagnosis and differential diagnosis of tuberculosis of the spine. T_2* mapping is a relatively novel approach to assessing cartilage composition, with similar imaging principles to the T2 relaxation time mapping. It adopts a multi-gradient echo time or ultrashort echo time (UTE) imaging technique [2].

1.3.4 Magnetic Resonance Diffusion Tensor Imaging

Magnetic resonance diffusion tensor imaging (DTI) is a DWI-based functional MRI technique. It can obtain the ADS reflecting the motion of water molecules, test the fractional anisotropy (FA) reflecting the diffusion of water molecules, show the changes of structure and function of tissue cells, and allow for the display of three-dimensional structure of fibrous tissues with the tractography.

At present, DTI is mainly used in the central nervous system to assess the structure of nerve fiber bundles and white matter. With the development of MRI scanning, DTI has been gradually applied to the musculoskeletal system and is expected to become a new hot area of research. For example, the 3D diagram of muscle fiber obtained with DTI-based fiber tractography allows for a visual display of the course direction and texture of muscle fibers. As such, the application of DTI in athletic injuries caused by trauma, exercise, or physical labor is of a certain value. When it comes to articular cartilage, DTI can be used to reflect the minor changes of the fibrous structure of type II collagen in the hyaline cartilage in the course direction and to evaluate cartilage damage in the early stage and cartilage repair. Some progress has been made in the studies involving the application of this technique in inflammatory injury, denervation injury, ischemia injury, hypoxia injury of the musculoskeletal system, and musculoskeletal tumor. Some early lesions which cannot be found with conventional MRI sequences may be detected by Quantitative analysis using ADC value and FA value. Yet, this technique is limited in clinical application as it is time-consuming and *b* value and signal-to-noise ratio (SNR) are mutually restricted.

1.3.5 ^{1}H-Magnetic Resonance Spectroscopy

^{1}H-magnetic resonance spectroscopy (^{1}H-MRS) can be used as supplementary imaging for conventional MRI [2]. It allows for direct in vivo and noninvasive detection of the status of metabolites in the physiological and pathological tissue cells. ^{1}H-MRS has been applied to the research of tumors of the musculoskeletal system, such as the diagnosis of osteosarcoma. For example, when it comes to the diagnosis of osteosarcoma, the main metabolites of normal musculoskeletal tissues detected by ^{1}H-MRS include choline (Cho), lipid (Lip), and creatine/phosphocreatine (Cr). Cho is the main metabolite of membrane phospholipid, with a peak at 3.22 ppm. It is involved in membrane transport and synthesis and is affected by cell proliferation and phospholipid metabolism. Active metabolism of the membrane and abnormal proliferation of tumor cells cause an abnormal increase of Cho content in the osteosarcoma. Therefore, auxiliary diagnosis can be performed by detecting the Cho content and Cho/Cr value in the osteosarcoma. ^{1}H-MRS is of limited value in the diagnosis of infectious diseases. According to some studies, ^{1}H-MRS showed an increase in lactic acid for both cystic tumors and abscesses within the skull. Lactic acid is a non-specific metabolite generated through anaerobic glycolysis. The increase in lactate, acetate, and succinate may result from the increased glycolysis and fermentation by microbial infection. It is known that amino acids such as valine and leucine are the end products of proteolysis by purulent neutrophils-released enzymes. It is vital to differentiate the amino acids (valine, leucine, and isoleucine; 0.9 ppm) from lipid (0.8–1.2 ppm) because lipid signals may be present in the cerebral tumor and abscess, while amino acids are absent in the in vivo proton spectrum of the cerebral tumor and can only be identified by in vitro detection. Therefore, multiple peaks may be observed in the spectrum of the cerebral abscesses, including peaks of amino acids (valine, leucine, and isoleucine), lipid, acetate, alanine, and lactic acid; while for cystic and necrotic tumors, the peak of lactic acid can only be visualized; sometimes the peaks of lactic acid and lipid may appear simultaneously, while the peak of amino acid is absent. Additionally, ^{1}H-MRS may be of a certain value in the evaluation of abscesses treated in the initial stage or abscesses treated without intervention.

1.3.6 Enhanced MRI and Dynamic Contrast-Enhanced MRI

When applied to the musculoskeletal system, MRI is highly sensitive to the changes of protein and water content, showing the good performance of displaying the contrast of soft tissue with high spatial resolution and at multiple planes. It can reflect the condition of the musculoskeletal diseases, especially the early pathological changes of infectious diseases and components of infectious lesions (e.g., abscesses and caseous substances). However, conventional MRI examination is limited in evaluating the lesions caused by spinal infection, degree of intervertebral disc involvement, epidural abscess, and spinal dura mater. The contrast agent is introduced for facilitating the detection and diagnosis of lesions. It can change the contrast of T_1 value or T_2 value between tissues and lesions, and increase the signal intensity contrast in T_1WI or T_2WI [6]. With the development of contrast agents and MRI techniques, contrast-enhanced MRI can be used in more indications, with a significant improvement in the accuracy of lesion detection. At present, dynamic contrast-enhanced MRI (DCE-MRI) has become the most valuable imaging examination technique in diagnosing infectious diseases of the musculoskeletal system and evaluating their sequelae. It can obtain additional information on complex osseous tissues and soft tissue infection (especially the range involved and necrosis). For example, when applied to the examination of a small abscess, it can show the scope of the abscess, the structure of the vomica, and the composition of the abscess wall, and clearly distinguish inflammatory edema from the abscess. Besides, DCE-MRI can be used to distinguish infectious lesions from tumors and assess joint involvement, joint injury, and postoperative joint status. A joint evaluation may be carried out with an intravenous injection of gadolinium-containing contrast agent (Gd-DTPA) (indirect arthrography) or access into the targeted joint (direct arthrography). MR arthrography has become an alternative to conventional MRI.

DCE-MRI is of great value in the differential diagnosis of various types of infectious lesions in the spine, as well as the differentiation of infectious and neoplastic lesions in the spine. For example, after a non-dynamic enhanced scan of the vertebral body, paravertebral soft tissue, and intervertebral disc that have been involved, tuberculosis of spine, pyogenic spondylitis, brucellar spondylitis, and other diseases show different patterns of enhancement [7]. For tuberculosis of the spine, after an injection of the contrast agent Gd-DTPA, an enhanced scan of the vertebral body involved may show enhancement, in which most vertebral body involved may present heterogeneous enhancement and a few may present homogeneous enhancement; the intervertebral disc involved may show heterogeneous enhancement and the paravertebral soft tissue may present heterogeneous, homogeneous, and circular enhancement. For pyogenic spondylitis, an enhanced scan of the vertebral body and intervertebral disc involved may show marked enhancement, in the form of homogeneous enhancement and heterogeneous enhancement; heterogeneous enhancement usually manifests as a homogeneous enhancement in the center of the lesion and a circular enhancement around the lesion, with long duration of enhancement; the paravertebral soft tissue mass shows plaque-like enhancement, with a few accompanied by abscess formation. For brucellar spondylitis, the conventional MRI shows no obvious or slight changes in the morphology of the vertebral body, and bone destruction and hyperostosis; in the involved area, the lesion appears hypointense on T_1WI and heterogeneous on T_2WI, the enhanced scan shows a significant enhancement of the lesion. The metastatic tumor usually appears as the involvement of multiple non-adjacent or different vertebral bodies, most commonly in the pedicle of vertebral arch and posterior part of the vertebral body, few in the intervertebral disc; lobulated soft tissue mass can be observed, and the mass shows irregular enhancement with the non-dynamic enhanced scan. When widespread metastasis causes spinal stenosis, injection of GD-DTPA can further show the contour of the tumor and determine the exact site that spinal cord compression occurs; when intramedullary spinal cord metastasis (ISCM) develops, after injection of Gd-DTPA, the tumor tissue shows the enhanced signal in a short TR and short TE sequence, while adjacent cerebrospinal fluid shows the black signal, thus the demarcation line between tumor and spinal cord can be precisely delineated.

With the development of the MRI technique, the increased scanning speed allows MRI to perform a dynamic enhanced scan of various parts of the body as multidetector computed tomography (MDCT). Through fast injection of contrast agent and image acquisition at multiple time points, DCE-MRI can obtain changes of lesions in enhancement at multiple time points, and then acquire dynamic information of the distribution of contrast agent in tissue space and capillary networks, obtain the changes of capillary permeability, microcirculation, and perfusion in the lesion, so as to provide more valuable information for the detection, qualitative diagnosis, and prognosis of lesions [8].

DCE-MRI is a noninvasive imaging examination method to evaluate physiological and pathological characteristics. Its quantitative analysis can be used to further study the changes of microstructure and blood flow of tissue, observe the patterns of dynamic enhancement in the lesion area, obtain the corresponding dynamic enhancement curve, calculate multiple quantitative parameters, and accurately assess the blood flow and permeation in the diseased tissue. The quantitative parameters, such as relative enhancement rate (RER), early enhancement rate (EER), max enhancement rate (MER), rate contrast (Kep), and transfer contrast (Ktrans) [8], can not only directly reflect the capillary permeability, perfusion change and blood supply of the diseased tissue but also detect the histological changes caused by the disease in the early stage.

For each DCE kinetic curve, the wash-in phase is referring to the increase of signal intensity within the first minute after injection of [Gd] contrast agents, which reveals the amount of [Gd] delivered to the lesion by blood perfusion. The peak enhancement indicates the highest amount of [Gd] contrast agents that are delivered and retained in the lesion at one post-Gd time point. Another important feature is the delayed phase after the peak point or after 1-min after injection, and it is usually classified into three DCE kinetic patterns: ① Wash-out pattern: the signal intensity reaches a peak before 1-min after injection, and shows wash-out with greater than 10% decrease from the peak intensity; ② Plateau pattern: the signal intensity does not reach a clear peak before 1-min after injection; ③ Persistent enhancement pattern: the signal intensity continues to enhance during the entire DCE period with a greater than 10% increase from the 1-min intensity.

For joint disease, the conventional plain film is first used for assessment; yet, generally, only advanced bone abnormalities in joint disease can be detected. MRI sequences can be used to detect cartilage changes in the early stage and to better depict the status of bone and soft tissue edema as well as the involvement of the synovial membrane. Usually, different planes of joint are usually subjected to scan with fast spin-echo (FSE) T_2WI sequence or non-enhanced spin-echo (SE) T_1WI sequence, and scan with fat-suppressed SE T_1WI sequence is applied after enhancement of the same plane. The non-dynamic enhanced scan is of great value for the differential diagnosis of joint effusion and tendon sheath effusion [9]. Generally, joint effusion and tendon sheath effusion appear homogeneously hyperintense in T_2WI, synovitis appears slightly lower hyperintense in T_2WI. As a result, it is often hard to distinguish before enhancement. After injection of the contrast agent, the synovial membrane may show a significant enhancement of signal in T_1WI and appear hyperintense, while the effusion does not show an enhancement of signal and appear hypointense; after enhancement, inflammatory changes of the synovial membrane may also be observed in T_1WI. DCE-MRI exploits differences in tissue vascularization. In this manner, this technique has been used to differentiate the etiology and synovial involvement in arthropathies according to the enhancement pattern and other quantitative derived biomarkers [10]. Features of synovial enhancement as well as the shape and distribution of bone edema are valuable for differential diagnosis.

In the early phase of brucellar spondylitis, it presents mild destruction of vertebral bone; conventional MRI often fails to show mild abnormalities of the vertebral body, and the pathological changes mainly manifest as injury and microstructural changes of vascular endothelial cells [11]. Yet, quantitative DCE-MRI can be used to show the aforesaid mild inflammatory changes, including microvascular changes, inflammatory cell infiltration, and cell destruction. Niu Heng et al. [12] conducted a retrospective study to analyze 56 patients with Brucellosis. It was found that Ktrans, Kep, and Ve are valuable for early diagnosis of the disease. In this study, 24 patients were identified as early Brucellosis as they have low back pain for less than 1 month and the enzyme-linked immunosorbent assay (ELISA) showed strong positive results of IgM. No obvious abnormalities were observed with a conventional non-enhanced MRI scan of the lumbar vertebra. However, quantitative DCE-MRI showed that the difference of Ktrans, Kep, and Ve between the normal vertebral bodies in the early lesion group and that in the lesion group was statistically significant, and the difference of Ktrans, Kep, and Ve between the normal vertebral bodies in the early lesion group and the diseased vertebral bodies in the lesion group was not statistically significant. The results indicate that brucellar spondylitis presents mild destruction of vertebral bone, which cannot be observed with conventional MRI. However, quantitative DCE-MRI can be used to show these mild inflammatory changes, including inflammatory cell infiltration, mild cell destruction, and microvascular changes. Therefore, quantitative DCE-MRI combined with conventional MRI plain scan is of great value in the diagnosis of brucellar spondylitis as well as its early diagnosis.

Among patients with diabetes, diabetic foot osteomyelitis is the most common complication, and one of the important factors for its occurrence and development is toe soft tissue infection and rupture. MRI has been widely used in the diagnosis and evaluation of diabetic foot due to its high resolution of the soft tissue of the foot and its ability to obtain fine anatomical structures and multidirectional images of the foot. However, the limitation of conventional MRI is that it fails to perform an objective and quantitative evaluation of osteomyelitis. The application of DCE-MRI allows for the acquisition of a dynamic contrast-enhanced curve of blood perfusion time-signal intensity as well as quantitative parameters of perfusion such as Ktrans, Kep, and Ve [13], which can be used to quantitatively reflect the blood perfusion of tissue in the lesion area.

DCE-MRI is also of great value in the differential diagnosis of tuberculosis of the spine and metastatic tumors. Both of the diseases have imaging manifestations of vertebral body destruction and single or multiple soft-tissue masses. Tuberculosis of the spine typically manifests as vertebral bone destruction, narrowing of the intervertebral space, involvement of intervertebral disc, and paravertebral abscess. It is easy to make a diagnosis if the patient presents with typical symptoms of tuberculosis. Metastatic spine tumors mainly manifest as vertebral bone destruction and soft tissue mass, with less involvement of intervertebral discs. For tuberculosis, when a tuberculous abscess has not developed or tuberculosis has not involved the intervertebral disc, paravertebral lesions manifest as solid masses and may be misdiagnosed as malignant lesions. When the lesion presents as vertebral bone destruction, local mass, non-involvement of the intervertebral disc, or abscess, it is difficult to distinguish tuberculous granuloma from metastatic soft tissue mass by simple pre-contrast scan and post-contrast non-dynamic enhancement. Yu Lang et al. [14] performed a DCE-MRI examination in 24 patients with tuberculosis of the spine and 22 patients with metastatic cancer in the spine. Studies have shown that the differences in the DCE kinetic patterns are of value in the differential diagnosis for tuberculosis of spine and metastatic cancer. In particular, DCE-MRI may provide additional information for differentiation between tuberculosis of spine and metastatic cancer when they show similar manifestations on conventional imaging. According to previous studies, although metastatic cancer and tuberculosis of spine showed similar features during the DCE wash-in phase, they had a significantly different delayed phase, suggesting that they have different vascular permeability and distribution space in the lesion. The typical granulomatous nodules under microscopy often showed necrosis in the center, including mycobacterium tuberculosis, surrounded epithelioid cells, Langhans giant cells, mycobacterium tuberculosis and a small number of fibroblasts proliferation, and peripheral infiltrating lymphocytes, suggesting that the organizational structure of tuberculosis has more interstitial space allowing the preservation of [Gd] MR contrast agents. The majority of tuberculosis cases showed the plateau and persistent enhancement patterns, and they even had a higher peak enhancement value compared to the metastatic cancer group. In histological examination, spinal metastatic cancers tend to show a high cellular density with little interstitial space for retention of [Gd] contrast agents. Therefore, contrast agents can quickly fill up this limited space, then rapidly diffuse back to the bloodstream for clearance. In addition, Maurya et al. [15] conducted a study for 80 cases of tuberculosis of the spine, in which, MR myelogram in coronal planes was done to evaluate the spine for the involvement of site and number of vertebral bodies. Early bone marrow edema is demonstrated as diffuse hypointensity on T_1WI and as hyperintensity on short TI inversion recovery (STIR) images. However, post-contrast images will demonstrate marrow enhancement of the affected vertebral body. Therefore, if a tubercular lesion is suspected during an MRI study, it is suggested that screening of the whole spine should be carried out with T_1WI fat-suppressed sequence.

1.4 Ultrasonography

1.4.1 Conventional Ultrasonography

Musculoskeletal ultrasound (MSKUS) refers to the application of high-frequency ultrasound to diagnose musculoskeletal diseases. In recent years, MSKUS has developed rapidly. High-frequency ultrasound is comparable to MRI in showing the lesions of soft tissues, except in some areas where reflections of the bone cortex prevent the access of ultrasound. In addition to clearly displaying the structure, motion state, adjacency relationship, and blood flow distribution of superficial soft tissues such as muscles, tendons, ligaments, and peripheral nerves, MSKUS can also accurately evaluate the anatomical variation, inflammation, degeneration, trauma, and tumor of the musculoskeletal system. Ultrasound scans are often used to assess fluid, such as soft tissue abscesses or joint effusions. When necessary, ultrasound-guided aspiration may be performed to identify the subperiosteal abscess. With guided aspiration, an ultrasound scan may be used in pediatric acute osteomyelitis. The ultrasound scan is widely used in the pediatric department as it is convenient, free from the sedation procedure, and, more importantly, free from ionizing radiation. Ultrasonography, an operator-dependent modality, is of limited value in adult osteomyelitis since it fails to penetrate the bone cortex.

Compared with other imaging examination techniques used in the skeletal muscles, MSKUS has the following advantages [16]: real-time and dynamic display of the motion of tissues (the main strength in the examination of the diseases of the skeletal muscles); real-time display of morphological changes of the bones, joints, muscles, and tendons under different active and passive statuses. For example, when there is a doubt in the clinical diagnosis of tendon disease and impingement disease (e.g., shoulder impingement syndrome), real-time ultrasonography shows obvious diagnostic advantages and may furnish guidance to the treatment. MSKUS has no contraindications to its use, does not use ionizing radiation, and does not require special preparation. It is easy to operate, featured by high repeatability and shorter examination time. Meanwhile, MSKUS can achieve convenient interaction and communication between physicians and patients. The above advantages make it readily accepted by the patients. In addition, MSKUS allows for contrast observation of bilateral joints and simultaneous examination of multiple joints. It has advantages in differentiating solid and cystic structures of musculoskeletal diseases and is superior to radiography in detecting soft tissue calcification. The MSKUS-guided interventional technique has been widely used in clinical practice. The anatomical structure of the limb is suitable for clear imaging of the puncture needle as the puncture needle should be parallel to the probe as much as possible. In this manner, the puncture needle can be clearly displayed, thus achieving "visualization" operation, and improving the puncture success rate and cure rate.

MSKUS examination has some limitations. MSKUS cannot show the complete and whole anatomical structure of the entire joint since ultrasound fails to penetrate the bone. When MSKUS is used for the examination of the musculoskeletal system, artifacts as interference may occur. An experienced operator is usually required to perform this examination and it is relatively difficult to carry out technical training.

1.4.2 Novel Ultrasound Techniques

1.4.2.1 Elasticity Imaging

Elasticity imaging is the imaging and quantification of the elasticity coefficient or stiffness of biological tissues. Evaluating the tissue elasticity by ultrasonography has been used as an adjunctive diagnosis in other radiological subspecialties, such as breast imaging. Studies have shown that this technique is also of a certain value in the musculoskeletal system. Ultrasound elasticity imaging provides an assessment of the stiffness of the tissue, which requires the operator to gently press the tissue to be evaluated which is under the probe. When the tissue is tightened or displaced, the measured change represents its stiffness or softness. Normal ligaments and tendons are resistant to stress, and tissue softening is common in degeneration and trauma. Ultrasound elasticity imaging can only be used as an assistant technique and cannot be an alternative to traditional B-mode ultrasound.

1.4.2.2 Contrast-Enhanced Ultrasound

Contrast-enhanced ultrasound (CEUS) is an ultrasound examination that introduces substances with significantly different acoustic impedance from human soft tissue or with markedly different characteristics of echo into the human body, this technique allows for increased visualization of viscera or living organ and dynamic observation of microcirculatory blood perfusion of the tissues. In musculoskeletal pathology, the growth of abnormal neovascularization is often accompanied by the formation of abnormal nerves, and these changes are well associated with pains. Therefore, early identification of neovascularization is essential for the diagnosis and targeted therapy of diseases. CEUS can be used to detect slow blood flow signals that cannot be detected by traditional ultrasound techniques. It has been widely used in the abdomen, blood vessels, and superficial organs. This technique can also reflect the activity of rheumatic diseases and provide a more accurate assessment of synovial vessels through intravenous injection of microbubble contrast agents. Further study is required to determine the application value of CEUS in the evaluation and follow-up of rheumatic diseases.

1.4.2.3 Interventional Musculoskeletal Ultrasound

Interventional MSKUS allows for real-time and dynamic observation of the position of the puncture needle in the body, showing a certain advantage in the interventional procedure of the musculoskeletal system. At present, the interventional procedures of the musculoskeletal system mainly include soft-tissue biopsy, effusion aspiration, injection of drugs into the articular cavity, tissues around the joints or muscles, tendons, nerve sheath. Real-time ultrasound guidance can significantly improve the puncture success rate of small joints and avoid the phenomenon of "dry tap" caused by a blind puncture in the process of puncture and aspiration of complex isolated effusion. In tendon and ligament injections, MSKUS can guide the needle tip in or out of the tendon. In addition, ultrasound-guided nerve block technique and artery and vein catheterization constitute the vital components of "visual anesthesia."

1.5 Nuclear Medical Imaging

Nuclear medical imaging is an imaging method that introduces radiopharmaceuticals into the body of a patient. Bone imaging is the most common nuclear medical technique for evaluating abnormalities of skeletal muscle. Single-photon emission computed tomography (SPECT) can be used to diagnose musculoskeletal diseases with radiopharmaceuticals similar to those used in traditional bone imaging. It has the strengths of multi-directional data collection and provision of a 3D image after reconstruction.

1.5.1 Three-Phase Bone Scan

In a three-phase bone scan, bone scintigraphy is performed with technetium-99m (^{99m}Tc) labeled diphosphonates. It can label the increased activity of osteoblasts and show metastatic bone lesions. This technique is highly sensitive to bone lesions as changes in bone metabolism predate morphological changes. In bone imaging, image acquisition is performed at three different time points after injection of the tracer, which are termed "flow phase," "blood pool phase," and "delayed phase" [17]. This examination is usually completed within 2–4 h and is especially sensitive to osteomyelitis. Bone imaging can be used for screening examination of periprosthetic joint infection; when the examination shows negative results, the possibility of infection can be basically ruled out.

1.5.2 ^{18}F-FDG-PET

18F-Fludeoxyglucose (^{18}F-FDG) is absorbed into cells by glucose transporters, yet, it is not metabolized further. The level of uptake is associated with cell metabolic rate and the number of glucose transporters, both of which are high in inflammatory cells, with low uptake in the normal bone marrow. FDG-PET allows for differentiation between degenerative disc disease and vertebral osteomyelitis and evaluation of chronic osteomyelitis. As a quantitative imaging method, it can be used to monitor efficacy.

1.6 Molecular Imaging

Molecular imaging was first proposed by Weissleder from Harvard University in 1999 and has been further developed in various medical sectors. At present, the main imaging techniques of molecular imaging include positron emission tomography (PET), CT, MRI, ultrasound imaging, optical imaging, and compound imaging. The molecular biological technique has achieved breakthroughs in some critical issues, which promotes the application of molecular imaging in clinical practice. Molecular imaging has also been gradually applied to the musculoskeletal system. It is believed that rapid progress will be made in the near future.

The molecular imaging of the musculoskeletal system serves as a tool to carry out a noninvasive visualization and quantitative evaluation of the molecular and cellular biology of the osseous tissues and soft tissues of the musculoskeletal system. The target organs in musculoskeletal imaging include bones, joints, muscles, and nerves [18]. Imaging techniques such as X-ray, ultrasonography, CT, and MRI are mainly used to visualize the anatomical changes in the development of musculoskeletal diseases. In musculoskeletal infection, molecular imaging allows for visualization of the physiological and pathophysiological changes in the early stage of infection as well as the detection of potential changes in tissues and molecular changes. Compared with traditional anatomical imaging, it furnishes valuable diagnostic information in the early phase of disease development or recovery. These strengths are expected to improve the diagnosis accuracy and predictive value of musculoskeletal imaging.

The molecular imaging of the musculoskeletal system today includes radionuclide imaging, optical imaging, and CEUS. Optical imaging contains fluorescence reflectance imaging and bioluminescence imaging. These formations are largely used in small animal models. The development of tomographic approaches using fluorescence-based optical techniques penetration to image superficial regions including joints. Although ultrasound is largely used in anatomical imaging of joints and soft tissue, advancements in microbubble contrast agents are expected to make molecular imaging with ultrasound a possibility. Radionuclide imaging is the merely in vivo molecular imaging technique that is far and widely used in clinical practice for infection and inflammation. Bone scan, especially a three-phase bone scan, is the most commonly implemented radionuclide procedure for the exploration of infection in intact bones. Ga-67 (^{67}Ga) scintigraphy is another imaging that is particularly effective and sensitive in spondylitis. In-111 (^{111}In) or Tc-99 m (^{99m}Tc) labeled leukocyte imaging has high characteristics for infection imaging. It has been resoundingly used in combination with bone marrow imaging for the diagnosis of osteomyelitis (OM). Antibiotics, radiolabeled biotin, and peptides have been used with diverse degrees of success, consistent results.

PET/CT with a first-rank combination of anatomical and functional imaging has new frontiers in clinical molecular imaging. Its role is well established in oncologic imaging and it is being explored for inflammation and infection imaging. FDG-PET/CT seems to be a hopeful tool in imaging various infective and inflammatory processes in the musculoskeletal system. It exceeds established diagnostic modalities with its high specificity, sensitivity, and whole-body imaging capability. Apart from FDG, FDG-labeled leukocytes, ^{18}F-NaF, and ^{68}Ga citrate may be used for infection/inflammation imaging. FDG-PET/CT not only in imaging of varieties of skeletal and joint infections but also for evaluation and diagnosis of various inflammatory diseases affecting nerves and muscles on the side. PET/MRI allows for imaging finer details of nerves, cartilage, and muscles. PET seems to be the front runner in imaging of musculoskeletal inflammation and infection.

1.7 Strategies and Preferred Options for Imaging Examination of Musculoskeletal Infection

Musculoskeletal infections have a relatively higher incidence and may occasionally cause death. The microorganisms that cause musculoskeletal infections encompass various types. The musculoskeletal diseases can be divided into suppurative (bacterial infection), granulomatous (mycobacterium tuberculosis, Brucella, and fungal infection), parasite, and AIDS-related musculoskeletal diseases according to the types of pathogens. Patients often present with fever, pain, and swelling of affected joints, and limitation of motion. Laboratory tests show accelerated erythrocyte sedimentation rate (ESR) and elevated C-reactive protein (CRP). Systemic symptoms are common in young patients. Therefore, during the acute onset, early diagnosis is vital to prevent the disease from developing into a chronic infection or to avoid the serious consequences (e.g., disabilities and deformities) caused by repeated attacks. In particular, timely diagnosis is required to prevent serious infections after operations such as internal fixation and implantation in children and orthopedics.

For pyogenic infection caused by a bacterial infection, plain X-ray examination helps to screen and rule out other diseases, such as fractures or malignant tumors. X-ray imaging is two-dimensional imaging, with image overlaps and limited density resolution. Therefore, it can only provide limited effective information when applied to sites with complex anatomical structures, soft tissues involved by lesions, or soft-tissue lesion-dominated diseases. X-ray imaging can only display the general location of lesions and skeletal changes, and cannot meet the requirements of clinical diagnosis and treatment. In this case, a CT examination may be performed. CT examination is an important examination approach of musculoskeletal infection, featured by fast scanning speed and wide scanning range. It allows for the isotropic multidirectional reconstruction and better visualization of bone details, mild bone destruction, periosteal proliferation, etc. For infection involving soft tissues or abscess forming within the soft tissues, enhanced CT examination can be used to evaluate the shape and extent of the abscess as well as its relationship with peripheral tissues. Additionally, CT is considered superior to MRI in the setting of chronic osteomyelitis for the demonstration of cortical destruction and gas. It also allows for better delineation of sequestrum, bone involucrum, and fistula, which helps in guiding the treatment. For periprosthetic infections, CT can reduce the interference caused by artifacts and improve the accuracy of diagnosis by expanding the CT window width, increasing kVp, reconstruction of maximum density projection (MIP), and iterative reconstruction that suppresses metal artifacts (Table 1.1). Yet, CT is limited in clearly displaying the bone marrow cavity and intraspinal lesions (Fig. 1.1).

Table 1.1 MR scan parameters of pyogenic infection (osteomyelitis) in long bone

No.	Pulse sequence	Plane	TR/TE/TI/FA (ms)	Number of slices	Slice thickness/ spacing (mm)	Intra-slice resolution	Number of excitations (NEX)	Fat-suppressed mode	Scan duration (min)
1	T_2WI	Coronal	4000/110/150	20	3/0.6	0.8 × 0.8	3		2′16″
2	T_1WI	Coronal	600/10/180	20	3/0.6	0.8 × 0.8	2		2′09″
3	T_1WI fat-suppressed	Coronal	600/10/180	20	3/0.6	0.8 × 0.8	2	Dixon	2′39″
4	T_2WI STIR	Coronal	3800/53/150	20	3/0.6	1.1 × 1.1	2	STIR	2′36″
5	T_2WI	Transverse	4000/110/150	25	3.5/0.7	0.8 × 0.8	3		2′04″
6	PD fat-suppressed	Transverse	3500/31/150	25	3.5/0.7	1.0 × 1.0			2′34″
7	T_1WI fat-suppressed (enhanced)	Coronal	600/10/180	20	3/0.6	0.8 × 0.8	2	Dixon	2′09″
8	T_1WI fat-suppressed (enhanced)	Sagittal	600/10/180	20	3/0.6	0.8 × 0.8	2	Dixon	2′09″
9	T_1WI fat-suppressed (enhanced)	Transverse	600/10/180	25	3/0.6	0.8 × 0.8	2	Dixon	2′09″

MRI provides good soft-tissue contrast resolution and is very sensitive to the changes in the content of different tissue components in the lesions of pyogenic infection of the musculoskeletal system. Compared with conventional X-ray and CT examinations, MRI allows for early detection of abnormal signals of the musculoskeletal system and is very sensitive to joint effusion and bone marrow edema, which is one of the earliest signs of osteomyelitis. Therefore, it is of great value for the diagnosis and differential diagnosis of acute and chronic musculoskeletal infections, and can better evaluate the involvement of soft tissue and abscess formation. In addition, DWI can be used as an auxiliary tool to diagnose the abscess without enhancement. MRI can also be used to evaluate whether chronic osteomyelitis is in the process of recurrence or persistent infection. Yet, the specificity of MRI is only 60% because the repaired fibrovascular tissue shows similar signal strength and enhancement characteristics as that of active infection and persists for 12 months. The diagnostic accuracy may be improved in combination with signs of secondary infections such as skin ulcers, sinuses, abscesses, and cortical destruction. The enhanced MRI is conducive to the diagnosis and evaluation of chronic osteomyelitis because the signal of active inflammation is enhanced and the sequestrum is surrounded by enhanced vascular granulation tissue, which helps the observation. Ultrasound is of a certain value in the diagnosis and treatment of acute pyogenic infection of the musculoskeletal system. In the setting of joint effusion and cellulitis, it allows for visualization of subcutaneous tissue edema and thickening. Ultrasound can be used to make a diagnosis when combined with corresponding clinical manifestations. Application of ultrasound-guided puncture and drainage of the effusion in the microscopic examination and culture also plays a role in diagnosis and treatment. PET/CT is rarely used in the diagnosis of chronic osteomyelitis, with sensitivity and specificity up to 95% and even 100%. FDG-PET allows for differentiation between aseptic fracture nonunion and osteomyelitis.

The spine is most often involved by the pathogens of granulomatous inflammation caused by mycobacterium tuberculosis, Brucella, etc. The lesions usually appear as narrowing of the intervertebral space, bone destruction, paravertebral abscess, and/or psoas abscess. MRI is highly sensitive and can detect abnormalities 1 week after infection, which is of great significance for the early diagnosis of spondylitis. MRI is able to perform multidirectional and multi-sequence imaging, without emitting ionizing radiation and with excellent soft-tissue contrast, which allows for better observation of vertebral bone destruction, intervertebral disc destruction, paravertebral or epidural abscess, periosteum changes, granuloma formation, and compression of the spinal nerve root. Therefore, MRI serves as an important examination means for the diagnosis of brucellar spondylitis. Meanwhile, MRI also helps to distinguish between pyogenic spondylitis and brucellosis spondylitis, providing a good basis for the differential diagnosis. In terms of MRI examination sequence, T_1-weighted or T_2-weighted SE sequence requires scanning in at least two directions (transverse plane and coronal/sagittal plane), so as to evaluate and locate intraspinal abscesses. STIR or T_2WI fat-suppressed sequence is of great value in the display of bone marrow edema, soft-tissue edema, and intervertebral disc abnormalities in the early stage. The fat-

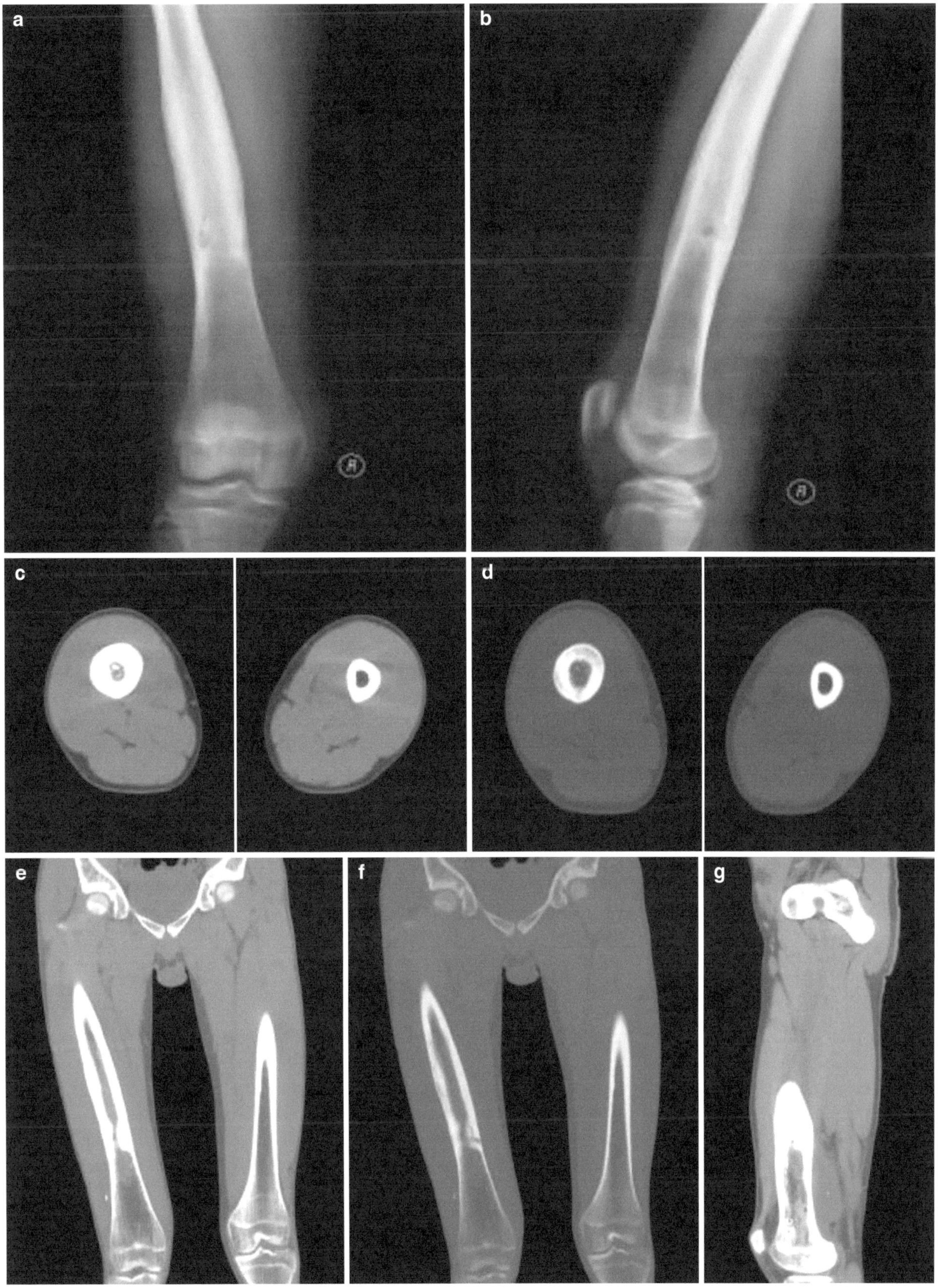

Fig. 1.1 Chronic suppurative osteomyelitis of the right femur with sinus. Plain DR: PA view and lateral view of the femur (**a**, **b**); Non-enhanced CT scan: transverse plane: soft tissue window (**c**), bone window (**d**); coronal plane reconstructed: soft tissue window (**e**), bone window (**f**); sagittal plane reconstructed: soft tissue window (**g**), bone window (**h**); MR scan: sagittal plane: T_1WI (**i**), T_2WI (**j**), T_2WI fat-suppressed (**k**); coronal plane: T_2WI fat-suppressed (**l**); transverse plane: T_2WI fat-suppressed (**m**)

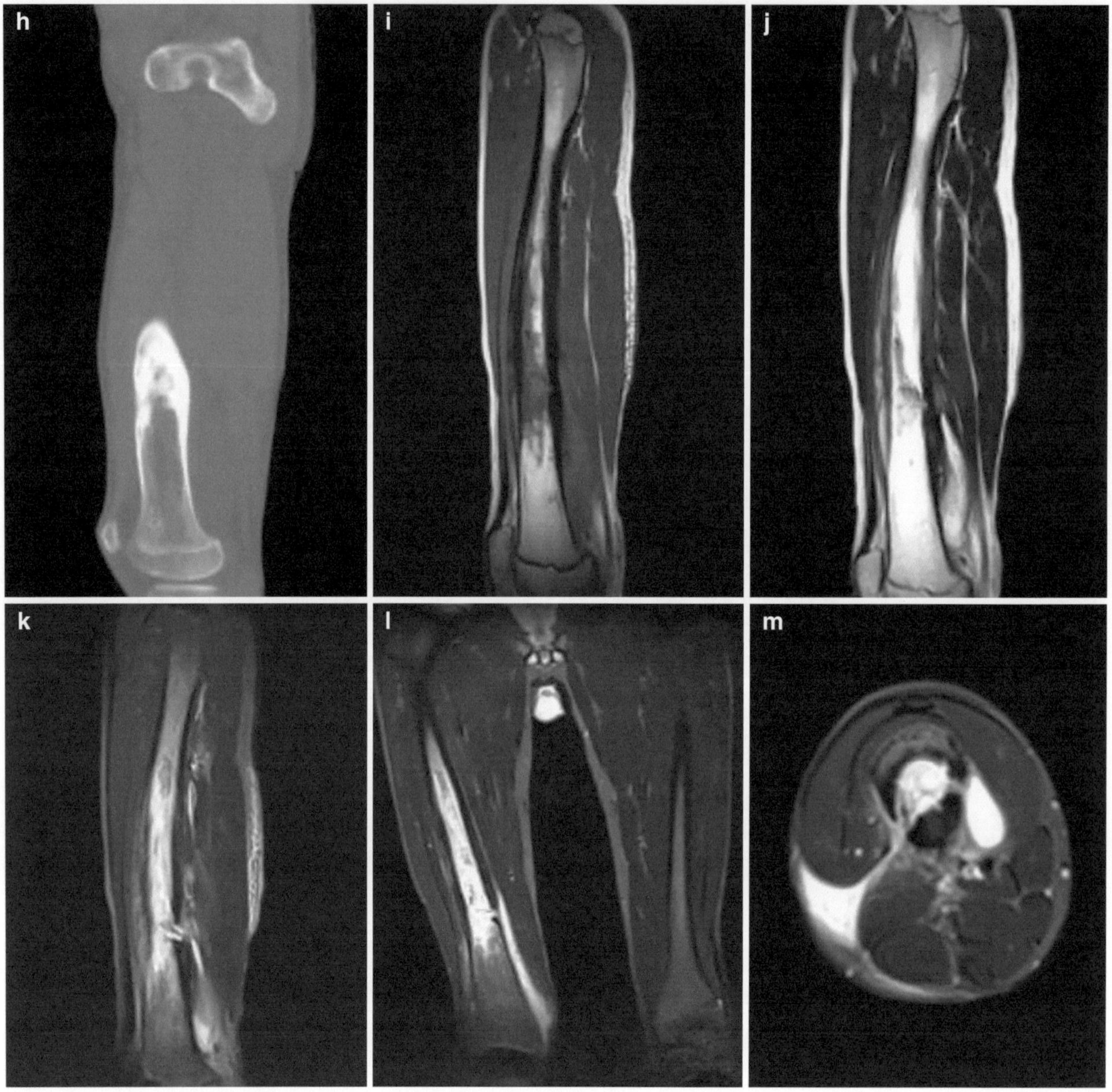

Fig. 1.1 (continued)

suppressed image attenuates the background signal of soft tissue and bone marrow, thus giving a clearer visualization of the lesion. Gadolinium-enhanced examination allows for further display of the enhancement of bone marrow edema in the involved vertebral body, and T_1WI fat-suppressed imaging before and after enhancement is conducive to the identification of abscesses in the vertebral or paravertebral soft tissues [19]. For example, a typical cold abscess shows homogenous enhancement of the abscess wall, although it has no significant inflammatory reaction around the lesion. Enhanced imaging also provides an accurate evaluation of the extent of the lesion and the degree of compression of the spinal cord. Gadolinium-enhanced examination is also of a certain value in identifying brucellar spondylitis at different phases. When the gadolinium-enhanced examination is applied to acute brucellar spondylodiscitis, the intervertebral disc and vertebral body show homogeneous contrast enhancement; When it is applied to chronic brucellar spondylodiscitis, the vertebral body shows heterogeneous enhancement. When a small joint is involved, the axial image using contrast enhancement combined with a fat-saturated technique can clearly show that the joint appears hyperintense. This may be because the involvement of the main joints caused by Brucellosis is a reactive and spontaneous fusion process (Figs. 1.2, 1.3, and Table 1.2).

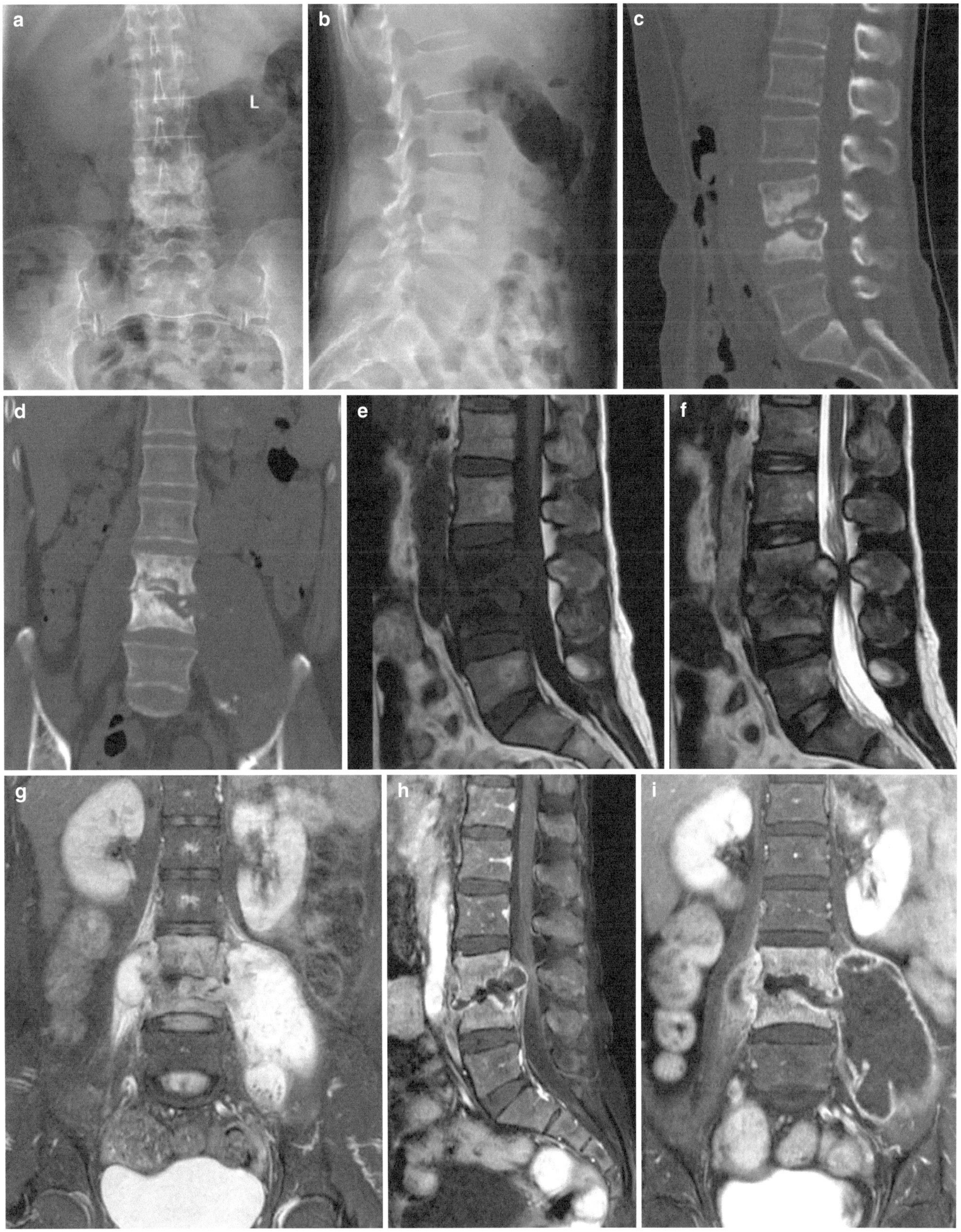

Fig. 1.2 Tuberculosis with bilateral psoas abscess in vertebral body of L_3 and L_4. Plain DR: PA view and lateral view of lumbar vertebra (**a**, **b**); CT scan: reconstructed images at sagittal plane and coronal plane (**c**, **d**); Non-enhanced MR scan: sagittal plane: T_1WI (**e**), sagittal plane: T_2WI (**f**), coronal plane: T_2WI (**g**); Enhanced MR scan: sagittal plane (**h**), coronal plane (**i**)

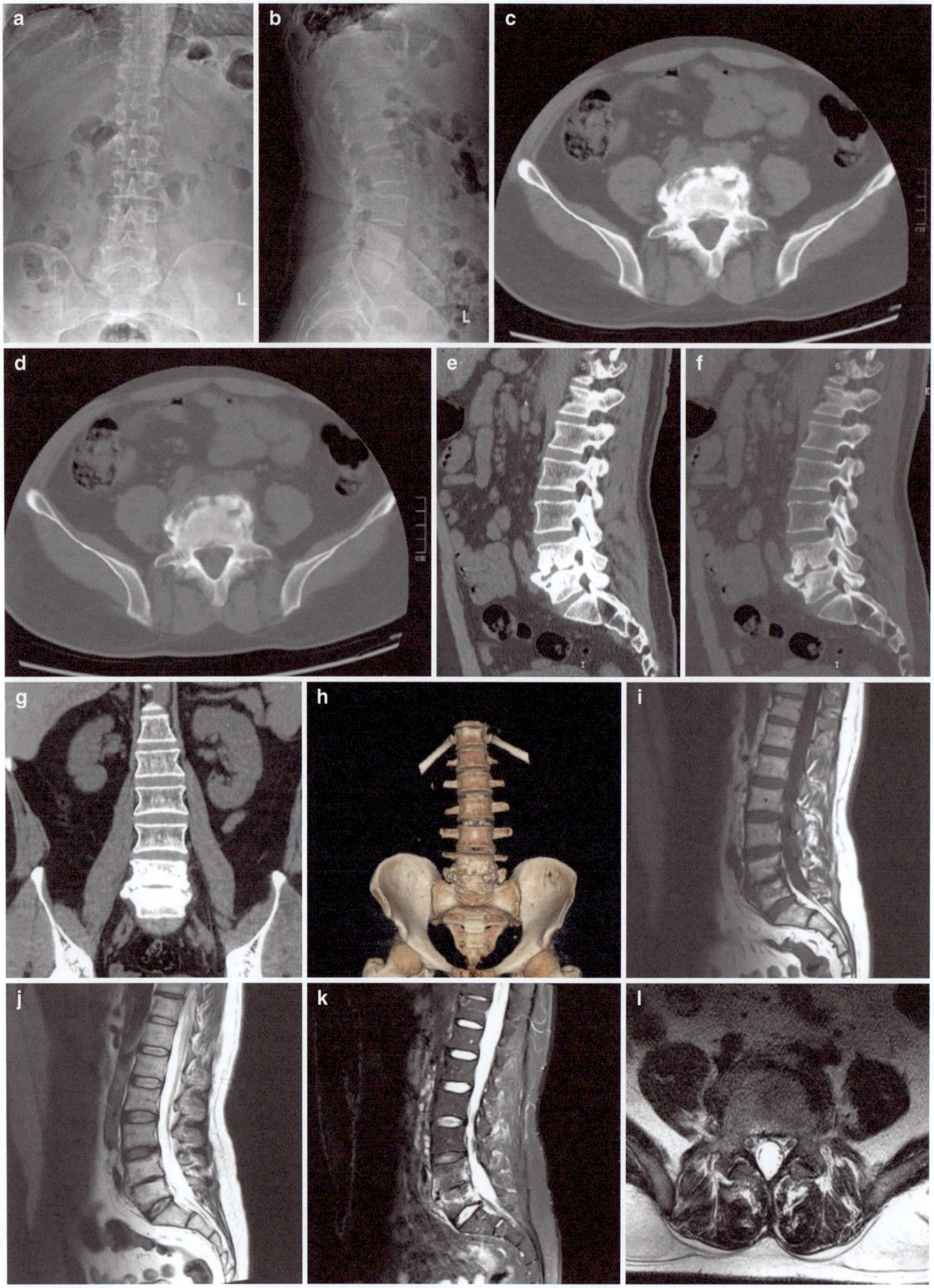

Fig. 1.3 Brucellar spondylitis in vertebral body of L_4 and L_5. Plain DR: PA view and lateral view of lumbar vertebra (**a**, **b**); Non-enhanced CT scan: transverse plane: soft tissue window (**c**), bone window (**d**); sagittal plane reconstructed: soft tissue window (**e**), bone window (**f**); coronal plane reconstructed: soft tissue window (**g**), VR (**h**); Non-enhanced MR scan: sagittal plane: T_1WI (**i**), T_2WI (**j**), T_2WI fat-suppressed (**k**); transverse plane: T_2WI (**l**)

Table 1.2 MR scan parameters of tuberculosis of spine and Brucellosis

No.	Pulse sequence	Plane	TR/TE/TI/FA (ms)	Number of slices	Slice thickness/ spacing (mm)	Intra-slice resolution	Number of excitations (NEX)	Fat-suppressed mode	Scan duration
1	T_1WI	Sagittal	500/8.6/150	11	3/0.3	0.7 × 0.8	1		1′09″
2	T_2WI	Sagittal	3000/93/150	11	3/0.3	0.8 × 0.8	2		1′16″
3	T_2WI STIR	Sagittal	2800/91/150	11	3/0.3	0.8 × 0.8	1	STIR	1′27″
4	T_2WI	Transverse	3100/87/150	12	3/0.3	0.7 × 0.7	1		1′33″
5	T_1WI fat-suppressed	Transverse	617/9.7/150	12	3/0.3	0.4 × 0.4	2	Dixon	2′13″
6	T_1WI fat-suppressed (enhanced)	Sagittal	500/8.6/150	11	3/0.3	0.7 × 0.8	1	Dixon	1′09″
7	T_1WI fat-suppressed (enhanced)	Transverse	617/9.7/150	15	3/0.3	0.4 × 0.4	2	Dixon	2′13″
8	T_1WI fat-suppressed (enhanced)	Coronal	500/8.6/150	11	3/0.3	0.7 × 0.8	1	Dixon	2′13″
9	DWI (B value = 0, 800)	Transverse	3700/108	18	5/0.5	1.8 × 1.8	1		2′06″

Early diagnosis is not common in bone infection caused by parasites as it is usually asymptomatic in the early stage. Patients visiting the hospital or clinic are generally in advanced stages of the disease or have developed pathologic fractures. For example, bone hydatid disease is a zoonotic parasitic disease caused by the larvae of Echinococcus parasitic on the human skeletal system. CT examination is sensitive to bone destruction and calcification of hydatid, which allows for clear visualization of the multilocular manifestations of hydatid. Yet, it is limited in the diagnosis and evaluation of alveolar hydatid [20]. Among all the imaging examinations, MRI provides the most valuable information in the diagnosis and evaluation of bone hydatid disease because it can not only comprehensively observe the relationship between the shape, extent, location of the cyst and the peripheral tissues and viscera from three planes (sagittal plane, coronal plane, and transverse plane) for the hydatid of the musculoskeletal system, but also reveal the characteristic signals and morphological changes of echinococcus cyst. When bone hydatid disease occurs in the vertebral body, ribs, and pelvis, MRI shows a hypointense osteosclerosis shadow and irregular or arc calcification shadow on both T_1WI and T_2WI. A hyperintense "vesicle" can be observed in the destruction area and soft tissue mass when using T_2WI or T_2WI fat-suppressed sequence. This is valuable for the diagnosis of alveolar hydatid [21] (Fig. 1.4 and Table 1.3).

Each imaging examination method has its own clinical application features, indications, and limitations. Therefore, it is a common challenge for clinicians and radiologists to select appropriate imaging examination procedures and methods according to the patient's condition, develop a patient-oriented personalized examination plan, and ensure sequence optimization (Figs. 1.5 and 1.6).

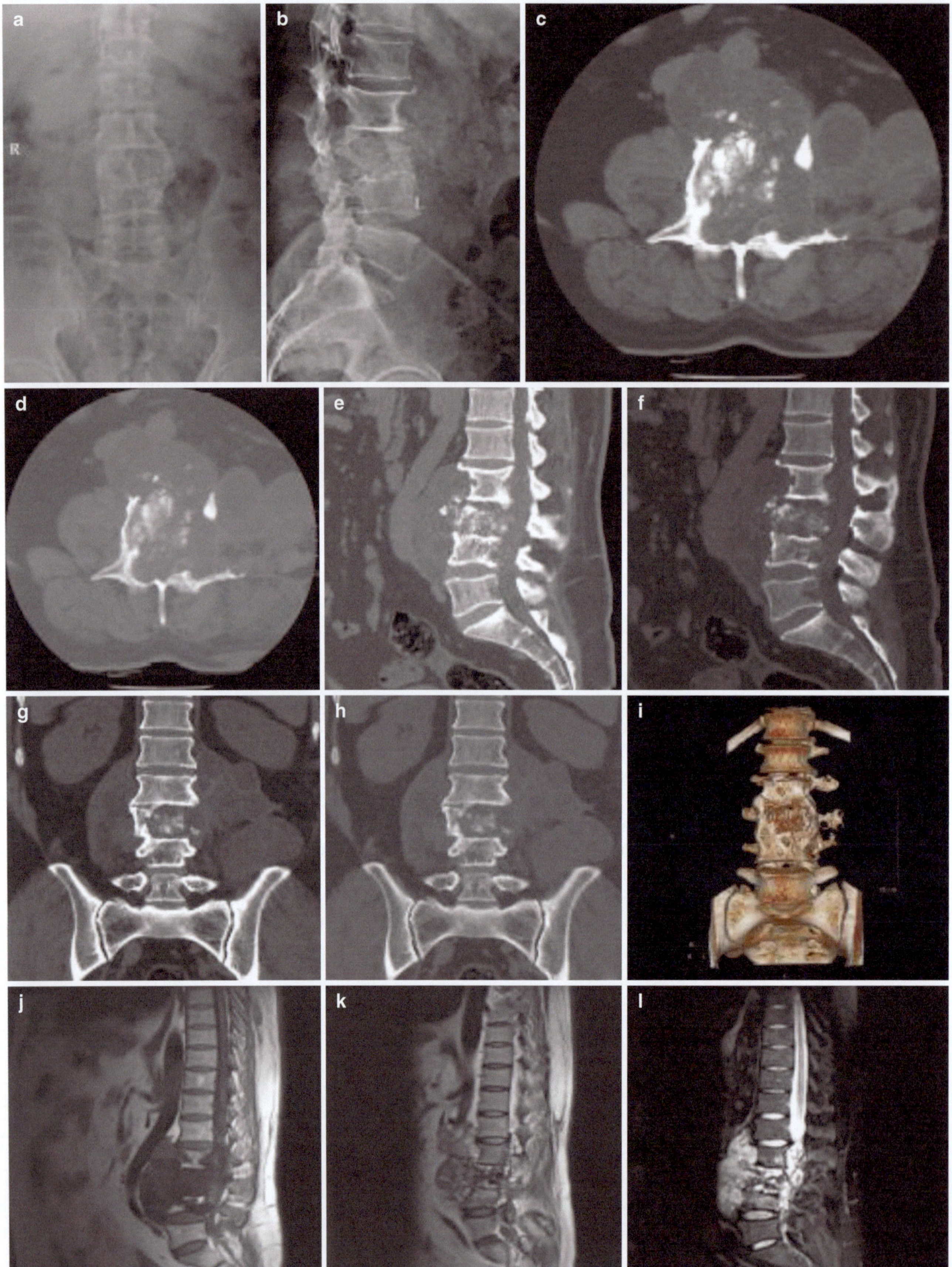

Fig. 1.4 Multiple hydatids in vertebral bodies of L_2–L_4, appendages and paravertebral areas. Plain DR: PA view and lateral view of lumbar vertebra (**a**, **b**); Non-enhanced CT scan: transverse plane: soft tissue window (**c**), bone window (**d**); sagittal plane reconstructed: soft tissue window (**e**), bone window (**f**); coronal plane reconstructed: soft tissue window (**g**), bone window (**h**), VR (**i**); Non-enhanced MR scan: sagittal plane: T_1WI (**j**), T_2WI (**k**), T_2WI fat-suppressed (**l**); coronal plane: T_2WI fat-suppressed (**m**); transverse plane: T_2WI fat-suppressed (**n**)

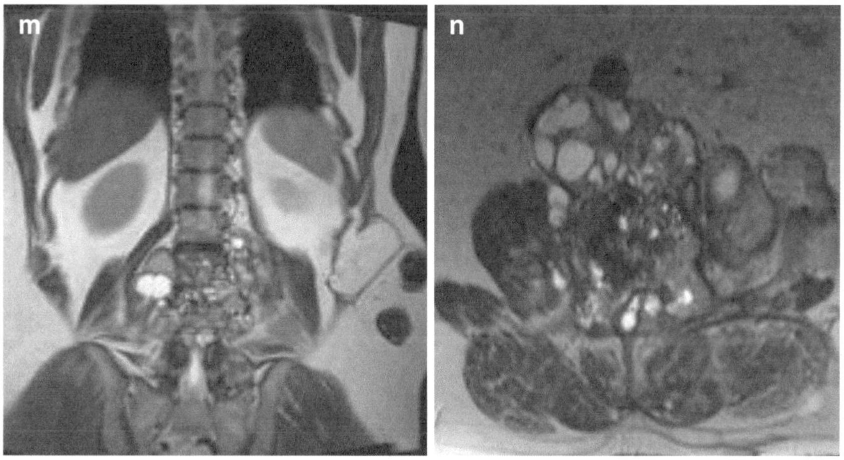

Fig. 1.4 (continued)

Table 1.3 MR scan parameters of hydatid

No.	Pulse sequence	Plane	TR/TE/TI/FAms)	Number of slices	Slice thickness/ spacing (mm)	Intra-slice resolution	Number of excitations (NEX)	Fat-suppressed mode	Scan duration
1	T_1WI	Sagittal	500/8.6/150	11	3/0.3	0.7 × 0.8	1		1′09″
2	T_2WI	Sagittal	3000/93/150	11	3/0.3	0.8 × 0.8	2		1′16″
3	T_2WI STIR	Sagittal	2800/91/150	11	3/0.3	0.8 × 0.8	1	STIR	1′27″
4	T_2WI	Transverse	3100/87/150	12	3/0.3	0.7 × 0.7	1		1′33″
5	T_1WI fat-suppressed	Transverse	617/9.7/150	12	3/0.3	0.4 × 0.4	2	Dixon	2′13″
6	T_1WI fat-suppressed (enhanced)	Sagittal	500/8.6/150	11	3/0.3	0.7 × 0.8	1	Dixon	1′09″
7	T_1WI fat-suppressed (enhanced)	Coronal	500/8.6/150	11	3/0.3	0.7 × 0.8	1	Dixon	2′13″
8	T_1WI fat-suppressed (enhanced)	Transverse	600/10/180	25	3/0.6	0.8 × 0.8	2	Dixon	2′09″

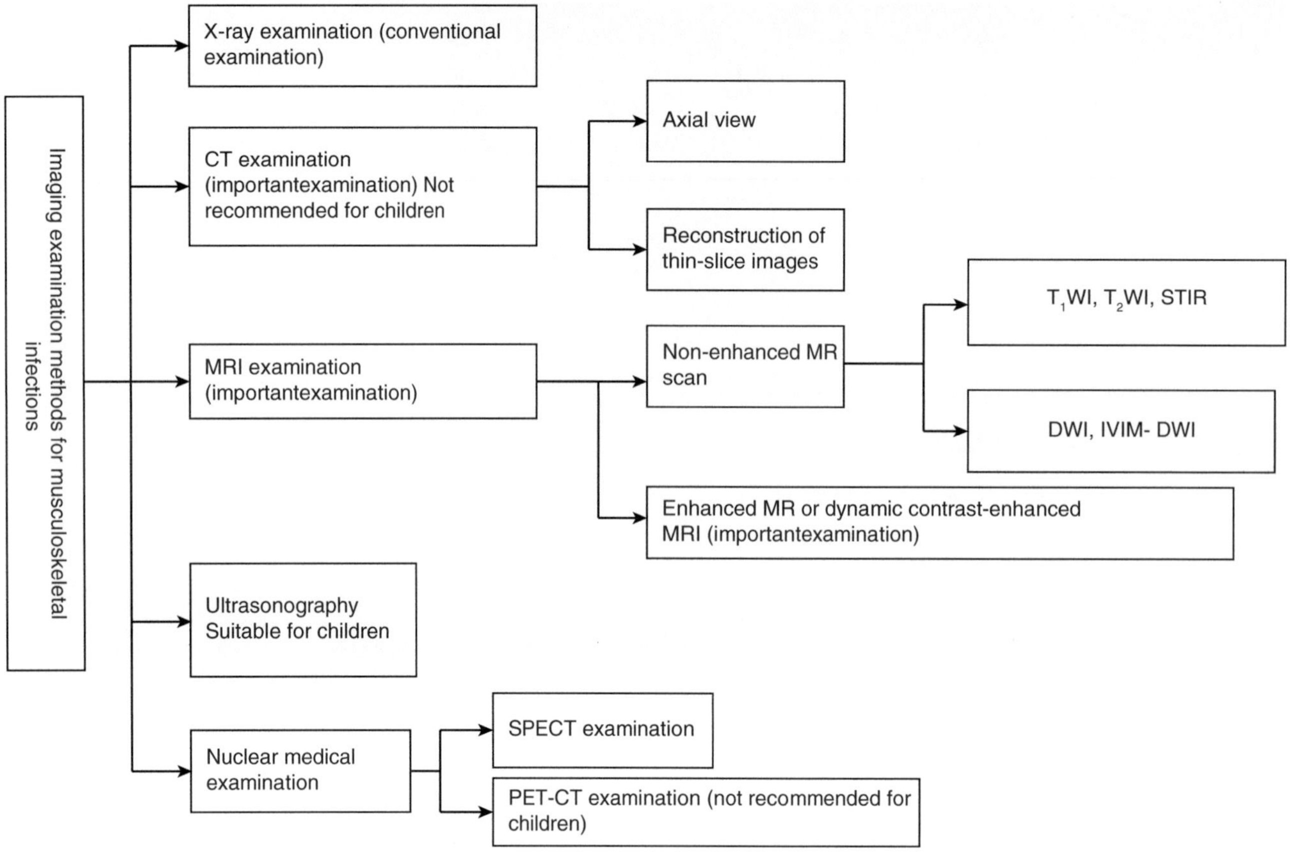

Fig. 1.5 Imaging examination methods for musculoskeletal infection

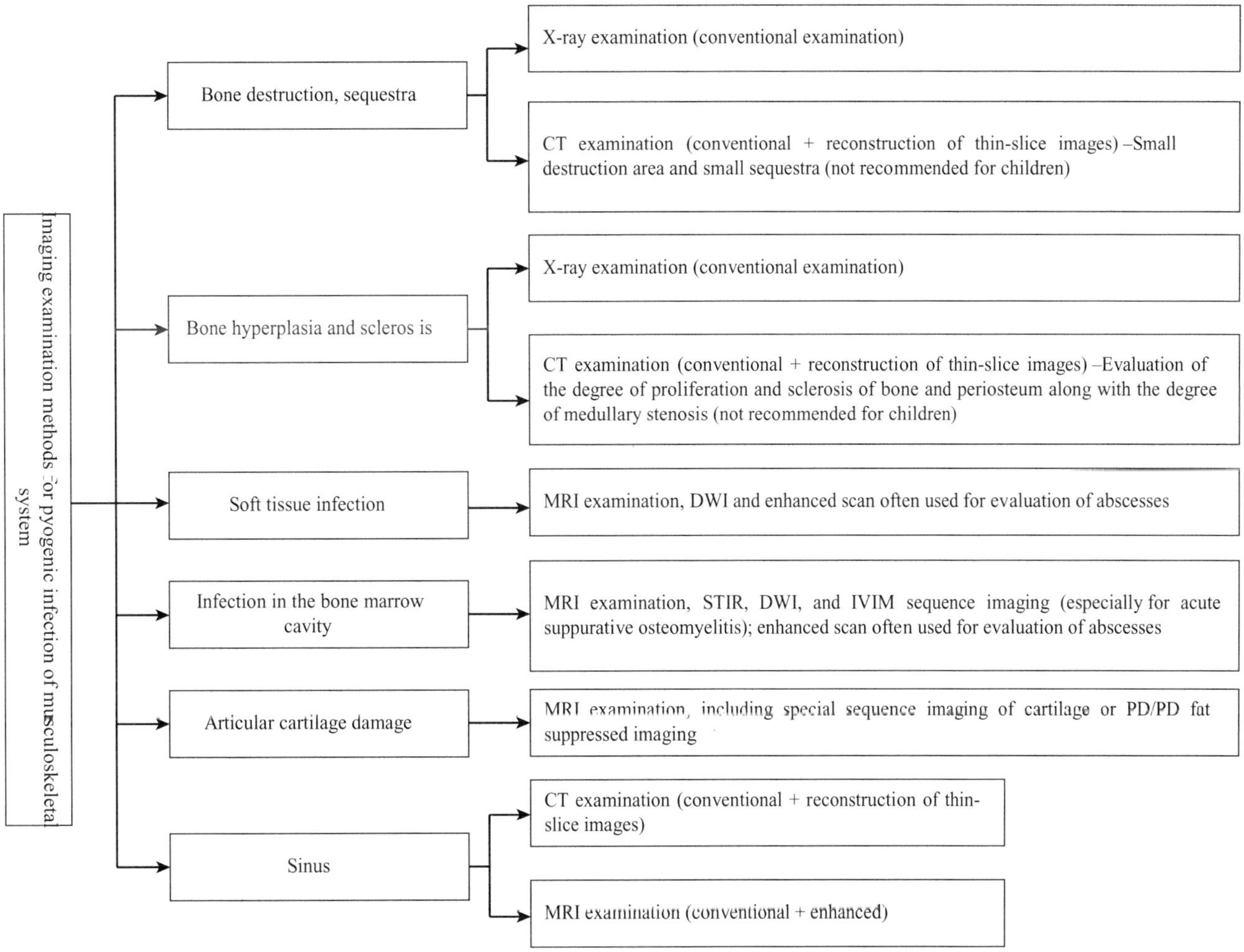

Fig. 1.6 Imaging examination methods for pyogenic infection of musculoskeletal system (Shinong Pan, Yuan Zhao)

References

1. Simpfendorfer CS. Radiologic approach to musculoskeletal infections. Infect Dis Clin N Am. 2017;31(2):299–324.
2. Minming Z. Grainger & Allison's diagnostic radiology. 6th ed. Beijing: People's Military Medical Press; 2015.
3. Huishu Y, Lisi L. Progress and clinical application of MR imaging on musculoskeletal system. 2015;6(2):81–5.
4. Ohno N, Miyati T, Kasai H, et al. Evaluation of perfusion-related and true diffusion in vertebral bone marrow: a preliminary study. Radiol Phys Technol. 2015;8(1):135–40.
5. Biffar A, Dietrich O, Sourbron S, et al. Diffusion and perfusion imaging of bone marrow. Eur J Radiol. 2010;76(3):323–8.
6. Sujlana P, Skrok J, Fayad LM. Review of dynamic contrast-enhanced MRI: technical aspects and applications in the musculoskeletal system. J Magn Reson Imaging. 2018;47(4):875–90.
7. Qiao P, Zhao P, Gao Y, et al. Differential study of DCE-MRI parameters in spinal metastatic tumors, brucellar spondylitis and spinal tuberculosis. Chin J Cancer Res. 2018;30(4):425–31.
8. Lohrke J, Frenzel T, Endrikat J, et al. 25 years of contrast- enhanced MRI: developments, current challenges and future perspectives. Adv Ther. 2016;33(1):1–28.
9. Yuming Y, Pan S. Clinical application of MR arthrography. Chinese J Radiol. 2012;46(3):197–202.
10. Martín Noguerol T, Luna A, Gómez Cabrera M, et al. Clinical applications of advanced magnetic resonance imaging techniques for arthritis evaluation. World J Orthop. 2017;8(9):660–73.
11. Esmaeilnejad-Ganji SM, Esmaeilnejad-Ganji SMR. Osteoarticular manifestations of human brucellosis: a review world journal of orthopedics. World J Orthop. 2019;10(2):54–62.
12. Heng N, Gao Y, Pengfei Q, et al. Dynamic contrast-enhanced MRI in the early diagnosis of brucellar spondylitis. Chin J Radiol. 2017;51(6):437–40.
13. Liao D, Xie L, Zhiwei Z, et al. The application value of dynamic contrast-enhanced MRI in diabetic foot osteomyelitis. J Clin Radiol. 2018;37(8):1347–51.
14. Lang N, Su MY, Yu HJ, et al. Differentiation of tuberculosis and metastatic cancer in the spine using dynamic contrast-enhanced MRI. Magn Reson Imaging. 2013;31(8):1285–91.
15. Maurya VK, Sharma P, Ravikumar R, et al. Tubercular spondylitis: a review of MRI findings in 80 cases. Med J Armed Forces India. 2018;74(1):11–7.
16. Guo R. Musculoskeletal ultrasound enters a new era. Chin J Med Ultrasound (Electronic Edition). 2015;12(1):3–5.
17. Palestro CJ. Radionuclide imaging of musculoskeletal infection: a review. J Nucl Med. 2016;57(9):1406–12.

18. Pawaskar A, Basu S, Jahangiri P, et al. In vivo molecular imaging of musculoskeletal inflammation and infection. PET Clin. 2019;14(1):43–59.
19. Pourbagher A, Pourbagher MA, Savas L, et al. Epidemiologic, clinical, and imaging findings in brucellosis patients with osteoarticular involvement. AJR Am J Roentgenol. 2006;187(4):873–80.
20. Raj DH, Dash PK. Hydatid disease of bone: a dangerous crippling disease. BMJ Case Rep. 2015;2015:bcr 2015211697.
21. Babitha F, Priya PV, Poothiode U. Hydatid cyst of bone. Indian J Med Microbiol. 2015;33(3):442–4.

2 Etiological Classification and Pathogenic Characteristics

Shinong Pan and Yuan Zhao

Musculoskeletal infections have a relatively higher incidence and may occasionally cause death. The musculoskeletal infections vary and may be caused by various pathogens, which may exist inside or outside the host body. The musculoskeletal diseases can be divided into suppurative (bacterial infection), granulomatous (mycobacterium tuberculosis, Brucella, and fungal infection), parasite, and AIDS-related musculoskeletal diseases according to the types of pathogens. The pathogens vary in growth characteristics, the way of infection, and body parts that they invade. Most musculoskeletal infections often manifest as the involvement of skeletons, limitation of motion of joints, muscular pain, and swelling, etc. Systemic symptoms may occur as well. In clinical practice, early diagnosis during the acute onset of infection of the musculoskeletal system is vital to prevent the disease from developing or evolving into a chronic infection or to avoid serious consequences (e.g., disabilities and deformities) caused by repeated attacks. Having a good command of the basic knowledge of the etiological classification and pathogenic characteristics of the musculoskeletal system plays an essential role in the image analysis and diagnosis of diseases in the advanced stage.

2.1 Pyogenic Infection

Pyogenic infection (bacterial infection) is most common in acute bone and joint infections. Bacteria evade the defense mechanism of the hosts by entering cells and slowing down metabolism. Infection can be classified into nonspecific infection and specific infection according to the type of inflammation caused by various bacteria. Nonspecific infection, also known as pyogenic infection, is featured by redness, swelling, heat, pain, and dysfunction. Among the patients with pyogenic infections of bone and joint at all ages, staphylococcus aureus is the most common pathogen. Pyogenic infections may be caused by primary bacteremia, or result from adjacent infected foci due to trauma and surgery, especially prosthesis implantation. According to statistics, chronic infections associated with orthopedic implants and approximately 90% of nail infections are triggered by coagulase-negative staphylococci such as staphylococcus epidermidis. In addition, pyogenic infections may be caused by Pseudomonas and Enterobacter [1].

Common pyogenic infection includes suppurative osteomyelitis, pyogenic arthritis, and pyogenic spondylitis. Suppurative osteomyelitis is a pyogenic inflammation involving bone marrow, bone, and periosteum. Pyogenic arthritis is a pyogenic inflammation involving the joint synovium. These diseases are collectively referred to as pyogenic infections. Staphylococcus aureus is the main pathogen in pyogenic infection involving the bone, accounting for 75% of pyogenic infection involving the bone tissues, followed by beta-hemolytic streptococcus, accounting for 10%. Antibiotics have been widely used in recent years, which significantly lowers the incidence of osteomyelitis and pyogenic infection of joints; no typical clinical manifestations are observed as well.

2.1.1 Suppurative Osteomyelitis

Suppurative osteomyelitis is most common in childhood and adolescence. The metaphysis of the long bone is the most common predilection site. The proximal tibia and distal femur are the most common sites, followed by the humerus and ilium. The main cause of suppurative osteomyelitis: (1) Tortuous and loop-shaped end-arteries and capillaries exist near the epiphyseal plate in children; (2) The blood flow is rich and slow; (3) Bacteria are easy to be lodged near the

S. Pan (✉)
Department of Radiology, Shengjing Hospital of China Medical University, Shenyang, Liaoning, China
e-mail: cjr.panshinong@vip.163.com

Y. Zhao
Department of Radiology, The First Affiliated Hospital of Xinjiang Medical University, Ürümqi, Xinjiang, China

H. Li et al. (eds.), *Radiology of Infectious and Inflammatory Diseases - Volume 5*,
https://doi.org/10.1007/978-981-16-5003-1_2

epiphyseal plate and metaphysis [2]. The most common pathogen is hemolytic staphylococcus aureus, followed by beta-hemolytic streptococcus. A few pathogens include Escherichia coli, pneumococcus, Haemophilus influenzae, Clostridium perfringens, and Staphylococcus albus. Potential risk factors that may cause suppurative osteomyelitis include diabetes, coronary artery disease (CAD), immunosuppression, in vivo implantation of an artificial prosthesis, alcoholism, cancer, or dialysis due to kidney failure.

Suppurative osteomyelitis can be acute or chronic, depending on its duration. In which, acute suppurative osteomyelitis mainly manifests as bone resorption and destruction; chronic suppurative osteomyelitis is featured by sequestra and new bone formation. Acute hematogenous osteomyelitis has a rapid onset and is often accompanied by symptoms of systemic poisoning (e.g., hyperpyrexia and chills), redness, swelling, heat, and pain of local skin, and limitation of motion. When the abscess breaks through the periosteum to form a soft tissue abscess, the pain is mitigated. In the early stage, the swelling is not obvious, and a few days later local edema may occur, which indicates the formation of a subperiosteal abscess. A pathologic fracture may occur when tenderness is present in the metaphysis after deep pressure.

Chronic hematogenous osteomyelitis occurs mainly due to failure to completely control the disease in the acute infection period, repeated attack, or bacterial infection of low virulence. It is characterized by pathological changes such as sequestrum, sinus, dead space, and involucrum. CT is able to better visualize the sequestrum and intraosseous abscess. MRI allows for a better demonstration of inflammatory tissue, abscess, sinus, or fistula, which helps to differentiate osteomyelitis from tumors [3].

Brodie's abscess, common in childhood and adolescence, is a form of subacute and localized suppurative osteomyelitis. Brodie's abscess has an insidious onset and mainly presents with tenderness, but with the absence of systemic inflammatory signs and symptoms. It is characterized by intramedullary abscess formation and is more common in the proximal tibia and distal femur. In children and adolescents, the capillaries and tiny end-arteries in the metaphysis bend and form a vessel loop. Therefore, the blood flow here is slow and bacteria are easy to be lodged and form foci. The main causes of the disease [4]: ① The low virulence of the pathogen and the strong immunity of the patient make the foci to be localized; ② Osteomyelitis is not cured completely and persists, which results in localized bone destruction in the lesion area.

Chronic sclerosing osteomyelitis, also known as Garre's sclerosing osteomyelitis, progresses depending on a series of comprehensive conditions. It is a rare chronic infectious disease, mainly in children and adolescents [5]. Chronic sclerosing osteomyelitis may occur in the mandible or metaphysis of the long bone. When it occurs in the mandible, this generally originates from an infection of low virulence, such as dental decay, mild periodontitis, or gingival herpes. Clinically, this reactive process accounts for the hard swelling of the jaw and the subsequent facial asymmetry with which patients may present. The lesion is usually asymptomatic with no accompanying general and local signs of inflammation, although the clinical picture may vary widely. In some patients, local pain may occur in the affected bone. This symptom has an episodic nonprogressive nature and may persist for several months [6].

2.1.2 Pyogenic Arthritis

Pyogenic arthritis is a joint pyogenic inflammation caused by bacterial infection of synovial membrane. It has a rapid onset. The affected joints often present with symptoms of redness, swelling, heat, pain, and dysfunction. The joints are often in a semi-flexed position. Deep joints involved by pyogenic arthritis are often in a position of flexion, abduction, or external rotation, with not obvious manifestations of redness, swelling, heat, and pain. Pyogenic arthritis is common in children. Staphylococcus aureus is the dominant pathogen, accounting for about 85%. Most pyogenic arthritis is caused by blood-borne transmission to the synovial membrane. The infection is easy to spread into the joint as the synovial membrane lacks a basement membrane. Large weight-bearing joints are common, mostly single. Pyogenic arthritis is most common in the knee joint, followed by the hip, shoulder, and ankle joints. Sternoclavicular joint infection often occurs in intravenous drug abusers.

Early diagnosis of pyogenic arthritis is essential to avoid limb dysfunction, any delayed diagnosis may cause permanent disability [7]. The imaging manifestations of pyogenic arthritis in the early stage are not specific. However, with the wide application of MRI, the diagnostic reliability of pyogenic arthritis has improved. MRI can reveal synovitis and joint exudate of pyogenic arthritis, identify the extent of inflammation involving the surrounding soft tissues, and show the destruction of the articular capsule, ligament, tendon, cartilage, and other structures, so as to improve the clinical prognosis.

2.1.3 Pyogenic Spondylitis

Pyogenic spondylitis is less common than suppurative osteomyelitis of the extremities, accounting for 2–4% of all osteomyelitis. Staphylococcus aureus is the most common pathogen causing osteomyelitis. Most of the bacteria invade through the hematogenous spread, while direct spread and spread with lymphatic drainage can also be seen. Pyogenic spondylitis is common in adult males. The lumbar vertebra is the most predilection site, followed by the thoracic vertebra. Almost all the infections of pyogenic spondylitis originate from the intervertebral disc, then invade the end plate from the intervertebral disc and spread along the ligament. When intervertebral disc-associated ischemia and necrosis occur, abscesses are formed with continuous destruction of end plate bone and abscess invasion into paravertebral soft tissue. Pyogenic spondylitis often has a rapid onset. Patients with pyogenic spondylitis may have aversion to cold, hyperpyrexia, or be forced to stay in bed due to severe back or waist pain, accompanied by localized pain of the spinous process at percussion. CT can clearly show the changes in bone destruction and soft tissues of the vertebral endplate. MRI is more sensitive than CT in demonstrating bone marrow edema and peripheral soft tissue lesions. When using STIR and fat-suppressed SE in the early stage, a patchy heterogeneous abnormal hyperintense area is observed in the vertebral body, and the upper and lower edges of the vertebral body and adjacent intervertebral discs show hypointense on T_1WI and hyperintense on T_2WI [8].

2.2 Granulomatous Infection

Granulomatous infection is a specific infection, and the common ones include mycobacterium tuberculosis infection and brucella infection.

2.2.1 Mycobacterium Tuberculosis Infection

Tuberculosis is a granulomatous disease caused by mycobacterium tuberculosis infection. Mycobacterium tuberculosis is rod-shaped or curved, with a thick cell wall composed of sugars and lipids. Its cell wall is rich in sugar, which makes bacteria resistant to decolorization with acid after being colored with phenol dyes, so it is called acid fast bacilli.

The main source of tuberculosis transmission is the excretion of bacteria from patients with open tuberculosis, and airborne transmission is the main route of transmission. The most common pathogenesis of bone tuberculosis infection is that mycobacterium tuberculosis reaches the bone or vertebra through blood circulation from the primary focus or reactivated focus in the body. Tuberculosis of bone and joint includes tuberculous spondylitis, tuberculous osteomyelitis, arthritis, dactylitis, multifocal bone tuberculosis, and soft tissue infections. Tuberculosis of the spine is the most common type, accounting for approximately 50% of musculoskeletal tuberculosis infections.

Tuberculosis of bone and joint is pathologically characterized by the formation of chronic granulomas, i.e., infiltration of the multinucleated giant cells, lymphocytes, and macrophages with central caseous necrosis.

2.2.1.1 Tuberculosis of Spine

Tuberculosis of spine, also known as Pott disease, is the most common type of musculoskeletal tuberculosis. It is most common in the lumbar vertebra, followed by the thoracic vertebra, and less common in the cervical vertebra. For children and adults, the predilection site of tuberculosis of the spine is the thoracic vertebra and lumbar vertebra, respectively. Mycobacterium tuberculosis may infect the vertebral body (tuberculosis before the spine) or various sites after the pedicle of the vertebral arch (tuberculosis after the spine), accounting for 90–95% and 5–10%, respectively. When tuberculosis is initially infected, it reaches the front of the vertebra through blood circulation, then spreads to the intervertebral disc, and finally to the paraspinous tissue. Typical manifestations of tuberculosis of the spine include pain, tenderness in deformed parts of the back, night crying, physical discomfort, weight loss, loss of appetite, night sweats, increased body temperature at night, and other systemic symptoms. Patients with advanced tuberculosis of the spine may have nerve damage.

2.2.1.2 Joint Tuberculosis

Tuberculosis of bone and joint accounts for 1.2% of tuberculosis, usually secondary tuberculosis. In most cases (80%), it may be hard to identify the site of primary tuberculosis, while the primary lesion is always present. Mycobacterium tuberculosis remains in bones and joints through hematogenous pathways. In tuberculosis of bone and joint, 50% of cases are accompanied by the affected spine. Joint tuberculosis is common in children and adolescents, involving large weight-bearing joints represented by hip and knee joints. Clinically, it has a slow onset and mild symptoms. During the active stage, systemic symptoms may occur, including night sweats, low fever, anorexia, gradual weight loss, joint swelling and pain, and limitation of motion.

2.2.1.3 Bone Tuberculosis

Bone tuberculosis can be divided into tuberculosis that affects the long bones or diaphyses of the short bones. Tuberculosis that affects the long bones is common in epiphysis and metaphysis. In the early stage of the onset, the adjacent joints present with the following symptoms: limitation of motion, soreness and discomfort, disease aggravation after weight-bearing and exercise, and local swelling. Tuberculosis that affects diaphyses of the short bones, also known as tuberculous dactylitis or spina ventosa, is common in children aged under 5 years. The lesions are usually bilateral, often in the proximal phalanges. Mild symptoms such as swelling may occur. Most of the diseases require no therapy, with occasional ulceration and sinus formation.

2.2.2 Brucella Infection

Brucellosis, an animal-derived infectious disease caused by Brucella, is a zoonosis that affects various organs and tissues throughout the body. It was first diagnosed in the

Mediterranean region and was initially named "Malta fever," also known as Mediterranean remittent fever, abortus fever, or undulant fever. It is widely distributed around the globe, especially in the Middle East and the Mediterranean region. In China, the main endemic areas include Inner Mongolia, northwest China, and northeast China. Brucellosis is more frequently seen in males and young adults.

Brucella spreads through: ① exposure to skin and mucosa; for example, veterinarian, butcher, or stockman may be infected via direct contact of affected animals or their secretions, excreta, or delivery; or via skin or conjunctiva during the process of feeding and slaughtering or when processing skin, wool, and meat products; ② Digestive tract, respiratory tract, flies as carriers, tick bites, etc. Studies have shown that human brucellosis can also be transmitted through breastfeeding, bone marrow transplantation, blood transfusions, and sexual activity.

Brucellosis lacks specificity in clinical manifestations, thus often being misdiagnosed. The disease has an incubation period of 1–3 weeks, up to several months. The average incubation period is 2 weeks. According to the course of the disease, the disease can be divided into three phases: ① Acute stage (0 ~ 3 months); ② Subacute stage (3–12 months); and ③ Chronic stage (>1 year). The musculoskeletal system is one of the most commonly affected sites of Brucellosis, accounting for 10–85% of the systemic brucellosis. Brucellosis of bones and joints is manifested as inflammation in bones and joints (such as swelling, pain, dysfunction, fever, tenderness, and redness). Brucellar arthritis often involves multiple joints, and the most commonly affected sites include the knee joint, sacroiliac joint, hip joint, and other large joints. When the spine is infected by the pathogen, it may lead to spondylitis. The lumbar vertebra is the most commonly affected site. Brucellar spondylitis is most common in the upper motor end plate with abundant blood supply. The local infection may subside and heal, or progress to the entire spine, intervertebral spaces, and adjacent bones. In general, the type of bone involvement depends on the age of the patient. As for children and adolescents, the disease is most common in the sacroiliac joint and knee joint; as for senior patients, the most commonly affected site includes vertebral columns, especially the lumbar vertebra. Brucellar osteomyelitis outside the spine is rare, in which the long bones (especially tibia, femur, humerus, or manubrium) may be involved, and bursitis, tenosynovitis, and subcutaneous nodules may also occur.

2.3 Fungal Infection

Fungal infections of the bones and joints are very rare and may be caused by various yeasts and molds. The symptoms are often subacute, similar to that of other common bone and joint infections, which may give rise to a high rate of misdiagnosis. The severity of the infection hinges on the inherent pathogenicity of the fungus, the immune status of the host, the anatomical location of the infection, and whether the infection involves foreign bodies. Patients usually receive surgical debridement combined with long-term antifungal therapy. At present, the incidence of fungal infection keeps rising. The main reasons include: (1) An increase in immunocompromised people, such as immunosuppressed HIV-positive patients, patients with severe underlying diseases, patients treated with glucocorticoid (GC), elderly patients with chronic diseases, and infants aged under 1 year whose immune systems are not fully developed; (2) Wide use of broad-spectrum antibiotics and use of immunosuppressive agents and corticosteroid hormones; (3) Application and implementation of invasive medical procedures such as organ (bone marrow) transplantation, interventional operation, endotracheal intubation [8]. Fungal infection is classified into superficial fungal infection and deep fungal infection. Superficial fungal infection is a frequently occurring and common disease, with low mortality. It involves hair, nail, surface skin, and other tissues. Deep fungal infection, also known as invasive fungal disease, is featured by great damage and high mortality. It is caused by a fungal infection involving deep skin structure, muscles, viscera, and blood below the epidermal stratum corneum.

While the type of conditionally pathogenic fungi that cause serious infections is increasing year by year all over the world, the principal one is still candida. Infections caused by cryptococcus, saccharomyces, trichosporon in addition to candida also do great harm, with a high fatality rate. The ways of infection include hematogenous spread, direct infection, and spread of adjacent infected tissues, among which hematogenous spread is most commonly seen. Fungal arthritis caused by the synovial thickening and chronic granulomatous has similar manifestations to tuberculosis of bone and joint. The common symptoms include chills, fever, joint swelling, and pain, which are common in the joints such as hip, knee, wrist, and elbow [9]. Most fungal osteomyelitis shows clinical symptoms within 4 weeks after the initial infection, but in a few cases, the occurrence of the symptoms may be delayed for several months or years. Later in the course of the disease, bone destruction may occur and subsequently lead to pathologic fracture, eventually causing the formation of chronic abscess and even sinus.

In fungal infections of the bones and joints, the spine is the most common infection site. The infection may also occur in other joints, appearing as multifocal osteomyelitis, pyogenic arthritis, and spondylodiscitis. For example, mycetoma tends to cause granulomatous infection of the plantar tissue, which further leads to chronic osteomyelitis, accompanied by pus and multiple sinuses. Madura foot is a chronic infection of the soft tissue and bone in the foot caused by fungi or actinomycetes due to a thorn prick [10], soft tissue abscess is characterized by multiple small vomicas.

2.4 Parasitic Infection

The larvae of echinococcus parasitic in the human body lead to echinococcosis, also known as hydatid disease. The most commonly affected sites include the liver and lungs. Bone hydatid disease is very rare, accounting for less than 1% of echinococcosis. Bone hydatid disease occurs in hematogenous infections or adjacent soft tissue lesions [11]. There are four types of hydatid parasitic on the human body: Echinococcus granulosus, Echinococcus multilocularis, Echinococcus oligarthrus, and Echinococcus vogeli.

Bone hydatid disease mainly occurs in pastoral areas and has two types of infection routes: direct infection and indirect infection. In China, most of the disease is found in Xinjiang, Qinghai, Tibet, Ningxia, and Inner Mongolia. Foxes and dogs are the main hosts and echinococcus parasites in their small intestines. The eggs are excreted with feces, polluted water sources, soil, pastures, livestock houses, and food, then humans, animals, and small mammals may be infected by eating the eggs. Bone hydatid disease prevailingly invades the spine (45%), pelvis (14%), femur (10%), ribs (8%), humerus (2%) [12], and less frequently other sites as the cranium, sternum, scapula, and the phalanges. In which, thoracic vertebra, lumbosacral vertebrae, and cervical vertebra account for 60%, 35%, and 5%, respectively. In long bones, primary echinococcus cyst may start from the diaphysis or metaphysis and cause multilocular cystic lesions and scallop-like changes in the cortex, but with no obvious expansion, sclerosis, or periosteal reaction. When the bone cortex is invaded, adjacent soft tissue may be involved [13]. Early diagnosis is not common in bone hydatid disease as it is usually asymptomatic in the early stage. As the disease progresses, pain, numbness, muscle atrophy of the limbs, nerves compressed by cysts in the spine and sacrum, symptoms and signs of nerve compression, and even paraplegia may occur. Patients visiting the hospital or clinic are generally in advanced stages of the disease or combined with pathologic fractures [14].

2.5 AIDS-Related Musculoskeletal Diseases

The pathogen of acquired immunodeficiency syndrome (AIDS) is called the human immunodeficiency virus (HIV), also known as the AIDS virus. HIV transmission occurs through sexual contact, blood, and vertical transmission from mothers to infants. It mainly invades $CD4^+$ T lymphocytes, which results in a cellular immune deficiency in the body and secondary opportunistic infections or tumors. Infection is usually caused by opportunistic pathogenic microorganisms such as Candida, Clostridium, and Mycobacterium avium. Initially, it was believed that musculoskeletal infection is relatively rare among HIV-infected patients. Yet, recent studies have shown that it is relatively common in these patients. In particular, the incidence of musculoskeletal infection among HIV-infected patients with intravenous drug use has increased year by year. In addition to musculoskeletal deformities such as painful articular syndrome and noninfectious arthritis, HIV-infected patients may also develop musculoskeletal infections, including infectious myositis, pyogenic arthritis, suppurative osteomyelitis, and tuberculous arthritis.

Musculoskeletal symptoms, especially musculoskeletal pain, are very common in AIDS patients. As the immune function recovers to near normal, HIV infected individual develops into rheumatic diseases. In addition, ischemic necrosis and osteoporosis are also common in AIDS patients. Relevant studies have shown that the proportion of AIDS patients with low bone mineral density is higher than that of the normal population control group, which may be related to the initiation of reverse transcription drug therapy. Even without the effect of antiretroviral therapy (ART), the increased risk of osteoporosis can be predicted, because HIV infected individual is prone to diseases related to low bone mass (such as hypogonadism, nephrosis, hepatopathy, diabetes, low body mass index, malabsorption, etc.). In addition, the HIV virus can affect the function of osteoblasts and osteoclasts, and HIV carriers are more prone to traumatic fractures than normal people. After antiretroviral therapy, hormones lead to hyperlipidemia, hypertrophy, and proliferation of adipocytes in bone marrow, gradually compressing and replacing bone marrow, aggravating intramedullary hypertension and forming a vicious circle. At the same time, the increase of prostaglandin E_2 and leukotriene B_4 in blood and bone all affect the arterial blood supply in osseous tissue and lead to avascular necrosis of the femoral head. AIDS patients show a decrease in the number of T lymphocytes and abnormal activation. The stimulation and inhibition of T lymphocytes on osteoblasts and osteoclasts are closely related to T lymphocyte subsets, cytokines, and local factors [15].

2.6 Syphilis of Bone

Syphilis is a chronic and systematic sexually transmitted disease caused by treponema pallidum infection, and the primary mode of transmission is by blood transfusion, sexual contact, or mother-to-child transmission. According to the different ways of infection, it can be divided into congenital syphilis and acquired syphilis. The former is transmitted from pregnant women with syphilis to the fetus through the placenta; the latter is a postnatal infection, of which more than 90% are directly infected by sexual contact, and a few are infected through indirect ways such as blood transfusion [16]. Syphilis of bone is found in muscles, bones, joints, tendons, tendinous sheaths, bursa, spine, spinal cord, etc. It often occurs in bones and joints and invades tibia, fibula, ulna, femur, skull, etc. Among them, tibia and fibula lesions are common, and long tubular bone diaphysis lesions are the most obvious. Early clinical manifestations include limb pain or local pain, joint soreness, obvious at night, and the pain aggravates during strenuous activities and tiredness. The skin is characterized by redness, swelling, heat, or local skin ulceration, and there is a history of unhygienic sex or syphilis infection among family members when asking for medical history.

Congenital syphilis of bone is caused by blood-derived infection of the fetus in the mother's body, and syphilitic osteochondritis and syphilitic periostitis often occur [17]. Syphilis of joint is less common clinically than syphilis of bone, with no joint redness and swelling and limitation of motion, less involvement of facet joints. Its symptoms are generally symmetrical joint soreness without migration, aggravation of symptoms at night, and relief after exercise. When syphilitic synovitis occurs, the larger joints have local soreness, and may with joint swelling and activity limitation; Syphiloma arthritis in patients with advanced syphilis is usually caused by large joints involvement such as knee joint. Bursa synovialis syphiloma or articular syphiloma ulceration enters into the joint, causing joint swelling and activity limitation. A few syphiloma can form fistula by ulceration. In addition, congenital or acquired syphilis can cause Charcot's arthropathy, often involving knees, hips, ankles, and lumbar vertebraes, etc., with obvious joint bone destruction and fragmentation, and decreased or disappeared perception and tendon reflex.

2.7 Novel Coronavirus

In December 2019, Novel Coronavirus-Infected Pneumonia occurred in Wuhan, Hubei Province. In 2020, China officially named it "Novel Coronavirus-Infected Pneumonia" (NCIP). On February 11, 2020, the International Committee on Taxonomy of Viruses named the novel coronavirus as SARS-Cov-2 virus, and WHO named pneumonia infected by SARS-Cov-2 virus as COVID-19. Its source of infection is the patients with COVID-19, and its transmission route is mainly through respiratory droplets and close contact. Whether it can be transmitted through fecal-oral and aerosol remains to be further studied. Epidemiological history refers to the patient's travel history in the affected area within 2 weeks before the morbidity of the disease, or contact with personnel from the affected area or other suspected and confirmed cases. The population is generally susceptible. The disease condition of the elderly and people with basic diseases worsens after infection. Children and infants can also suffer from the disease, and the symptoms are milder than those of adults. Fever, fatigue, and dry cough are the main symptoms. Severe cases often have dyspnea, and may rapidly progress to acute respiratory distress syndrome, septic shock, refractory metabolic acidosis, coagulopathy, renal failure, and even death. SARS-Cov-2 nucleic acid antibody detected in biochemical specimens is taken as the diagnostic gold standard.

Imaging findings: ① In the early stage, ground-glass opacities (GGO) mainly distribute in a subpleural or adjacent interlobar fissure in one or both lungs, with thickened microvascular shadow and primary interlobular septum thickening, form grid-like changes on HRCT, especially the very weak ground-glass opacities and small nodule shadow, which are usually atypical and easy to be misdiagnosed. In the progressive stage, it is characterized by mixed GGO and consolidation, with enlarged and fused focus range, and is parallel to the pleura, patchy, not distributed according to the lobes and segments; As the number of focuses increased, the lesions gradually expand from the lung edge to the central lobe; Imaging findings in the repair stage: fibrosis hyperplasia to the focus is obviously reduced, the boundary becomes clear, and in the absorption stage, the consolidation focuses gradually change to ground ground-glass opacities. ② Symmetrical swelling of bilateral intercostal muscles can be found on CT in some confirmed cases. Whether this change is muscle edema or compensatory change caused by virus infiltration requires pathological confirmation.

2.8 Rheumatic Immune Diseases

Rheumatic disease refers to a kind of connective tissue disease that affects bones, joints, muscles, bursa, tendons, blood vessels, etc. It can invade multiple systems, with pain as the main symptom, and the etiology and pathogenesis are unclear. Many studies suggest that pathogen infection, genetic factors, environmental factors, endocrine dyscrasia, etc. are all related to pathogenesis. Rheumatic skeletal muscle diseases include rheumatoid arthritis, ankylosing spondylitis, reactive arthritis, systemic sclerosis, etc.

2.8.1 Rheumatoid Arthritis

Rheumatoid arthritis (RA) is a systemic immune disease characterized by multiple and nonspecific chronic arthritis. It is characterized by symmetrical invasion of facet joints of hands (feet) and gradual invasion of multiple joints of the whole body, eventually leading to joint deformity and dysfunction, of which axial bone involvement is rare. As rheumatoid arthritis is a systemic disease, it can also have many extra-articular manifestations, such as fever, fatigue, rheumatoid nodules, lung involvement, pericarditis, peripheral neuropathy, blood system involvement, vasculitis, etc. Among them, 15–25% of cases have rheumatoid nodules, which are more common near elbow joints. The disease can occur in all ages, with a prevalence of about 0.3%, and the incidence gradually increases, with a male-female ratio of 1:3. It is commonly found in the age group of 45–54.

Synovitis is the basic pathological change of rheumatoid arthritis. In the early stage, the symptoms are synovial membrane congestion, edema, thickening, capillary hyperplasia, increased permeability, and articular cavity effusion. In the chronic stage, synovial membrane cells proliferate actively, granulation tissue hyperplasia and pannus formation occur, the latter erodes and destroys articular cartilage and osseous tissue; and in the advanced stage, a large number of fibrous tissue hyperplasia and calcification lead to joint deformity, tonic, and dysfunction. The specific pathological changes of rheumatoid arthritis mainly include synovial membrane tissue hyperplasia, pannus, and granulation tissue formation.

2.8.2 Ankylosing Spondylitis (AS)

Ankylosing spondylitis (AS), whose etiology is unknown, is a systemic disease mainly characterized by progressive and chronic inflammation of axial joints. Seronegative spondyloarthropathy (SPA) is a general term for a class of arthritic diseases with negative serum rheumatoid factor and positive HLA-B27, of which ankylosing spondylitis is the most common. Almost all cases of ankylosing spondylitis show sacroiliac joint involvement and extensive ossification of spinal ligaments, eventually leading to bony ankylosis. AS is more common in young males with the ratio of male to female (2–3):1. The age of attack is usually 15–30 years old, and the disease is closely related to HLA-B27. The prevalence rate of AS has ethnic differences. At present, it is believed that it is related to many factors such as heredity, environment, infection, immunity, etc. The attack of the disease is hidden with slow progress and is a mostly dull pain in the buttocks, sacroiliac joints, or thighs. The pain develops from unilateral to bilateral, intermittently to persistent, with bilateral alternation of pain and aggravation in the morning. There may be obvious morning stiffness in the early stage, relief after activity, the disappearance of pain in the late stage, spinal ankylosis, and even deformity. Extra-articular manifestations include conjunctivitis, uveitis, pulmonary fibrosis, ascending aortic inflammation, aortic valve disease, nerve involvement, kidney disease, etc. Severe osteoporosis and vertebral body compression fracture are often accompanied in the advanced stage.

References

1. Lanjuan L, Wang Y. Infectious diseases. 3rd ed. Beijing: People's Health Publishing House; 2015.
2. Renju B. Medical imaging diagnostics. 3rd ed. Beijing: People's Health Publishing House; 2010.
3. Minming Z. Grainger & Allison's diagnostic radiology. 6th ed. Beijing: People's Military Medical Press; 2015.
4. van der Naald N, Smeeing DPJ, Houwert RM, et al. Brodie's abscess: a systematic review of reported cases. J Bone Joint Infect. 2019;4(1):33–9.
5. de Moraes FB, Motta TM, Severin AA, et al. Garré's sclerosing osteomyelitis: case report. Rev Bras Ortop. 2014;49(4):401–4.
6. Suma R. Garre's sclerosing osteomyelitis. J Indian Soc Pedod Prev Dent. 2007;25(Suppl):S30–3.
7. Zijun L. Bone and joint pathology. Beijing: People's Health Publishing House; 1992.
8. Weissleder R. Primer of diagnostic imaging. 4th ed. Mosby Elsever: Philadelphia; 2007.
9. He Y, Ting S, Dong T, et al. A case of fungal osteomyelitis of the left femur. Chin J Radiol. 2016;50(1):73–4.
10. Theil C, Schmidt-Braekling T, Gosheger G, et al. Fungal prosthetic joint infection in total hip or knee arthroplasty: a retrospective single-centre study of 26 cases. Bone Joint J. 2019;101(5):589–95.
11. Tianyun L, Haining F, Bao H. Imaging features of bone metastasis in hepatic hydatid disease. Chin J Radiol. 2018;52(3):209–12.
12. Monge-Maillo B, Olmedo Samperio M, Pérez-Molina JA, et al. Osseous cystic echinococcosis: a case series study at a referral unit in Spain. PLoS Negl Trop Dis. 2019;13(2):e0007006.
13. Raj DH, Dash PK. Hydatid disease of bone: a dangerous crippling disease. BMJ Case Rep. 2015;2015:bcr2015211697.
14. Monge-Maillo B, Chamorro Tojeiro S, López-Vélez R. Management of osseous cystic echinococcosis. Expert Rev Anti-Infect Ther. 2017;15(12):1075–82.
15. Walker-Bone K, Doherty E, Sanyal K, et al. Assessment and management of musculoskeletal disorders among patients living with HIV. Rheumatology (Oxford). 2017;56(10):1648–61.
16. Rothschild BM. History of syphilis. Clin Infect Dis. 2005;40(10):1454–63.
17. Tabák R, Tabák A, Várkonyi V. Congenital syphilis. Orv Hetil. 2010;151(2):54–61.

Imaging Characteristics and Analysis Strategies

3

Shinong Pan and Hui Guo

Bone and joint infection refers to the invasion of bacteria, viruses, fungi, parasites, and other pathogens into human bones and muscles, their growth and reproduction in bones and muscles, resulting in abnormal functions and metabolism of the body, destruction of tissue structure, and injury lesions and systemic inflammatory reactions in bones and muscles. Pathological changes and imaging findings of bone, joint and soft tissue are various. Changes in bone, joint, and soft tissue caused by different pathogens have their own characteristics on imaging images.

3.1 Skeletal Change

Skeletal changes include bone destruction, bone marrow abnormality, periosteal reaction, osteonecrosis, bone deformity, osteoporosis, abnormal ossification, and abnormal calcification.

3.1.1 Bone Destruction

Overview

Bone destruction is a local bone structure loss caused by local osseous tissue being replaced by pathological tissue.

Bone destruction can be caused by periosteum lesions, bone cortex, medulla, and periosseous soft-tissue lesions. Osteolysis and absorption are caused by bone destruction caused by enzymes produced by inflammatory cells or changes in bone dynamic balance caused by pathological changes.

S. Pan (✉)
Department of Radiology, Shengjing Hospital of China Medical University, Shenyang, Liaoning, China
e-mail: cjr.panshinong@vip.163.com

H. Guo
Department of Radiology, The First Affiliated Hospital of Xinjiang Medical University, Ürümqi, Xinjiang, China

Imaging Findings

1. **X-ray and CT.** It is manifested as decreased bone density, blurred and disappeared bone trabecula, bony defect, the bone defect is replaced by diseased tissue, with clear or unclear edge, with or without sclerotic edge, moth-eaten, etc. Pyogenic bacteria infect bones, and lesions can involve most or even all of the bones, but generally, they do not involve epiphysis across the epiphyseal plate or invade joints through articular cartilage. In the acute phase, the lesion is sieve-shaped and moth-eaten, with unclear boundaries and no sclerotic edges (Figure 3.1a and b); In the chronic phase, the lesion is a patchy bony defect with a clear boundary and sclerotic edge. Chronic recurrent multifocal osteomyelitis is characterized by multifocal and osteolytic bone destruction with sclerosis at the edge [1]. SAPHO syndrome is a chronic inflammation involving the bone cortex and bone marrow cortex, which is characterized by the coexistence of osteolysis and sclerosis or complete sclerosis [2]. For the bone infected by mycobacterium tuberculosis and brucella, the early imaging of vertebral body lesions is very similar. The defect area of infectious lesions is localized with a relative clear edge. Mycobacterium tuberculosis infection lesions can sclerosis to a certain extent, and then diffuse damage intensifies, which is easy to spread to the marrow cavity and form tuberculous osteomyelitis. Bone destruction is easy to occur at the epiphysis and metaphysis, and defects can be formed at the center or edge of the bone. Usually, the epiphysis and metaphysis are destroyed at the same time, forming a unified destruction area that is not limited by the epiphyseal plate (Fig. 3.2). Brucella infection has obvious hyperostosis and osteosclerosis with the development of pathological changes, and its bone density reduction changes are lighter than tuberculosis. The hydatid infected bones showed the round or irregular cystic radiolucent area with sharp edges, no erosive damage, and no obvious sclerosis edge.

H. Li et al. (eds.), *Radiology of Infectious and Inflammatory Diseases - Volume 5*,
https://doi.org/10.1007/978-981-16-5003-1_3

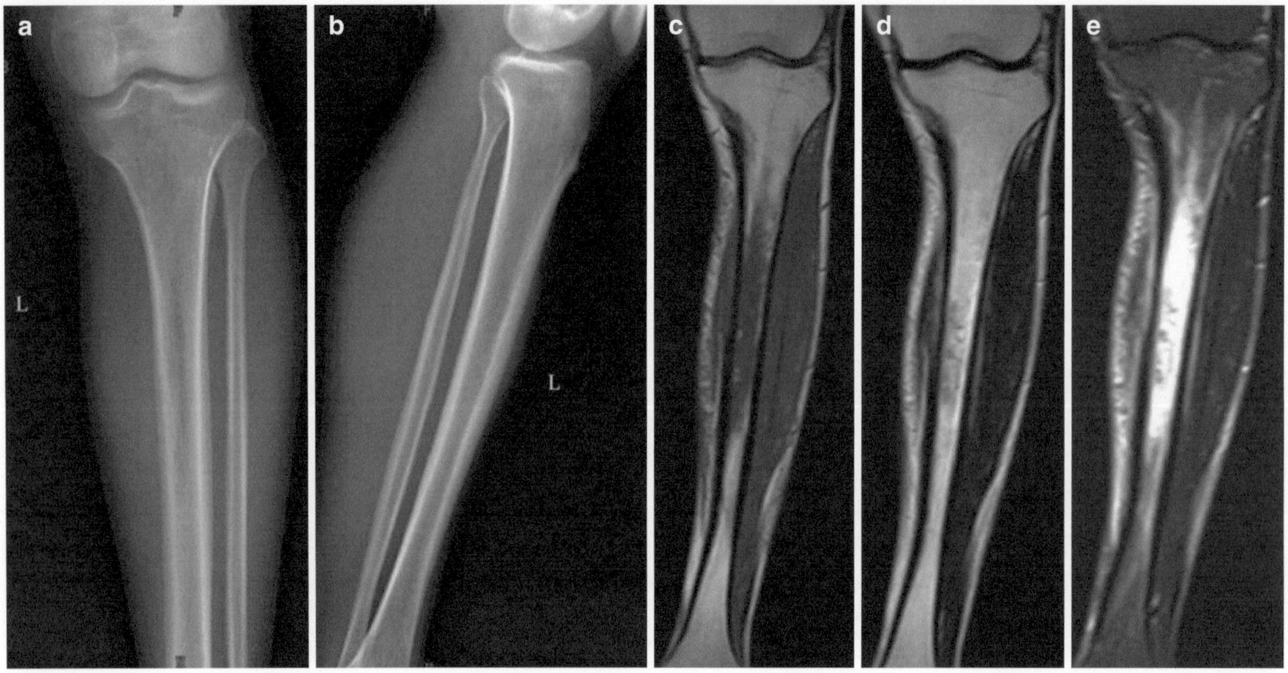

Fig. 3.1 Acute suppurative osteomyelitis of left tibial diaphysis. (**a**, **b**) DR PA & LAT views showed moth-eaten bone destruction with unclear boundary in the diaphysis of the middle and upper segment of the left tibia. (**c**–**e**) MRI coronal plane T_1WI, T_2WI, and STIR showed abnormal signals in the diaphysis of the middle and upper segment of the left tibia, with unclear boundaries and inflammatory edema in the surrounding soft tissue

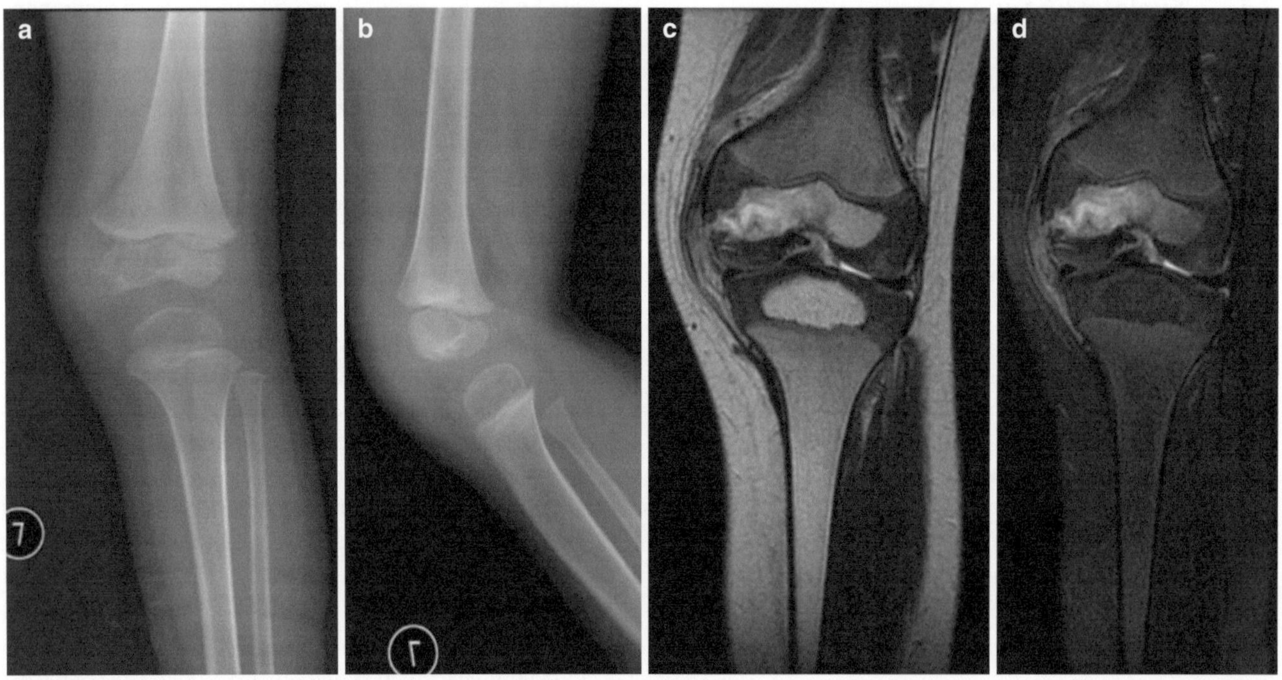

Fig. 3.2 Epiphysis tuberculosis of left distal femur. (**a**, **b**) DR PA & LAT radiographs showed cystic bone destruction on the medial of the left femoral epiphysis and swelling of soft tissue around the joint. (**c**, **d**) MRI coronal planeT_2WI and STIR showed irregular hyperintense in the medial of the left femoral epiphysis, and inflammatory edema around the medial joint

Most of the pathological tissues that destroy bone are low density, with soft tissue, pus, cystic fluid, calcification, and sequestrum, etc., and with uniform or nonuniform density.

The observation and analysis of bone destruction signs should be based on the changes of its region, shape, scope, edge, periosteum, soft tissue, as well as clinical, pathological, and dynamic changes.

2. **MRI.** Its display of bone structure is not as good as X-ray and CT, but it has great value in displaying the characteristics of pathological tissues of bone destruction. Most of the lesions in the defect region of bone destruction showed hypointense on T_1WI, hyperintense on T_2WI, and hyperintense on T_2WI FS sequence (Figure 3.1c–e). However, the changes of signals are complex and affected by lesion components, and analyzing the pathological tissues represented by these signals is valuable for diagnosis. More characteristic signs or pathological tissue contents: liquid-containing cystic cavity and abscess, granulation tissue, fibrous tissue, hemorrhage, and hemosiderin deposition [3, 4]. Liquid-containing cystic cavity and abscess are found in bone hydatid disease cyst, pyogenic abscess, tuberculous abscess, and brucella abscess. Hydatid contains a liquid cystic cavity, and bone abscess, it is the most sensitive on MRI.

Because the abscess wall is granulation tissue with abundant blood vessels, CT and MRI enhanced scans show ring enhancement, while the central pus is not enhanced. The vomica contains water and necrotic substances, it shows hyperintense on T_2WI. Necrotic tissue can limit the diffusion of water molecules, so it shows hyperintense on DWI, and decreased ADC value. The caseous necrotic vomica of the tuberculous cold abscess has less water content and shows isointensity or slightly hypointense on T_2WI, while the restriction of diffusion movement is smaller than that of pyogenic infection pus, so it shows slightly hyperintense or isointense on DWI.

Mature fibrous tissue shows hypointense on T_1WI and T_2WI and can be enhanced.

For internal hemorrhage or hematoma of lesions, subacute manifestations of different signals in different periods are typical T_1WI hyperintense, and all sequences of hemosiderin deposition are hypointense. Internal hemorrhage in infectious lesions is generally rare.

3.1.2 Abnormal Bone Marrow

Overview

Bone marrow abnormalities include bone marrow edema, bone marrow infiltration, and bone marrow replacement.

Pathophysiology

Bone marrow edema is found in inflammation, trauma and other pathological changes, it is the increase of local bone marrow interstitial water content caused by congestion and exudation. Both bone marrow infiltration and bone marrow substitution refer to the invasion and substitution of marrow cavity by abnormal cells or substances, such as infected inflammatory cells, tumor cells, etc. Bone marrow infiltration refers to an incomplete replacement, there are some residual normal adipocytes. Bone marrow replacement refers to the complete replacement of local bone marrow tissue by lesions.

Imaging Findings

1. **Bone marrow edema.** X-ray and CT cannot show bone marrow edema (Fig. 3.3a), only MRI can show it. STIR or T_2WI fat-suppressed sequence show patchy, lamellar, or feathery hyperintense images with unclear boundaries in bone marrow, and hypointense on T_1WI (Fig. 3.3b–d). An enhanced scan can have mild enhancement.
2. **Bone marrow infiltration and bone marrow replacement.** It cannot be displayed by X-ray and CT, but only by MRI. It shows moderate hypointense on T_1WI, hyperintense on T_2WI, which is equivalent to that of red bone marrow. Fat does not disappear completely, and the boundary between the affected region and normal fatty bone marrow is unclear. Bone marrow replacement shows hypointense on T_1WI, which is equivalent to muscle or intervertebral disc, and the fat disappears completely. It can be single, multiple, or diffuse multiple foci with normal bone marrow, also known as intramarrow saltatory focus. Single and multiple focuses show hypointense on T_1WI, which is significant compared with the hyperintense of normal bone marrow. T_2WI FS and STIR are hyperintense and are enhanced after enhancement [5, 6].

3.1.3 Periosteal Reaction

Overview

Periosteal reaction is a proliferative reaction that occurs after the periosteum is stimulated by inflammation, trauma, and tumor. In the past, only X-ray plain film showed a proliferative reaction after periosteum was stimulated, and periosteal ossification could determine the periosteal reaction. At present, MRI can observe periosteal proliferation before periosteal ossification.

Outcome of periosteal reaction: (1) edema, hyperplasia, thickening-improved after absorption -return to normal (only visible on MRI); (2) edema, hyperplasia, thickening-mineralization-periosteal proliferation-lesion improvement

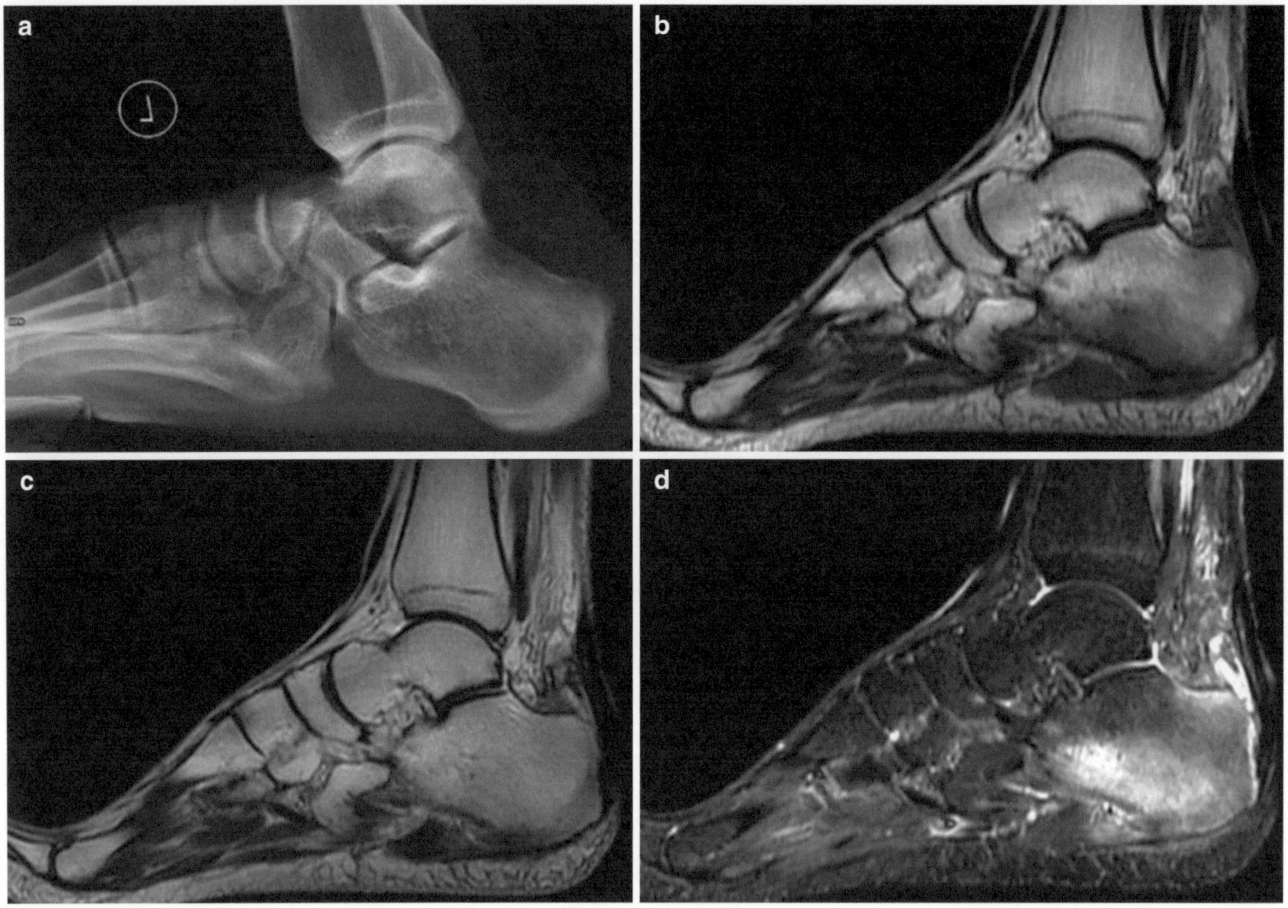

Figure 3.3 Bone marrow edema (left calcaneus infection). DR PA view showed unremarkable in the left calcaneus (**a**); MRI sagittal plane T_1WI (**b**) and T_2WI (**c**) showed abnormal signals in the left calcaneus, while STIR (**d**) showed obvious bone marrow edema signals in the left calcaneus and posterior and inferior inflammatory edema

and absorption, local bone cortex thickening caused by fusion of periosteal proliferation and bone cortex; (3) edema, hyperplasia, thickening-mineralization-periosteal proliferation-local bone cortex thickening caused by fusion with bone cortex-persistent existence of intraosseous lesions, destruction of bone, even new bone cortex, and then periosteal re-hyperplasia (mineralization)-re-destruction-expansive bone destruction, mostly benign or chronic changes; (4) edema, hyperplasia, thickening-mineralization-periosteal proliferation-intraosseous lesions rapidly destroy bone and bone cortex, periosteal proliferation-lesions break through periosteal proliferation-periosteal proliferation interruption-periosteal triangle (Codman triangle), mostly malignant bone tumors, and a few acute inflammatory lesions.

Imaging Findings

Periosteum edema or periosteum thickening cannot be displayed by X-ray and CT before ossification. MRI T2WI FS or STIR shows perimeter or strip-like hyperintense close to bone cortex, which is periosteal proliferation. After mineralization, it shows hypointense on both T_1WI and T_2WI, and the surrounding lesions mostly show hyperintense on T_2WI. X-ray plain film and CT show high density shadow, which is linear or strip-like high density shadow in the early stage, locating outside the bone cortex, and there is a narrow transparent line between it and the bone cortex. The ossified periosteum has a variety of manifestations, which can be layered, scallion skin-like, lace-like, parallel to the bone cortex, or sunlight-irradiated, radial perpendicular to the bone cortex, or the above periosteal proliferation is destroyed again by the lesion, forming a central interruption, leaving triangular periosteal proliferation on both sides, i.e., periosteal triangle. Acute osteomyelitis can present homogeneous, continuous, and dense periosteal reactions, while chronic osteomyelitis can present lace-like periosteal reaction, but these signs have no specificity. Most lesions of the long bone such as mycobacterium tuberculosis infection, brucella infection, and bone hydatid disease have no periosteal reaction, and only a few lesions have a periosteal reaction.

3.1.4 Osteonecrosis

Overview

Osteonecrosis is mainly due to the termination of local osseous tissue metabolism caused by blood supply interruption. The necrotic bone is also called sequestrum.

The sequestrum is prone to fracture and bone collapse due to the cessation of metabolism, loss of organic components, decrease in strength, and increase in brittleness. Subchondral bone is prone to fracture collapse and cause secondary osteoarthritis. Osteonecrosis can be found in suppurative osteomyelitis, tuberculosis, etc. After osteonecrosis, the surrounding spongy bone will edema and congestion, or the surrounding will have pus or newly formed granulation tissue. In large sequestrum caused by osteomyelitis, metabolism stops, especially blood supply is interrupted and cannot be absorbed for a short time. Due to body repair, osteoblasts form bone on the original bone trabecula, which makes the relatively high bone mineral density of sequestrum.

Imaging Findings

1. **X-ray and CT.** CT is the most sensitive for sequestrum formed by osteomyelitis and tuberculosis with high specificity. Osteomyelitis sequestrum is often manifested as a strip-like abnormal high-density shadow along the long bone, while the surrounding pus and granuloma are obviously low-density shadows. Most of the sequestrum of tuberculosis are gravel-like and mostly fragmented high-density shadows (Fig. 3.4).

   X-ray plain film shows that ischemic osteonecrosis is insensitive and can be completely normal in the early stage. Later, density reduction zone or cloud-like density increase shadow appears, or density reduction and increase are mixed, and the edge is usually unclear. X-ray plain films are usually blurred or even difficult to determine. CT shows more clearly than X-ray plain films. In the later period, subchondral bone often collapses, which is manifested as abnormal and irregular curvature of the bony articular surface.
2. **MRI.** MRI can sensitively display ischemic osteonecrosis, which is mainly bone marrow necrosis and local moisture increase caused by edema, and shows hypointense on T_1WI and hyperintense on T_2WI. Then the necrotic fat is partially decomposed, edema gradually disappears, and shows hyperintense on both T_1WI and T_2WI. Granulation tissue and bone proliferative reaction zone around the sequestrum show both hyperintense and hypointense, especially typical double-line signs can be found in T_1WI and T_2WI FS, which is a typical pattern on the whole. MRI manifestations of osteomyelitis and tuberculosis sequestrum are not as clear as X-ray plain film [7], and all show various sequences of hypointense.

3.1.5 Bone Deformity

Overview

Bone deformity refers to abnormal changes in bone contour and morphology or abnormal bone shaping due to pathological changes.

In infectious diseases, bone destruction such as bone tuberculosis and osteomyelitis can usually cause bone thinning, periosteal proliferation in chronic osteomyelitis can

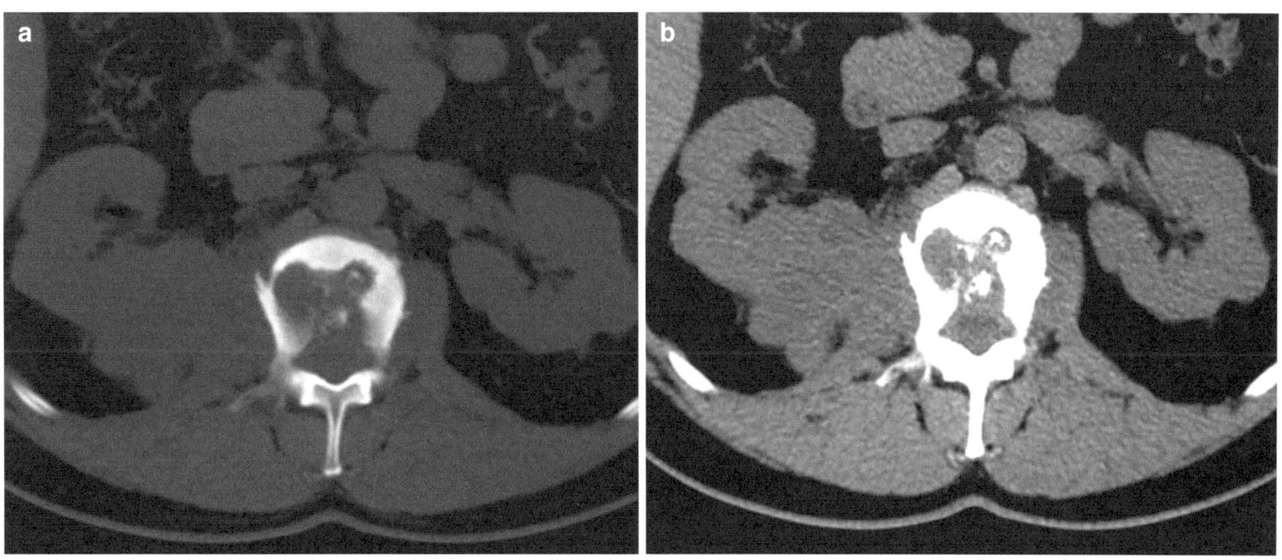

Figure 3.4 L_1 ~ L_2 vertebral tuberculosis. (**a**) CT showed osteolytic bone destruction in L_1 vertebral body with sequestrum in it; (**b**) The right psoas major muscle was thickened, and a soft tissue shadow was found between the thickened greater psoas muscle and the right kidney

thicken bone shape, and bone swelling and destruction in long bone echinococcosis can cause bone shape thickening and change.

Imaging Findings

X-ray and CT can clearly display bone morphological changes, and X-ray plain film is of great value. CT and MRI can be used as supplementary examinations for fine anatomical structures and complex regions.

3.1.6 Osteoporosis

Overview

Osteoporosis refers to the reduction of mineralized bone mass per unit volume and the proportional reduction of organic matter and calcium salt.

Bone is a living organ, and bone absorption and formation maintain a dynamic balance. Weakened osteogenic activity or enhanced osteoclast activity can break this balance and cause osteopenia, while the ratio of organic matter to inorganic matter in bone is normal, i.e., osteoporosis is formed. Histological manifestations include thinning of bone cortex, enlargement of Haversian canal, reduction, thinning, or disappearance of bone trabecula.

Osteoporosis is divided into systemic and localized categories. Etiology of systemic osteoporosis: (1) senile and postmenopausal osteoporosis; (2) endocrine disorders, such as hyperparathyroidism; (3) iatrogenic, long-term hormone therapy; (4) congenital diseases, such as osteogenesis imperfecta; (5) nutritional or metabolic disorders, such as vitamin C deficiency; (6) alcoholism; (7) unknown reasons, such as adolescent idiopathic osteoporosis. Localized osteoporosis is caused by local lesions, such as post-fracture, inflammation, tumor, and limb apraxia. Osteoporosis reduces bone strength, increases brittleness, and is prone to fracture. Infectious diseases are mainly localized osteoporosis, which is common in bone tuberculosis.

Imaging Findings

1. **X-ray and CT.** It shows that the bone density is decreased, the bone trabecula is sparse with a widened gap, the bone cortex becomes thinner and layered, but the margins of the bone cortex and bone trabecula are clear. The vertebral body can be double concave, even compressed and flattened, and the intervertebral space widens.
2. **Bone mineral density quantificatio**n It can help clinically formulate treatment plans for osteoporosis and prevent fracture. Dual-energy X-ray absorptiometry (DXA) is a commonly used technique for the quantitative examination of bone mineral density in a clinic. The T value of DXA < -1, but > -2.5 refers to osteopenia, and ≤ -2.5 refers to osteoporosis.

3.1.7 Abnormal Ossification

Overview

There are two kinds of abnormal ossification: one is the body's response to pathological changes, namely hyperostosis; The other is tumor bone, which is abnormal bone formed by mineralization of matrix secreted by bone tumor cells. Matrix mineralization is mainly the deposition of hydroxyapatite into osteoid tissue. Hyperostosis is common in infectious diseases.

Hyperostosis is an increase in bone mass per unit volume. The histological manifestations include thickening of bone cortex and thickening and increase of bone trabecula. Most of them are repair reactions caused by abnormal stimulation of pathological changes, including inflammation, acute and chronic trauma, tumor, etc. Chronic stage of pyogenic spondylitis, hyperostosis, and osteosclerosis around the focus of chronic osteomyelitis, and chronic stage of brucellar spondylitis can form "lacelike vertebrae" and bird's beak-like proliferation and sclerosis changes at the anterior margin of the vertebral body. Hyperostosis can also be osteosclerosis caused by endocrine and metabolic abnormalities, toxic bone development disorders or tumors, such as renal osteosclerosis, skeletal fluorosis, osteoporosis, and lead poisoning.

Imaging Findings

1. **X-ray and CT.** Hyperostosis and osteosclerosis are characterized by increased local bone density, thickening of cortex, thickening and increase of bone trabecula. Lumbar spine diseases are often accompanied by bird's beak-like and lace-like proliferation and sclerosis (Figure 3.5a–e). It can also be extensive bone cortex thickening sclerosis, which is found in osteopathy, skeletal fluorosis, renal osteopathy, etc. Infectious diseases are generally localized hyperostosis and osteosclerosis.
2. **MRI.** Hyperostosis and osteosclerosis show hypointense on conventional sequence T_1WI and T_2WI (Figure 3.5f, g).

3.1.8 Abnormal Calcification

Overview

Abnormal calcification is the abnormal deposition of calcium salt in tissues. Abnormal intraosseous calcification is mostly found in bone tuberculosis, bone hydatid disease, intraosseous cartilaginous lesions, and bone infarction.

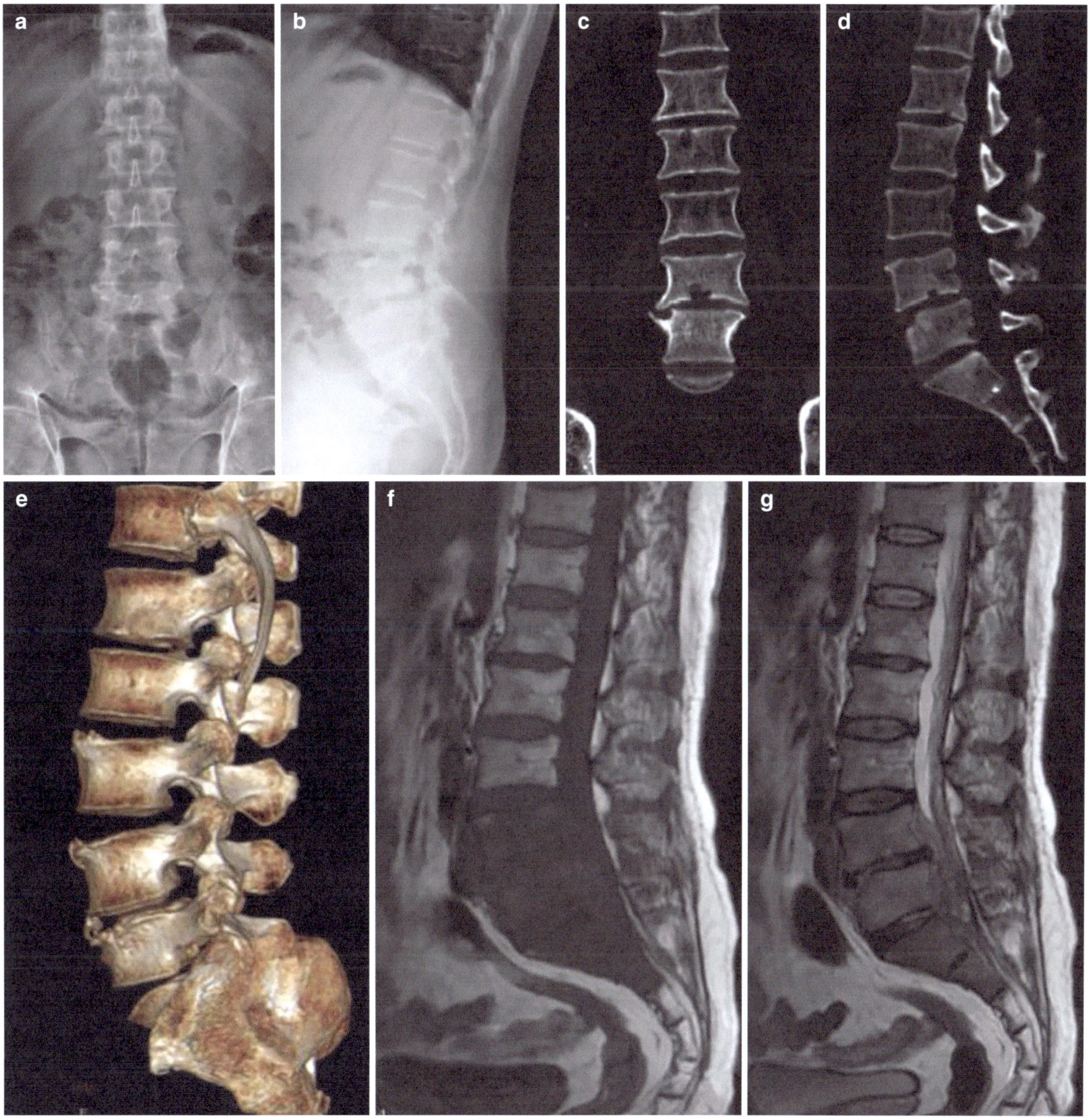

Fig. 3.5 Brucellar spondylitis. (**a**, **b**) DR PA&LAT radiographs showed that the $L_4 \sim L_5$ anterior margin of the vertebral body showed moth-eaten bone destruction, and accompanied by bird's beak-like hyperostosis and osteosclerosis; (**c**–**e**) CT reconstruction showed bird's beak like hyperostosis and osteosclerosis at the edge of multiple vertebral bodies; (**f**, **g**) MRI sagittal plane T_1WI and T_2WI showed proliferation and sclerosis at the anterior margin of the vertebral body, both showing hypointense

Calcification after tissue necrosis is such as calcification in caseous lesions of bone tuberculosis, eggshell-like calcification of cystic echinococcus, gravel-like, amorphous calcification of alveolar hydatid cyst, calcification of bone infarction, etc.

Imaging Findings

X-ray and CT showed scattered and amorphous high-density shadows, showing various shapes such as dots, strips, sheets, rings, arcs, and lumps, with no bone trabecular structure (Fig. 3.6). The density is high and the CT value varies greatly,

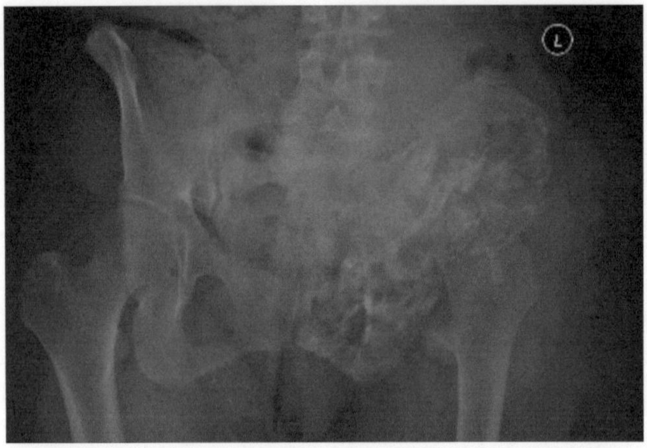

Fig. 3.6 Bone hydatid disease with left hip joint dislocation. DR PA view showed osteolytic bone destruction of left ilium, ischium, and pubis, and spotted and irregular calcification could be found under ischium

which may occur in 100 ~ 1000 HU. If typical central spongy bone and superficial bone cortex are formed, ossification can be distinguished from calcification, and it is not easy to distinguish from calcification when ossification is atypical.

3.2 Abnormal Joint Changes

Abnormal joint changes include joint swelling, joint destruction, degeneration of joint, ankylosis, joint dislocation, intra-joint masses, and periarticular cystic lesions.

3.2.1 Joint Swelling

Overview

Joint swelling is a common term in clinical and common X-ray plain films, joint thickening can be called joint swelling. It is common in inflammation, trauma, and hemorrhagic diseases. Joint effusion, joint empyema, soft-tissue edema around the joint, hemorrhage, and inflammation can all lead to local thickening of the joint.

Joint effusion refers to the increase of fluid in the articular cavity, it can be an increase in synovial membrane secretion caused by inflammation, synovial membrane injury, etc., or intra-articular cavity hemorrhage caused by trauma and hemorrhagic diseases.

Imaging Findings

1. **X-ray and CT.** The soft tissue around the joint is swollen with slightly increased density, the structural layer of soft tissue is unclear, and the fat pad and intermuscular fat layer are displaced, deformed, blurred, or disappeared. It can be found that the joint space is widened with a large amount of joint effusion and joint empyema. CT is superior to X-ray plain film, besides the above soft-tissue swelling, it can also directly show articular cavity effusion.
2. **MRI.** The specific causes of clinical joint swelling can be clearly distinguished, i.e., surrounding soft-tissue edema, mass, or joint effusion. Basic lesions of soft-tissue edema and mass around joints. Joint effusion is characterized by enlargement of the articular capsule and articular cavity with liquid signal shadow in it. If the effusion is bloody, can find hyperintense on T_1WI, and sometimes fluid-fluid level can be observed. Its sensitivity and specificity are the highest.

3.2.2 Joint Destruction

Overview

Joint destruction is the destruction and replacement of articular cartilage and its underlying bone by pathological tissues. It can cause joint dysfunction and even disability, and is common in pyogenic arthritis, joint tuberculosis, rheumatoid arthritis, and rheumatic arthritis, etc., rarely found in brucella arthritis, viral hepatitis arthritis, etc.

Imaging Findings

1. **X-ray and CT.** If only articular cartilage is involved in the destruction, there may be no abnormality or only narrowing of joint space. If the articular surface bone is involved, the corresponding articular surface is blurred, with small aggressive destruction foci, or large local bone destruction and defect. Severe cases can cause joint subluxation, deformation, and rigidity. CT can show fine bone destruction and soft tissue changes. CT can show fine bone destruction and soft tissue changes.
2. **MRI.** It can directly show cartilage destruction, which is manifested as rough, thinning, fracture, and disappearance of articular cartilage. Bone destruction showed hypointense, interruption, or disappearance of bone cortex continuity on T_2WI FS, and enhanced scanning showed abnormal intra-articular enhancement and continuation of bony defect foci. It can clearly show soft tissue abnormalities causing bone destruction. Bone destruction on the weight-bearing surface: Cartilage destruction begins on the weight-bearing surface of the joint or invades subchondral bone from the edge of the joint. Cartilage and bone destruction is rapid and extensive and is common in acute pyogenic arthritis [8, 9]. Marginal bone destruction: Cartilage destruction starts at the edge of the joint and gradually involves the bone. It is

manifested as moth-eaten destruction of the marginal part. Generally, it progresses slowly. It is common in joint synovial membrane tuberculosis, rheumatoid arthritis, etc., mostly the thickened synovial membrane pannus, and hyperplastic granulation tissue erodes and destroys the end bone at the attachment of capsular ligament.

3.2.3 Degeneration of Joint

Overview

Degeneration of joint refers to the change of joint aging and degeneration with age. At the late stage of joint infection, degeneration of joints can also be caused.

Early changes begin with cartilage, which is cartilage damage. The content of water and proteoglycan gradually decreases, and cartilage degenerates and exfoliates. Extensive cartilage exfoliation can cause stenosis of joint space, leading to hyperostosis and osteosclerosis of bony articular surface, osteophyte formation at bone edge, hypertrophy of articular capsule, and calcification of ligament. Primary joint degeneration is more common in the elderly, with the weight-bearing spine, hip joint, and knee joint being the most obvious. Secondary joint degeneration can be found in chronic injury, bone and joint ischemia and necrosis, arthritis, etc. Long-term excessive weight-bearing of joints, exercise can also accelerate joint degeneration, which is found in athletes, porters, and other groups.

Imaging Findings

1. **X-ray and CT.** In the early stage, X-ray plain film may have no abnormality, or show slight osteophyte formation at the edge of the bone end and blurred bony articular surface. In the middle and late stage, the manifestations are stenosis of joint space, formation of subchondral bone pseudocyst, and formation of osteophyte at the edge of bony articular surface, and joint deformation may also occur in severe cases. CT is more sensitive to show subarticular capsular degeneration area.
2. **MRI.** Conventional sequences can show abnormal signals in the cartilage at an early stage, which can be limited to the surface layer of cartilage or involve the whole layer. PDWI and 3D dual-echo steady-state sequences (3D-DESS) show better. The increase of signal may be related to cartilage edema and abnormal arrangement of collagen fibers, while the decrease of signal may be related to chondrocyte reduction. After that, the cartilage surface is rough and uneven, with small defects, and in serious cases, it is completely stripped. In recent years, there have been some quantitative techniques for cartilage composition, such as the T_2 relaxation time mapping technique for quantitative water composition in cartilage.

3.2.4 Ankylosis

Overview

Joint ankylosis is that after the joint is obviously destroyed, the bone end of the joint is connected by osseous tissue or fibrous tissue, and the joint is stiff and unable to move.

Joint ankylosis is divided into bony ankylosis and fibrous ankylosis. Bony ankylosis is that after the bone destruction of the joint, the two bone ends that make up the joint are connected by osseous tissue, which is more common in acute pyogenic arthritis and ankylosing spondylitis. Fibrous ankylosis is also the consequence of joint destruction. The bone end of the joint is connected by fibrous tissue, which is common in joint tuberculosis and rheumatoid arthritis.

Imaging Findings

1. **X线和CT.** Bony ankylosis is characterized by the disappearance of joint space and bone trabecula penetrating the joint to connect the bone ends on both sides. For fibrous ankylosis, joint activity disappears, but X-ray plain film still shows narrow joint space and no bone trabecula penetrates. The diagnosis of fibrotic ankylosis should be combined with clinical manifestations, not only by X-ray plain film.
2. **MRI.** When bony ankylosis occurs, it can show that articular cartilage is completely destroyed, joint space disappears, spongy bone connects the bone ends on both sides of the joint, and completely fuses with the spongy bone of both bones; When fibrous rigidity occurs, the joint space still exists, but there is destruction to the bone end of the joint, and abnormal signals mixed with hyperintense and hypointense can be found between the bone ends.

3.2.5 Joint Dislocation

Overview

Joint dislocation refers to the loss of normal involution of the bones that make up the joint.

According to the etiology, it can be divided into traumatic, congenital, pathological, and habitual dislocation, with traumatic being the most common. According to the degree of articular surface separation, it can be divided into complete dislocation and subluxation.

Imaging Findings

1. **X-ray and CT.** It can show the position change of the bone end of the joint, abnormal joint space, and joint dislocation caused by the destruction of the joint by bone hydatid disease (Fig. 3.7). CT can remove the influence of structural overlap, and the display of dislocation of com-

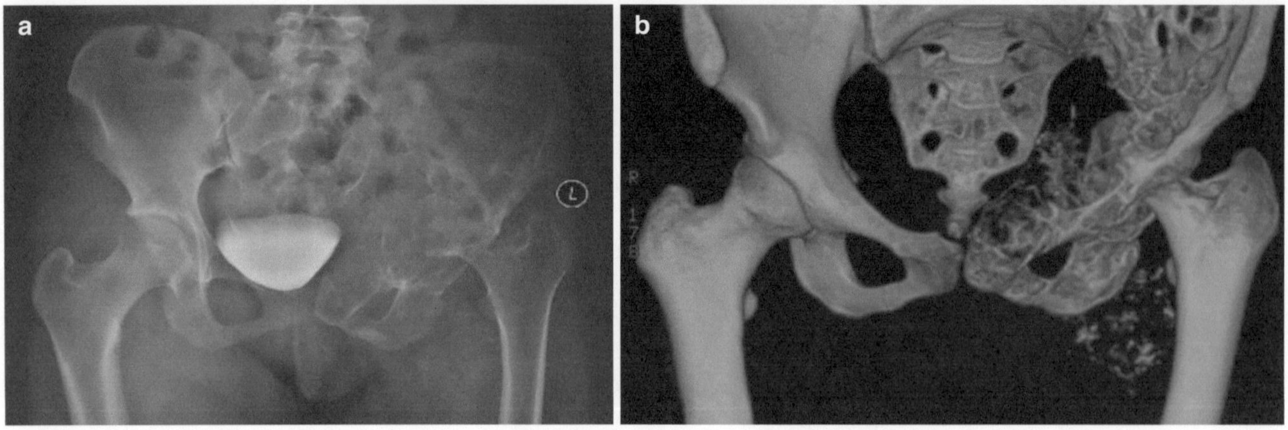

Figure 3.7 Bone hydatid disease with left hip joint dislocation. (**a**) DR PA view showed osteolytic bone destruction of left ilium, ischium, and pubis and central dislocation of the femoral head; (**b**) VR image visually and stereoscopically displayed joint dislocation.

plex parts, such as sternoclavicular joint and spinal intervertebral joint, is better than X-ray plain film. SSD, VRT, or three-dimensional reconstruction can show joint dislocation more intuitively and stereoscopically.

2. **MRI.** It can not only directly show the positional relationship of the joint bone end, but also intuitively show the damage of the joint stable structure combined with dislocation, such as the damage and tear of the glenoid labrum, articular cartilage, ligament, tendon, etc.

3.2.6 Intra-Articular Mass

Overview

Intra-articular masses are common in synovial osteochondromatosis, pigmented villonodular synovitis, synovial hemangioma, and other diseases, and sometimes tumor-like changes can be found in infectious diseases such as joint tuberculosis, rheumatoid arthritis, gout, and so on.

Imaging Findings

1. **X-ray and CT.** The display of the mass is generally insensitive, and when the mass is large, it is displayed as a soft-tissue mass shadow. Sometimes destruction and/or sclerosis of adjacent bones can be found. When secondary osteoarthritis occurs, joint space stenosis can be found. CT has a higher density resolution, is more sensitive and specific to the display of calcification, fat, and other components in the mass, and has more advantages than plain film in the display of lesion edge and tiny bone erosion.
2. **MRI.** It has good soft-tissue resolution and bone marrow imaging advantages. Multidirectional imaging can clearly display different signals and reflect different histological components in lesions, such as synovial tissue hyperplasia, hemosiderin, fat, fibrous tissue, and joint effusion, which is helpful for differential diagnosis.

3.2.7 Periarticular Cystic Lesions

Overview

Bursitis in infectious diseases can cause cystic lesions in soft tissues around joints. The wall of bursitis is synovial tissue, which is full of liquid. The contents of bursitis may be purulent liquid caused by infection, the most common being inflammatory exudate, or the increased intra-articular liquid is directly injected into the bursa communicating with it.

Imaging Findings

1. **X-ray and CT.** X-ray generally does not show (Figure 3.8a). CT can show cystic liquid density shadow when the lesion is large, and the relationship with the surroundings is clearly or poorly shown (Figure 3.8b).
2. **MRI.** The most sensitive and clear, with high specificity. It is manifested as a liquid-containing capsule cavity, mostly with typical water signals with clear and sharp margins, but the composition changes of some capsule contents have corresponding signal characteristics; Echinococcosis showed hypointense on T_1WI, hyperintense on T_2WI, and higher hyperintense on STIR. The cyst in the cyst of hydatid cyst has typical characteristics (Figure 3.8c–e). When the protein content increased, it showed isointensity and hyperintense on T_1WI; If the cyst is complicated with infection, cyst wall thickening can be found, and moderate enhancement can be found when enhanced scanning the thickened cyst wall [10, 11].

Bursitis is the anatomical position where the bursa is located. Sometimes it can be found that it is communicated

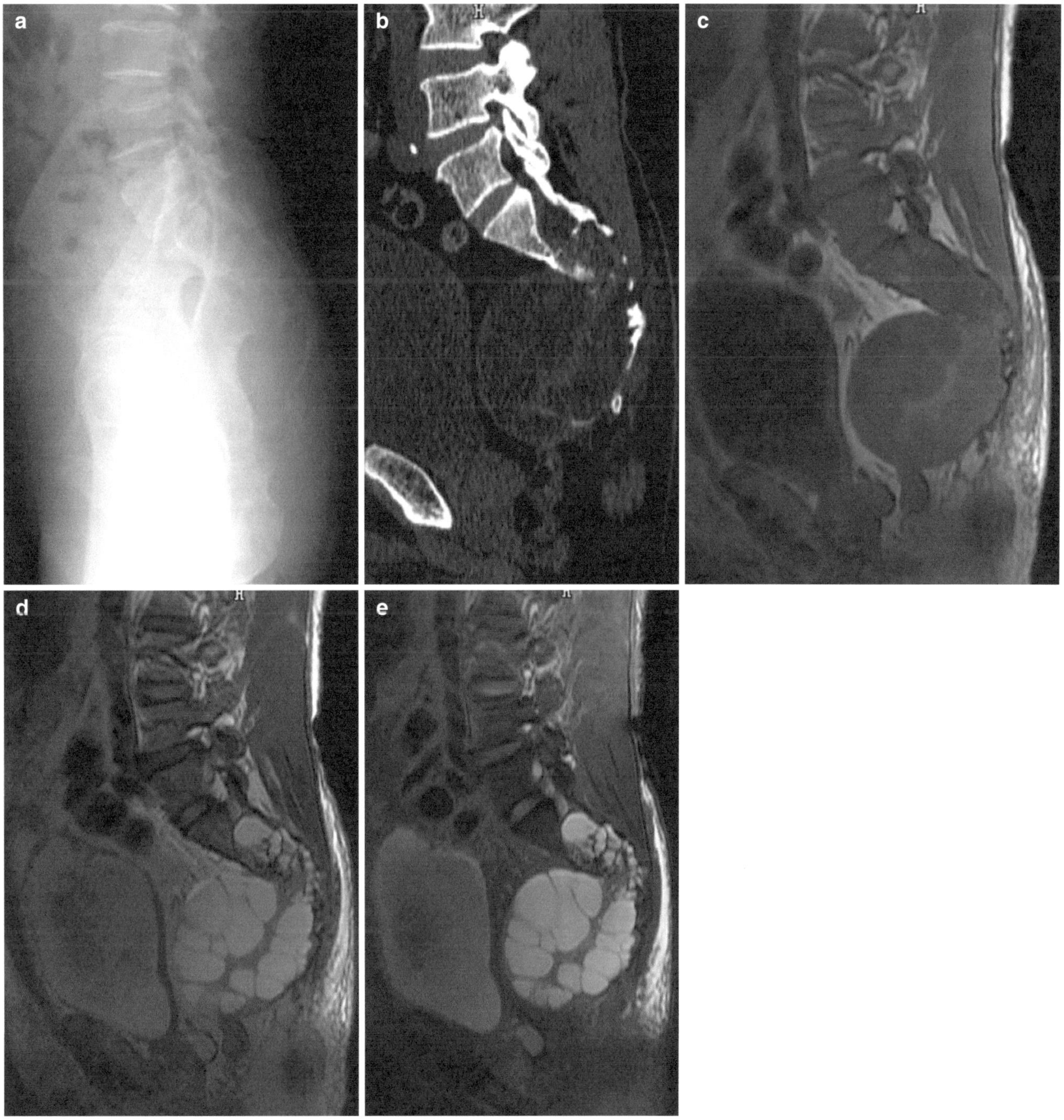

Fig. 3.8 Echinococcus cyst in the sacrum and surrounding regions. (**a**) DR LAT radiograph showed cystic bone destruction of the sacral vertebral body; (**b**) CT sagittal plane showed cystic bone destruction of the sacral vertebral body, with a large polycystic lesion in front; (**c**–**e**) MRI sagittal plane T_2WI, T_2WI and STIR showed S_2 ~ S_5 cystic bone destruction, with a large cystic echinococcus cyst in front of it

with the knee joint cavity, but most bursa is not communicated with the articular cavity. Popliteal cyst, meniscus cyst, synovial membrane cyst, and ganglion cyst are usually identified by the anatomical location and structure of the focus, but the diagnosis needs a histopathological basis.

3.3 Abnormal Soft Tissue Changes

Abnormal soft tissue changes include soft-tissue edema, calcification and ossification in soft tissue, gas in soft tissue and soft tissue abscess, etc.

3.3.1 Soft-Tissue Edema

Overview

Soft-tissue edema can be caused by soft tissue inflammatory reaction, exudation, hemorrhage, etc. caused by various infections that increase tissue space fluid.

Imaging Findings

1. **X-ray and CT.** It showed that the density of soft tissue increased, subcutaneous fat showed grid-like changes, the boundary line between muscle and muscle was blurred, and the fat line between muscle and intermuscular space was blurred or disappeared. CT display is slightly better than X-ray plain film, but it is difficult to make a definite diagnosis.
2. **MRI.** It can clearly define soft tissue edema with obvious advantages in showing edema and distinguishing it from abscess and hematoma. The water content of soft tissue increased, showing patchy hypointense on T_1WI and diffuse hyperintense on T_2WI. The boundary was unclear, expanding along with the intermuscular space, and the volume of soft tissue increased. Because edema and fat show hyperintense on T_2WI, in order to determine whether it is edema, STIR or T_2WI FS is generally used to remove fat signal. Diffuse hyperintense combined with the etiology of edema in clinical manifestations can mostly determine edema.

3.3.2 Calcification and Ossification in Soft Tissue

Overview

Calcification in soft tissue is an abnormal deposition of calcium salt in soft tissue. However, ossification is that cells secrete bone matrix and calcium salt deposits from bone, mostly trabecular bone. In case of a long time, lamellar bone can be formed on the periphery.

Infectious diseases such as tuberculosis and parasitic infection are the causes of calcification, which can occur in muscles, intermuscular spaces, tendons, articular capsules, lymph nodes, and other tissues. Mature ossification is similar to normal bone structure and consists of bone cortex and marrow cavity containing bone trabecula. Soft tissue calcification is often an amorphous high-density structure. Accurate distinction between calcification and ossification is valuable for disease diagnosis, but it is often difficult to distinguish between calcification and ossification when the lesion volume is small, and partial calcification can develop into ossification with the passage of time.

Imaging Findings

1. **X-ray and CT.** Calcification is an amorphous, scattered punctate, strip, annular or semi-annular high-density shadow in soft tissue, with unclear edges (see Fig. 3.6); However, typical ossification can show the cortical density of bone trabecula and even peripheral bone cortex, with clear and smooth edges, but it is often difficult to completely distinguish the two. Annular or semi-annular cartilage is often calcified, with certain characteristics. CT is superior to X-ray plain film and MRI in showing calcification and ossification.
2. **MRI.** Most lesions show hypointense in each sequence. Under special circumstances, the combination of calcified particles and proteins has paramagnetism, which can lead to hyperintense on T_1WI. It is often impossible to determine calcification and ossification by MRI alone. However, large typical ossification can show bone marrow-like signals in the central bone and a cortical-like signal-free band in the periphery, which may be defined as ossification in combination with plain film.

3.3.3 Gas in Soft Tissue

Overview

Gas usually exists in soft tissues and is usually caused by aerogenic bacteria infection.

Imaging Findings

1. **X-ray and CT.** CT has the highest diagnostic value, showing low-density gas shadow in soft tissue, bubble-shaped or tape-shaped translucent shadow. The gas distribution is consistent with the long axis of the muscle bundle, sometimes setting off the contour shape of muscle bundle, and local tissue can swell and thicken. The CT value is generally less than -100HU, with a clear margin. Whether it is gas can be determined by measuring the CT value.
2. **MRI.** There is no signal in each sequence, which is sometimes difficult to distinguish from calcification and is not as clear as CT.

3.3.4 Soft-Tissue Abscess

Overview

Soft tissue abscess is soft tissue infection, and the central liquefactive necrosis forms vomica, which can be nonspecific bacteria or specific bacterial infection. The common ones are staphylococcus aureus, mycobacterium tuberculosis, or brucella infection.

Imaging Findings

1. **X-ray.** It is not sensitive to display soft tissue abscess, which is manifested as soft tissue swelling. It is better when there are structures with large density differences around it to form a contrast. For example, tuberculosis abscess is paravertebral, and soft tissue swelling can be found in the iliac fossa.
2. **CT.** It shows a soft tissue mass with unclear boundary, circular, quasi-circular, or irregular shape. Some borderlines can be clear. Compared with muscles, the abscess wall is of isodense or slightly hypodense, and the central pus is of hypodense (Figure 3.9a). Enhanced scanning is of great value in determining abscess, which shows moderate irregular enhancement of abscess wall. The wall of the tuberculous abscess is relatively regular, thin and uniform, and mild enhancement.
3. **MRI.** It is the most sensitive and specific in displaying abscess, showing heterogeneous hypointense on T_1WI, slightly higher signal on abscess wall than central pus, hyperintense on T_2WI, and slightly lower signal on abscess wall than pus. The mature abscess shows hyperintense on DWI (Figure 3.9b–d). Hypointense rings are often found at the edge of lesions. Its pathological basis may be tissue fibrosis under long-term stimulation of chronic inflammation. The boundary is relatively smooth and uniform in thickness, and edema can be found in surrounding soft tissues [10]. The enhancement characteristics of enhanced scanning are similar to those of CT.

3.4 Analysis Strategies of Musculoskeletal Infections

When bone joints or soft tissues find lesions in examination, the location of the lesions should be determined first, and whether the lesions are infectious lesions, neoplastic lesions or other diseases should be further distinguished. When analyzing pathological changes, attention should be paid to analyzing whether the pathological changes are single-site, multi-site, systemic diseases, single osteoarticular system diseases, or two or more system diseases. Attention should also be paid to the analysis of whether it is a primary lesion or secondary lesion.

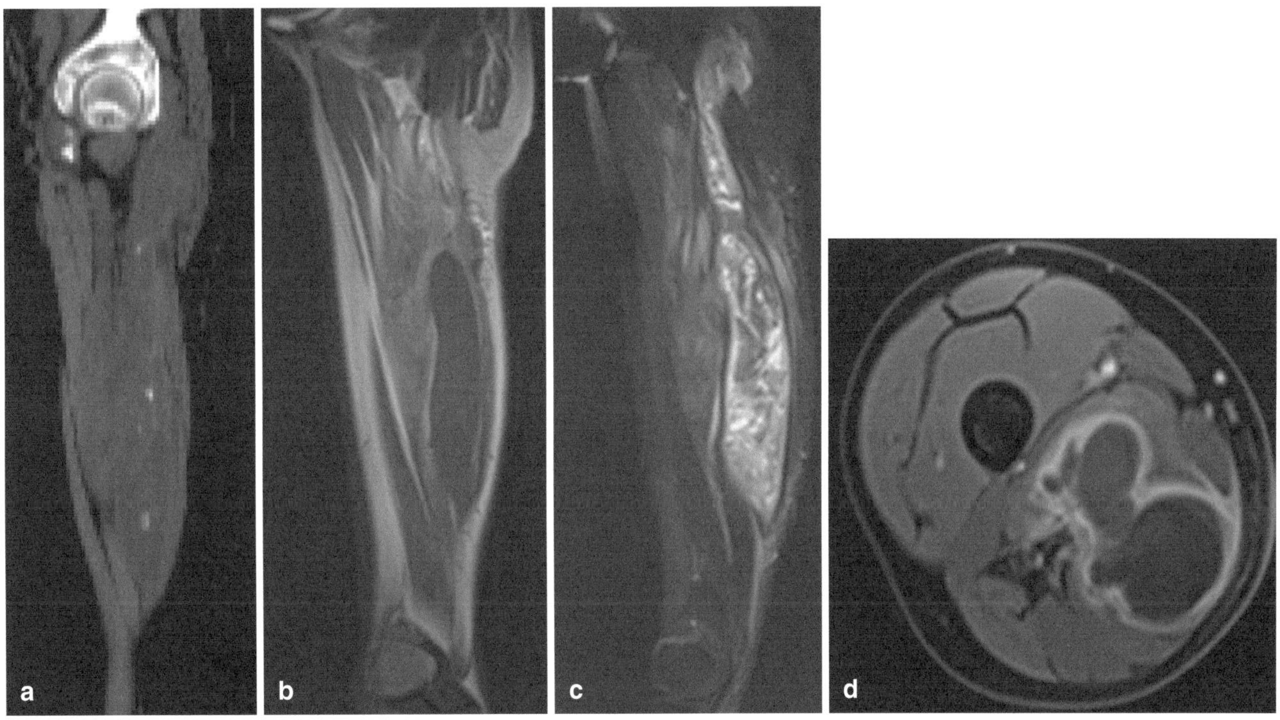

Fig. 3.9 Tuberculosis abscess in right femoral medial and posterior muscle group. (**a**) CT sagittal reconstruction showed deep multiple abscesses low-density shadow in the medial and posterior muscle group of the right femur, there were stippled calcification foci with a thick wall; (**b**, **c**) MRI sagittal plane T_1WI and STIR showed abnormal signals in the right femoral medial and posterior muscle groups; (**d**) MRI enhancement showed marked enhancement of the annular thick wall, and the pus in the annular thick wall was not enhanced

There are many kinds of musculoskeletal infectious diseases, and the clinical manifestations of different infectious diseases are often similar. Therefore, the correct diagnosis of musculoskeletal infectious diseases depends on the comprehensive analysis of clinical, imaging, and flora culture. Musculoskeletal infectious diseases are lack of specific clinical manifestations; The culture of flora is affected by factors such as the location and quantity of materials, and has certain limitations; Imaging examination can locate and quantitatively measure musculoskeletal infectious diseases, and is also helpful for qualitative analysis. Mastering the basic pathological changes of musculoskeletal infectious diseases, carefully analyzing the imaging signs, and combining with clinical and flora culture are the basic ideas for diagnosing musculoskeletal infectious diseases. Imaging of musculoskeletal infectious diseases is analyzed from the following issues: (1) whether it is normal; (2) the location of the lesion; and (3) origin, bone, joint, or surrounding soft tissue [12].

3.4.1 Whether the Image Is Normal

After observing the image carefully and comprehensively, it is necessary to determine whether the image is normal, which is also the most critical problem in image diagnosis. Familiarity with the imaging anatomy of bones and joints is the key to correct judgment, and the limitations and characteristics of various imaging examinations should also be clearly understood. Early bone marrow infiltration may not be shown by X-ray plain film and CT. Bone destruction can only be shown when bone destruction reaches a certain degree. When analyzing images, we should carefully observe whether bone trabecula is clear, whether density is normal, and whether bone cortex has clear and sharp margins. Some structures have more overlapping sites, and plain films may cover smaller lesions, it should be combined with CT scanning. On X-ray plain film, intestinal gas sometimes overlaps with pelvis and lumbar spine, which is like bone destruction. CT scan can be performed when it cannot be well distinguished. Mild swelling of soft tissue and a small amount of effusion in articular cavity may not be shown on X-ray plain film and CT. If clinically highly suspected abnormality and X-ray plain film and CT are normal, an MRI scan can be performed. Bone marrow edema, early stage of acute osteomyelitis, mild swelling of soft tissue, and a small amount of effusion in articular cavity can be scanned by MRI, which is more sensitive than X-ray plain film and CT.

3.4.2 Origin of Lesion

There are few diseases with a simple bone infection, such as bone hydatid disease. Diseases accompanied by bone infection and soft tissue infection include suppurative osteomyelitis, tuberculous osteomyelitis, brucellar spondylitis, and bone hydatid disease. Diseases accompanied by bone infection include tuberculous arthritis and brucellar arthritis. There are many diseases of simple joint infection, including single joint involvement, which are mostly found in pyogenic arthritis and tuberculous arthritis. Multiple joint involvement is common in inflammatory arthropathy, connective tissue disease, crystalline arthritis, etc. Symmetrical distribution of facet joint involvement is common in rheumatoid arthritis and psoriatic arthritis. Among them, rheumatoid arthritis often involves the proximal interphalangeal joint, metacarpophalangeal joint, and wrist joint. In the foot, rheumatoid arthritis mostly involves the metatarsophalangeal joint, especially the fifth metatarsophalangeal joint. Gouty arthritis mostly involves the first metatarsophalangeal joint, tarsometatarsal joint, distal hand joint, and wrist joint. Asymmetric involvement of facet joints is found in degenerative osteoarthritis, which is easy to involve distal interphalangeal joint and the first carpometacarpal joint. Large joint involvement is mostly found in rheumatoid arthritis, ankylosing spondylitis, pigmented nodular synovitis, gouty arthritis, and infectious arthritis. Sacroiliac joint involvement is mostly found in ankylosing spondylitis, psoriatic arthritis, Reiter syndrome, and enteritis arthritis. Involvement of spine atlantoaxial joint is mostly found in rheumatoid arthritis and ankylosing spondylitis. Involvement of thoracolumbar segment spine is mostly found in tuberculous spondylitis. Involvement of spine and lumbar spine is mostly found in brucellar spondylitis.

1. Changes in bone structure
    a. **Joint dislocation.** Joint dislocation and subluxation are found in advanced rheumatoid arthritis, gouty arthritis, etc., and hip joint hydatid can cause hip joint subluxation.
    b. **Changes in bone density.** It includes osteosclerosis/osteoporosis. Periarticular osteoporosis is mainly found in rheumatoid arthritis, tuberculous arthritis, and ankylosing spondylitis. Hyperostosis and osteosclerosis are mostly found in pyogenic spondylitis and brucellar spondylitis.
    c. **Bone erosion.** It is the main imaging findings of bone infection. Almost all bone infections have bone erosion at a certain stage of development. Bone erosion can be divided into marginal type, central type, and periarticular type. Marginal bone erosion refers to bone erosion in non-cartilage protected areas at the attachment of articular capsules at the edge of joints, which is more common in early rheumatoid arthritis, brucellosis spondylitis, and synovial joint tuberculosis. Central bone erosion, i.e., bone erosion on the weight-bearing surface of joints, is more common in pyogenic arthritis and tuberculous spondylitis. Periarticular bone erosion occurs outside the articular capsule and is caused by

tophus or lump in soft tissue. It is mostly found in gouty arthritis. Sclerosis can be found at the edge of bone erosion, showing a typical hanging edge or spur-like outward protrusion. Extraarticular bone erosion can also occur near ligament tendon attachment or bursa, which is manifested as proliferative marginal bone erosion, mostly occurring in calcaneal tuberosity, ischial tuberosity, femoral trochanter, and other parts, and found in ankylosing spondylitis, Reiter syndrome, psoriatic arthritis, and so on.

2. Changes in joint space

X-ray cannot show articular cartilage, showing changes in joint space, mainly including widening, narrowing and disappearance.

1. **Narrowing of joint space.** (1) homogeneous narrowing of joint space: it is found in infectious arthritis, rheumatoid arthritis, and seronegative spondyloarthropathy; (2) Non-homogeneous narrowing of joint space: it is found in osteoarthritis, including primary and secondary osteoarthritis. Secondary arthritis is common in traumatic arthritis, neuroarthritis, mineral deposition, and hemophilic arthritis.
2. **Widening of joint space.** Early widening is due to articular cavity effusion, which can be found in all arthritis. Late widening is due to embedding fibrous tissue or debris, such as distal interphalangeal joint widening, which is more common in psoriatic arthritis, and bone resorption can also lead to joint space widening, such as neuroarthropathy.
3. Soft-tissue changes

Soft-tissue swelling around joints is the most common manifestation of arthropathy, the etiology of which can be articular capsule effusion, joint synovial hyperplasia, and soft-tissue edema around joints. In arthropathy, articular cavity effusion is a common but non-characteristic manifestation, arthritis shall be considered first after traumatic factors are eliminated. For unexplained joint effusion of a single joint without trauma and obvious degeneration, purulent focus accompanied by synovial hyperplasia should be considered first. MRI is very sensitive to articular cavity effusion, synovial hyperplasia, and soft-tissue edema, and can distinguish synovial hyperplasia from simple effusion. Dynamic contrast-enhanced MRI (DCE-MRI) can not only accurately display the range of synovial hyperplasia, but also judge the type of synovial hyperplasia according to the characteristics of the time-signal intensity curve of hyperplasia synovial enhancement, which is valuable for early diagnosis, monitoring the changing trend of diseases and evaluating the curative effect. Proliferative synovium showed moderate to hypointense and nodular hyperplasia on T_2WI, which can be found in gout, synovial osteochondromatosis, rheumatoid arthritis, etc. Scattered or large amounts of hypointense can be found in proliferative synovium. In particular, the gradient echo sequence indicates hemosiderin deposition or hemorrhage, which is found in pigmented villonodular synovitis, hemophilia, etc. Arthritis and inflammatory arthropathy also often cause a large amount of joint effusion.

At the same time of mastering imaging characteristics, clinical history is very important for the diagnosis of infectious diseases. If there are symptoms of redness, swelling, heat, and pain, it strongly indicates acute suppurative osteomyelitis or pyogenic arthritis. If there are symptoms of low fever and night sweat, it strongly indicates bone tuberculosis, tuberculous arthritis, or tuberculous spondylitis. Patients in pastoral areas with intermittent high fever and contact history of cattle and sheep strongly suggest brucellar arthritis or brucellar spondylitis. If there is a history of echinococcosis in pastoral areas, it strongly indicates bone hydatid disease. If the female facet joint has multiple symmetrical swelling and pain and recurs for more than 3 months, it strongly indicates rheumatoid arthritis. Such as young men, low back pain or hip joint pain, it strongly indicates ankylosing spondylitis.

References

1. Hofmann SR, Kapplusch FZ, Girschick HJ, et al. Chronic recurrent multifocal osteomyelitis (CRMO): presentation, pathogenesis, and treatment. Curr Osteoporos Rep. 2017;15(6):542–54.
2. Nguyen MT, Borchers A, Selmi C, et al. The SAPHO syndrome. Semin Arthritis Rheum. 2012;42(3):254–65.
3. Pineda C, Espinosa R, Pena A. Radiographic imaging in osteomyelitis: the role of plain radiography, computed tomography, ultrasonography, magnetic resonance imaging and scintigraphy. Semin Plast Surg. 2009;23(2):80–9.
4. Cheung WY, Luk KD. Pyogenic spondylitis. Int Orthop. 2012;36(2):397–404.
5. Rahmouni A, Chosidow O. Differentiation of necrotizing infectious fasciitis from nonnecrotizing infectious fasciitis with MR imaging. Radiology. 2012;262(2):732–3.
6. Collins MS, Schaar MM, Wenger DE, et al. T1-weighted MRI characteristics of pedal osteomyelitis. Am J Roentgenol. 2005;185(2):386–93.
7. Ferrer MF, Torres LG, Ramirez OA, et al. Tuberculosis of the spine. A systematic review of case series. Int Orthop. 2012;36(2):221–31.
8. Shemesh S, Heller S, Salai M, et al. Septic arthritis of the knee following intraarticular injections in elderly patients report of six patients. Isr Med Assoc J. 2011;13(12):757–60.
9. Kim EY, Kwack KS, Cho JH, et al. Usefulness of dynamic contrast- enhanced MRI in differentiating between septic arthritis and transient synovitis in the hip joint. AJR Am J Roentgenol. 2012;198(2):428–33.
10. Song X, Liu D, Wen H. Diagnostic pitfalls of spinal echinococcosis. Spinal Disord Tech. 2007;20(2):180–5.
11. Hualu C, Baiyan L. Imaging findings of bone hydatid disease. Journal of Practical Radiology. 2009;25(4):586–8.
12. Cheng X, Jianling C. Radiologic diagnosis of musculoskeletal system. Beijing: People's Health Publishing House; 2018.

Part II

Monographs on Infection and Inflammatory Diseases of Skeletal Muscles

Infectious Lesions in Bones and Joints

4

Hongjun Fu, Liwei Xie, and Ping Wang

4.1 Anatomy of Bones and Joints and Imaging Anatomy

Hongjun Fu and Liwei Xie

Bone is the movement tissue of human body. It originates from the mesenchyme in the embryonic period and differentiates from the mesenchyme around the notochord at about the eighth week of embryo. It first forms membranous bone, then develops into cartilage, and then gradually ossifies. Some osseous tissues are also directly derived from membranous bone. From outside to inside are periosteum, bony substance, and internal bone marrow, the distribution of blood vessels and nerves can be found in all of them [1].

4.1.1 Anatomy of Bone

4.1.1.1 Composition of Skeletons

1. **Bony substance.** It includes compact bone substance and spongy bone. Compact bone substance is distributed on the surface of bone and consists of multiple layers of dense bone plates with strong compression resistance. Spongy bone is composed of bone trabeculae, which are distributed inside the bone and interwoven with each other to form a three-dimensional network in a spongy shape. The arrangement of bone trabeculae is consistent with the direction of pressure and tension borne by the bone, so its texture is light and it can bear large weight.
2. **Periosteum.** It is a connective tissue membrane covering the bone surface and is divided into inner and outer layers. The outer layer is dense and the inner layer is loose. It contains osteoblast and osteoclast with the functions of osteogenesis and osteoclast.
3. **Bone marrow.** Children's bone marrow cavity is red bone marrow with the hematopoietic function. With the growth of age, it is gradually replaced by adipose tissue and loses hematopoietic function. It is called yellow bone marrow and has no hematopoietic function. However, some spongy bone of flat bone still has hematopoietic ability (such as skull, sternum, ribs and ilium, etc.). In case of chronic excessive blood loss or severe anemia, yellow bone marrow can be converted into red bone marrow to restore hematopoietic ability.

4.1.1.2 Morphology of Skeletons

1. **Long tubular bone.** Most of them are located in limbs and are long tubular in shape. Their length is much larger than their width and they can be divided into two ends of a whole body. The diaphysis refers to the body, the periphery of which is compact bone substance, called bone cortex, and the center is spongy bone and bone marrow. The swelling at both ends is epiphysis. The surface of epiphysis is articular cartilage, which is not covered by periosteum and forms a joint with the articular surface of adjacent bones. The adjacent part of diaphysis and epiphysis is metaphysis. Epiphyseal cartilage can be found in children and adolescents and degenerates in adulthood.
2. **Short tubular bone.** It is a short columnar or cuboid bone block and is mostly distributed in groups in hands, wrists, feet, and spine, often has multiple articular surfaces and forms amphiarthrosis with adjacent bones. The bone cortex is thin and the spongy bone is located in the middle.
3. **Flat bone.** It is plate-shaped, thin and curved, and the middle layer of spongy bone is sandwiched by two parallel dense bones. It mainly forms the walls of cranial cavity, thoracic cavity, and pelvic cavity, plays a protective role, and also provides an attachment surface for muscle attachment.

H. Fu (✉) · L. Xie · P. Wang
Department of Radiology, The Tenth People's Hospital of Shenyang, Shenyang, Liaoning, China
e-mail: xkyyfhj@126.com

H. Li et al. (eds.), *Radiology of Infectious and Inflammatory Diseases - Volume 5*,
https://doi.org/10.1007/978-981-16-5003-1_4

4. **Irregular bone.** Its shape is irregular, and some bones have air-containing holes, called air-containing bones, such as maxilla and sphenoid bone that constitute paranasal sinus.

4.1.1.3 Blood Supply to Bones

The vein of bone accompanies the artery of the same name, and the blood supply of bone mainly comes from the following 4 sources.

1. **Nutrient artery.** It enters the diaphysis through the nutrient foramen of the bone cortex, divides into ascending branch and descending branch, and then divides into many small branches, which are distributed in the marrow cavity and the inner 2/3 of the bone cortex.
2. **Epiphyseal artery.** It mainly comes from the branches of soft tissue artery outside the joint.
3. **Metaphyseal artery.** It penetrates into the bone at the metaphysis and anastomoses with the branches of nutrient artery. The epiphyseal artery anastomoses with the metaphyseal artery after the union of the epiphysis and the trunk.
4. **Periosteal artery.** It sends out multiple branches at different levels to form a periosteal artery network to supply periosteum and enter the bone cortex to supply 1/3 of the outer bone cortex.

4.1.2 Anatomy of the Joint

The joint is the connecting part between two or more bones. The bones are connected through the joint to form the scaffold of the human body and play a role in supporting and protecting the internal organs of the human body. According to the nature and activity of the connecting tissue, the joint can be divided into diarthrosis, amphiarthrosis, and synarthrosis. The former is also called indirect connection, while the latter two are collectively called direct connection [2].

4.1.2.1 Diarthrosis

Diarthrosis includes limb joint and spinal facet joint, and its structure mainly includes three parts: articular surface, articular capsule, and articular cavity. In order to meet the functional needs, some joints differentiate ligament, articular disc, articular labrum, synovial fluid bursa and synovial fold, etc., which are collectively referred to as auxiliary structures of synovial joints.

1. **Articular surface.** Its surface is smooth and elastic, with the main function to reduce friction and buffer the impact and oscillation during movement, and with a thickness of less than 5 mm. It is composed of cells, matrix, and fibers and is divided into three layers: surface layer, middle layer, and deep layer. The collagen fibers of surface cartilage are closely arranged tangentially. The middle layer is oblique and arcuate. The deep layer is vertically arranged, and the calcification zone and bone plate are located below the deep layer. The nutrition of articular cartilage comes from the penetration of articular fluid in cartilage matrix and the blood of subchondral bone tissue. Articular cartilage is amitosis, it will have no regeneration ability and be replaced by fibrous tissue once damaged or injured.
2. **Articular capsule.** It is divided into inner and outer layers. The outer layer is fibrous layer, which is relatively tough and strengthens the stability of the joint together with the surrounding ligaments. The inner layer is synovial layer, which consists of loose connective tissue and is rich in blood vessels and can secrete synovial fluid. Synovial fluid can lubricate joints and nourish articular cartilage. There is often a synovial sac at the contact between tendon and bone surface to reduce friction, which contains a small amount of synovial fluid.
3. **Articular cavity.** It is a closed space surrounded by the bone end and synovial membrane of the joint, with a small amount of synovial fluid in it. Some joints also have ligaments in the articular cavity, such as knee joint and shoulder joint.

4.1.2.2 Amphiarthrosis

Amphiarthrosis has no articular capsule and is a transitional connection between diarthrosis and synarthrosis. It is characterized in that the two bones are directly connected by cartilage tissue, and there are cracks in the cartilage, with a small range of movement, such as pubic symphysis.

4.1.2.3 Synarthrosis

The two bones of the synarthrosis are connected by dense connective tissue, and there is no gap in the middle, also known as no lacunar connection, such as the bony combination of skull bone slices, sacral vertebrae, and acetabulum.

4.1.3 Imaging Anatomy of Bone and Joint

4.1.3.1 X-ray

1. **X-ray anatomy of tubular bone.**
   Tubular bone consists of periosteum, bone cortex, spongy bone, bone marrow cavity, epiphysis, and epiphyseal line (Fig. 4.1).
   (a) Periosteum: The inner and outer sides of the bone cortex are covered with periosteum, which is not developed by X-ray under normal conditions. If developed, it is a pathological phenomenon, which can be found in the new bone formed by periosteal proliferation, such as bone tumor, inflammation, posttraumatic healing period, etc.
   (b) Bone cortex: It has high calcium content, compact bone substance with uniform density. The bone cortex

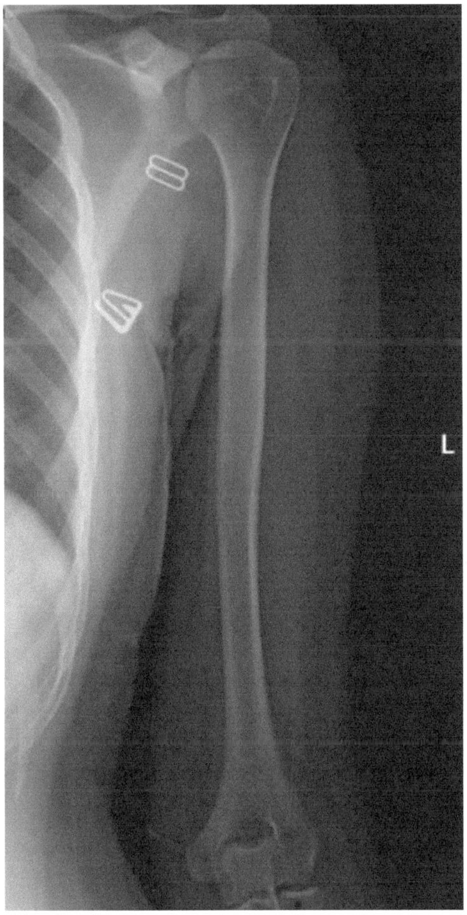

Fig. 4.1 Humerus PA view

in the middle part of the diaphysis is the thickest, with both ends gradually thinning, and only a thin layer when reaching the epiphysis. On X-ray, it shows a dense shadow with uniform density, with smooth and neat edges, and local unevenness at the attachment of muscles and tendons. The nutrient artery foramen obliquely passes through the bone cortex in the upper 1/3 or lower 1/3 of the diaphysis, showing a small round or oval radiolucent area with smooth edges. Do not mistake it for bone destruction or defect.

(c) Spongy bone: It consists of staggered bone trabeculae arranged according to the specific weight-bearing and tension directions of each bone. On X-ray, it shows a fine and neat net-like bone texture structure with a density lower than that of bone cortex.

(d) Bone marrow cavity: It is located in the center of the diaphysis. X-ray shows that it is an unstructured translucent tissue surrounded by the diaphysis cortex with an unclear boundary, which is often difficult to display due to the cover of bone cortex and spongy bone, and shows a band-shaped bright area in the diaphysis segment. When the number of bone trabeculae increases or thickens, the bone marrow cavity becomes narrower or disappears.

2. **X-ray anatomy of joints**

The joint consists of bony articular surface, joint space, and articular capsule.

(a) Bony articular surface: The opposite surface of the bone that makes up the joint is cartilage, which is not shown on X-ray. The bony articular surface seen is composed of subchondral calcification zone and dense bone of thin layer, showing smooth and sharp "linear" dense shadow.

(b) Joint space: It is the transparent space between two opposite bony articular surfaces. The width of the joint space shown on X-ray plain film is wider than the actual space width, because the density of articular cartilage on X-ray is similar to that of soft tissue and cannot be distinguished. When observing the joint space, the medial and lateral sides should be compared.

(c) Articular capsule: Its density is the same as that of the surrounding soft tissue, and is often not shown. Sometimes its border can be seen against the foil layer outside the articular capsule.

(d) Joint accessory structure: Ligaments around some large joints, such as knee, hip, and ankle joints, can be displayed against the background of adipose tissue. The fat layer outside the joint is located between the articular capsule and the surrounding muscles, with clear layers, which can sometimes set off the outline of the articular capsule.

3. **X-ray anatomy of some bones and joints**

(a) Upper limbs

(i) Phalanges of fingers: There are 14 phalanges on each side, all of which are short tubular bones. Except for the thumb, there are only 2 phalanges, and the other 4 fingers have 3 phalanges, which are, respectively, called proximal, middle, and distal phalanges, with only epiphysis at the basilar part. The distal phalanges end is swollen shadow. Usually, PA & OBL radiographs are taken, while LAT radiographs are not used because of obvious overlap of each bone (Fig. 4.2).

(ii) Metacarpal bones: There are 5 metacarpal bones, which are short tubular bones. The first metacarpal bone is the thickest and shortest, and the second metacarpal bone is the longest. The epiphysis of the first metacarpal bone is located at the basilar part, while the other epiphyses are located at the distal end. The proximal end of the metacarpal bones and the carpal bones form the carpometacarpal joint, while the distal end forms the metacarpal joint with the proximal phalanges of each finger, respectively. On X-ray, the basilar of metacarpal bones is slightly square and the metacarpal bone is spherical. In the PA view of both hands, the tangent extension line passing through the

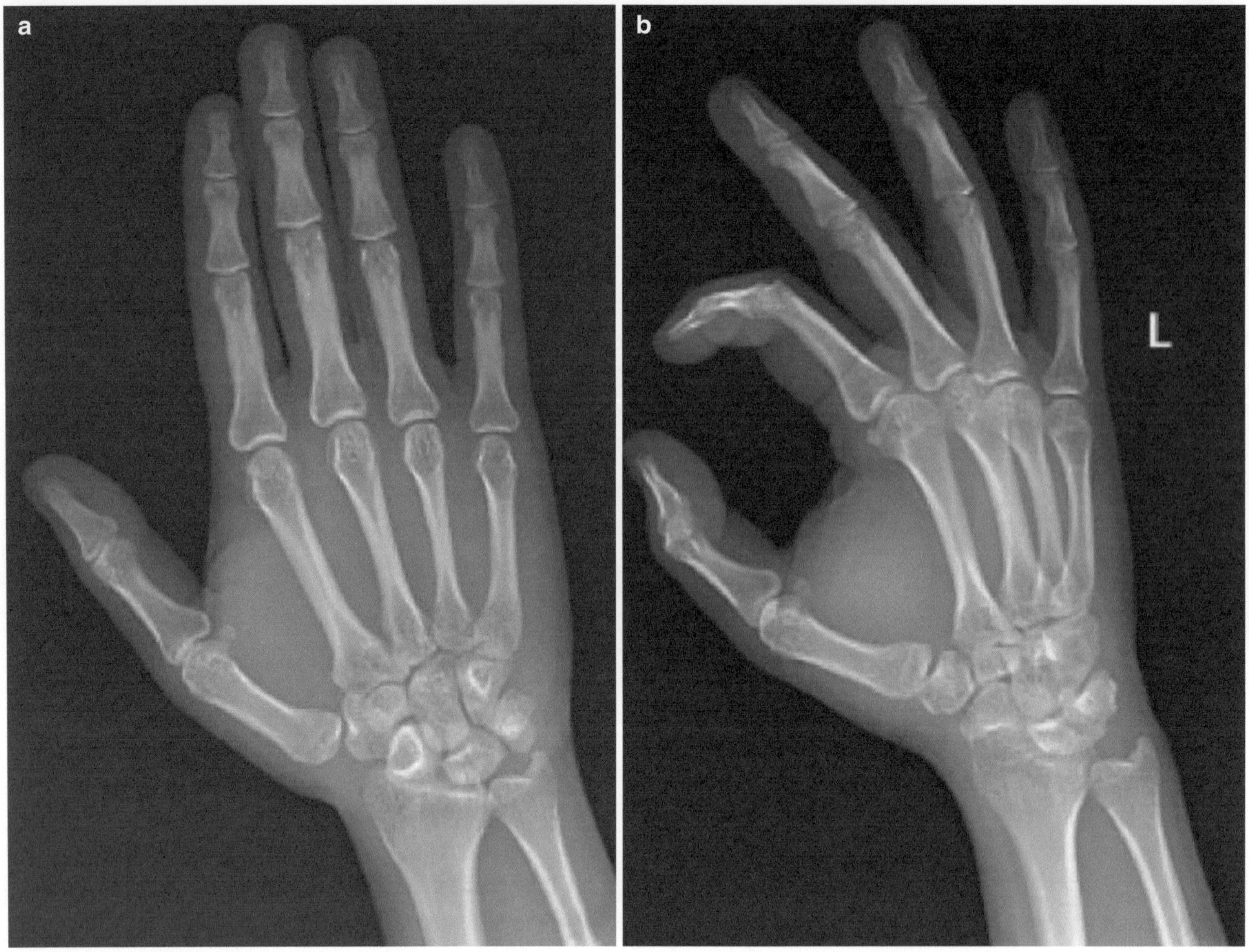

Fig. 4.2 Hand PA & OBL

fourth and fifth metacarpal bones should be tangent to the third metacarpal bone. If it intersects with the third metacarpal bone, it is positive for metacarpal bone sign, which is common in some patients with gonadal hypoplasia and also in normal people.

(iii) Carpal bones: The 8 carpal bones are divided into two rows, the proximal row is scaphoid bone, lunar bone, triangle bone, and pisiform bone from radial to ulnar, and the distal row is trapezium bone, trapezoid bone, capitate bone, and hamate bone. Each bone forms an intercarpal joint with each other. The wrist joint consists of the proximal row of scaphoid bone and lunar bone and the articular surface of the distal radius. The carpometacarpal joint consists of distal carpal bones and metacarpal bones. Conventional X-ray radiographs take PA & LAT.

(iv) Radius: Located on the lateral of the forearm, the upper part is small and the lower part is large. The superior extremity is called the radius shaped like an annular small disc. Its joint concave is related to the capitulum humeri, and the medial also forms the proximal radioulnar joint with the radial notch of the ulna. The relative margin of the ulnar and radius diaphysis has crista interossea, and the radial styloid process is the part that protrudes downward from the lateral of the lower border of the radius. The distal end of the radius expands and forms an articular surface, which forms a radiocarpal joint with scaphoid bone and lunar bone.

(v) Ulna: The upper part is thick and the lower part is thin. The distal end is the capitulum ulnae. It forms the distal radioulnar joint with the ulnar notch at the distal end of the radius, but does not form a joint with the carpal bones. The medial still has a downward extending protrusion, which is the styloid process of the ulna. There is a semicircular deep concave in front of the ulna superior extremity, called trochlear notch, which forms brachioulnar joint with trochlea of humerus. The larger structure on the back is olecranon, and the shorter structure on the front is coronoid process (or processus coracoideus), which is prone to avulsion fracture during trauma. The lower segment is the ulnar bone. Under normal circumstances, the ulnar styloid process is about 1 cm higher than the radial styloid process. The conventional radiography positions of ulna and radius are PA & LAT (Fig. 4.3).

(vi) Humerus: It is the thickest long tubular bone of the upper limb. The upper segment of the diaphysis is cylindrical, and the lower segment gradually widens, showing a front-back flat shape. The hemispherical eminence of humerus at the superior extremity and the glenoid cavity of the scapula together form the shoulder joint. In order to observe the superior extremity of the humerus, it is often needed to take the LAT radiographs of the shoulder. The annular superficial sulcus around the eminence of humerus is the anatomical neck. There are raised greater tubercles and lesser tubercles on the lateral and anterior sides of the eminence of humerus, and the junction of the diaphysis superior extremity and the greater and lesser tubercles of the humerus is slightly thinner, which is the surgical neck of the humerus and is the predilection site of fracture. There is a shallow groove in the middle of the back, which is oblique from inside to top to outside, called sulcus for radial nerve. It courses through nervus radialis and deep brachial artery, and may be damaged when humeral shaft is fractured. The inferior extremity is the capitulum of humerus, which forms the elbow joint with ulna and radius. Conventional photography positions are PA & LAT.

(vii) Elbow joint: It consists of three groups of joints: brachioulnar joint composed of trochlea of humerus and ulnar semilunar notch, brachioradial joint composed of capitulum of humerus and head of radius, and the proximal radioulnar joint composed of head of radius and radial notch of ulnar coronoid process. The conventional radiography positions of elbow joint are PA & LAT (Fig. 4.4).

(viii) Shoulder joint: It is the joint with the greatest mobility in human body. The acromioclavicular joint consists of the acromial end of the clavicle and the acromion of the scapula. The shoulder joint consists of the glenoid cavity of the scapula and the caput humeri. The clavicle is horizontal and "S"-shaped, and the middle bone cortex is 2–3 mm thick. On the PA view, the anterior margin of the glenoid cavity is medial, the posterior border is lateral, and the posterior border partly overlaps with the caput humeri, and the overlapping part is biconvex or spindle-like. The medial

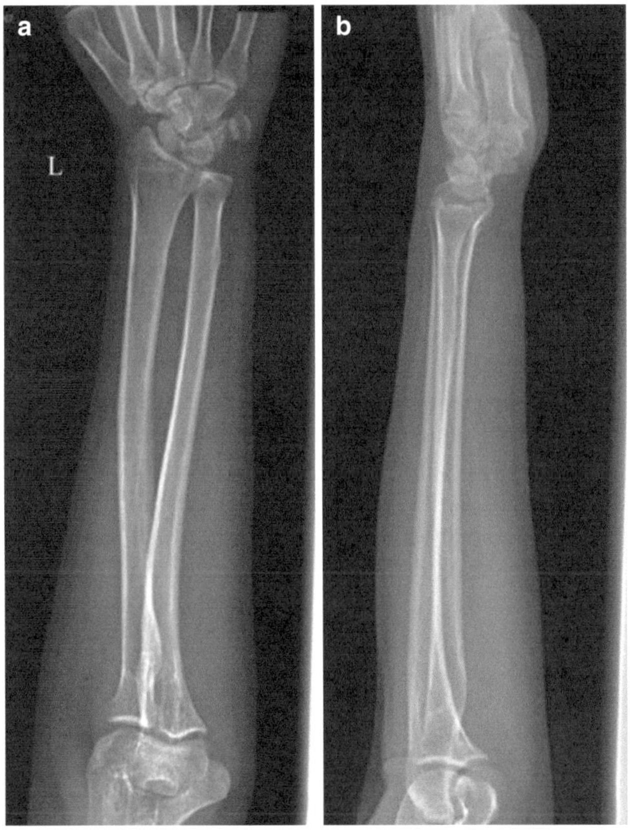

Fig. 4.3 Left ulna and radius PA & LAT

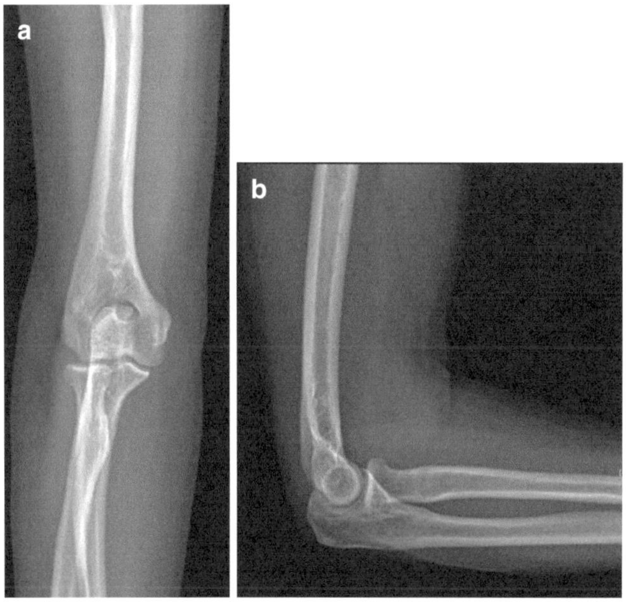

Fig. 4.4 Right elbow joint PA & LAT

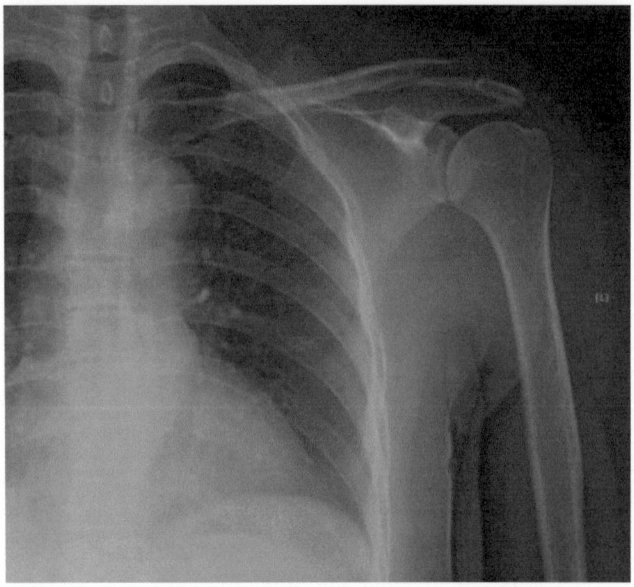

Fig. 4.5 Left shoulder joint PA

border of glenohumeral joint is 4–6 mm, the space of acromioclavicular joint is 2–5 mm, and the space between the lower border of acromion and the upper border of caput humeri is 6–14 mm in adults (Fig. 4.5). X-ray films are usually taken anteroposterior.

(b) Lower limbs

   (i) Foot: Foot bones include phalanges, metatarsals, and tarsus. There are 14 phalanges on each side: the hallux toe has 2 segments and the rest has 3 segments each. There are 5 metatarsal bones, the first metatarsal bone is the thickest and shortest, the second metatarsal bone is the longest, its base is wedge-shaped, and its head is hemispherical. Except the epiphysis of the first metatarsal bone is located at the base, the epiphysis of the other 4 metatarsal bones are all located at the distal end. There are 7 tarsi: calcaneus, talus, scaphoid, cuboid and cuneiform 1, 2 and 3, respectively. There may be multiple articular surfaces covered with articular cartilage. Small sesamoid bone is often seen at the distal end of the first metatarsal bone. The accessory scaphoid is often seen at the medial of navicular bone. Conventional photography positions are PA & OBL (Fig. 4.6). LAT is less used and is mainly used to judge the direction and degree of fracture displacement.

   (ii) Ankle joint: It is composed of tibia, fibula inferior extremity, and trochlea of talus. The corresponding surfaces of the articular surface are parallel to each other, and the joint space is regular and equal in width. The joint space between tibia and talus is clear, with a normal width of 3–5 mm. The conventional radiography positions are PA & LAT (Fig. 4.7).

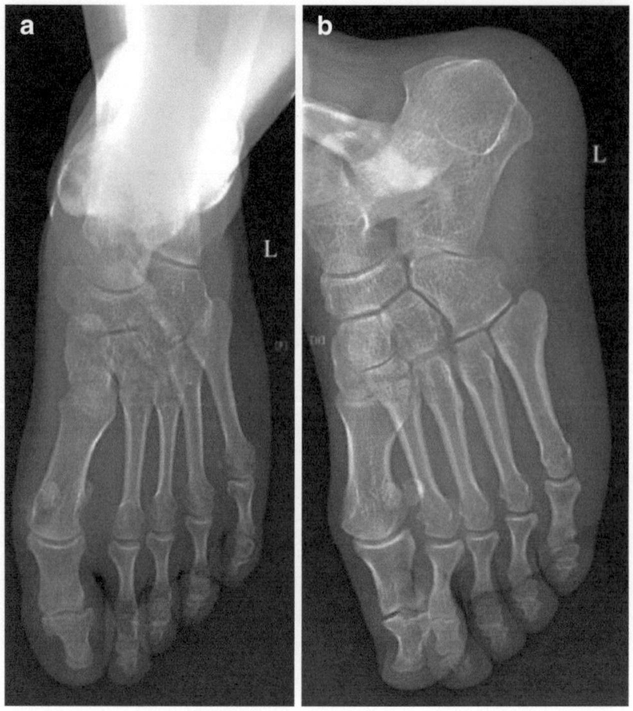

Fig. 4.6 Left foot PA & OBL

   (iii) Tibia: long tubular bone. The tibia is a long bone on the medial of the lower leg. The lateral of the diaphysis and the adjacent border of the fibula have interosseous ridge, which is divided into two ends. The superior extremity has medial and lateral condyles, corresponding to the medial and lateral condyles of the femur, respectively, to form the knee joint. The ridge between the two condyles at the superior extremity of the tibia is intercondylar ridge, and the anterior and lower part is tibial trochanter, which is the attachment of patellar ligament. The distal end of the tibia expands and participates in the formation of the ankle joint. The medial is the medial malleolus, which protrudes downward and participates in the formation of the ankle joint. The outer side has a concave surface and is associated with the fibula.

   (iv) Fibula: It is a long and slender long tubular bone, attached to the lateral of the tibia, and plays an auxiliary and supporting role. The superior extremity is slightly expanded and spherical, called the caput fibulae. The internal bony substance is relatively loose, and sometimes there may be a local density reduction area. The pro-

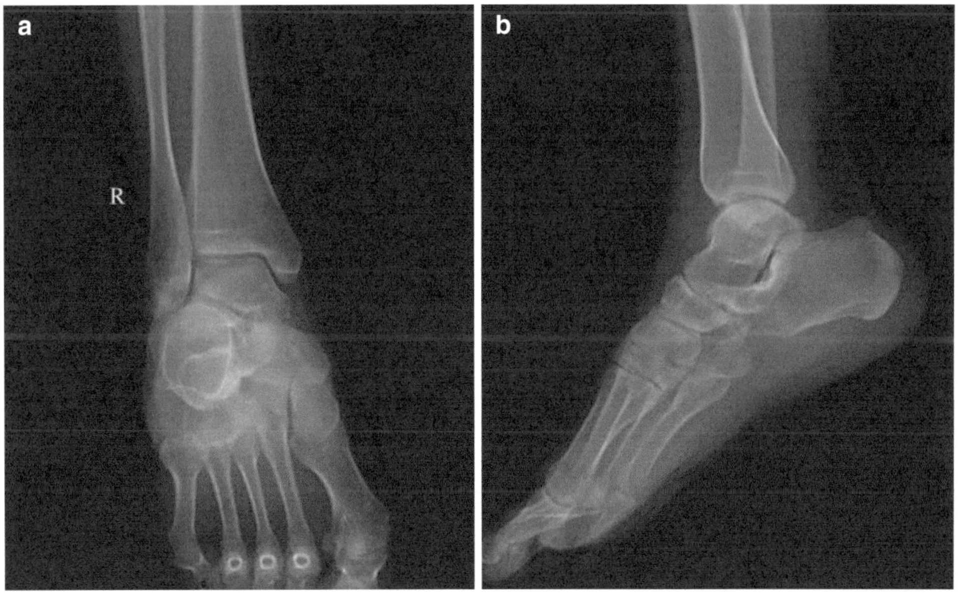

Fig. 4.7 Ankle joint PA & LAT

truding tip above is styloid process and is related to the adjacent tibia. The swollen part at the inferior extremity is the lateral malleolus, and the medial of the lateral malleolus is smooth and forms a joint with the trochlea of talus. The conventional radiography positions are PA & LAT (Fig. 4.8).

(v) Knee joint: It is the largest and most complicated mobile joint in human body, which consists of inferior extremity femur, superior extremity tibia, patella, intra-articular meniscus, ligament, and bursa. Small sural bones are often found behind the lateral femoral condyle. Patella is the largest sesamoid bone in the whole body, which is located in the tendon of quadriceps femoris. Its front bone is not complete, with the cartilage covered back, smooth surface, forming an articular surface with femur. There is an infrapatellar fat pad under the patella, which shows a lower density translucent area under the patella on the LAT film. Under normal circumstances, it is taken PA & LAT radiographs (Fig. 4.9). The medial femoral condyle is larger than the lateral condyle on the lateral views of the knee joint. If the patella requires to be observed, the transverse plane radiograph of patella should be taken.

(vi) Femur: It is the longest and largest long tubular bone in the human body, slightly bent inward and backward, and divided into two ends. The superior extremity of femur has structures such as femoral head, neck, greater and lesser trochanter, etc., forming hip joint together with acetabulum. The inferior extremity of femur has medial and lateral condyles and other structures, forming the knee joint together with tibia and patella. The conventional radiography positions are PA & LAT (Fig. 4.10). On X-ray, the bone cortex is a uniform and compact strip-shaped shadow with high density, sharp and smooth outer border and unsmooth inner border. The bone end is only a thin layer of bone cortex, and X-ray shows thin line shadow, with reticular shadow formed by the intersection of many bone trabeculae below. The

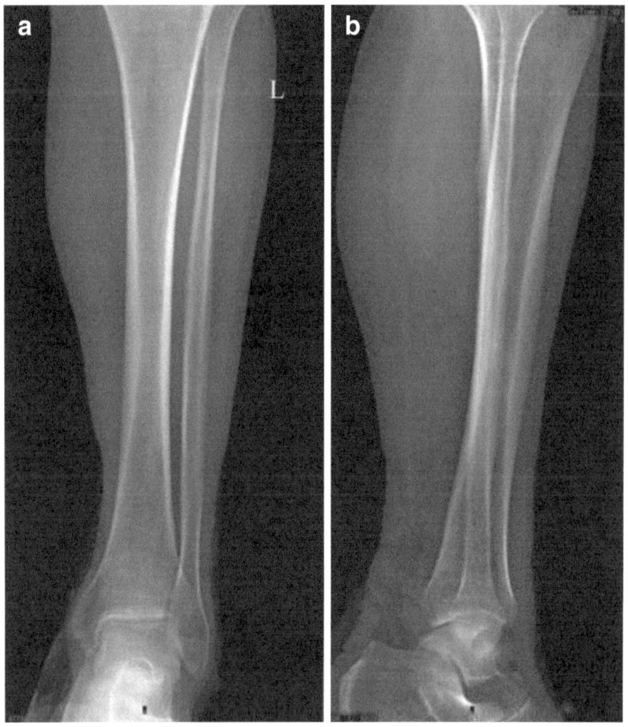

Fig. 4.8 Tibia and fibula PA & LAT

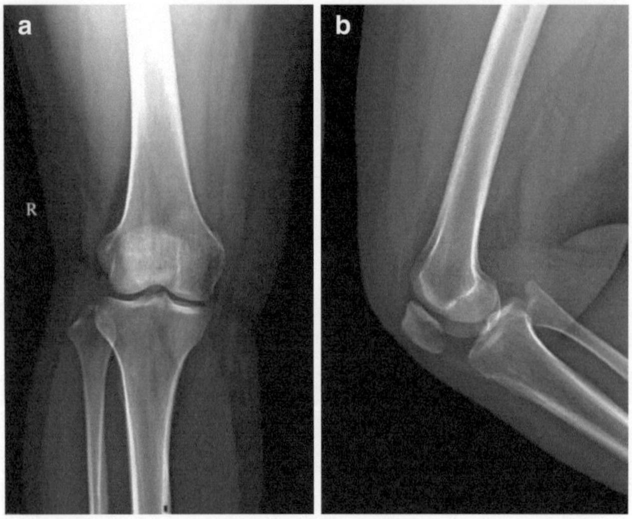

Fig. 4.9 Knee joint PA & LAT

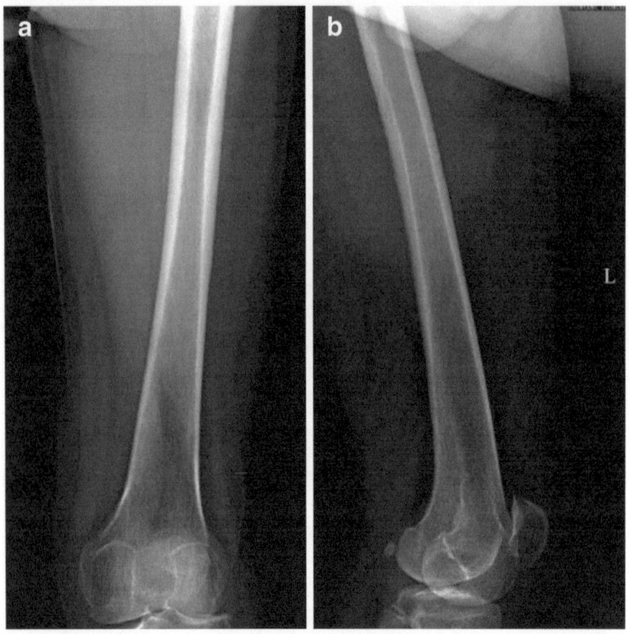

Fig. 4.10 Femur PA & LAT

middle part of the diaphysis is the bone marrow cavity, which is a relatively bright area with fuzzy reticular structure.

(vii) Hip joint: Both hip joints are symmetrical, and Shenton line and Calve line are continuous. The acetabulum is 30–50 mm in diameter and consists of ilium, pubis, and ischium. It can accommodate 2/3 of the articular surface of the femoral head with the thickness of articular cartilage of about 2 mm. The femoral head is spherical, facing inward and upward, with smooth surface. There is a small femoral head concave in the center of the head, which is attached by the round ligament. The femoral neck is located below the head, the upper and outer bulge is the greater trochanter, and the lower and inner bulge is the lesser trochanter. The inferior extremity of femur is medial condyle and lateral condyle, forming knee joint with the superior extremity of tibia. Conventional PA view (Fig. 4.11).

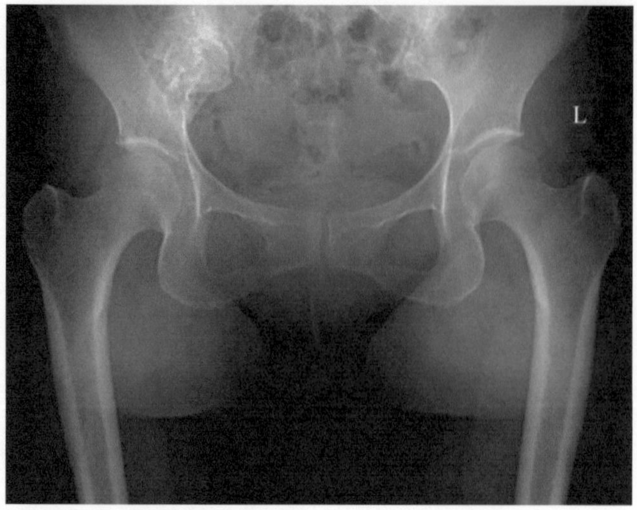

Fig. 4.11 Hip joint PA

4.1.3.2 CT

CT is a transverse plane imaging, avoiding the overlap of various anatomical structures in X-ray imaging. The display of anatomical structures is clearer with a high-density resolution. It can display fine lesions and soft tissue changes that are difficult to be found by X-ray [3]. Through CT enhanced examination, the blood supply of lesions can be further understood and normal and diseased tissues can be distinguished (Fig. 4.12).

1. **Bone.** On the bone window of CT, bone cortex and bone trabecula can be clearly observed. The former shows dense linear or banded shadows, while the latter shows reticular shadows. The bone marrow cavity is hypodense due to the fat composition in bone marrow.
2. **Joint.** The bone end and bony articular surface of the joint can be clearly displayed. The latter shows "linear" hyperdense shadow, but articular cartilage usually cannot be displayed. When the window width and position are appropriate, the sections of articular capsule, surrounding muscles and ligaments inside and outside the capsule can be seen, and these structures all show isodense shadow. A small amount of liquid in normal articular cavity is difficult to identify on CT, the joint space is a low-density shadow between articular bone ends, and articular cartilage and meniscus cannot be displayed.

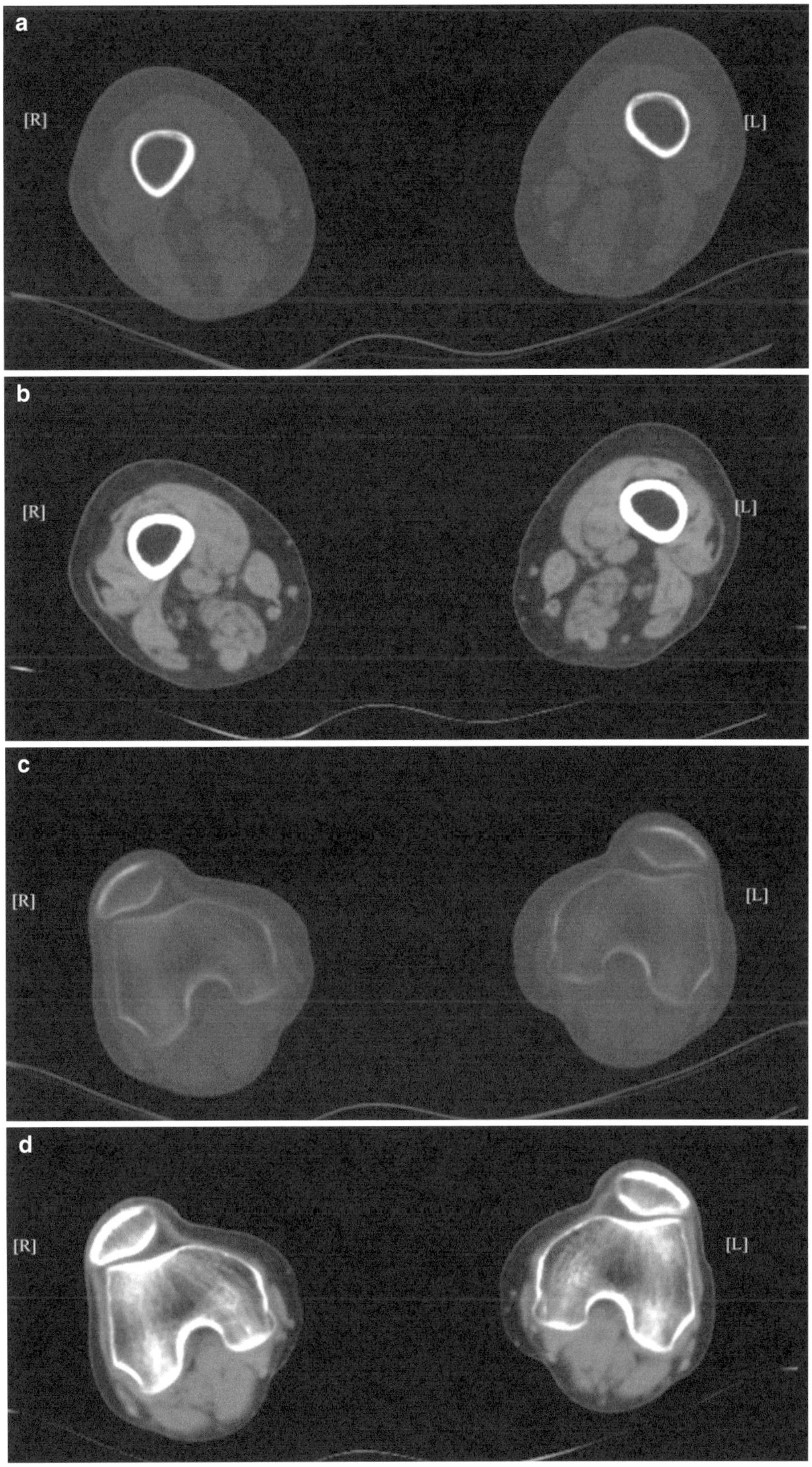

Fig. 4.12 Bone joints CT. (**a**, **b**) Femoral diaphysis bone window and soft tissue window; (**c**, **d**) Normal knee joint bone window and soft tissue window; (**e**, **f**) Sagittal plane three-dimensional reconstruction of knee joint, showing anterior cruciate ligament and posterior cruciate ligament. Unless there is obvious rupture, it cannot show whether the ligament is injured or not and the degree of injury, which is of little clinical significance

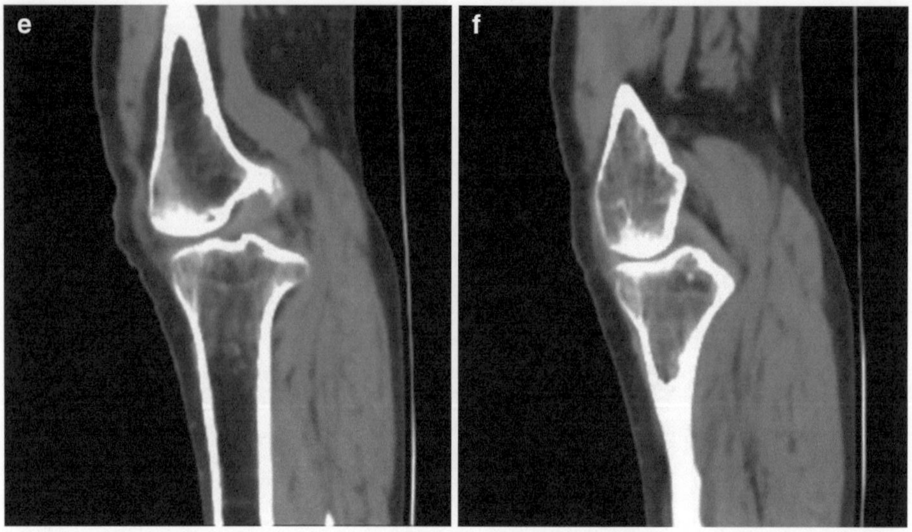

Fig. 4.12 (continued)

3. **Soft tissue.** On the soft tissue window, due to the existence of fat space between various structures, medium density muscles, tendons, and epiphyseal cartilage can be clearly displayed against the background of low-density adipose tissue. Fat, blood vessels, and nerves can be seen in the intermuscular space. The latter two show isodense small quasi-circular or stripe shadow against the background of low-density adipose tissue, and course continuously at all levels. And the enhanced scanning of blood vessels shows hyperdense shadow. The articular capsule and tendons and ligaments near the joint all show isodense shadow. On CT transverse plane images, from the outermost layer to the inner layer, there are "linear" isodense skin, hypodense subcutaneous fat and isodense muscle in turn.

4.1.3.3 MRI

MRI has extremely high resolution, as well as a variety of imaging sequences and parameters, which can well display the anatomical morphology of bone, joint, and soft tissue, and can display the tissue structure that X-ray plain film and CT cannot display or display not good, such as articular cartilage, ligament and bone marrow, etc. The detection rate of MRI for joint effusion can reach 100%, which is significantly higher than X-ray and CT [4, 5]. MRI contrast-enhanced examination can also provide information such as blood supply, enhancement degree and blood vessels, and is more and more widely used in bone and joint diseases. In many cases, MRI contrast-enhanced examination is the preferred examination method (Fig. 4.13).

1. **Bone marrow.** Because the proportion of fat contained in yellow bone marrow is higher than that in red bone marrow, its T_1WI shows hyperintense, similar to subcutaneous fat, and the signal of red bone marrow is between subcutaneous fat and muscle. T_2WI signals of yellow bone marrow and red bone marrow are similar, both higher than muscle and lower than water.
2. **Bone cortex.** Its free water content is very small, so it shows hypointense in any sequence.
3. **Periosteum.** It is a thin layer of membrane that clings to the surface of bone cortex except articular surface and cannot be displayed under normal circumstances.
4. **Articular cartilage.** It shows isointense between muscle and fat on T_1WI and PDWI, and relatively hypointense on T_2WI. T_1WI fat-suppressed sequence is an ideal sequence for observing articular cartilage, which can increase its comparison with adjacent structures. In this case, articular cartilage shows hyperintense, joint effusion shows isointense, and subchondral bone plate and bone marrow show hypointense.
5. **Intra-articular fluid.** It shows hypointense lower than muscle on T_1WI and hyperintense on T_2WI and STIR images.
6. **Synovial membrane.** Normal synovial membrane is usually very thin and cannot be displayed on conventional MRI. Generally, no enhancement or only mild enhancement will occur after enhancement.
7. **Fibrocartilage.** Meniscus and articular labrum are composed of fibrocartilage, which show hypointense in most sequences. The section of meniscus is triangular or arched, and the glenoid labrum of shoulder blade is triangular.
8. **Tendons and ligaments.** The components of the two are similar, showing uniform hypointense in all sequences, with smooth borders and usually round, oval or flat sections.
9. **Muscle.** There are fatty connective tissue septa between muscle bundles and muscle bundles, and between muscle

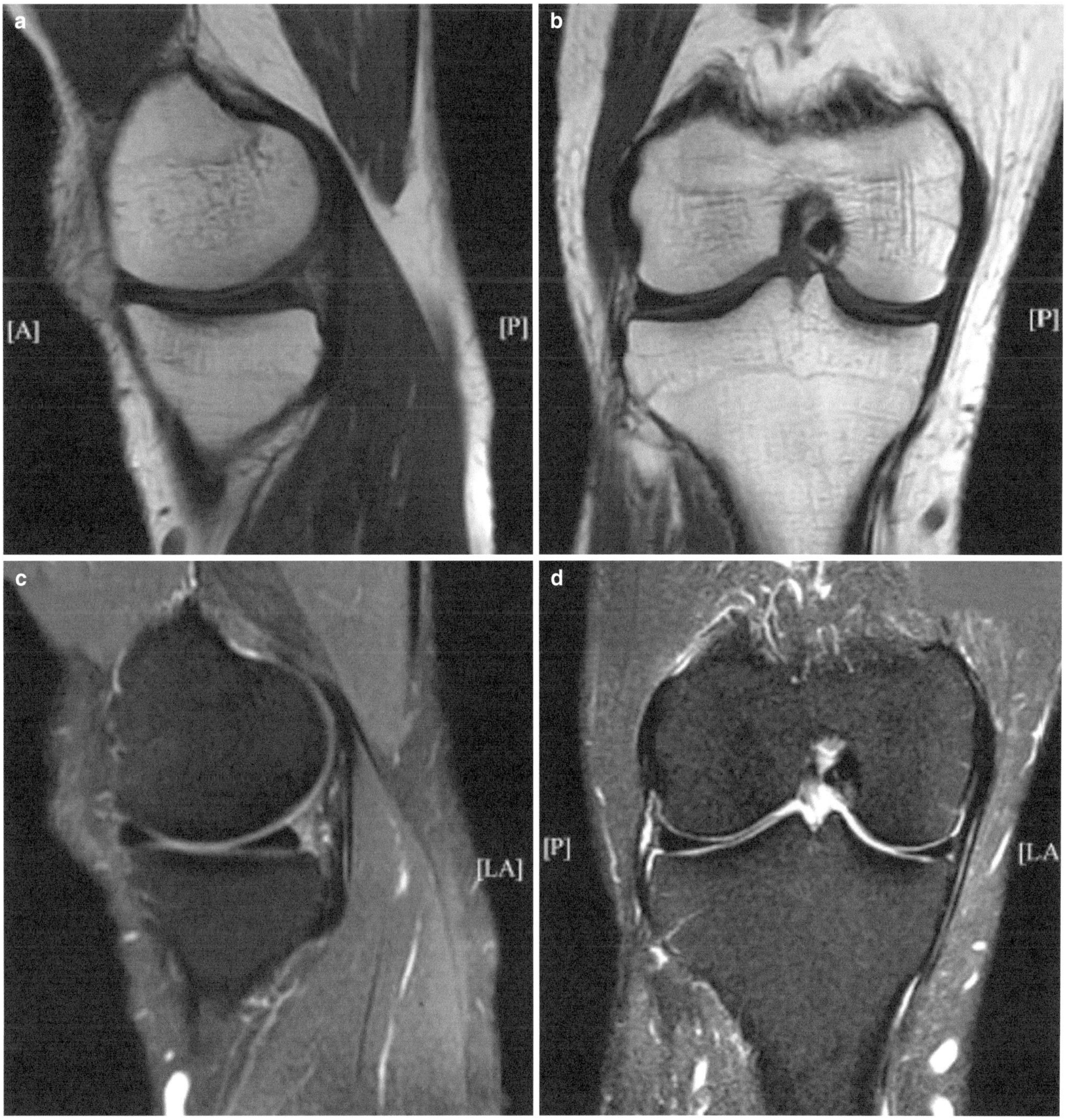

Fig. 4.13 Knee joint MRI. (**a**, **b**) On sagittal plane and coronal plane T_1WI, knee joint cartilage showed isointense, meniscus showed hypointense, and subchondral bone cortex showed hypointense; (**c**) On sagittal plane PDWI, signal intensity of articular cartilage was between muscle and fat, and meniscus was still hypointense; (**d**) On coronal plane T_2WI fat-suppressed sequence, the articular cartilage showed isointense, while the meniscus was still hypointense, showing clearly under the background of intra-articular fluid; (**e**, **f**) On sagittal plane T_1WI and T_2WI fat-suppressed sequence, the anterior cruciate ligament showed slightly hyperintense on T_2WI due to its thin and affected by surrounding substances showing slightly hyperintense on T_2WI; (**g**, **h**) On sagittal plane T_1WI and T_2WI fat-suppressed sequence, all the posterior cruciate ligaments were hypointense with a small amount of articular cavity effusion in the anterior part

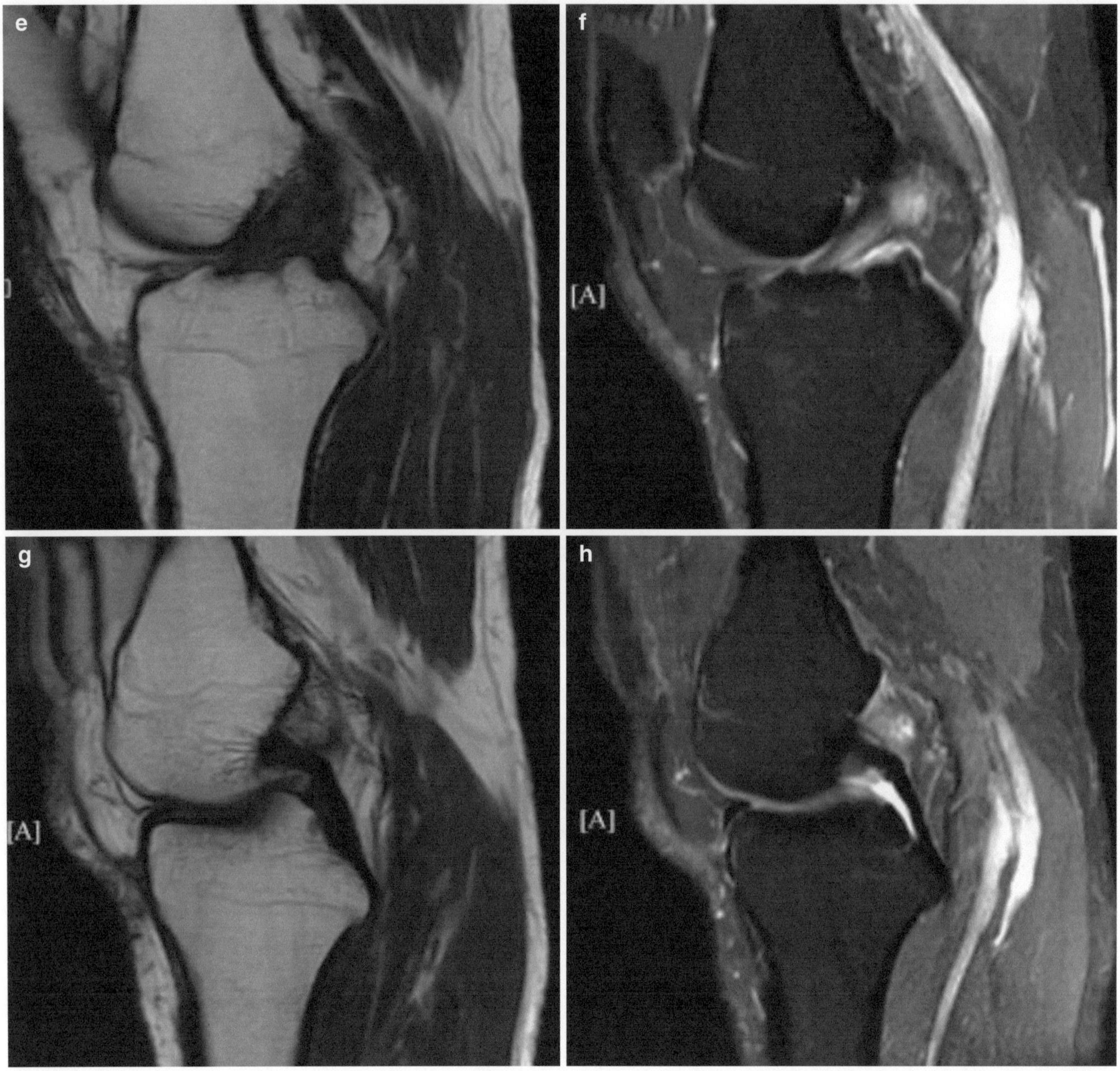

Fig. 4.13 (continued)

and muscle. The hyperintense fat interval on T_1WI is in sharp contrast to the hypointense muscle, which can distinguish different muscles and shapes.

4.2 Characteristics and Pathophysiological Changes in Common Pathogen Infection

Hongjun Fu, Ping Wang, and Liwei Xie

Common pathogens causing infectious lesion of bones and joints mainly include bacteria, fungi, parasites, and spirochetes (Table 4.1). Among them, the most common pathogens of suppurative osteomyelitis and arthritis are Staphylococcus aureus, occasionally enterobacterium, streptococcus, Pseudomonas aeruginosa, and typhoid bacillus. The second is tuberculosis of bone and joint caused by Mycobacterium tuberculosis infection. In addition, infectious lesions of bones and joints also include some rare infections, such as fungal infections of the bones and joints, the pathogens mainly include aspergillus, Coccidioides immitis, candida, cryptococcus, sporotrichosis, etc. Osteoarticular parasitic infection is mainly bone hydatid disease, and osteoarticular spirochete infection is most common syphilis of bone.

Table 4.1 Composition of common pathogens in bone and joint infection

Gram positive bacteria	Gram-negative anaerobic bacteria
Gram-positive aerobic coccus	Bacteroides fragilis
Staphylococcus	Produce melanin bacteroides
Nostoc foliaceum	Fusobacterium
Micrococcus	Gram-negative facultative anaerobic rod
Gram-positive anaerobic coccus	Enterobacter
Peptococcus	Escherichia
Peptostreptococcus species	Klebsiella
Gram-positive sporeless bacterium	Citrobacter spp.
Listeria	Proteus
Corynebacterium	Salmonella
Gram-positive bacillus-producing anaerobic	Serratia
Clostridium perfringens	Yersinia
Actinomycetes	Saprospira gigantea
Actinomyces	Bacterium atrosepticum
Nocardia	Streptobacillus
Streptomyces	**Fungi**
Ehrlichia ovina	Aspergillus nidulans
Mycobacterium tuberculosis complex	Blastomycete
Mycobacterium tuberculosis	Candida
Mycobacterium leprae	Cryptococcus
Atypical bacterial form	Coccidioides
Gram-negative bacteria	Histocytoplasmic bacteria
Gram negative aerobic bacteria	Sporotrichum
Brucella	**Parasites**
Pseudomonas aeruginosa	Hydatid
Acinetobacter	**Helicoid**
Gonococcus	Syphilis

Note: Mycobacterium and Nocardia are not easy to color due to their special cell wall structure, although Gram staining is positive, and acid-fast staining is commonly used

4.2.1 Staphylococcus aureus

There are many species of staphylococcus, most of them are not pathogenic. Staphylococcus aureus is the most common purulent pathogens in clinic. Gram-positive cocci can cause a variety of diseases, it is also the most common pathogen in bone and joint bacterial infection [6]. It is spherical or oval with a diameter of about 1.0 μm, and is named because of often stacked into grape clusters. It has no flagella, no spores and most strains have no capsules.

The pathogenicity of Staphylococcus aureus is related to its toxin and invasive enzyme. ① Hemolytic toxin: exotoxin, according to different antigenicity, it can be divided into four kinds: α, β, γ, δ. Among them, α-hemolysin plays a major role in hemolysis of red blood cells, destruction of platelets and lysosomes, contraction of small blood vessels, leading to local ischemia and necrosis of the body. ② Leukocidin: it contains fast (F) and slow (S) two kinds of protein, requiring the cooperation of both to increase the permeability of cell membrane, thus destroy polymorphonuclear granulocyte and macrophage, aggravating tissue damage. ③ Plasma coagulase: Coagulase enables fibrin in blood or plasma to be coagulated on the thallus surface, thus preventing the bacteria from being phagocytized by phagocyte or damaged by antibacterial substances. Coagulase also makes infection localized, thus causing thrombosis. It is immunogenic and can stimulate the production of antibodies for cross-protection. ④ Thermonuclease: Resistant to high temperatures, the enzyme can be tested to determine whether Staphylococcus aureus is pathogenic. ⑤ Toxic shock syndrome toxin-1 (TSST-1): An exotoxin produced by Staphylococcus aureus. It can cause fever and systemic multisystem disorders and shock by increasing vascular permeability of blood capillaries. The formation of biofilm also plays a key role in pathogenicity of Staphylococcus aureus [7].

Staphylococcus aureus generally causes localized pyogenic infection of body parts, primarily in the form of abscesses. It also can cause pneumonia, enteritis, pericarditis, even general infections such as septicopyemia and septicemia, and food poisoning and toxic shock syndrome. Staphylococcus aureus is highly resistant to sulfonamides, penicillin, erythrocin, and other antibiotics. Methicillin-resistant Staphylococcus aureus (MRSA), also known as superbacteria, is resistant to all existing antibiotics except vancomycin.

4.2.2 Streptococcus

Streptococcus widely exists in nature, human and animal feces, and the nasopharynx of healthy people. It is second only to Staphylococcus aureus in terms of bone and joint infections. The bacterium is arranged in chain-like conformation of different length, among which group A streptococcus and Streptococcus pneumoniae are mostly pathogenic. Streptococcus is divided into three types based on its capacity to lyse erythrocyte: ① α-hemolytic streptococcus, also known as Viridans streptococci. This type of streptococcus, mostly opportunistic pathogens, do not completely lyse the erythrocyte in α-hemolytic rings. ② β-hemolytic streptococcus, also known as hemolytic streptococcus, completely lyse erythrocyte in β-hemolytic rings. This type of streptococcus are highly pathogenic, accounting for the majority of pathogens. ③ γ-hemolytic streptococcus, also known as streptococcus non-hemolytics. This type of streptococcus do not produce hemolysin and are barely pathogenic.

According to its antigenic structure, streptococcus is divided into 20 groups from A–H and K–V. Ninety percent of streptococcus pathogenic to mankind are in group A and mostly are β-hemolytic, which are also known as pyogenic streptococcus. Streptococcus are Gram-positive, aerobic, or facultative anaerobic, some of which are anaerobes. The bacterium is spherical or oval in shape, with a diameter of 0.6–1.0 μm, arranged in chains, on which capsules made of hyaluronic acid can be seen, without spore or flagellum.

4.2.2.1 Pathogenic Substance

Pathogenic substances include cell wall constituents (adherin, M-protein and peptidoglycan), exotoxins (pyrogenic exotoxin and streptolysin), and invasive enzymes (hyaluronidase, streptokinase, and streptodornase). Streptolysin can lyse erythrocytes, kill leukocytes, destroy blood platelets, and produce "O" and "S" hemolysins, with cardiotoxicity. Streptolysin O (SLO for short) has a strong antigenicity. More than 85% of patients develop anti-"O" antibodies 2–3 weeks after infection, which is an indicator of streptococcal infection in recent days. Streptolysin S (SLS), without antigenicity, can be more destructive to leukocytes and blood platelets.

4.2.2.2 Diseases Caused

Group-A streptococcus can cause a variety of purulent inflammations (infections of skin tissues, meningitis, pyogenic arthritis, and the like), toxicosis (scarlatina and streptococcal toxic shock syndrome) as well as allergic diseases (rheumatic fever and acute glomerulonephritis). Streptococcal toxic shock syndrome (STSS) is one of the most deadly complications caused by streptococcus infection, with death rate as high as 30%–64% [8]. Viridans streptococcus and Group-B streptococcus are opportunistic pathogens that can cause infection only when the body immunity is compromised.

4.2.3 Meningococcus

Meningococcus, also known as *N.* meningitidis, can cause epidemic cerebrospinal meningitis. It is mainly spread via droplets and respiratory secretions of patients. Patients often suffer from infection of upper respiratory tract first. As the body immunity drops, meningococcus in nasopharynx multiply rapidly and enter blood circulation, causing septicemia and bacteremia, and may stagnate in the bone and joint system via the blood flow, thus resulting in suppurative osteomyelitis, osteoarthritis, and other purulent diseases. Meningococcus is a Gram-negative diplococcus, kidney-shaped, arranged irregularly in pairs, with opposite concave surfaces and a diameter of 0.6–0.8 μm. The bacterium has weak resistance and can be easily killed by cold, dry, sunlight, UV, and general disinfectants. Meningococcus can be found in pharyngonasal cavity of healthy people. Pathogenic substances are mainly capsules, fimbriae, lipo-oligosaccharide, and IgA1 protease. The IgA1 protease is a kind of extracellular enzyme produced by the bacterium, which can specifically lyse human IgA1, enabling the bacterium to adhere to the surface of cell mucosa, thereby destroying the immunity.

4.2.4 Klebsiella

Klebsiella is an important pathogen causing hospital-acquired infection. It is Gram-negative, short and thick, ball rod-shaped, with a size of (0.5–0.8) μm × (1–2) μm. Klebsiella has no spore or flagellum, most of which have fimbriae and a thick polysaccharide capsule. Klebsiella is divided into 7 genera, among which the Klebsiella pneumoniae is highly pathogenic to human, with virulence associated with its capsule. The bacterium primarily targets people with low immunity, causing urinary tract infections, trauma infections, and pneumonia, which may be very severe, accompanied by extensive pulmonary hemorrhage and necrotic lung consolidation.

4.2.5 Pseudomonas aeruginosa

Pseudomonas aeruginosa (P. aeruginosa), one of pseudomonas, a Gram-negative bacillus with a size of (0.5–1.0) μm × (1.5–3.0) μm. The bacterium has a straight or slightly curved rod shape, without spore, most of which have fimbriae and 1–3 flagella at one end of their thallus. It moves actively. With a stronger resistance than other Gram-negative bacteria, it is resistant to many chemical disinfectants and antibiotics. Pseudomonas aeruginosa has O-antigen and H-antigen. O antigen is composed of endotoxin lipopolysaccharide and endotoxin protein. The latter is a good cross-protection antigen. Traumatic osteomyelitis is mostly caused by mixture of two pathogens, while Pseudomonas aeruginosa can also be isolated in some cases. As traffic accidents occur frequently in recent years, purulent inflammations of bones and joints caused by Pseudomonas aeruginosa have also increased. Since the bacterium is intrinsically resistant to a variety of antibiotics, and may become mutant and drug-resistant during treatment, drug sensitivity test should be referred during medication.

4.2.6 Brucella

Brucella is a zoonosis pathogen first isolated by David Bruce, a British military doctor, in 1886. For this reason, it was named brucella. Based on hosts, biochemical characteristics, metabolic ways, and immunology gaps, WHO Brucellosis Expert Committee divides brucella into 6 species and 19 biotypes, among which the Brucella abortus, Brucella melitensis, Brucella suis, and Brucella canis are pathogenic to human [9]. These bacteria vary in pathogenicity, among which the Brucella melitensis can cause severe infection and evolve into caseous granuloma.

Brucella is a Gram-negative micrococcus or Curtobacterium without flagellum or spore. It is motionless, and smooth-type strains have microcapsule. Due to its strong resistance, the bacterium can survive for several weeks to even several months in soil, fur, organs, secretions, meat, milk, and dairy products of sick animals. It can be killed at a hot & humid condition above 60 °C or direct sun exposure for 20 min. It is sensitive to general disinfectants and broad-spectrum antibiotics. The major pathogenic substances of Brucella are endotoxins, capsules, and invasive enzymes. It is believed that human are occasional host of Brucella. Generally, the bacteria first spread among the same species of infected animals, making the animals carry the bacteria and suffer from infections. After directly touching the sick animals or their secretions/feces, or eating/using the products of the animals, humans are thereby infected with the bacteria via their skin and mucous membranes, respiratory tracts as well as digestive tracts [10]. The latency of brucellosis is 1–6 weeks. After entering the human body, it repeatedly results in bacteremia, with clinical manifestation of undulant fever. The infection is prone to become chronic, involving multiple organs and tissues throughout the body, causing fever, joint swelling & pain and hepatosplenomegaly.

4.2.7 Mycobacterium Tuberculosis

Mycobacterium is a kind of slender bacillus, slightly curved, characterized by the following main features. ① The cell wall contains a lot of lipids. The special structure of the bacterium makes it difficult to be stained during general Gram staining. However, after being stained, the red bacterium cannot be discolored with acidic ethanol, thereby it is called acid-fast bacilli [11]. ② It is motionless, without spore or flagellum and cannot produce endotoxin or exotoxin. ③ A variety of species. ④ The infection is a chronic process that can be long evolved into destructive tissue lesions.

Mycobacterium tuberculosis can be divided into human Mycobacterium tuberculosis, bovine Mycobacterium tuberculosis, and Mycobacterium microti, among which the first one is mainly pathogenic to human [12]. Mycobacterium tuberculosis grows slowly and usually forms colonies after 4–6 weeks of cultivation. The bacterium body contains lipoids, proteins, and polysaccharides, among which the lipoids account for 50%–60% of the total weight. This makes the bacterium highly tolerable, resistant to dryness, strong acid & strong base and coldness, able to long live in the external environment, and susceptible to drug-resistant variation with production of L-type bacterium. But it is barely resistant to hot and humid condition, ethyl alcohol, and UV. The pathogenicity of Mycobacterium tuberculosis also depends on the above bacterium compositions, in particular the large amount of lipids contained in the cell wall, whose amount is in proportion to the virulence of Mycobacterium tuberculosis. This means that the larger the lipid amount, the stronger the toxicity. The lipid is mainly composed of phospholipid, fatty acid, and waxiness D, among which the phospholipid can stimulate the proliferation of monocytes while inhibiting the decomposition of proteases, resulting in insufficient tissue dissolution, thereby forming tubercle and caseous necrosis; The cord factor (6, 6-dimycocyl-a, a'-D-trehalose) can suppress the neutrophil migration to form chronic granuloma; Waxiness D, combined with tuberculin in protein, can cause delayed hypersensitivity.

Mycobacterium tuberculosis is mainly transmitted via respiratory tracts, and a small number of bacteria enter the body through digestive tracts and infected skin wounds, thus infecting multiple systemic tissues and organs, such as lung, brain, bones & joints, intestinal tracts, and urogenital system, among which tuberculosis is the most common disease. Human are generally susceptible to Mycobacterium tuberculosis. The incidence among infants, post-pubertal teenagers, and the elderly is high. After infected, low immunity groups, such as AIDS patients, are prone to cause hematogenous disseminated pulmonary tuberculosis in case of severe conditions. The immunity and pathogenicity of Mycobacterium tuberculosis are both related to the cellular immunity and delayed hypersensitivity mediated by T-lymphocytes, which are produced by the body after Mycobacterium tuberculosis infection. In most cases, tuberculosis of bone and joint occurs secondary to tuberculosis. Through hematogenous dissemination, Mycobacterium tuberculosis tends to stay in the spongy bone and red bone marrow, where the blood supply is sufficient, and joints, such as synovial membrane of vertebral body, long bone metaphysis, knee, hip and other large joints, which are heavy-loaded and highly active.

4.2.8 Hydatid Cyst

There are different species of hydatid cysts, among which the Echinococcus granulosus, alveolar (multilocularis) echinococcus, Echinococcus vogeli, and Echinococcus oligarthrus are parasitized in human body. The Echinococcus granulosus is the most common cause of human echinococcosis [13]. Echinococcosis, distributed in vast pastoral areas around the globe, spreads between humans and animals. The adult parasite has a thin, tiny body, 2–7 mm in length, living in the small intestine of the definitive host. It is composed of scolex, neck, immature proglottid, mature proglottid, and gravid proglottid. The gravid proglottid accounts for 1/2 of the parasite body, in which the uterus is filled with eggs. After the eggs become mature, the gravid proglottid will be expelled via the host's intestinal tracts. Before or after this, the eggs are discharged as the uterus ruptures to the host's intestinal tracts and expelled from the body along with feces, thus contaminating water and grassland. Cattles, sheep, and human will be infected after eating the contaminated food, vegetables, and water, thus becoming an intermediate host. In the stomach or duodenum of the intermediate host, the eggs hatch oncospheres with the action of the digestive juice. The oncospheres develop into a hydatid cyst in the liver after passing through the intestinal wall and entering the portal vein circulation. When the definitive host (such as a dog) eats internal organs of the intermediate host, the scolex inside the cyst develops into an adult in the host's small intestine after 3–10 weeks, thus completing the life cycle [14].

The hydatid cyst wall is divided into outer and inner layers. The former is a cuticle layer that can absorb nutrients and protect the germinal layer; The latter is a germinal layer with proliferation ability. Cells at germinal layer bud inwards and form numerous bulges, which gradually develop into brood capsules. After shedding, the germinal cysts become daughter cysts, in which several scoleces can be generated, called protoscolex. Protoscolex breaks the cyst wall and enters into the cyst fluid, which is called cyst sand. The structure of the daughter cyst is the same as that of hydatid cyst (mother cyst), which can keep producing new brood capsules and granddaughter cysts after shedding [15]. Cyst fluid, derived from the host's blood, has antigenicity, which can cause the allergic reaction of the peripheral tissues after the rupture of the cyst wall.

4.2.9 Aspergillus

Aspergillus widely exists in the nature and has a wide variety of species. This type of fungus, however, has a low pathogenicity to human, and basically only affects individuals with low immunity. The most common strain is Aspergillus fumigatus. By encroaching on multiple body parts, aspergillus can cause diseases including direct infection, hypersensitivity, and aspergillosis poisoning. Mostly, the skeletal system is infected via direct diffusion from lung to adjacent vertebrates, intervertebral disc and ribs, or via blood. Due to the fact that aspergillus is a common contaminant in culture, direct biopsy for deep tissues should be adopted during pathogenic diagnosis. Under the microscope, pathogen on the fresh tissue, which is made into a smear, can be found. Galactomannan, which has been confirmed as a surrogate marker for invasive aspergillosis, is suitable for the specific diagnosis of aspergillus infection [16].

4.2.10 Candida

Candida, with circular or oval body and a diameter of 3–6 μm, is Gram-positive and reproduced by budding. It is easy to form blastospores and pseudohyphae in tissues, a few can form chlamydospore and fungal mycelium, but Candida glabrata cannot form mycelium. Candida is an opportunistic pathogen. The most common disease caused by the bacterium is Candida albicans infection, which is more common in the patients with body dysbacteriosis or decreased immunity, hematological malignant tumor, long-term administration of steroid pills, prosthesis implantation, long-term use of broad-spectrum antibiotics, and the like [17]. Candida can cause infections of skin, mucous membranes, and systemic & local deep layer tissues [18]. It normally exists in the gastrointestinal tracts of human and animals. Candida infections are mostly caused by endogenous rather than exogenous exposure. Candida infections in orthopedic patients are mostly seen in those who long use antibiotics for open injuries.

4.2.11 Cryptococcus Neoformans

Cryptococcus neoformans, one species of cryptococcus, is a circular or oval-shaped bacterium with a diameter of 5–20 μm. Different from other yeast-like fungi, it reproduces by budding and does not produce pseudo mycelium. It is surrounded by a wide, thick polysaccharide capsule, which serves as a main virulence factor to inhibit the phagocytosis of phagocytes and lower the body's immunity. The microscopic examination after negative staining with ink shows that the bacteria body is circular, oval-shaped, and transparent under the black background. Cryptococcus neoformans is ubiquitous in the nature. It can be separated from fruits, soil, and skin, mucous membranes and feces of healthy human, especially abundant in pigeon feces. As for human, Cryptococcus neoformans is an opportunistic pathogen. Like many other pathogenic fungi, infections caused by cryptococcus usually start from the lungs, where subclinical symptoms are often shown. In many clinical cases, patients complain of neurological involvement, a manifestation of chronic meningitis. Bone and joint infections are caused by hematogenous dissemination, more common in osteomyelitis. Joint involvements are mostly aroused by spread of adjacent osteomyelitis [19]. It is not easy to distinguish the changes in Cryptococcal osteomyelitis from osteomyelitis and metastatic tumor of bone caused by other pathogens. Synovial tissues are mainly manifested as acute and chronic synovitis, with multinucleated giant cell, granulomas, and a large number of budding yeasts stained by special colors found under the microscope.

4.2.12 Coccidioides

Coccidioides, a dimorphic fungus, presents as yeast type and mycelium type, respectively, in a 37 °C tissue and a 28 °C culture medium. It can rupture into arthrospores. Coccidioidomycosis mainly occurs in the arid areas of southwestern America [20], mostly caused by inhalation of arthrospores in contaminated soil. The coccidioides in the soil presents as mycelium. Once invading tissues, it transforms into an ablastemic spherule with a diameter of 2–200 μm, containing many endospores. The ruptured non-blasto sphere releases endospores, which are transmitted to other parts of the body via lymph or blood. Each spore can become an ablastemic spherule again and start a new lifecycle. Like other fungal infections, coccidioidomycosis causes more bone infections than joints. Joint infections are mostly caused by the spread of adjacent osseous tissue. Based on etiology, the definite diagnosis can be made if sporangium is seen under the microscope after treating the collected specimen with potassium hydroxide.

4.3 Bacterial Infection

Hongjun Fu and Liwei Xie

Osteomyelitis refers to the acute or chronic inflammation of bone and its accessory tissues caused by direct or indirect infections. It can be divided into three types: acute, subacute, and chronic. It can be further divided into purulent and nonpurulent (granulomatous) according to host's response to pathogen infection.

One can be infected with osteomyelitis via three ways. ① Hematogenous infection, the most common way, wherein primary purulent focus is located in other parts of the body, and pathogens spread to osseous tissues via blood circulation. The primary infection focuses, such as furuncle, carbuncle, tonsillitis, and otitis media, are mostly located in the skin and mucosa. ②. Posttraumatic infection, a direct infection, which is caused by open fractures after trauma, wound contamination, infection aroused by untimely and insufficient debridement, or secondary infection after bone and joint surgery. Osteomyelitis caused by posttraumatic infection is called traumatic osteomyelitis. ③ Direct spreading of adjacent soft tissue infection, also known as extraneous osteomyelitis, such as whitlow. It can cause phalangeal osteomyelitis if not treated in time. The latter two infection ways are more common in adults.

4.3.1 Acute Suppurative Osteomyelitis

Overview

Suppurative osteomyelitis, common in children and adolescents, are mostly caused by hematogenous infection. The most common pathogen is Staphylococcus aureus, followed by Streptococcus pyogenes. In addition, Haemophilus influenzae, Escherichia coli, Streptococcus pneumoniae, and methicillin-resistant Staphylococcus aureus are also pathogenic.

Acute purulent osteomyelitis refers to an acute purulent inflammation involving bone marrow, bone, and periosteum. It is a common clinical acute bone infectious disease, whose severity is associated with various factors such as the patient's own immunity, species of infected bacteria, lesion site, and destruction of peripheral tissues. Without effective and timely treatment during acute stage, it may develop into a chronic, recurrent disease that is difficult to heal and seriously affect the prognosis. The disease can occur at any age, mostly common in children and adolescents at the age of 2–10 years. The disease may attack any part of the bone, among which the localized, fastest-growing bones, and the highly vascularized metaphysis are most susceptible. It is common in upper and lower limbs of long bone, such as tibia, fibula, femur, humerus, and radius. The metaphysis and diaphysis of long tubular bone are, respectively, predilection sites for children and adults [21].

1. **Hematogenous osteomyelitis.** When the primary focus is not timely treated or the body's immunity drops, bacteria will enter the blood circulation and then colonize the osseous tissue to cause disease. However, only around 20% of patients have a clear history of infection or visible primary infection during infection. Risk factors include trauma, premature delivery, urinary tract infection, vascular built-in pipe operation, and immunodeficiency. As bumping often occurs on children, the significance of trauma is unknown. The disease may be prone to occur followed by trauma and bleeding of tissues caused by a local trauma. The first clinical manifestations are systemic infection, sudden onset, high fever, chills, and even coma and septic shock under severe circumstances. The patient may suffer from soft tissue swelling, increased skin temperature, obvious tenderness at affected part, and partially inflected limbs, muscle spasm, refusal to move, and even diffuse swelling of soft tissues and more obvious pain. At this time, a subperiosteal abscess has already formed. After the periosteum ruptures and the abscess flows into the peripheral soft tissues, pressure is lowered and pain is relieved. Reactive joint effusion may be produced if the focus is adjacent to the joint. The natural course of acute osteomyelitis may last for 3–4 weeks. Failing to control the lesion and prevent further deterioration can result in that the abscess penetrates the soft tissue and forms a sinus, thus causing chronic osteomyelitis.

   In some cases, acute osteomyelitis caused by some pathogens with weak virulence (in particular the Staphylococcus albus) may show highly atypical clinical manifestations, lacking high fever and poisoning symptoms, and showing weak signs, thus making the diseases difficult to be diagnosed, resulting in missed diagnosis and misdiagnosis [22].

2. **Traumatic osteomyelitis.** In recent years, contingencies including traffic accidents have occurred frequently, raising the incidence of traumatic osteomyelitis year by year. The diseases are more common in patients with open fracture, who have a higher specificity and are more likely to be infected by rare bacteria. Generally, the disease is caused by insufficient, untimely debridement after trauma. However, osteomyelitis may still occur in spite of sufficient and timely debridement; In addition, closed bone injury may be caused by deficient aseptic operation during surgery, direct infection, injury of blood vessel, postoperative infection, host immunodeficiency, or postoperative wound contamination. The vast majority of pathogens are Staphylococcus aureus, Gram-negative bacillus anaerobic, and Pseudomonas aeruginosa. Among them, a small number of pathogens come from the environment where the injury occurs. Predilection sites are mostly located at the wound. The local trauma damages the blood circulation and protective barriers, thus remarkably lowering the local immunity. For this reason, any infection will cause severe, extensive damage, resulting in massive osteonecrosis, merged sinus formation, necrotic soft tissues and stiff adjacent joints [23]. Unlike long tubular bones, calcaneus, a key structure in supporting weight, is mainly composed of spongy bones. With the thin bone cortex at the lateral side, it is vulnerable to vertical strike forces, which can cause comminuted fracture. As marrow cavity opens, any infection occurred may be spread and concurrent with various degrees of soft- tissue defects. At the heel, bones are wrapped with skin. Due to such a special structure, the heel lacks rich muscle, fat, and other soft tissues, thus may lead to poor postoperative wound healing, bacterial infection, and even spread of infections in case of pathogen entering marrow cavity.
3. **Exogenous osteomyelitis.** Failing to effectively control the soft tissue infection makes the adjacent osseous tissues involved. Phalanx osteomyelitis is generally related to prick of foreign matter and cut, which is prone to involve adjacent joints. Mandible is an osseous tissue that is most susceptible to osteomyelitis in head and neck region. Mandible osteomyelitis is mostly odontogenic. Pseudomonas aeruginosa infection is also common in mandible, unlike other parts involved.

The latter two types of osteomyelitis are complicated, wherein clinical symptoms are easily masked by the original disease and imaging findings are delayed, which may lead to missed diagnosis. At present, acute suppurative osteomyelitis is mainly treated by surgical drainage, to timely relieve the high pressure around the focus, prevent pus from further damaging the osseous tissue, and effectively avoid the development of sequestrum. In addition, antibiotics specific to the pathogen are used to treat the infection, thus weakening the pathogenicity of bacteria and relieving the systemic poisoning. Once diagnosed, the empirical antibacterial therapy will be provided immediately, and then the sensitive antibiotics according to findings of bacterial culture. Antibiotics are better selected according to findings of bacterial culture and drug sensitive test. In case of failed culture, drugs can be selected based on experience, preferring to use broad-spectrum antibiotics during a treatment course of 4 to 6 weeks.

Surgery needs to completely remove infected and inactivated tissues, which is built on effective preoperative imaging examinations, clarification of the surgery scope, and a complete surgical plan. The disease can be fully healed with early diagnosis and effective treatment. To this end, patient should receive diagnosis as early as possible.

Pathophysiology

The disease can evolve into bone destruction and sequestrum, accompanied by different degrees of bone hyperostosis.

Most cases begin with the focal infection of the metaphysis bone marrow. When the primary focus is not treated properly or the body's resistance is lowered, pathogen will enter the blood circulation, reach the bone marrow through the nutrient artery, and stay in spongy bone area of metaphysis adjacent to the epiphyseal plate. This area is characterized by rich blood supply, slow blood flow, and discontinuous endothelium, which makes the pathogens easy to remain and reproduce here, thus rapidly causing osteomyelitis infiltration. The micro terminal arterioles and blood capillaries adjacent to children's epiphyseal plate are bent into vascular loops, where the blood flow is slow and pathogen is easy to deposit. For this reason, long bone metaphysis is a predilection site of acute suppurative osteomyelitis for children. Thanks to the barrier function of the epiphyseal plate, the disease rarely involves joints. As for adults, epiphyseal plate has fused, wherein blood vessels at diaphysis and joints ends continue, thus enabling abscess to directly enter articular cavity. For this reason, osteomyelitis focus can occur in any part of bones.

The course of the disease can be divided into 4 stages: ① Osteomyelitis infiltration stage within 2–3 days after the onset, during which the venous sinuses are damaged and a small amount of pus blood presents. At early stage, the focus is small, with hyperemia, exudation, and infiltration of a small amount of neutrophil. If the pathogen virulence is weak, with strong body immunity and timely treatment, the patient can heal after infection is controlled and pathogens are eliminated. If the disease deteriorates, exudates and necrosis can cause suppuration, vascular congestion, and intravascular thrombosis, thereby resulting in increased intramedullary pressure. In some cases, multiple infected focuses may exist and eventually merge into a larger abscess. In addition to general infection, the clinical manifestations also include local swelling of the affected limb and obvious, localized tenderness. At this stage, conservative treatment with antibiotic is usually adopted. ② Subperiosteal abscess stage within 3–4 days after the onset, during which the inflammation further diffuses, with such infection spreading in the marrow cavity. As the pus in the bone marrow cavity increases, the pressure rises, thus transmitting the infection to the subperiosteal space through the Haversian canal in the cortex, causing subperiosteal abscess and stimulating periosteal proliferation. Due to the peeled periosteum, nutrient artery branches of periosteal vessels into the bone are completely interrupted, thereby forming a vast amount of sequestra. The clinical manifestation at this stage is diffuse swelling. The surgery should be performed as early as possible to expel pus for decompression. With timely treatment, the patient can have good prognosis. ③ Periosteum destruction stage within 5–8 days after the onset, during which the subperiosteal pus increases and penetrates the periosteum to infect the adjacent soft tissues, thus resulting in varying degrees of periosteum necrosis and extensive damage to blood supply in bones. At this stage, extensive bone and soft tissue necrosis may occur, which is very likely to cause septicopyemia. The clinical manifestations include extensive swelling and tenderness of the affected limbs, obvious fluctuations in the affected area, and formation of sequestrum of varying sizes. Undesirable prognosis at this stage may result in permanent deformity. ④ Sequestrum formation stage, during which the osseous tissue become sequestrum due to loss of blood supply, forming inflammatory granulation tissue in the surrounding area, and the margins of the sequestrum are gradually absorbed, separating the sequestrum from the adjacent viable bone tissues. During the formation of sequestrum, stimulated by the inflammatory congestion and pus, the periosteum around the focus keeps producing new bones that wrap the outer layer of the diaphysis to form an involucrum, on which several small holes are communicated with the skin sinus. Inside the involucrum, there are sequestrum, pus, and inflammatory granulation tissues, causing inadequate drainage and thereby forming a dead space. Small pieces of sequestrum can be cleared or absorbed by phagocytes, or be expelled from the body through the sinus. By contrast, large pieces of sequestrum can seldom be absorbed or expelled, thus long remaining in the body, making the sinus unhealed for a long time and evolving into the chronic osteomyelitis.

Imaging Findings

The early diagnosis of acute suppurative osteomyelitis is very important, while the development of the disease is affected by many factors. In particular, with the extensive use of antibiotics and changes in bacterial virulence, atypical osteomyelitis has seen a gradual increase, along with more difficult diagnosis and differential diagnosis. For this reason, MRI examination is more effective than X-ray in early diagnosis.

1. **X-ray**
   (a) Soft tissue swelling: Usually occurs within 1–2 days after infection. The clinical manifestations include swelling & enlargement of affected limb and blurred boundary between subcutaneous fat layer and muscle. The subcutaneous fat layer is thickened due to edema, forming a large, thick reticular structure. Intermuscular fat may be moved, blurred, or disappeared. During early stage, X-ray can only show swelling of soft tissues at infected site, generally without obvious bone change. The focus is limited to a certain part of the bone, but may involve all the surrounding soft tissues therein. Generally, joints are not involved in the early stage.
   (b) Bone destruction: Bone destruction cannot be found until 10–14 days after the onset, and this time may be delayed to around 1 month if the patient has used antibiotics. Bone trabecula in spongy bone of metaphysis is blurred and disappeared, accompanied by localized osteoporosis. Subsequently, a number of scattered, moth-eaten, different-sized patchy bone destruction areas are formed, with blurred margins and rapid disease progression, thus causing pathologic fracture. Besides, hyperostosis happens along with the bone destruction, manifested as localized proliferation and sclerosis surrounding the destruction area. All the above changes occurring simultaneously point to a typical sign of acute suppurative osteomyelitis. In severe cases, most of diaphysis, or even the entire diaphysis, can be involved, and epiphyseal plate may be bypassed to involve epiphysis, thus forming suppurative osteomyelitis accompanied by epiphysitis. What's more, the disease may destruct bony articular surface, encroaching on joints, thus resulting in pyogenic arthritis.
   (c) Periosteal proliferation: It occurs when periosteum is stimulated by inflammation and proliferated. Periosteal proliferation can form onion-peel, linear, layered, lace-like, radial, and other patterns of compact shades. As the disease progresses, periosteum becomes thicker with a higher density, and compact new bone with irregular margin is then formed (Fig. 4.14). The thick proliferated periosteum may surround all or most of sequestrum in diaphysis, thus forming an involucrum, some of which are similar to a layer of solidified wax next to a candle.

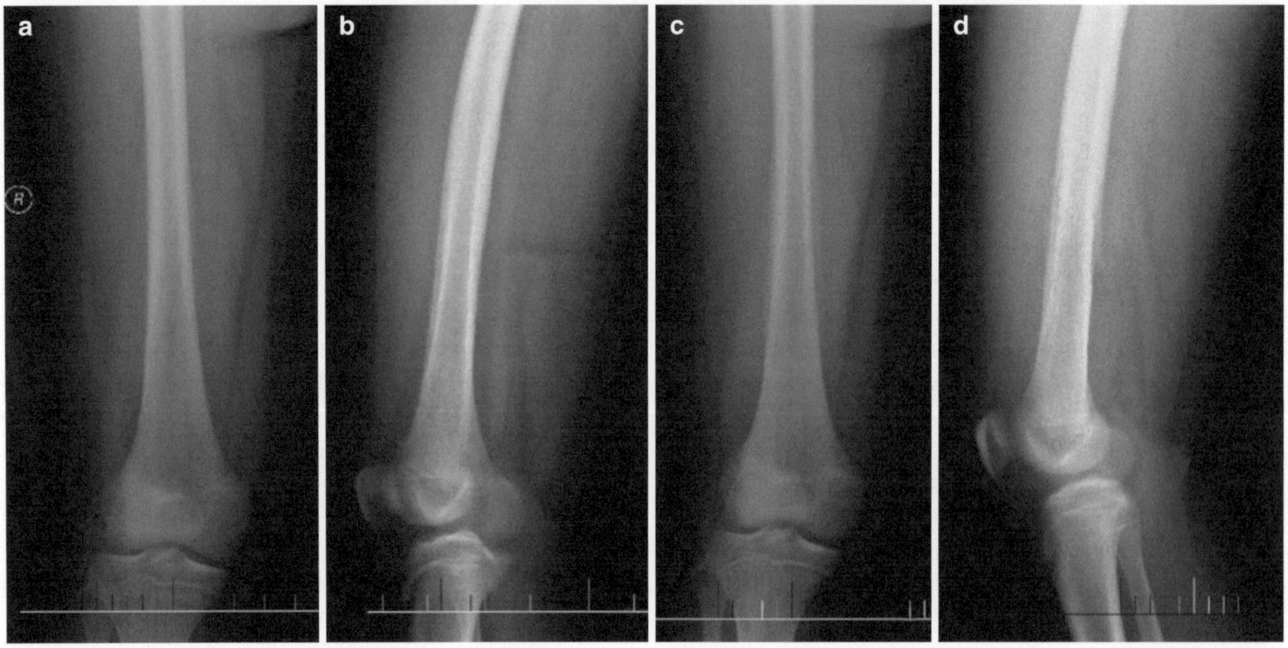

Fig. 4.14 Early changes in middle & lower segments of right femur with acute suppurative osteomyelitis. (**a**, **b**) show that periosteum of middle & lower segments of right femur has layered proliferation, with heterogeneous bone mineral density of femur and swollen surrounding soft tissues. As shown in (**c**, **d**) DR reexamination performed 11 days later shows that the periosteal proliferation is more obvious than before

(d) Formation of sequestrum: About 2 weeks after the onset, the blood supply of the bone cortex is interrupted due to the peeling of the periosteum, nutrient interruption, vascular thrombosis, and pus pressure, thus forming the sequestrum. It manifested as different-sized patchy and stripy bone shadows, with clear boundaries and a high density. Compared with the surrounding bone substances, which gradually are absorbed and become loose, the sequestrum has a higher density because it stops metabolism and cannot be absorbed. In case of an extensive destruction, large, long strips of sequestrum pieces can be formed along the long axis of diaphysis, which represents a characteristic manifestation of acute suppurative osteomyelitis. Mostly, there are abscess cavities with lower density surrounding the sequestrum.

2. **CT.** It is better than ordinary X-ray examination and is more sensitive to soft tissues swelling, which is characterized in that the gap between intermuscular fats has a higher density, or becomes blurred or disappeared. CT can clearly show the high-density strip- or grid-shaped shadow in the subcutaneous fat. Muscles surrounding the focus are swollen, manifested as irregular patchy muscles in lesion area with a decreased density. In the diaphysis, since the normal bone marrow has a relatively high content of fat, the density of pus and granulation tissue is higher than that of normal yellow bone marrow. Destruction of spongy bone in metaphysis is manifested as low-density small patchy shadow; Compared with MRI and radionuclide scan, CT can better show the small destruction area and small sequestrum, which is manifested as the free, high-density shadow in vomica. The large sequestrum has an increased bone mineral density, with no bone trabecula structure formed therein. CT can clearly show the location and spreading range of abscess in the early stage, as well as the gas in bones or soft tissues (Fig. 4.15). The tiny bone abscess, however, is still difficult to be found through CT.

3. **MRI.** It is better than general X-ray and CT. Thanks to its superior contrast of soft tissue, MRI is extremely sensitive to hyperemia and edema of bone marrows and soft tissues in the early stage. It can detect changes in bone marrow within 2–3 days after infection, clearly distinguish intraosseous lesions from lesions of parosteal soft tissues, and also distinguish abnormal bone marrow from the normal one. Normally, yellow bone marrow in marrow cavity, which is similar to a fat signal, shows hyperintense on both T_1WI and T_2WI, while the bone cortex shows obvious hypointense due to its low water content. Due to inflammatory infiltration and edema, bone marrow cavity at the lesion shows hypointense or isointense on T_1WI, which is in stark contrast to the hyperintense of normal bone marrow, and hyperintense on T_2WI and fat-suppressed sequence, thus clearly showing the range of involved marrow cavity. Bone marrow vomica and subperiosteal abscess show hyperintense on T_2WI, while periosteum shows hypointense “linear” structure

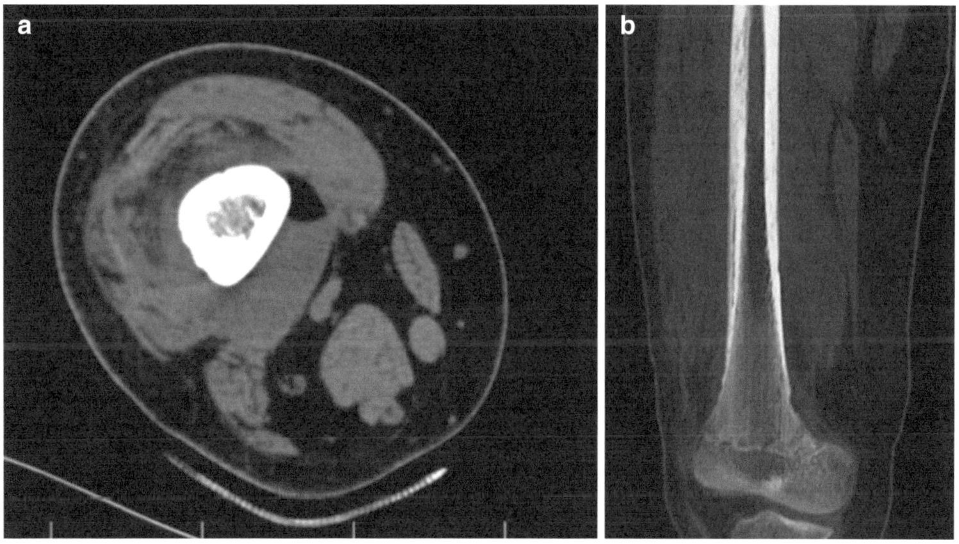

Fig. 4.15 Acute suppurative osteomyelitis in the middle & lower segments of right femur. Same case as that shown in Fig. 4.14. (**a**) CT imaging in soft tissue window shows that an abscess is formed around the focus, with visible gas density shadow therein. (**b**) 3D reconstruction of sagittal plane shows visible layered periosteal proliferation

(Fig. 4.16). With Gd-DTPA contrast agent, the granulation tissue surrounding the abscess shows hyperintense, while the abscess shows hypointense. The location & size of abscess and sinus stretching into soft tissues can be clearly displayed on T_2WI sequence. This provides guidance for both clinical treatment and surgery [24].

4. **Radionuclide bone imaging**. Characterized by extremely sensitive to inflammation, radionuclide scan can provide positive result within 48 h after onset. Patients under suspicion of osteomyelitis usually receive ^{99m}Tc-MDP radionuclide bone scanning, through which the ^{99m}Tc are massively gathered around the focus in the early stage due to the dilated and increased blood vessels there. For this reason, the nuclide uptake around the abscess is high, with concentration of radioactive substances (Fig. 4.17), while the abscess is manifested as a cold spot without radioactive uptake. Having said that, the radionuclide bone scan can only show the position of the lesion and support the early diagnosis. It cannot be used as a basis for qualitative diagnosis [25].

Key Points of Diagnosis

1. With acute onset, patients suffer from systemic poisoning, local acute inflammation, and persistent, sharp pain at a certain area of the body. Children tend to be inactive.
2. Metaphysis of long tubular bone is a predilection site, and the affected area has obvious tenderness.
3. Count of leukocyte, neutrophil and C-reactive protein increase, with a higher erythrocyte sedimentation rate.
4. X-ray plain film shows that swelling of surrounding soft tissues within 10 days of onset is an early change. Ten days later, bone destruction and sequestrum may appear, accompanied by hyperostosis. Due to delayed manifestations, the X-ray findings cannot serve as the basis for early diagnosis.
5. According to CT plain scan, vomica has a low density and abscess wall has an equal or slightly higher density. Periosteum new bones and different-sized sequestra can be seen, wherein the bone destruction is dominated, accompanied by bone repair and hyperostosis which begin almost simultaneously, with increased bone mineral density around destruction area as the main feature.
6. MRI is helpful in early diagnosis. Pus shows hypointense on T_1WI and hyperintense on T_2WI. Abscess wall shows isointense or slightly hypointense on T_2WI. The enhanced scan shows marked enhancement of the abscess wall.
7. Pathogens can be obtained via blood culture, but the positive rate is not high. In particular for those who have used antibiotics, all the pathogens obtained should be tested for drug sensitivity.
8. Layered puncture for local abscess in early stage is of great significance for diagnosis and treatment. If the patient is highly suspected of suppurative osteomyelitis according to clinical and imaging findings, aspiration biopsy and culture should be performed as early as possible to determine types of pathogens and their sensitive antibiotics. It should be noted that the results of bacterial culture for sinus tissues are often different from that of bone biopsy.

Differential Diagnosis

1. **Eosinophilic granuloma.** It can be found on infants, children, and young people. Without systemic symptom, the disease accelerates erythrocyte sedimentation rate and increases the count of eosinophilic granulocyte. Any bone can be involved. The focus originates from the marrow cavity and spreads to the surrounding area. The early man-

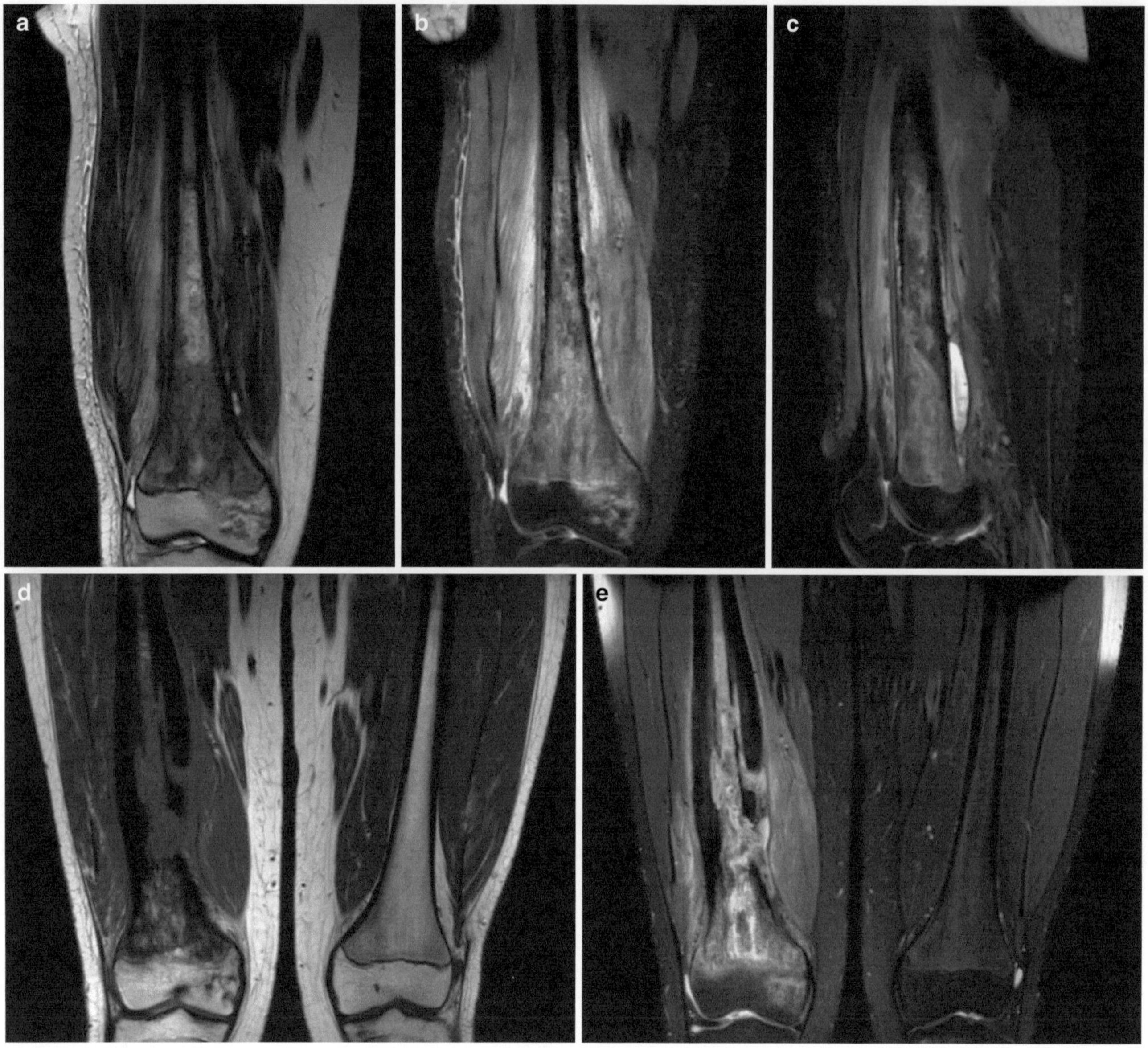

Fig. 4.16 Acute suppurative osteomyelitis in the middle & lower segments of right femur. Same case as that shown in Fig. 4.14. (**a–c**) According to MRI, the middle & lower segments of right femur show heterogeneous hypointense on T_1WI and hyperintense on T_2WI, and the peripheral soft tissues are obviously swollen. (**a** T_1WI; B and C: T_2WI fat-suppressed sequence); In (**d**, **e**) the MRI reexamination after 15 days shows that the diseases progresses rapidly and forms sinus (**d** T_1WI; E. T_2WI fat-suppressed sequence)

ifestation is cyst. In the middle stage, the count of histiocyte increases. The lesion evolves into a gray connective tissue in the late stage, and can finally be ossified, with non-obvious soft tissue swelling or mass. The focus located in long bone shows unicystic or polycystic osteolytic destruction. The focus's long axis is often parallel to the diaphysis, with clear boundary and expansive, thinned cortex. Irregular linear and layered periosteal proliferation can be seen around the lesion. Most of the periosteum is intact, with smooth outer margins, no damage or rupture. CT shows patchy bone fragments in the lesion; As for lesion located in skull, the bone destruction area shows punched-out pattern, involving both inner and outer plates. In addition, patchy bone destruction may also exist, with a soft tissue mass formed laterally. As for lesions located in ribs, shoulder blade, pelvis, or sternum, the bone destruction areas are mostly geographic or oval-patterned, with mild proliferation and sclerosis of edges, and periosteal proliferation as well as soft tissue mass; The disease progressed more rapidly than acute osteomyelitis.

2. **Ewing sarcoma.** It is common in adolescents below 25 years old, and occurs preferably in the middle section of long bones (tibia, diaphysis, and humerus). Patients usually show systemic symptoms, such as increased body temperature, leukocytosis, and accelerated erythrocyte sedimentation rate. Early clinical manifestations and

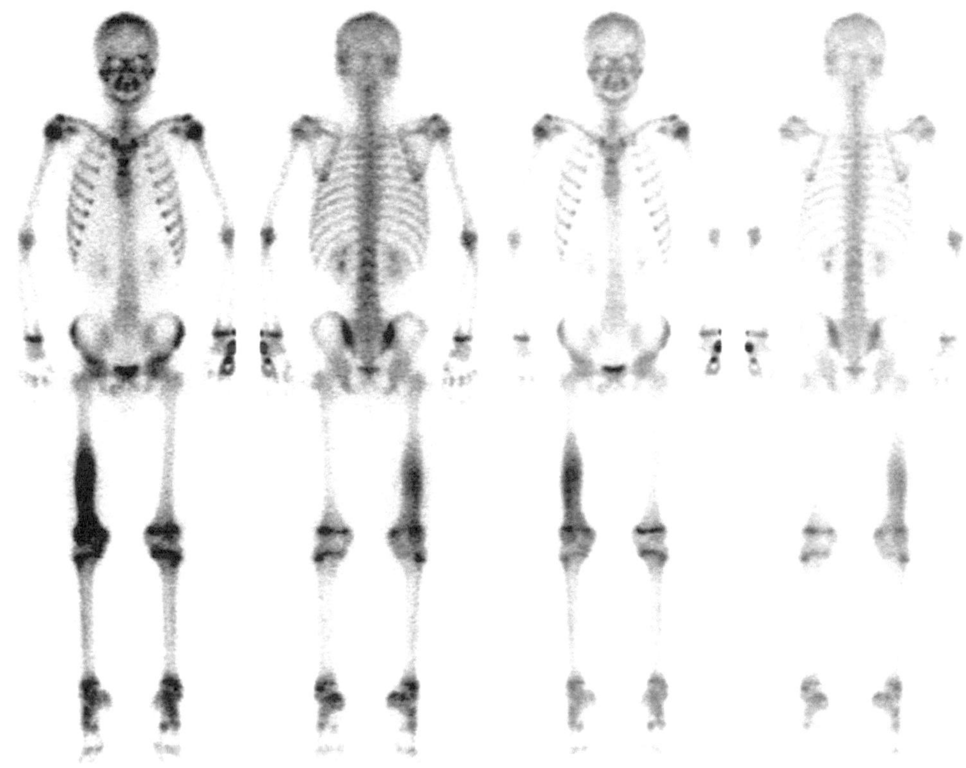

Fig. 4.17 Acute suppurative osteomyelitis in the middle & lower segments of right femur. Same case as that shown in Fig. 4.14. The concentration of nuclide in the lower section of right femur indicates that the disease is still in the advanced stage

imaging findings are similar to that of osteomyelitis. Compared with the acute suppurative osteomyelitis, Ewing sarcoma has a slightly longer course, measured on a monthly basis. Onset time is not well-defined, and there is no sequestrum. Surrounding destruction area is blurred, and soft tissue swelling is usually localized. According to the basic X-ray and CT findings, Ewing sarcoma is manifested as spot-like and moth-eaten osteolytic destruction areas, which may be accompanied by a small amount of hyperostosis and osteosclerosis. The surrounding bone cortex shows cribriform or lace-like defects and destruction, with clear boundaries between the soft tissue mass and slightly dilated marrow cavity. No sequestrum is formed. Periosteal proliferation shows localized onion-peel pattern. Since it is highly invasive and destructive, the tumor often grows through the periosteum to form a Codman triangle. Tiny, slender spicules can be found at the rupture of periosteal proliferation. The periosteal proliferation of osteomyelitis, most of which are laminated, involves a wider range. It is clear from MRI findings that the soft tissue mass shows heterogeneous hypointense on T_1WI and hyperintense on T_2WI, with clear boundaries, often accompanied by hemorrhage signals. The soft tissue mass is large, disproportionate to the bone destruction area. A few cases show intraosseous skip metastasis. Osteomyelitis, however, due to its particularity of inflammation, has no obvious boundary, and the surrounding edema is obvious. The cyst cavity formed by necrotic tumor tissues should be differentiated from the abscess-like cyst cavity. The latter is more regular in shape and shows obvious hyperintense on DWI, while the former is mostly irregular and shows hypointense on DWI. Soft tissue swelling caused by early acute osteomyelitis shows diffuse distribution, forming annular or C-shaped structures at the transverse plane. By contrast, soft tissue mass caused by Ewing sarcoma is localized.

3. **Bone tuberculosis.** It mainly refers to long tubular bone tuberculosis, characterized by mild symptoms, slow progress, systemic tuberculosis poisoning symptoms, local swelling, and dull heat sensation. Epiphysis and metaphysis are predilection sites. The disease rarely occurs in the diaphysis, but more frequently in the superior extremity of femur, proximal ulna, and distal radius, manifested as moth-eaten, cystic osteolytic bone destruction area, without obvious reactive proliferation and sclerosis at the edge. Adjacent osseous tissues have osteoporosis and may be accompanied by grit-like sequestrum, marrow cavity expansion, lamellar periosteal proliferation, thinning of bone cortex, spina ventosa of quasi-short tubular bone tuberculosis, and fusiform swelling of surrounding soft tissues, which is different from the diffuse swelling of soft tissues in acute osteomyelitis. Typical changes in concentric circular intensity can be seen on MRI T_2WI. The center is a caseous necrosis zone with homogeneous hyperintense, and the outer layer is a thin hypointense fibrous tissue strip, and the outermost layer is a hyperintense edema zone of varying widths. Besides, the focus often crosses the epiphyseal line and may evolve

into joint tuberculosis without timely treatment, which is the characteristic of epiphyseal and metaphyseal tuberculosis.

4. **Congenital syphilis of bone.** It is common in long bone, typically manifested as symmetrical, polyostotic focal bone destruction. The main pathological changes are periostitis, osteitis, and osteomyelitis, forming moth-eaten loose area, or bringing extensive destruction and proliferative changes, which is similar to acute suppurative osteomyelitis. To distinguish the two diseases, the presence of sequestrum and isolated focus can be used as a main basis. Congenital syphilis of bone can form linear or layered periosteal proliferation, with marrow cavity expanded in a fusiform shape. The periosteal proliferation involves expansive range, but the destruction area is localized.

Status Quo and Progress of Research

Currently, more and more cases are caused by methicillin-resistant Staphylococcus aureus. Patients may have taken antibiotics prior to the collection of culture specimens, resulting in that the leukocyte count and inflammatory markers from the laboratory test are not reliable, thus changing the results of laboratory test.

1. **X-ray.** Within 10 days of infection, X-ray plain film can barely detect the bone destruction, while is insensitive to the swelling of soft tissues. The reports indicate that even the positive diagnosis rate after 2 weeks is only 20%. In addition, the wide use of antibiotics conceals the typical symptoms, making it difficult to diagnose the disease in the early stage.
2. **CT.** It boasts a higher sensitivity to sequestrum, capable of detecting the silt-like sequestrum, which cannot be shown by X-ray and MRI. In addition, compared with MRI, X-ray and CT can better show the morphologic changes in periosteal proliferation and distinguish periosteal reaction osteogenesis. Enhanced CT displays the focus area more clearly, with a faster scanning speed and fewer contraindications, in spite of a higher radiation dose than X-ray. Radionuclide bone scanning is also widely applied in osteomyelitis diagnosis. All these three methods are radioactive, so their application is limited in some patients.
3. **MRI.** It boasts a high resolution to soft tissues and extremely high sensitivity to changes in moisture, and can deliver multi-parameter and multi-orientation imaging without radiation hazards. Thanks to these features, it is of great significance to the early detection of the disease. General sequences include T_1WI, T_2WI, and fat-suppressed sequence. Scanning methods include transverse plane, coronal plane, and sagittal plane. With fat suppression technology, it can provide the clearest display for bone marrow and soft tissue inflammatory edema. A number of clinical practices have proven the overall advantages of MRI in osteomyelitis assessment. It is recognized as the preferred imaging method for detecting osteomyelitis and infections related to extraosseous soft tissues [26]. In a word, the best existing imaging method for detecting suspected osteomyelitis is X-ray plain film, and then followed by MRI.

People remain divided over the timing of providing gadolinium-containing contrast agent to patients with suspected osteomyelitis. Latest researches indicate that intravenous injection of gadolinium-containing contrast agent cannot improve the sensitivity and specificity of osteomyelitis diagnosis. If fluid-sensitive images (such as fat-suppressed sequence STIR and T_2- FS) are normal, gadolinium enhancement has no additional value for diagnosis. In case of abnormal fluid-sensitive images, however, gadolinium enhancement is of great clinical significance to the diagnosis of abscess and planning of abscess suction and drainage. In addition, osteomyelitis involving epiphyseal plate can only be shown on gadolinium-enhanced T_1WI sequence, rather than on the non-contrasted T_1WI, fluid-sensitive sequence, X-ray, or PET scanning. The infected epiphysis is manifested as an area where one or multiple epiphysis cartilages are reduced or not enhanced, otherwise the epiphysis should be uniformly enhanced. As mentioned above, infection of the epiphyseal plate in infancy may cause growth disorder, so it is recommended to use gadolinium in this age group [4, 27–29].

Currently, MRI scanning uses standard T_1WI and T_2WI, and sometimes adds contrast enhancement sequences. DWI, DCE, magnetic resonance spectroscopy, and other more advanced imaging techniques can also be used, in spite of their undefined roles. As for DWI, one potential application is to describe the fluid accumulation associated with osteomyelitis, since abscess is characterized by limited spread on DWI. Further researches are required to figure out roles of these imaging technologies in the disease.

Beyond that, when applied to children, MRI also shows obvious shortcomings, including long scanning duration and susceptibility to motion artifacts. What's more, patients with metal foreign bodies and certain types of implants are prohibited from MRI.

4.3.2 Chronic Osteomyelitis

Overview

Incurable, persistent acute suppurative osteomyelitis may evolve into chronic osteomyelitis. In addition, when the virulence of the pathogen is weak or body immunity is good, the disease can be a chronic process from the very beginning, characterized by insidious onset, mild symptoms, and atypical signs, thus making diagnosis difficult [30, 31]. Amidst the widespread use of antibiotics and changes in bacterial virulence, the incidence of chronic osteomyelitis is ever-growing.

Presence of sequestrum and involucrum is a characteristic sign of chronic osteomyelitis. The disease is caused by the following four reasons: ① Evolved from the acute hematogenous osteomyelitis; ② Primary disease; ③ Traumatic disease; ④ Spread of infection in adjacent tissues.

Patients typically have a clear history of acute suppurative osteomyelitis. Systemic symptoms are mild when the intraosseous focus is inactive; However, acute onset may recur when body immunity is decreased, manifested as swelling and pain in the affected area, a higher body temperature, opened sinus orifice with discharged pus, and sequestrum. After treatment, as the inflammation subsides and the sinus closes, the disease re-enters the chronic phase, with lasting course up to decades of years. The disease may occur repeatedly, and the sinus may be long incurable. Long-term recurrence can result in enlarged, twisted, and deformed affected limb, pathologic fracture, contraction deformation of adjacent joints, pigmented, thin skin, several cicatrices, long incurable sinus, with proliferation of granulation tissue and discharged pus surrounding the sinus orifice and even cancer. The bone destruction can affect children's bone development, making the affected limb shortened and deformed.

Since it is difficult to completely remove the focus and eliminate the dead space, pathogens cannot be wiped out, thus causing recurrent infection. This is the main reason why chronic osteomyelitis is difficult to cure.

Pathophysiology

The pathogenesis and pathologic manifestations of chronic osteomyelitis are similar to that of acute suppurative osteomyelitis, with a focus on the formation of sequestrum, dead space, and sinus. Infiltration of plasma cell, lymphocyte, and macrophage can be seen in the focus. The granulation tissue enables the necrotic spongy bone to be gradually absorbed, wherein the compact bone substance located in the junction area is absorbed first, and finally falls off into a sequestrum. The synergy between osteoclasts and proteolytic enzymes makes the sequestrum fallen off and its surface rough. After that, when the body's immunity is reduced or other diseases occur concurrently, the disease may recrudesce due to the pathogens remaining in the cavity. Irritated by the inflammation, endosteum and periosteum cause reactive osteogenesis, resulting in thickening of bone cortex and forming a bone shell on the outer edge of the bone cortex. Long irritated by the inflammation, soft tissues on the surface of the focus are severely damaged, while the surface skin is easily injured, thus forming cicatrices and making sinus unhealed within a long term.

Imaging Findings

As the most basic examination means, X-ray can deliver valuable findings. By contrast CT, MRI, and radionuclide imaging are more conducive to observing details inside the focus due to their clear display, especially for the active focus. These examination methods mainly aim to find the active focus remaining in chronic osteomyelitis focuses, especially to observe the following signs: any soft tissue swelling, periosteal reaction, proliferation and sclerosis structure, bone destruction area, and sequestrum in the lesion, and any invasion of epiphyseal cartilage. Special attention should be paid to young patients, as they may suffer from osteogenesis disorders, thus affecting their development.

1. **Chronic Osteomyelitis**
   (a) X-ray
      (i) Soft tissue swelling: Soft tissues of the site acutely attacked by chronic suppurative osteomyelitis are mainly dominated by inflammatory exudate, manifested as localized swelling of soft tissues, and streak and reticular shadows in subcutaneous fat (Fig. 4.18). In the chronic phase, the lesion is mainly manifested as repair of soft tissue hyperplasia, forming localized soft tissue masses with clear margins. Since then, the soft tissue mass shrinks gradually, thus forming partially defective soft tissue atrophy or fistula.
      (ii) Bone destruction and proliferation and sclerosis: Osteolysis of adjacent metaphysis changes, and then a sclerosis strap gradually appears in the surrounding area, sometimes showing the destruction area and sequestrum in the osteosclerosis [32]. Damages to osteolysis by pus, manifested as blurred margins, are usually active focuses. Homogeneous osteosclerosis without bone trabecula structure indicates active focus therein. On the contrary, osteosclerosis with bone trabecula structures indicates that inflammation has been absorbed and new bones are being rebuilt. Proliferation and sclerosis is a reaction during the repair of chronic osteomyelitis. The hyperostosis around the bone abscess involves a wide range, manifested as homogeneous or heterogeneous density without bone texture. In severe cases, the marrow cavity can be narrowed or occluded, mostly accompanied by extensive periosteal proliferation, which may be associated with the species and virulence of pathogen.
      (iii) Periosteal proliferation: Periosteal proliferation caused by chronic suppurative osteomyelitis is extensive and obvious, and endosteum proliferation can make the marrow cavity narrowed or

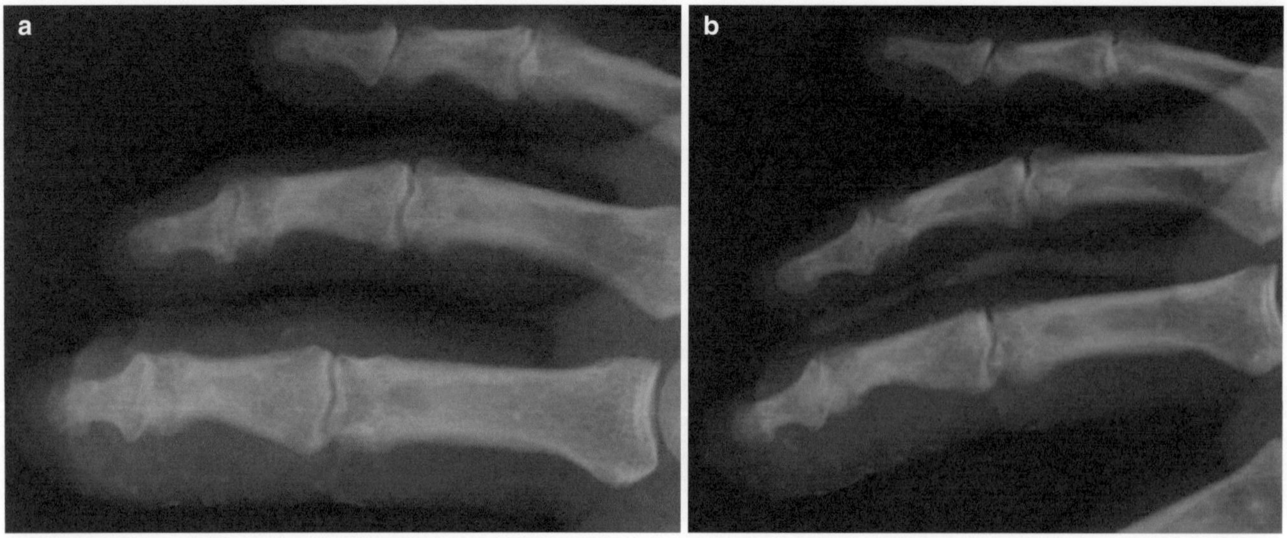

Fig. 4.18 Chronic osteomyelitis in right middle finger. (**a**) Right middle finger PA; (**b**) Right middle finger OBL. The middle phalanx of right middle finger is characterized by uneven bone density, swollen surrounding soft tissues, and increased subcutaneous fat density, with no obvious bone destruction area noted

even disappeared. Periosteal proliferation is usually multi-layered, lace-like, intermittent, irregular-shaped or shell-wrapped. The proliferated periosteum is often fused with the diaphysis cortex, which is difficult to distinguish, making the affected bone thickened and deformed, with a bone mineral density remarkably increased. Periosteal proliferation occurring in the long bone, called involucrum, is generally fusiform.

(iv) Formation of sequestrum and dead space: The disappearance of sequestrum and dead space marks the healing of chronic suppurative osteomyelitis. That said, since hyperostosis and osteosclerosis surrounding vomica and the extensive proliferation of endosteum & periosteum significantly increase the bone mineral density, thereby often concealing the sequestrum or vomica therein, doctors may be misled to believe the chronic suppurative osteomyelitis has healed, causing recurrence of the disease. For this reason, special attention should be paid to look for the sequestrum and dead space, which are the main basis for the imaging diagnosis of chronic suppurative osteomyelitis. Sequestrum may be intraosseous or extraosseous, or exists in the soft tissues. Sequestrum often exists in the dead space and sinus, manifested as high-density free bone shadows that are different-sized, irregularly shaped, free from bone trabecula and located in osteolytic destruction area and soft tissues. In case of extensively destroyed periosteum, the necrotic diaphysis caused by ischemia can form large pieces of sequestrum (Fig. 4.19).

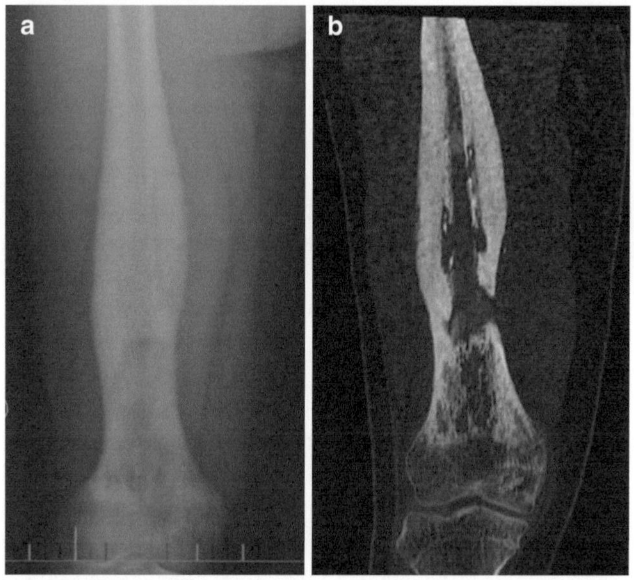

Fig. 4.19 Osteomyelitis in the middle & lower segments of right femur after focus cleaning. (**a**) DR PA; (**b**) According to CT coronal plane reconstruction, diaphysis shows fusiform thickening, bone cortex significantly thickens, with visible irregular bone substance defect areas and formed sinus. Besides, marrow cavity changes after recanalization

Also, abscesses are often formed in the focus. The different-sized osteolytic destruction areas are dead spaces. The chronic vomica is regular in shape, mostly circular or quasi-circular, with smooth and clear margins. Bone substances surrounding the vomica show obvious proliferation

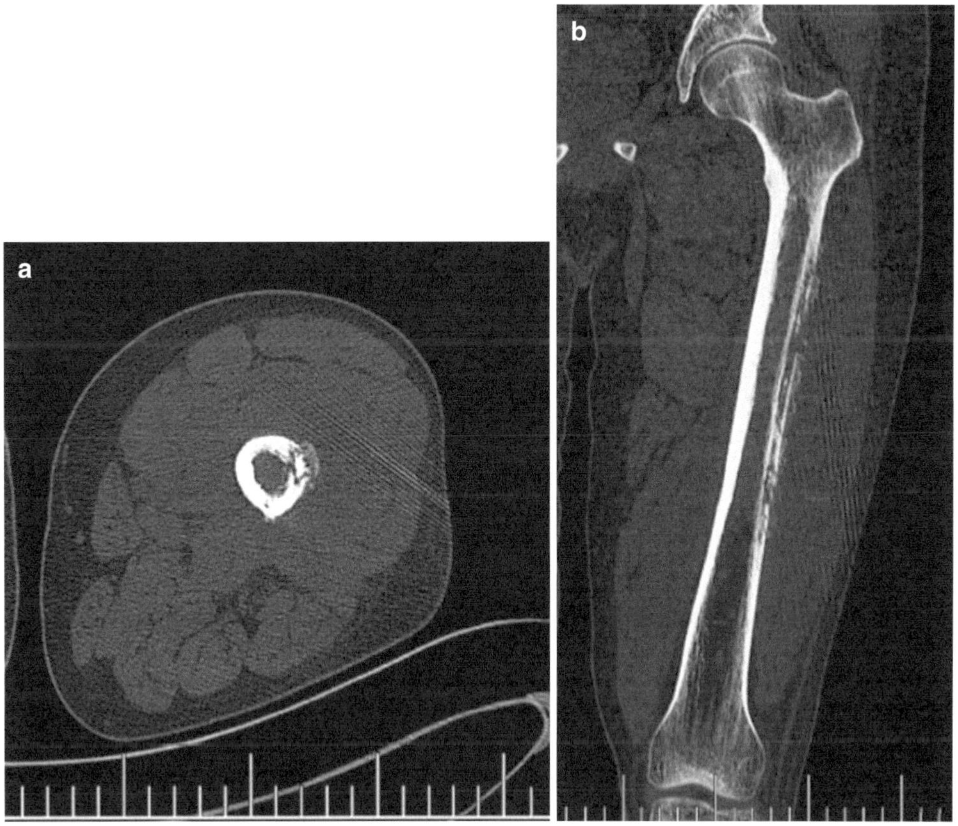

Fig. 4.20 Chronic osteomyelitis in the middle segment of left femur. (**a**) CT transverse plane; (**b**) According to CT coronal plane reconstruction, middle and upper segments of left femur show bone destruction, periosteal proliferation, and formed sequestrum seen in destruction area. Among them, the bone mineral density of sequestrum is higher than that of normal osseous tissue

and sclerosis, with density gradually decreasing from the edge of the focus to the surrounding area [33]. The active focus of chronic suppurative osteomyelitis has the following characteristic signs: ① There is no bone texture structure in proliferation and sclerosis area; ② There is visible destruction area in osteosclerosis area; ③ There is sequestrum in the destruction area; ④ Bone destruction focuses are often seen adjacent to the periosteal reaction; ⑤ Focus is located adjacent to the swelling of soft tissue or ruptured fistula.

(b) CT: X-rays cannot accurately show the residual focus in chronic osteomyelitis. By contrast, CT can better display the bone destruction and surrounding structures of the lesion. Hyperostosis and osteosclerosis are manifested as thickened and blurred bone trabecula, thickened bone cortex, narrowed marrow cavity, increased density, chronic sinus, gas inside the marrow cavity, and other manifestations of chronic osteomyelitis. Sequestrum appears as isolated, irregular thick bone shadows, surrounded by liquid density, with clear margins. Intraosseous abscess focus is manifested as low-density focus in sclerosis zone, with less regular margins and quasi-circular or irregular cross-sections, in which sequestrum can be noted (Fig. 4.20).

(c) MRI: It can deliver desirable tissue contrast through multi-sequence and multi-position imaging. Especially in the early stage of the disease, MRI can detect the focus earlier than X-ray and CT, and accurately display the position and scope. It is currently the most valuable imaging method for the diagnosis of chronic osteomyelitis [34]. MRI provides high resolution of soft tissues, capable of distinguishing inflammatory reactions of periosteum and soft tissues, as well as epiphysis lesions. These are difficult to achieve by X-ray and CT. Besides, MRI is more sensitive than bone imaging. Through MRI, chronic osteomyelitis is manifested as the follows.

(i) Soft tissue swelling: Boundaries between the focus of chronic suppurative osteomyelitis and normal bone marrows & soft tissues are usually clear. During acute attack:

Fibrous tissue, edema, inflammatory lesions, granulation tissue, and pus in focus show hypointense on T_1WI, while inflammatory focus, pus, and edema show hyperintense on T_2WI. The focus shows hyperintense on STIR sequence, while with suppression of fat signal, focus can be shown best. The display of anatomical details, however, is not good enough.

(ii) Bone destruction and proliferation and sclerosis: destruction area shows hypointense on T_1WI and heterogeneous intense dominated by hyperintense on T_2WI. Bone destruction area is irregular, surrounded by visible hypointense sclerosis ring,

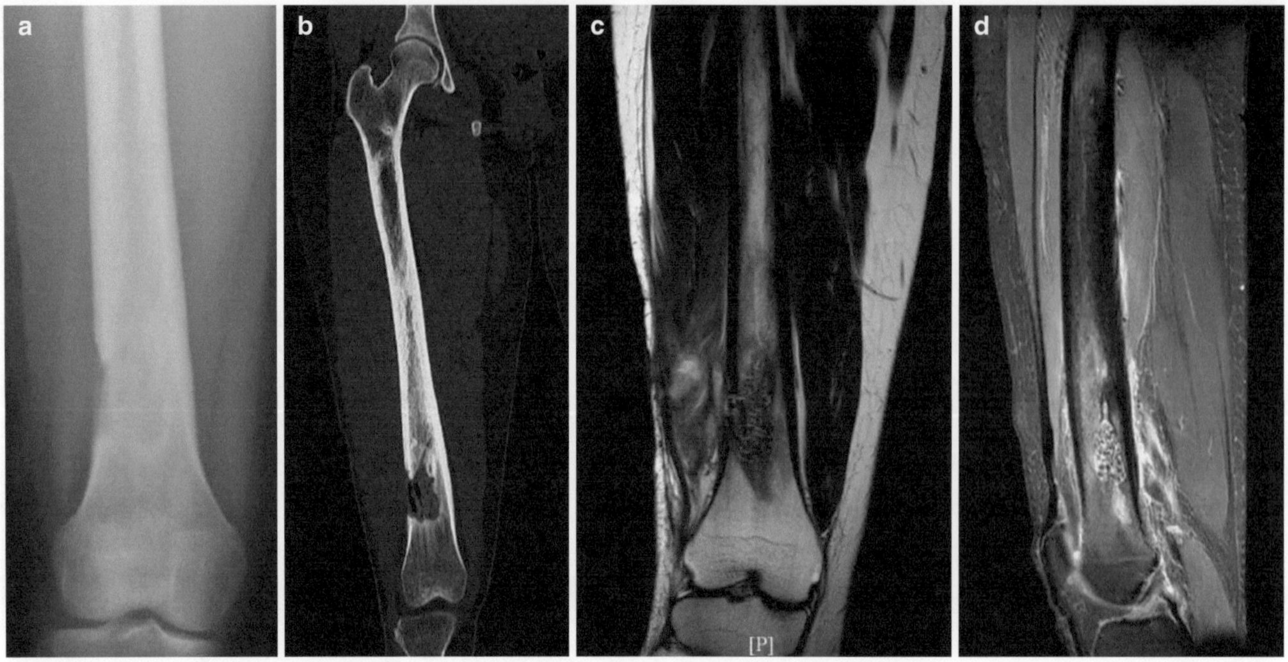

Fig. 4.21 Chronic osteomyelitis (sinus formation) in right femur. (**a**) According to the PA X-ray of the middle and lower segments of right femur, area of osteolytic bone destruction can be seen on the lateral margin of lower femur, lateral margin bone cortex is defective, edged with visible osteosclerosis margin. (**b**) The clearer picture provided by CT 3D reconstruction indicates thickened bone cortex, narrowed marrow cavity, and formed sinus; (**c**, **d**) MRI T_1WI indicates that the focus shows heterogeneous hypointense on T_1WI, with localized defect of skin and formation of sinus. The focus shows heterogeneous hyperintense on T_2WI fat-suppressed sequence, and the surrounding soft tissues show hyperintense

with relatively clear boundaries. Heterogeneously thickened bone cortex shows hypointense on both T_1WI and T_2WI (Fig. 4.21).

(iii) Sequestrum and dead space: Sequestrum mostly shows hypointense on T_1WI and T_2WI. However, if it has a lot of bone marrow, it shows hyperintense. Dead space shows hypointense on T_1WI and hyperintense on T_2WI.

(iv) Sinus: Manifested as a local defect of bone cortex and soft tissue, communicated with the intra & extra marrow cavity, generally showing isointense on T_1WI and hyperintense on T_2WI. However, MRI cannot accurately distinguish the reactive bone marrow edema from the bone marrow edema caused by osteomyelitis, both of which show the same intensity.

(v) With Gd-DTPA contrast agent, granulation tissue shows marked enhancement and abscess wall shows rim-like enhancement, while necrosis and pus show hypointense with no enhancement. For this reason, MRI enhancement can best display the active focus or residual inflammatory lesion in chronic osteomyelitis and show bone cloaca and soft tissue sinus, playing a key role in the diagnosis and differential diagnosis of osteomyelitis. What's more, MRI enhancement helps to distinguish atypical osteomyelitis from tumors and can clearly show the range involved by osteomyelitis, thus providing guidance for the scope of focus removal in surgery.

(d) SPECT: Chronic osteomyelitis can lead to rich blood supply, increased leukocytes, and enhanced osteogenic activity at the site of inflammation reaction. Based on these pathological and physiological changes, certain biological radioactive tracers can be introduced into the human body. After entering the blood circulation, these tracers gather around the involved bone, thus forming a hotspot of radioactive concentration. Different tissues vary in activity intensity (Fig. 4.22). Common tracers include ^{99m}Tc-MDP, ^{67}Ga, and ^{111}In-leukocyte, whose motions are traced by ray detector to outline the metabolic profile of osseous tissues. These tracers have low specificity in spite of high sensitivity.

(e) Positron emission tomography (PET): One of the most effective examination methods for bone infection diagnosis, which can reflect the nature of the lesion from the perspective of molecular metabolism and functional status. 18F-fluorodeoxyglucose, namely ^{18}F-FDG, is the most common tracer cur-

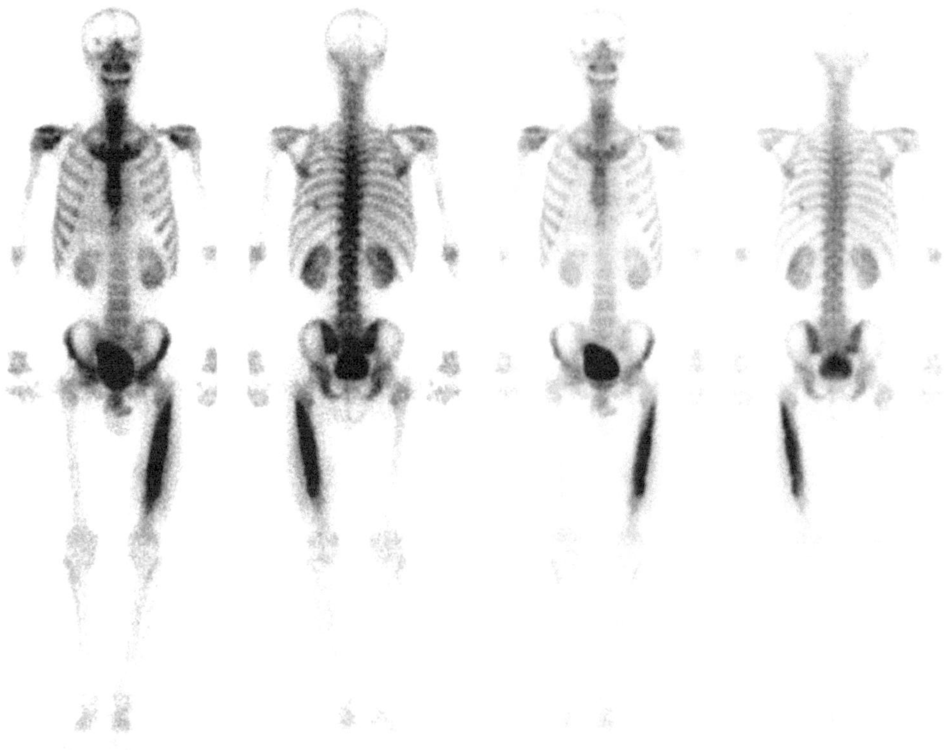

Fig. 4.22 Chronic osteomyelitis in left femur diaphysis. Left femur diaphysis shows abnormal concentration of tracers in full length, indicating that the area has a high metabolic rate

rently used. It reflects changes in metabolism according to the uptake of glucose by diseased tissues. FDG is a small molecule that can quickly enter the infusion area, making the examination process relatively short; The imaging is not affected by adjacent metal objects; Spatial resolution is high; The focus can be positioned more accurately because of the two back-facing photons emitted simultaneously. ^{18}F-FDG PET can distinguish bone infection from bone repair [35]. Having said that, the high cost of PET may bring financial burdens to patients, so it is not recommended as a routine examination item. But it can be used as appropriate when it is difficult to distinguish bone infection from tumor diseases (Fig. 4.23).

2. **Traumatic osteomyelitis:** Generally occurs after trauma or orthopedic surgery, especially after open fracture surgery. Pathogens can be common clinical pathogens or pathogens specific to the environment where the injury occurs. Lesions are mostly located at the fracture site and can be divided into intra-marrow cavity infection and skin/muscle infection at the wound. The former progresses rapidly and may be accompanied by chills, high fever, and other toxemia symptoms. The latter can result in necrosis of infected soft tissue at the wound, exposed deep osseous tissue, and dry necrosis. Imaging findings are unhealed bone fractured end, bone destruction area, proliferation, and sclerosis of margin and swelling of surrounding soft tissues (Fig. 4.24).
3. **Diabetic osteomyelitis**. This special type of osteomyelitis has a different cause and onset mode from other types of osteomyelitis. As population ages and incidence of diabetes remains high, diabetic osteomyelitis has also become more and more common. It occurs frequently in metatarsal-phalangeal bone, with only 54% sensitivity and 58% specificity to X-ray diagnosis. Furthermore, early manifestations are often negative [36]. Through MRI, the preferred method of inspection, the disease is manifested as lack of fat signal in normal soft tissues, accumulation of fluid in soft tissues, and thick-walled ring enhancement, with lesion adjacent to the bone. The key imaging finding indicated by MRI is the change in signal intensity of bone marrow, which shows hypointense on T_1WI and heterogeneous intense or hyperintense on T_2WI. In the STIR sequence, the infection degree may be overestimated, especially when accompanied by adjacent arthritis.
4. **Chronic osteomyelitis of jaw.** The disease is usually caused by bacterial infections (infection of oral cavity or bacteremia derived from adjacent focus), vascular defects (local endarteritis), autoimmune diseases or trauma; Sources of infection are generally periodontal and may also be a tooth extraction surgery, a maxillo-facial injury, or the subsequent complications. Thanks to the improvement of residents' oral cavity hygiene and introduction of new technologies, the incidence of the disease has dropped sharply. That said, certain groups of patients are

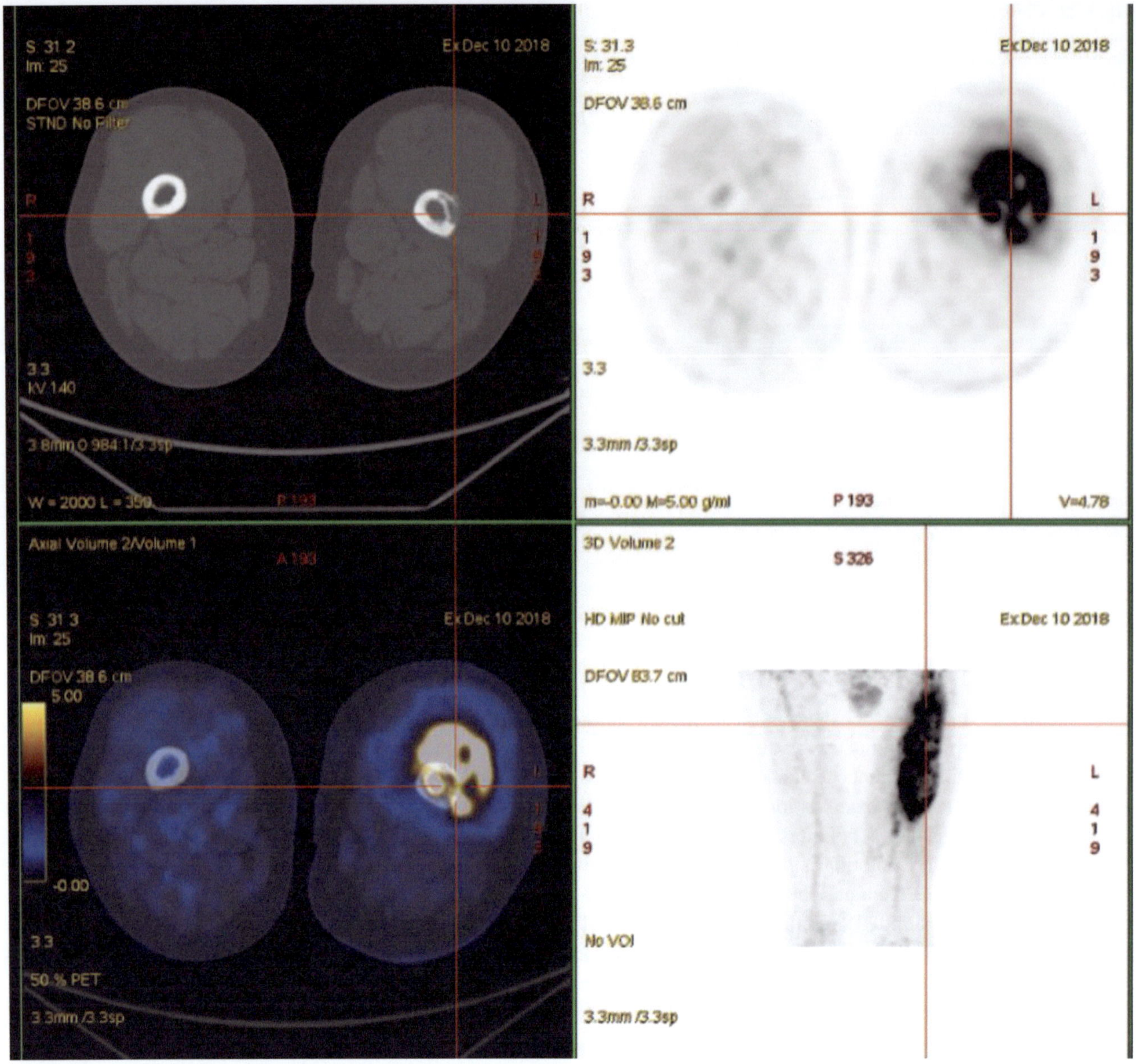

Fig. 4.23 Chronic osteomyelitis in left femur. Focus of left femur, where tracers are concentrated, has a relatively high metabolic rate

still facing an increased risk of osteomyelitis. Different from other osseous tissues of the body, jaw is in direct contact with teeth, thus providing a direct access to inflammatory infections, which are manifested as purulent sinus draining in the oral cavity, bone destruction, adjacent teeth defect, and the like. Pathogens are mostly Staphylococcus aureus, Staphylococcus epidermidis, actinomycetes, Prevotella, and Eikenella. The latter two are more common in refractory osteomyelitis of jaw [37]. Hyperbaric oxygen therapy can improve oxygen tension during hypoxia, thus enhancing blood vessel proliferation, fibroblast activity, osteoclast activity as well as the capacity of cell to kill bacteria. Imaging findings are teeth absence affiliated with bone destruction, with proliferation and sclerosis and periosteal reaction that are generally less obvious than long tubular bone (Fig. 4.25).

Key Points of Diagnosis

1. Most patients have a history of acute suppurative osteomyelitis or trauma.
2. Metaphysis of long tubular bone is a predilection site, and the scope involved may be enlarged. In case of formed sinus, unhealed sinus can be found in the affected limb.
3. X-ray and CT mainly show extensive hyperostosis and osteosclerosis, periosteal proliferation and sclerosis, thickening of bone cortex, thickening and deformation of

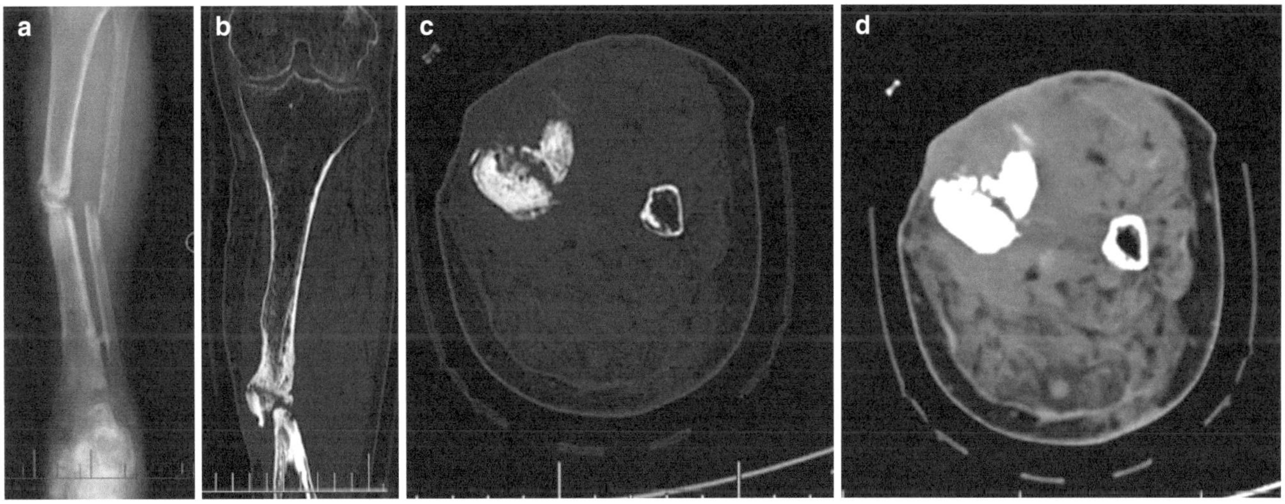

Fig. 4.24 Traumatic osteomyelitis in left lower limb. Chronic osteomyelitis concurrent with unhealed traumatic fracture of left leg. Area of osteolytic bone destruction and sequestrum are seen at the fractured end, with obvious hyperostosis and osteosclerosis, swelling of surrounding soft tissues and disappeared subcutaneous fat space. (**a**) Left tibia & fibula PA X-Ray. (**b**) CT coronal plane 3D reconstruction. (**c**, **d**) CT transverse plane bone window and soft tissue window

Fig. 4.25 Chronic osteomyelitis of jaw. (**a**) CT shows area of osteolytic bone destruction and proliferation and sclerosis on the left margin of the maxilla; (**b**) CT shows bone destruction on the left margin of the mandible, slight proliferation, and sclerosis on margins and teeth absence

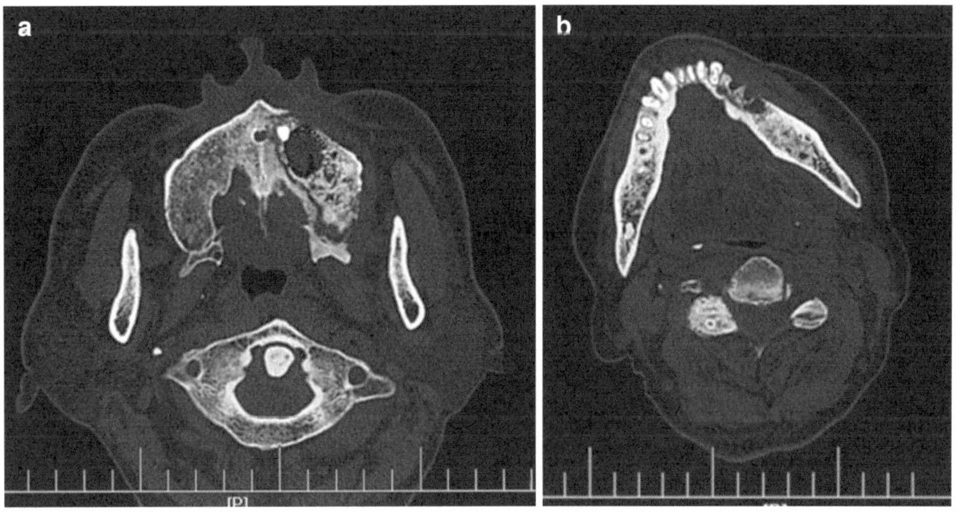

the involved bone, wherein varying degrees of liquefactive necrosis of soft tissue, and formation of sequestrum, bone abscess, and sinus can be observed.

4. MRI shows the formation of dead space and sinus and soft tissue swelling or atrophy.

Differential Diagnosis

1. **Acquired syphilis of bone.** It occurs in multiple bones, mainly manifested as lamellar or lace-like periosteal proliferation involving most of the diaphysis, thickened and enlarged bone cortex, and proliferation and sclerosis of spongy bone and marrow cavity, which is similar to chronic suppurative osteomyelitis. However, the disease is not associated with history of acute suppurative osteomyelitis and does not involve surrounding soft tissues. It causes no soft tissue swelling & atrophy or fistula formation, which can be used as a basis for distinguishing the disease from chronic osteomyelitis. When necessary, Kehn serologic test for syphilis can be performed for distinguishing.
2. **Long bone diaphysis tuberculosis.** This disease is rare, mostly occurring in children below 10 years old, more common in femur, tibia, radioulna, humeral shaft and fibular shaft, and often complicated by pulmonary tuberculosis or other bone tuberculosis. Imaging findings show circular or oval osteolytic destruction areas in the affected bone, most of which are single. Hyperostosis and osteosclerosis are not obvious, and the sclerosis is milder than

that of chronic osteomyelitis. Slight lamellar periosteal proliferation, which is smooth and regular, with swollen surrounding soft tissues, can be noted in peripheral area.

3. **Ewing sarcoma.** It is a malignant primary myelosarcoma originated from bone marrow of diaphysis and metaphysis. Patients are usually accompanied by localized pain, low fever, weight loss, and other symptoms. The disease is more common in children and young people, among which male outnumbers female. It can occur in almost any bone, most common in long bone diaphysis and metaphysis, and mainly manifested as osteolytic destruction, with cribriform or lace-like defects on surrounding bone cortex. If the patient has no history of acute suppurative osteomyelitis, it can be differentiated from chronic suppurative osteomyelitis. Whole-body bone scanning can detect multiple focuses and CT can indicate metastasis focus. Periosteal proliferation shows onion-peel pattern. It is slender with low density, easy to be ruptured, thus forming a Codman triangle. No sequestrum is formed in the destruction area; Codman triangle can also occur in osteomyelitis. Even so, osteomyelitis is characterized in that its periosteal reaction is more obvious and diaphysis tends to be thickened and deformed, with smooth and sclerotic margins partially in communication with cortex. By contrast, malignant bone tumors are the opposite.
4. **Osteosarcoma.** It is a malignant osteogenic tumor that occurs in children and young people, more common in male. It frequently occurs in metaphysis of long bones, in particular knee joint adnexa. The tumor grows very fast, making knee joints and other large joints painful. It is characterized in that a hard mass with tenderness will be formed 1–3 months later, on which the surface skin shows phlebectasia. Extensive proliferation and sclerosis and periosteal proliferation can occur in osseous lesions caused by osteogenic osteosarcoma, and osteolytic destruction area can be formed in the hyperostosis and osteosclerosis zone of mixed osteosarcoma, which is not easy to be distinguished from chronic suppurative osteomyelitis. Bone destruction area shows moth-eaten pattern, with indistinct margins. The periosteal reaction, which is most prominent on periosteum, can be divided into lamellar, Codman triangle, and sunburst. These periosteal reactions can produce abundant irregular tumor bones. Periosteal reaction caused by chronic osteomyelitis is mild. In the late stage, the bone destruction area shows clear boundary, wherein sclerosis margin can be seen, bone cortex is remarkably thickened, periosteum is intact and smooth, the new bone mineral density is high and bone trabeculae are increased and concentrated. The bone trabeculae mentioned here refer to those that are normally differentiated, different from the poorly differentiated and structure-less tumor bones.

Status Quo and Progress of Research

1. MRI has a higher sensitivity to chronic suppurative osteomyelitis than bone imaging. When using MRI and combined bone imaging to monitor chronic traumatic osteomyelitis patients, researchers found, after comparison, that the sensitivity of MRI and combined bone imaging are, respectively, 100% and 77%, demonstrating that MRI boasts a higher sensitivity to chronic suppurative osteomyelitis than combined bone imaging. The diagnostic specificity of MRI to chronic osteomyelitis is only 60%, and that of leukocyte imaging and PET are, respectively, 77% and 91% [30, 34]. Radionuclide: Research conducted by Harmer et al. [38] indicates that the sensitivity of ^{99m}Tc-MDP bone imaging can reach 90%, with a specificity of only 27%. ^{67}Ga can also be applied concurrently. In case of normal findings of ^{67}Ga bone imaging, chronic osteomyelitis can be excluded. In addition, several combined methods have also achieved desirable sensitivity and specificity.
2. With double-exponential model multi-*b*-value DWI, IVIM imaging can evaluate the water molecule diffusion and microvascular perfusion of the lesion, providing a new method for the diagnosis and differential diagnosis of inflammatory bone lesions. Indirectly evaluating the morphology of microcirculation with IVIM may provide a non-invasive tool for monitoring the growth and degeneration of tissue microvessels. Besides, when using traditional diffusion technologies, the impact by perfusion on signal direction may affect the quantification of diffusion anisotropy in tissues.
3. Among all the above imaging methods, PET/CT has the highest accuracy in the diagnosis of chronic osteomyelitis [39]. After internal fixation, metal artifacts may result in poor display of lesion on CT and MRI. By contrast, PET/CT can effectively avoid the influence of metal. Research [34] shows that the sensitivity and specificity of PET/CT to bone infection after internal fixation are, respectively, 85.7% and 100%, with positive/negative predictive values of 100% and 75%, respectively. This demonstrates that PET/CT is a promising method for suspected infection regarding implants.

4.3.3 Chronic Abscess of Bone

Overview

Chronic abscess of bone is a special type of chronic osteomyelitis. It was first described by British scholar Brodie in 1832 as a rare subacute or chronic localized intraosseous purulent inflammation with mild toxicity, thus also known as Brodie abscess. The disease has a slow onset and can be caused by local trauma or systemic blood dissemination.

Due to the weak virulence of the pathogen, when the body immunity is strong, the focus of suppurative osteomyelitis will be long confined to a small area, thus resulting in the chronic abscess of bone. Moreover, the disease may recur as the patient's body immunity decreases [40]. It may also occur when antibiotics are used in the early stage of osteomyelitis, but the infection has only been limited without further progress, rather than been completely controlled. The disease has a long course and lacks specific clinical symptoms [41], thus is difficult to be distinguished from other bone diseases. It is featured with paroxysmal, short pain, accompanied by local tenderness and swelling and pain of adjacent joints. It can be relieved through antibiotics, but is difficult to be cured and tend to recur. It occurs frequently in children and teenagers, among which male outnumbers female. Predilection sites include spongy bone and metaphysis of limb long tubular bone, wherein metaphysis of tibia, femur, and humerus are the most common site. According to clinical recommendations, treatment is mainly based on surgery, supplemented by antibiotics, thus completely removing bone abscess focuses and sclerosis walls, to achieve optimal curative effect. [42]

Pathophysiology

Brodie abscess is generally caused by hypotoxic pyogenic bacteria entering and staying in bone via blood circulation, thus forming infection focuses, most of which are localized in spongy bone of long tubular bone and involve metaphysis.

The most common pathogens are Staphylococcus aureus and Streptococcus [43]. The low virulence of pathogens and the strong immunity of the patient prevent the focus from spreading, thus becoming localized; In addition, if antibiotics used during acute infection prevent the lesion from spreading to the subperiosteum or diaphysis marrow cavity, but fail to completely control the disease, bone destruction and bone abscess will be localized in the lesion area. The purulent exudate filling the destruction area of the lesion in the early stage is gradually replaced by granulation tissue. And then the fibrous capsule wall is formed due to the collagenization around granulation tissue, in which fibrous tissue gradually appears. The fibrous tissue may be replaced by osseous tissue and healed, and the lesion is surrounded by hyperplastic and sclerotic bone substance.

The pathological features include osteocyte necrosis, bone trabecula defect, inflammatory cell infiltration, multinucleated cell reaction, fibrous and purulent exudate, and hyperplasia of granulation tissue. Inflammatory exudates and hyperplastic granulation tissues fill the abscess, in which piecemeal sequestrum may be found. Long irritated by inflammation, surrounding normal bone substances appear reactive hyperostosis and osteosclerosis, as well as periosteal reaction.

Imaging Findings

1. **X-ray.** Generally, the focus is small, with a diameter of 1–3 cm, and it was common in single-cystic lesions and occasionally multiple lesions were seen. The focus is mostly located in the localized area of osteolytic bone destruction, which is at or slightly off the center of long tubular bone spongy bone area. The focus is circular, oval, or lobulated with low density, showing low-density shadows on X-ray. In the early stage of the lesion, the margin of the destruction area is often indistinct, surrounded by no obvious osteosclerosis. As the lesion progresses, a clear and smooth sclerosis margin gradually forms on the edge. Reactive osteosclerosis may be formed in the surrounding area and gradually disappears from the normal bone substances. Periosteal reaction and sequestrum occur rarely. Fine granular sequestrum can be seen occasionally in the low-density bone destruction area. In case of periosteal reaction in the metaphysis margin and diaphysis cortex, periosteal proliferation can be observed. The proximal soft tissues are basically normal or slightly swollen (Fig. 4.26). The lesion may involve growth plate. Bone abscesses are often beyond rather than confined to the epiphyseal plate [44, 45]. Large abscess may occasionally be found in the marrow cavity of long bone diaphysis. As the lesion relieves, the abscess will be absorbed by the granulation tissue, while the bone destruction area will be shrunk or even disappeared, which marks the disease is cured.
2. **CT.** It can better display the small destruction area and sequestrum therein and show more clearly the pathological condition of atypical cases or cases with extensive proliferation and sclerosis. Therefore, CT is superior to

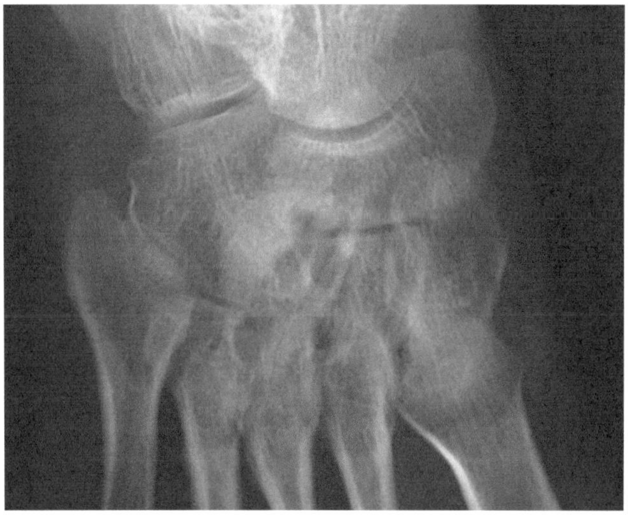

Fig. 4.26 Abscess in tarsus of right foot. Right foot PA X-ray plain film indicates that cystic bone destruction area can be seen in lateral wedge bone, with hyperostosis and osteosclerosis on margins

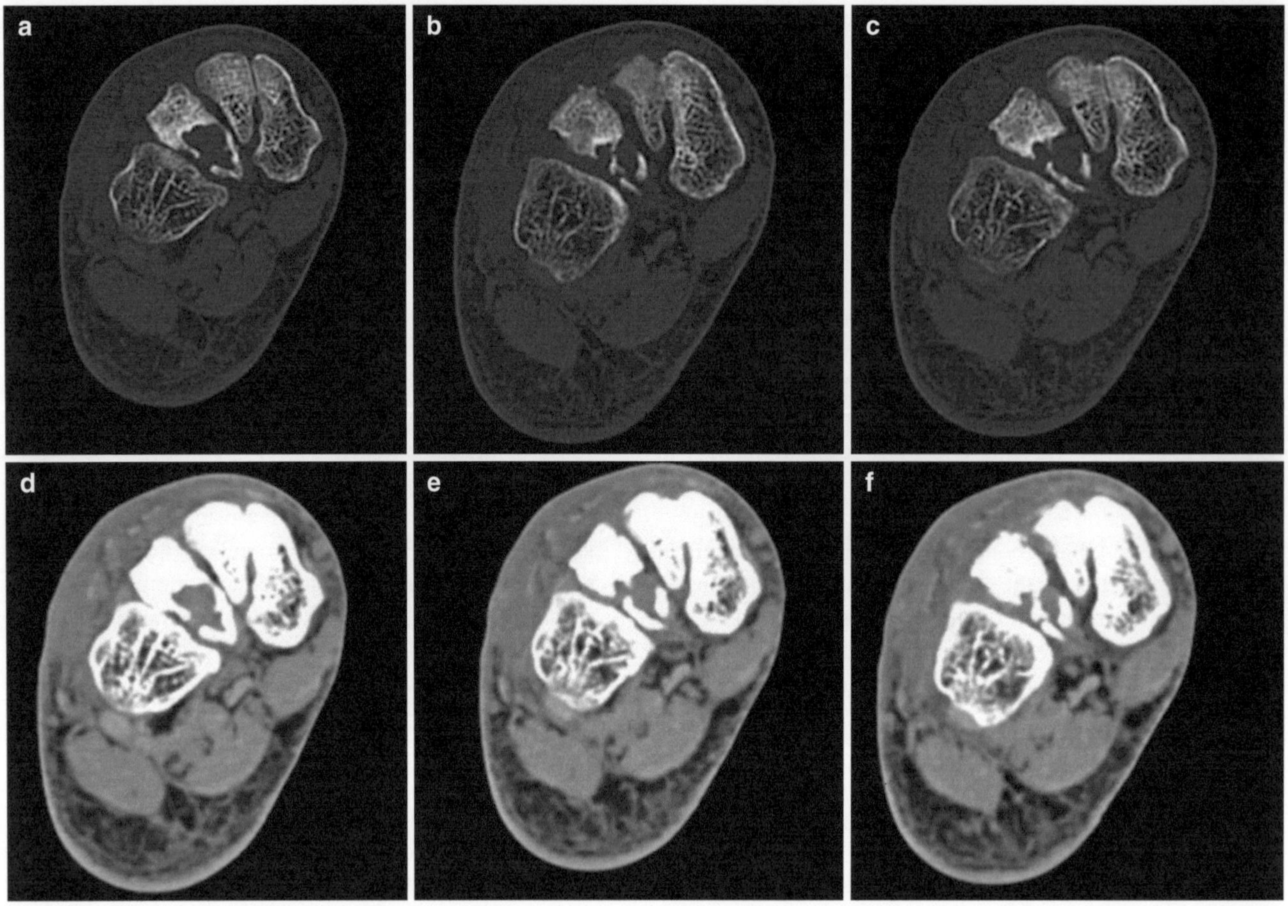

Fig. 4.27 Abscess in right foot lateral wedge bone. The same case as Fig. 4.26. (**a–c**) According to CT plain scan bone window, oval osteolytic destruction focus is found in spongy bone area of lateral wedge bone, with a slightly high density of abscess, surrounded by discontinuous osteosclerosis ring. No obvious periosteal reaction is observed; (**d–f**) CT plain scan soft tissue window indicates that surrounding soft tissues are slightly swollen

regular X-ray. CT feature is localized area of osteolytic bone destruction with clear boundary, manifested as circular, quasi-circular, dumbbell, lobulated or irregular-shaped low-density focus, surrounded by dense sclerosis strap. Part of the contents in destruction area are liquid density shadows with uniform density, and piecemeal sequestrum can also be observed therein (Fig. 4.27). Slight periosteal reaction, mostly ring-shaped, can be noted; Soft tissue around the focus has no obvious or slight swelling.

3. **MRI.** Center focus shows hypointense on T_1WI and hyperintense on fat-suppressed sequence and T_2WI. Surrounding osteosclerosis ring shows hypointense on T_1WI and T_2WI (Fig. 4.28). A ring-shaped granulation tissue wall can be noted around vomica of the active focus. At this time, the characteristic manifestation is the "target sign" or "halo sign" in bone marrow cavity of the metaphysis: (from the inside out) the vomica shows hypointense on T_1WI, and hyperintense on fat-suppressed sequence and T_2WI; Surrounding is a ring-shaped abscess cyst wall, which shows slight hyperintense on T_1WI and hyperintense on T_2WI; Peripheral region is surrounded by a thin layer of sclerosis strap, which shows hypointense on T_1WI and T_2WI; Due to bone marrow edema, adjacent bone substance may show diffuse hypointense on T_1WI and hyperintense on T_2WI [46] (Fig. 4.29).

Periosteal reaction is manifested as strip-shaped isointense shadows around cortex. Soft tissues around the focus may have varying degrees of inflammatory edema, which shows slightly hypointense on T_1WI and hyperintense on T_2WI [47].

4. **SPECT/CT.** It is highly sensitive to inflammatory bone lesions. The imaging is based on blood supply and active degree of bone metabolism around the lesion area, because increased blood flow and extremely active bone metabolism can lead to the concentration of developer. According to fusion imaging, the bone destruction area shows an obvious "halo-like" and extremely high concen-

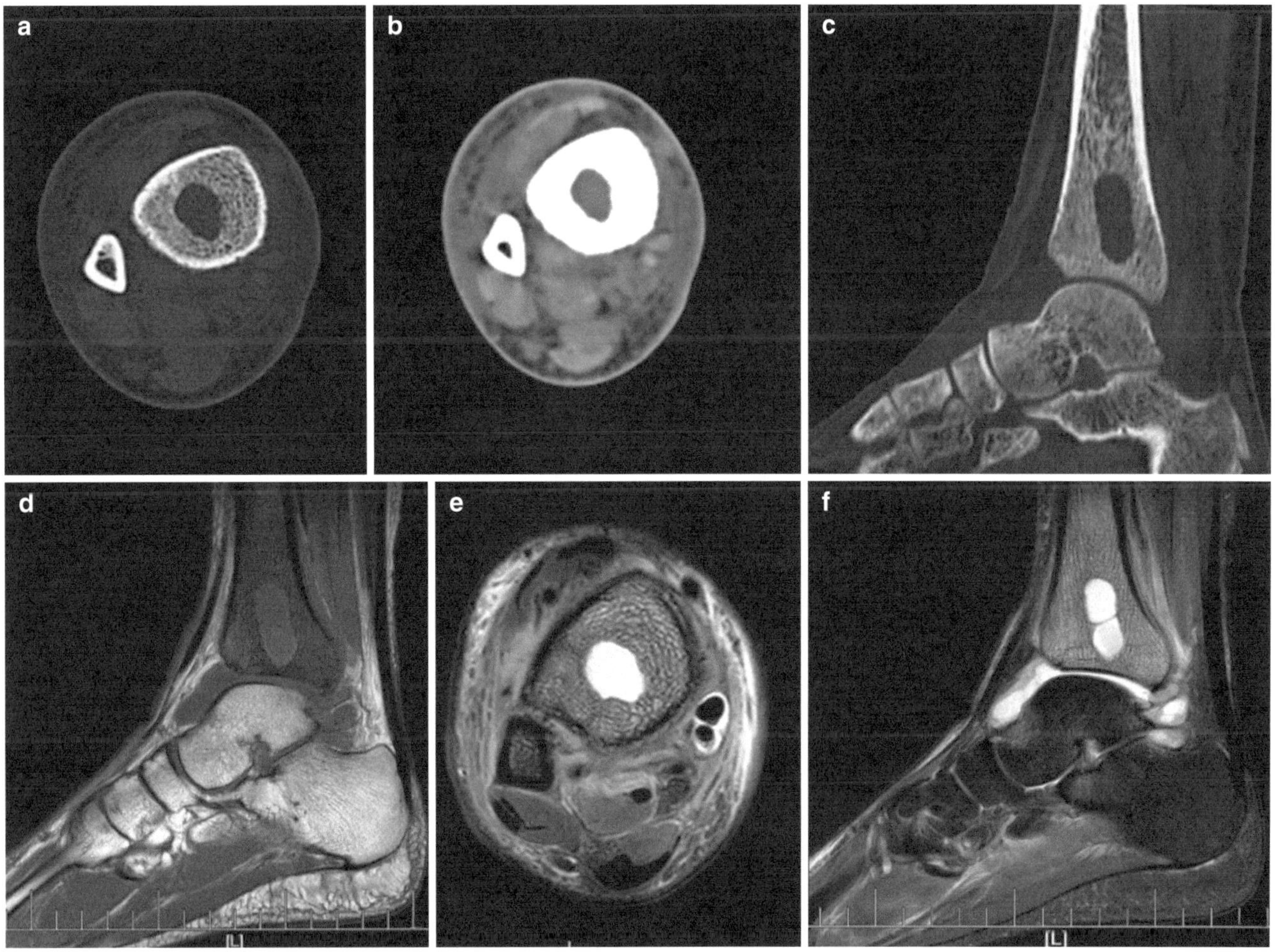

Fig. 4.28 Bone abscess in distal right tibia. Male, 23-year-old, suffering from fever, pain, and subsequent swelling in distal right leg since 90 days ago, without obvious predisposing cause. (**a**, **b**) CT shows that in the distal right tibia spongy bone there is an oval, low-density bone destruction area, wherein bone trabecula and sequestrum are not seen, the boundary is clear, surrounding soft tissues are slightly swollen, subcutaneous fat space is blurred and grid-shaped with an increased density, and no periosteal reaction occurs. (**c**) CT MPR shows that the bone destruction area reaches below the bone end articular surface, the density of abscess is uniform, and no sequestrum is formed. (**d**) The abscess shows hypointense on MRI T_1WI; (**e**, **f**) The abscess shows hyperintense on T_2WI fat-suppressed sequence. Most of surrounding soft tissues show hyperintense

tration of radionuclides. These radionuclides are most concentrated in the osteosclerosis area around focus, where the blood supply is rich and bone metabolism is vigorous; and less concentrated in central destruction area, since the focus is filled with inflammatory exudate, with a low active degree of bone metabolism [48, 49].

Key Points of Diagnosis

1. Characterized by insidious onset, slow progress, atypical symptoms, and mild pain.
2. Spongy bone area of long tubular bone metaphysis is a predilection site.
3. X-ray plain film indicates that the focus is quasi-circular and low-density, edged with sclerosis margin, and the boundary is clear.
4. X-ray indicates that vomica has a low density, abscess wall has an equal or slightly high density, and reactive proliferation and sclerosis can be seen on margins.
5. According to MRI plain film, pus shows hypointense on T_1WI and hyperintense on T_2WI, and abscess wall shows isointense or slightly hypointense on T_2WI.

Differential Diagnosis

1. **Bone tuberculosis.** It occurs frequently in epiphysis or metaphysis, manifested as localized osteoporosis in the early stage, and then scattered bone absorption destruction spots. These spots are gradually enlarged and merge together, forming a circular, oval, or irregular-shaped destruction area. The boundaries of tuberculosis focus are often clear, surrounded by no obvious sclerosis margins,

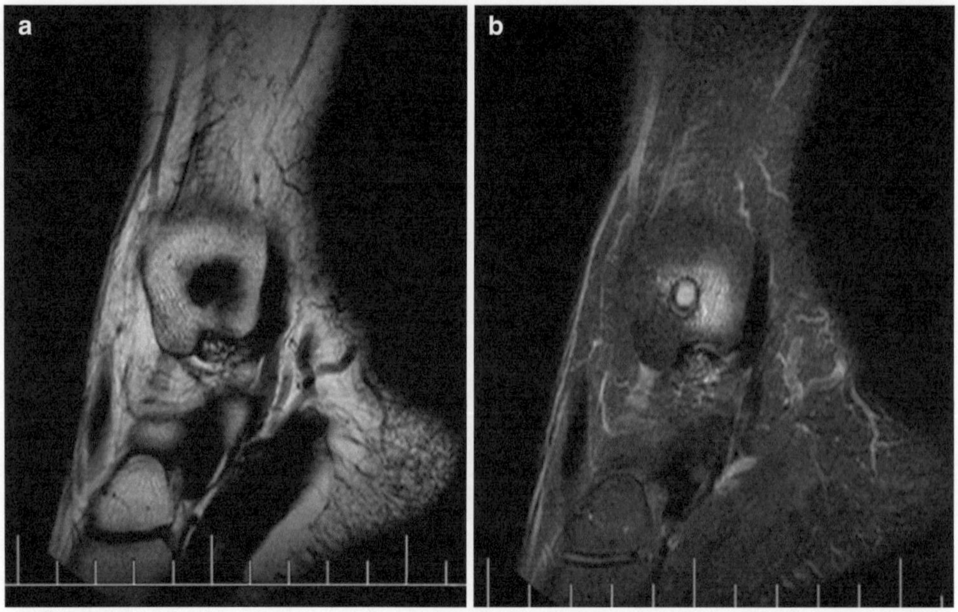

Fig. 4.29 Bone abscess in inferior right tibia. Male, 36 years old, suffering from pain caused by left ankle injured half year ago. (**a**, **b**) On the inferior margin of left tibia, there forms a quasi-circular bone destruction area, which reaches below the bone end articular surface and is surrounded by visible sclerosis ring. No obvious swelling is noted in surrounding soft tissues (**a** T_1WI; **b** T_2WI fat-suppressed sequence)

with mild periosteal reaction. Unlike Brodie abscess, sand-like sequestrum can be seen in the focus, and the lesion often extends beyond the epiphyseal line, which is the characteristic of epiphyseal and metaphyseal tuberculosis. The disease tends to involve epiphyseal plate and joints, showing "straddle" sign.

2. **Bone cyst.** It is also manifested as a bright area of metaphysis, most of which are irregular cyst-like quasi-circular. Inside the bright area, there may be a few slender strip intervals. The local cortices are thinned, and the surrounding sclerosis margins are thin. There is no periosteal proliferation or soft tissue swelling, and pathologic fracture is prone to occur. By contrast, Brodie abscess shows obvious hyperostosis, with increasingly intensified sclerosis as history prolongs.
3. **Eosinophilic granuloma of bone.** It is more common in children below 10 years old and may occur singly or collectively. Single eosinophilic granuloma occurs frequently in skull and femur, while multiple eosinophilic granulomas occur frequently in vertebral body, with pathological features of granuloma formed by reticular cell proliferation and eosinophilic granulocyte infiltration. Long bone lesions mostly involve metaphysis and diaphysis, manifested as a single irregular bone destruction area, which is usually located in the marrow cavity, growing in an expansive way with clear margins. Small, patchy dense osteosclerosis may be observed in the destruction area, accompanied by lamellar periosteal reaction and hyperostosis and osteosclerosis, and surrounded by soft tissue masses. The eosinophilic granuloma is similar to Brodie abscess, except that the periosteal proliferation is less common. Diagnosis can be based on the lesion site in conjunction with increased eosinophilic granulocytes from laboratory test.
4. **Osteoid osteoma.** It is common in teenagers with slow onset, manifested as pain at the site, which can be aggravated at night and relieved after taking salicylic acids and the like. It is a benign osteogenic tumor, composed of new osteoid tissues and arranged in a radial, reticular manner. The tumor is surrounded by dense reactive hyperplastic bone. Imaging findings include small (typically less than 1.5 cm), circular or oval bright area in the focus, and irregular calcification or ossification shadows observed in tumor nidus, surrounded by obvious proliferation and sclerosis rings, thickened bone cortex and periosteal reaction. According to MRI, the non-calcified part of the tumor shows hypointense or isointense on T_1WI and hyperintense on T_2WI, whereas the calcified part always shows hypointense. With the scan enhancement, the tumor shows marked enhancement. Osteosclerosis surrounding the tumor nidus shows hypointense. Hyperemia is prone to occur in bone marrow and soft tissue surrounding the tumor, showing hypointense on T_1WI and hyperintense on T_2WI.
5. **Non-ossifying fibroma.** It is common in teenagers at the age of 8–20 years, typically located in the metaphysis of the limb long bone 3–4 cm away from the epiphyseal plate, especially the tibia, femur, and fibula. It is a benign tumor derived from bone connective tissues. If the focus is located in metaphysis or epiphysis of long bone, the single or multiple cystic radiolucent areas, which grow in a central, expansive manner in bones, can encroach on the bone along the most or entire transverse diameter, with homogeneous density and sclerosis margins, edged with

thin shell of sclerotic osseous tissue that tends to grow outwardly. Proliferation and sclerosis are not as significant as Brodie abscess.

Status Quo and Progress of Research

1. X-ray plain film remains the preferred method for examination of bone and joint diseases. It is good in identifying the location of the lesion, observing its shape, and displaying the bone destruction area and surrounding hyperostosis and osteosclerosis. X-ray can be used in follow-up observation of the disease.
2. CT boasts high resolution for soft tissue, without image overlap. Compared with plain X-ray plain film, it can better observe the lesions located at the site with complex structures. In particular, the thin-slice 3D CT, which can clearly show the relationship between the bone abscess focus and the peripheral tissues, is the most sensitive way to display sequestrum in vomica.
3. Compared with X-ray plain film and CT, MRI is more sensitive to early bone destruction, capable of detecting periosteal reactions and soft tissue swelling more timely. Since the incidence of Brodie abscess is low, various latest MRI scanning methods have not been used widely. What's more, there is a lack of relevant literature and reports.

4.3.4 Sclerosing Osteomyelitis

Overview

Chronic sclerosing osteomyelitis is a type of chronic osteomyelitis also called periostitis ossificans and Garré's sclerosing osteomyelitis. It was first reported by Garré in 1891. It is generally believed that such a rare disease is a chronic bone inflammatory change of periosteum osteogenetic reaction caused by infection of hypotoxic pathogen, and it is difficult to cultivate pathogens in the focus [50]. The disease has a slowly progressive course with unknown etiology, which is typically related to trauma, in particular subperiosteal hemorrhage after trauma. Main manifestations include hyperostosis and osteosclerosis that are obviously diffuse, usually accompanied by bone destruction. The disease does not cause hypotoxic infectious osteomyelitis of osseous tissue mainly manifested as abscess and sinus.

It is common in young people with strong immunity and occurs frequently in long bone diaphysis, such as tibia, fibula, ulna, and metatarsus. According to recent literature and reports, it is not uncommon that the disease occurs in irregular bones (such as jaw and tarsus). Compared with maxilla, mandible is more susceptible to the disease, which frequently occurs on the inferior margin of the mandible in the first molar region and is mostly caused by odontogenic infection [51]. The patient tends to have mild systemic symptoms, usually characterized by swelling of local soft tissues, pain, and recurrent episodes. Secondary lesions can reoccur in other parts many years later since the initial onset. Joints are generally not involved. Laboratory tests are basically normal, except that C-reactive protein is slightly increased and erythrocyte sedimentation rate is mildly accelerated, making the disease easy to be confused with limb symptoms caused by muscle strain, lumbar intervertebral disc herniation, and other similar diseases [52]. The widely used antibiotics inhibit the pathogenicity of bacteria to a certain extent, slowing down the progress of the lesion. Having said that, the recurrent lesion involves diaphysis, resulting in poor blood supply. Besides, since bone marrow cavity is narrow and occlusive, antibiotics are difficult to reach the affected site, thus delivering a poor therapeutic efficacy for such a refractory, persistent disease. Usually, surgery is needed to completely and thoroughly remove the focus and necrotic, swollen granulation tissues, while reopen the narrow, occlusive marrow cavity, reducing the pressure in the marrow cavity based on sufficient drainage, with a view to improving bone blood supply and oxygen metabolism of osseous tissue. In this way, recurrence of the disease can be effectively avoided, with desirable prognosis [53]. However, to avoid potential risk of recurrence and multifocus, it is recommended to remove bones with no important functions, such as ribs, through surgery [54].

Pathophysiology

Sclerosing osteomyelitis is a progressive, extensive, and sclerosing inflammation of the bone, with pathogenesis similar to that of acute and chronic suppurative osteomyelitis. Through the bloodstream, pathogens stagnate in the lesion area, and the infection focus is localized due to low virulence pathogen and strong immunity of body. Diaphysis, a compact bone substance, has a relatively poor blood supply, with restricted bacterial growth and reproduction. Bone changes are mainly manifested as periosteal reactive hyperplasia, causing sclerosing osteomyelitis of diaphysis.

Persistent irritation by inflammation can result in a series of pathological changes, including extensive and irregular thickening of bone trabecula, replacement of bone marrow with fibrous tissue, narrowed or even occluded marrow cavity, reactive thickening of the endosteum, active osteoblast, formation of new bone, and bone cortex thickened in a fusiform shape [55]. Unlike general purulent inflammation, chronic sclerosing osteomyelitis typically causes no visible purulent focus. In addition, the disease may occasionally form fistula on skin and does not result in abscess, sinus, or sequestrum. A small amount of inflammatory cell infiltrations and capillaries can be detected in bone through pathological examination. In the early stage of osteomyelitis, a thin shell-like raised layer appears on the cortex. As the disease progresses, constantly deposited new bone makes the cortex thickened, forming mixed structures, including sclerosis area, normal area, and osteolytic destruction area in sclerosis area, on adjacent spongy bone [56]. The disease shows chronic non-specific osteomyelitis according to histological examination, with negative blood and tissue culture, wherein a little pus and granulation tissue may appear on a small number of wounds, with Staphylococcus aureus growing in the culture vessel [57]. Unfortunately, there is still a lack of bacterial culture result to prove that whether sclerosing osteomyelitis of jaw is caused more by odontogenic infections or by hematogenous infections.

Imaging Findings

1. **X-ray.** Chronic sclerosing osteomyelitis occurs preferably in diaphysis of long tubular bone, typically characterized by localized lesion and slow progress, without abnormal X-ray findings within 1 month since the initial onset. As the disease progresses, it manifested as localized or extensive thickening and sclerosis of the bone cortex in the lesion, dense bone substance, increased density of the spongy bone area, and long bone diaphysis thickened in a fusiform shape, with smooth, neat, and ivory-shaped outer margin. The focus is migratory, and there is no obvious boundary between the focus and normal bone substances. Periosteal proliferation is typically lamellar, fused with thickened bone cortex, without obvious boundary. No periosteum is lifted off, and marrow cavity is remarkably shrunk or even occluded. Soft tissues around the focus may have varying degrees of swelling or free from swelling. Generally, osteosclerosis area is free from or only has extremely slight irregular spot-like bone destruction area. In most cases, there is no sequestrum or sinus formed (Fig. 4.30a, b).
2. **CT.** The affected bone is obviously thickened, the bone cortex is extensively proliferated and sclerous, the density of bone trabecula is increased, and the marrow cavity is narrowed, or even occluded. Generally, no bone destruction, sequestrum, pus, sinus, or soft tissue mass is formed. Compared with X-ray plain film, CT can better display and more precisely locate the low-density osteolytic focus in sclerosis area. It is the preferred method for examination of irregular bone sclerosing osteomyelitis. Taking mandible as an example, a low-density channel in connection with the focus in bone can be seen on the inferior margin of affected root apex of tooth, manifested as irregular-shaped focus. Osteolytic destruction area with indistinct edges can be noted in osteosclerosis area, accompanied by periosteal reaction or absorption of outer bone plate (Figs. 4.30c–e and 4.31a–d).
3. **MRI.** The boundary of the lesion is not clear enough, bone cortex and diaphysis are thickened. Heterogeneous hypointense is shown on T_1WI and T_2WI. Marrow cavity becomes smaller or disappeared, and it is ideal to show the coronal plane or sagittal plane. In case of any existing destruction area, hypointense and hyperintense are, respectively, shown on T_1W and T_2WI, which can be used to judge the whether the focus is active. MRI can clearly display the range of soft tissue involved (Fig. 4.31e–g).

Key Points of Diagnosis

1. The patient typically has no history of acute suppurative osteomyelitis. The symptom is atypical, the affected area is swollen and painful, and the local skin is free from redness and swelling.
2. Diaphysis of long tubular bone is a predilection site.
3. X-ray plain film shows thickening of diaphysis and obvious hyperostosis and osteosclerosis of bone substance.
4. According to X-ray plain film, bone cortex is thickened, marrow cavity is narrowed and disappeared, and usually there is no bone destruction area.
5. MRI shows thickened bone cortex, hypointense on T_1WI and T_2WI, shrunk or even occluded marrow cavity, and non-swollen or slightly swollen surrounding soft tissue.

Differential Diagnosis

1. **Osteoid osteoma.** It is a benign osteogenic tumor, typically occurring in bone cortex of long tubular bone. The tumor nidus is composed of new osseous tissues, accompanied by irregular calcification and ossification shadows. Sclerosis rings, thickened cortex, and periosteal reaction can be noted around the focus. According to MRI, the non-calcified part of the tumor shows hypointense or isointense on T_1WI and hyperintense on T_2WI, while calcified and ossified parts show hypointense on both T_1WI and T_2WI. Edema may appear in the bone marrow and soft tissues around the focus, which will be marked enhanced after imaging enhancement. New osseous tissues will not turn into mature lamellar bones. Bone cortical hyperplasia forms at superior extremity of diaphysis, with a small, nest-like bright area in the middle, which is manifested as a sclerosis ring with thinned bone cortex, and rarely forms periosteum new bones. Osteosclerosis on diaphysis caused by chronic sclerosing osteomyelitis is manifested as thickened endosteum and periosteum, accompanied by thickened diaphysis and narrowed marrow cavity.
2. **Osteosarcoma.** It is a primary bone-derived malignant tumor, common in teenagers. Early atypical sclerosing osteosarcoma is not easy to be distinguished from sclerosing osteomyelitis. Both are similar in patient group,

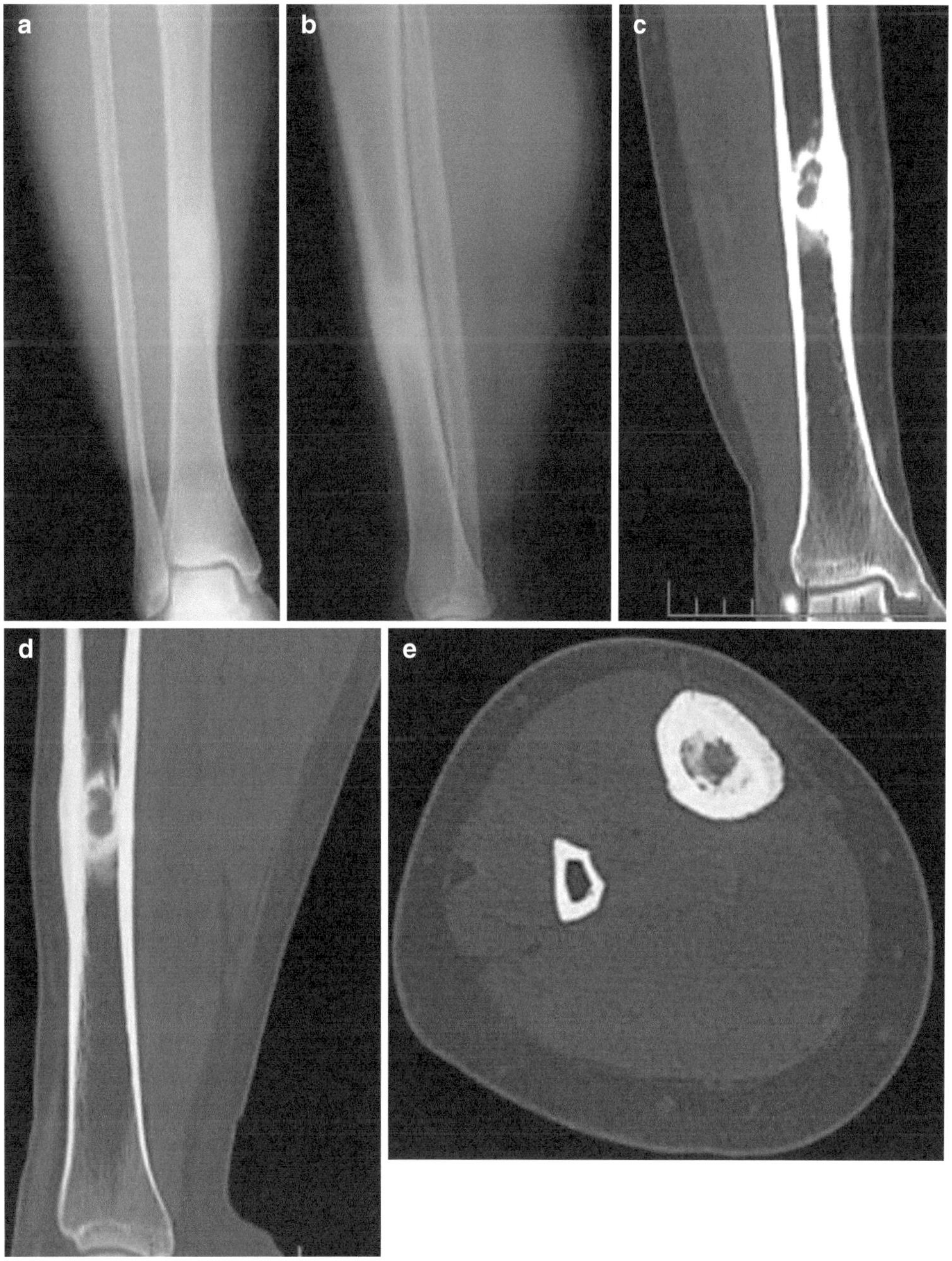

Fig. 4.30 Sclerosing osteomyelitis in the middle segment of right tibia. (**a**, **b**) X-ray plain film shows that diaphysis at the middle segment of right tibia is thickened in a fusiform shape, bone cortex is thickened, marrow cavity is narrowed, density is increased, with visible low-density focus in sclerosis area; (**c**–**e**) Boundary between the thickened bone cortex and surrounding normal bone substance is not clear, and low-density bone destruction area can be seen in the sclerotic marrow cavity, without obvious swelling of the surrounding soft tissue

clinical symptoms and imaging manifestations. The tumor cells are well differentiated, with high degree of ossification. The lesion is manifested as patchy ossification in the early stage and gradually expands as disease progresses, encroaching on the entire metaphysis, dense as dentin. In the advanced stage, the tumor destroys cortex and forms extra-cortical radial tumor bone, accompanied by radial hyperplasia and Codman triangle, while forms a mass by encroaching soft tissues. Metastasis may occur in the advanced stage, whereas chronic sclerosing osteomyelitis preferably occurs in diaphysis.

3. **Fatigue fracture**. It is also known as stress fracture, preferably occurring in tibia, fibula, and metatarsus and common in athletes and long-range walkers. The disease is caused by repeated, relatively mild sudden force acting on fracture site, thus constantly breaking bone trabecula, and eventually leading to fracture due to the slow local repair. X-ray films typically show indistinct fracture lines 2 weeks later, and then the formation of periosteum new bone and the growth of callus.
4. **Osteitis deformans** (Paget disease). It is common in senior patients, with extensive and multiple lesions frequently occurring in long tubular bone and skull. The disease is chronically progressive, and the cause is still unclear. Imaging findings show thickened and layered bone cortex, with a density lower than that of bone

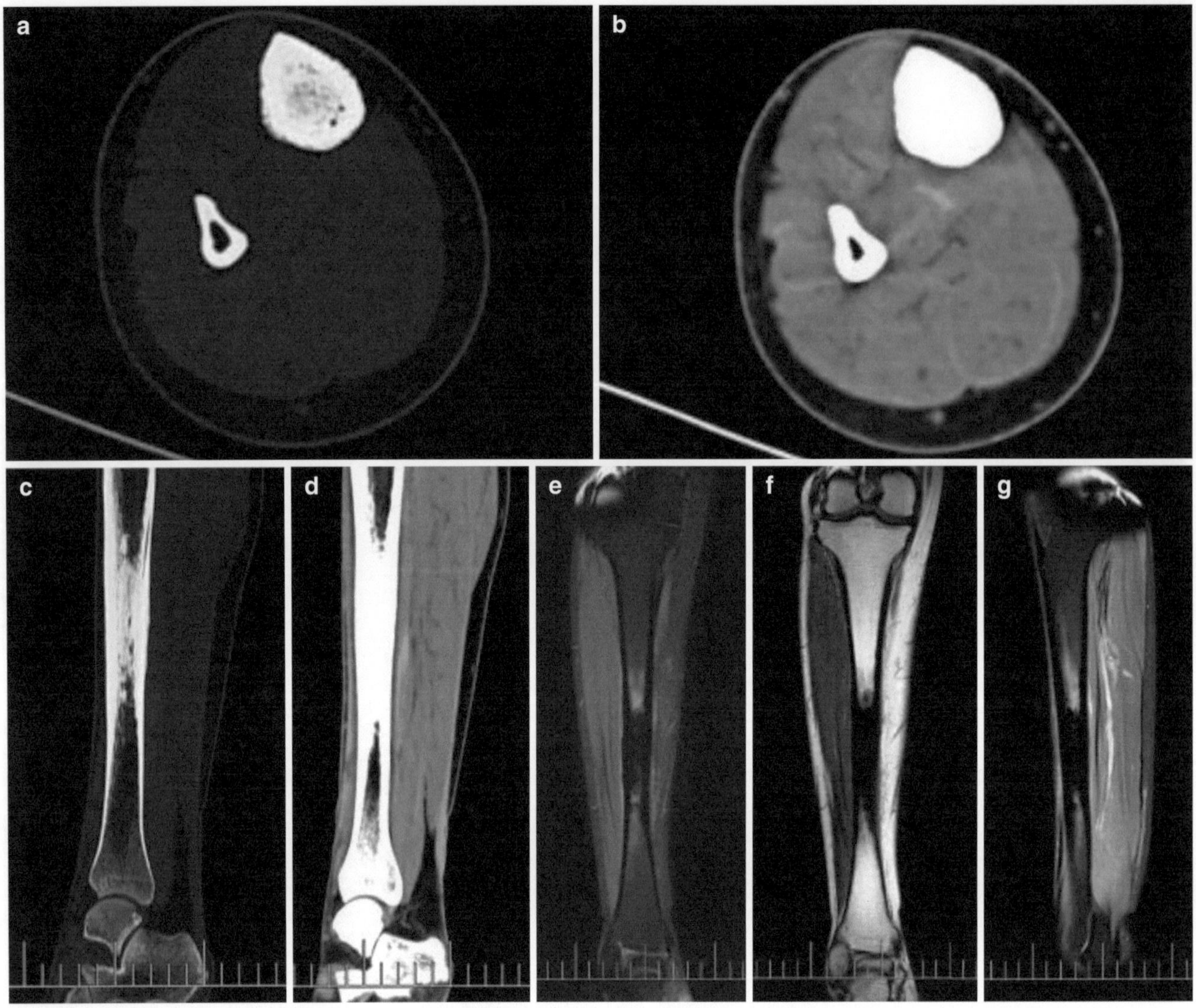

Fig. 4.31 Sclerosing osteomyelitis in right tibia. (**a**, **b**) CT transverse plane indicates that bone cortex of tibia is thickened, density of spongy bone is increased, marrow cavity is occluded, and the surrounding soft tissue is not swollen; (**c**, **d**) Coronal plane 3D reconstruction indicates that bone cortex in middle segment of right tibia is significantly thickened, diaphysis is slightly thickened, bone trabecula is thickened, marrow cavity is narrowed and occluded, adjacent marrow cavity shows hyperintense, and soft tissue around the focus is not swollen; (**e–g**) MRI shows that bone cortex in the middle segment of tibia is thickened, hypointense is shown on T_1WI and T_2WI fat-suppressed sequence, marrow cavity is disappeared, and no abnormal signal shadow is noted in the surrounding soft tissue

substance in sclerosing osteomyelitis. In osteitis deformans, bone cortex is proliferated and sclerosed based on osteoporosis, wherein the cystic low-density focus, thickened, curved, deformed, and even fractured diaphysis, and narrowed marrow cavity can be seen.

Status Quo and Progress of Research

1. Focus of sclerosing osteomyelitis is mostly located in the diaphysis, with thickened bone cortex and occluded marrow cavity, making it difficult for drugs to enter the focus via blood circulation or infiltration, thus resulting in poor efficacy of drugs. For these reasons, the disease requires surgery. Surgery mainly aims to remove focuses and reopen marrow cavity, typically including clearance of abscess and focus, fenestration and decompression, beans relief, and the like. Generally, the curative effect is desirable and symptoms can be obviously alleviated, with low recurrence rate [58, 59].
2. X-ray plain film can provide high spatial resolution, displaying the subtle bone structure of bones and joints. As a basic inspection method, it adopts simple, low-cost, and low radiation way to find lesions and identify the scope and extent of the lesions, thus making qualitative diagnosis. CT provides performance similar to that of X-ray, and it has significant advantages in identifying the narrowing

and blockage of marrow cavity, periosteal reaction, and formation of sequestrum. CT is typically used for irregular bone, among which the thin-slice 3D CT can display the relationship between focus and peripheral tissues & structures in a clear and three-dimensional manner through multi-aspect reconstruction.

3. MRI has a limited effect. Since the hyperostosis and osteosclerosis are obvious, and the lesion shows hypointense on both T_1WI and T_2WI, MRI is mainly used for identifying active focus and involved marrow cavity and defining the range of soft tissue swelling.

4.4 Fungal Infection

Overview

Fungal infections of the bones and joints are a rare complication of systemic invasive fungal infection with insidious clinical manifestations. It is easy to cause misdiagnosis and delayed diagnosis, thus resulting in grave consequences. It is mostly caused by primary infection focus (especially focus in lung) spreading to bones and joints via hematogenous dissemination. It occurs frequently in patients under immunosuppression (malignant tumor and drug therapy). In addition, overuse or misuse of antibiotics, abuse of diabetes drugs, anti-tuberculosis drugs and intravenous drugs, trauma, artificial joint replacement, and arthrocentesis also raise the risk of fungal infections of the bones and joints [60].

There are a wide variety of fungus species, and about 100,000 species have been found so far, among which more than 270 known species are pathogenic fungi that can cause bone and joint infections of human (based on WHO statistics). The fungal infection is usually disseminated via spore inhalation, direct colonization of wound or double infection after application of antibiotics. It does not spread between human and human, or between human and animal. The main pathogens of fungal infections of the bones and joints include Coccidioides, Blastomycetes dermatitidis, Candida, Aspergillus, Cryptococcus neoformans, Sporotrichum schenckii, Blastomyces brasiliensis, Histoplasmosis capsulati and other rare fungi, such as Pseudallescheria boydii, Curvuloria lunata, Fusarium, Exophiala jeanselmei, and Talaromyces marneffei [61]. Invasive fungus can be divided into infectious pathogen and opportunistic pathogen. Coccidiodes and blastomycete are infectious pathogens, most of which exist in nature and can cause exogenous infections. Fungal arthritis or osteomyelitis caused by infectious pathogens often occurs in patients without obvious immunodeficiency and occasionally occurs in those with immunodeficiency. Opportunistic pathogens, such as candida and cryptococcus, are mostly non-pathogenic, resulting in endogenous infection in case of lowered body immunity. For this reason, patients with hematological malignancies, organ transplant recipients who receive immunosuppression therapy, and patients long receiving corticosteroid therapy are particularly susceptible to opportunistic pathogens. It has been reported that severe, acute disseminated fungal infection, whose pathogens include candida, aspergillus, and cryptococcus neoformans, can occur in patients receiving tumor necrosis factor-α inhibitors and receptor antagonist of human interleukin-1 [62]; AIDS patients are particularly prone to be infected by Cryptococcus neoformans and Histoplasmosis capsulati, and cryptococcosis is the second most common cause of fatal infection in AIDS patients [63]. Children and newborns suffering from chronic granulomatous diseases are most susceptible to candida and aspergillus infections, while the former rarely affects in bones and joints of adults. A small number of infected adults are individuals with obvious susceptible factors, such as patients long inserted with central venous catheter (usually related to long-term antibiotic therapy and parenteral nutrition), patients receiving hemodialysis and abusers of injecting drugs [19]. Fungous tenosynovitis may be caused by blood transmission or direct infection. It may result in infection of joint space and is related to juxta-articular osteomyelitis. Candida and non-candida yeasts, including Cryptococcus neoformans and Sporotrichum schenckii, are the most common pathogens of tenosynovitis.

Fungal osteomyelitis is typically caused by hematogenous dissemination. Bone lesion may exist individually or as a part of multisystem disease [64]. Most of fungal osteomyelitis and arthritis are insidious and chronic, without obvious clinical symptoms in early stage. Fungous arthritis usually occurs in a single joint, especially knee joint. It is often manifested as local pain and limitation of motion in the affected limb. Severe cases may suffer from erythema, joint swelling, joint effusion accompanied by a sense of fluctuation and obvious tenderness. Chronic infections, such as coccidioidomycosis or blastomycosis, can cause cold abscess of soft tissue and sinus, accompanied by systemic symptoms of varying degrees, including fever, fatigue, appetite decrease, and loss of weight.

The golden standard for diagnosing fungal infections of the bones and joints is to achieve tissue culture of pathogen. The diagnosis may require biopsy of synovial membrane. Compared with synovial fluid, synovial tissues culture can offer a higher positive rate but takes a longer time. It has been reported that the positive rate of synovial membrane cultivation in arthritis caused by Candida glabrata can reach 92%. However, this kind of bacterium cannot grow in vitro until 6 weeks later [18]. Improvement on biopsy techniques may contribute to diagnosis. Synovial membrane fluid, leukocyte count, and culture results vary in different fungal infections and individual cases, which may be misleading. In addition to synovial tissues culture, blood culture, bone marrow examination and culture, antibody tests (such as serum coccidioides antibody or histoplasmosis antibody), and inspection of fungal antigens in body fluids (such as serum cryptococcus antigen, urine tissue cytoplasmic antigen) can be used as auxiliary diagnosis methods. It has been proved that Galactomannan (GM) is a surrogate marker for invasive aspergillosis. Detection of GM by enzyme immunoassay (EIA) can serve as a diagnosis method specific to aspergillus infection. In addition, detection of 1,3-β-D-glucan (BG), which widely exists on fungal cell walls with high specificity, can also provide basis for the diagnosis of invasive fungal infections. However, this method can only indicate whether there is an invasive fungal infection, rather than identify species of fungus.

Pathophysiology

Pathological changes in fungal infection lack specificity. Pathogenic fungi do not produce any toxins and mainly cause allergy. Common pathological changes include mild non-specific inflammation, purulent inflammation, necrotizing inflammation, and granulomatous inflammation. Changes mentioned above may exist individually or collectively. Different pathogens and allergic reactions caused vary from each other. Even the same pathogen has different tissue responses in different phases. For example, necrotizing granulomas are often associated with histoplasmosis, while coccidioidomycosis can cause necrotizing and purulent granulomas. Pathogenesis of fungal osteomyelitis and arthritis is still unknown and it may be similar to that of bone infection caused by bacteria. Most of fungi have weak pathogenicity. As body immunity reduces, they invade tissues and multiply quickly to cause disease. Fungal pathogen can cause direct implant infections or enter the synovial membrane via blood circulation, thus forming granulomas (such as coccidioidomycosis) or microabscesses (such as candida, aspergillosis, and the like). After that, the fungal pathogens infect synovial membrane fluid and are phagocytized by phagocytes and lining cells of synovial membrane, in which the fungal pathogens are proliferated, thereby resulting in inflammatory reaction and exudative joint effusion. At the same time, collagenase and other proteolytic enzymes are released, damaging the surface of joints. In case of chronic granulomatous synovitis, such as coccidioidomycosis, synovial hyperplasia is vigorous. The joint swelling is mainly caused by thickening of synovial membrane, rather than joint effusion, wherein the vasculitis caused may erode articular cartilage and even the bones under the joints.

Imaging Findings

1. **X-ray and CT**
   (a) Imaging of fungal infections of the bones and joints, which can involve the whole skeleton, lacks specificity. Different pathogens can involve different body parts. Fungous arthritis typically attacks unilateral large joints, most common in knee joints, followed by elbow joints, ankle joints, and wrist joints. A small number of pathogens can cause multiple joints, including small joints of hands and feet. Fungal osteomyelitis occurs preferably in tubular epiphysis, especially some projecting parts, such as tubercle of tibia, ankle, acromion, and rib. (Fig. 4.32)
   (b) According to X-ray plain film, the lesion is manifested as limited osteolytic bone destruction or absorption with clear margins. No new bone is formed in the early stage, and regular-shaped sclerosis edges can be seen in the late stage occasionally. Periosteal reaction rarely occurs or does not occur, with no sequestrum formed. A saucer-shaped erosion of bone cortex can be seen in long bone [19]. Sometimes, if the pathogen is highly virulent with rapid destruction

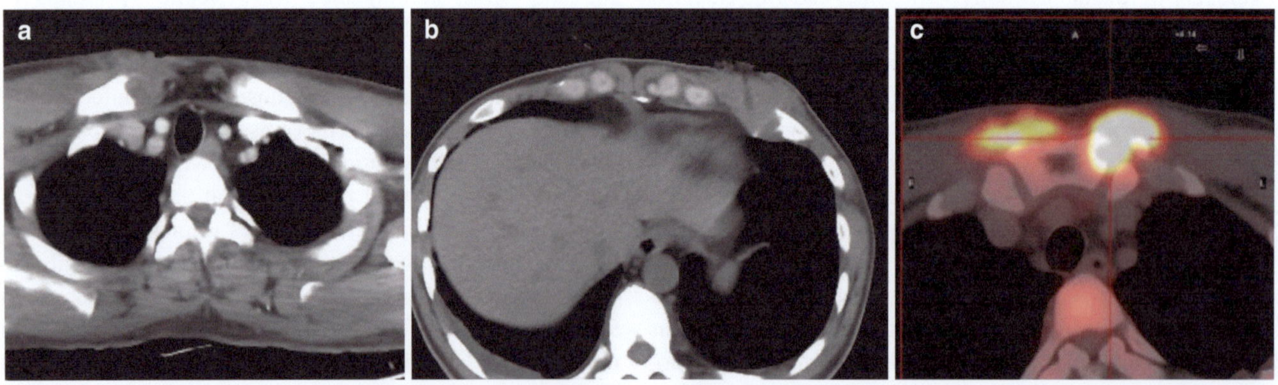

Fig. 4.32 Multiple fungal infections in rib and clavicle. Fungal infection involves multiple bones throughout the body. Coccidiodes is cultured through soft tissue needle biopsy. (**a**) CT shows a limited quasi-circular bone destruction area at right extremitas sternalis claviculae, with clear, sharp boundary, swollen surrounding soft tissues, and thickened adjacent skin; (**b**) A limited bone destruction area forms in left rib, surrounding soft tissues are swollen, the subcutaneous tissue is involved, and adjacent skin is thickened; (**c**) ^{18}F-FDG PET/CT indicates that bone destruction area at bilateral sternocostal joints and adjacent soft tissues have hypermetabolism

speed, the bone destruction can be moth-eaten, which is difficult to be distinguished from tuberculosis and bone malignant tumors only based on imaging findings.

(c) In the early stage, joint spaces may be normal. However, as the disease progresses, 1/3 of joint spaces can be narrowed, accompanied by swollen surrounding soft tissues, which is usually caused by joint effusion or thickening of synovial membrane. Baker cyst may appear if knee joint is involved.

(d) Lesion of vertebral body, similar to tuberculosis, progresses slowly and mostly destroys intervertebral disc and anterior vertebral body, wherein abscess inferior to ligament is formed [65] (Fig. 4.33). Generally, aspergillus osteomyelitis is caused by pulmonary lesion directly invading adjacent vertebral bodies, intervertebral discs, and adjacent ribs.

(e) Sporotrichosis often infects a single joint or multiple joints in equal proportions, and frequently involves knee joints, wrist joints, hands, elbow joints, and shoulder joints. The disease usually occurs in hands and wrist joints, which can be distinguished from other fungal bone infections [66].

(f) Sporotrichosis or blastomycosis can invade the soft tissues surrounding bones, thus forming soft tissue cold abscesses and subcutaneous sinus (Fig. 4.34).

(g) Actinomycosis of bone is usually secondary to infection of peripheral soft tissues. The disease often involves mandible, manifested as limited bone destruction on X-ray, and rarely forms new bone. When the actinomycotic infection of chest wall involves ribs, it is manifested as bone destruction and formation of periosteum new bones, with thickening of rib.

2. **MRI.** With a higher sensitivity and resolution than traditional radiography, MRI can provide more comprehensive and complete images of joints, thus identifying inflammatory changes, such as bone marrow edema, in the early stage. MRI can clearly display joint effusion and thickened synovial tissues, which show hypointense on T_1WI, hyperintense on T_2WI, middle intensity and hypointense on T_1WI and STIR, similar to muscle signal intensities [67].

Key Points of Diagnosis

1. Common in immunocompromised patients.
2. Fungal osteomyelitis frequently occurs in tubular epiphysis of limbs. Fungal osteomyelitis usually invades single, large joint, especially knee joint.
3. There are limited osteolytic bone destruction or absorption with clear margins. No new bone is formed in the early stage. Periosteal reaction rarely occurs or does not occur. Generally there is no sequestrum, joint spaces may be narrowed, and joint effusion may appear, accompanied by synovial thickening.
4. The diagnosis can take histological culture of fungal pathogen as a golden standard, supplemented by fungal antibody and antigen tests.

Differential Diagnosis

1. **Suppurative osteomyelitis and arthritis.** Clinically, the disease has an acute onset, manifested as local redness, swelling and fever, and severe pain during movement. The disease is common in people with normal immune functions, progressing rapidly. It may result in bone destruction within 8–10 days since the early stage, sclero-

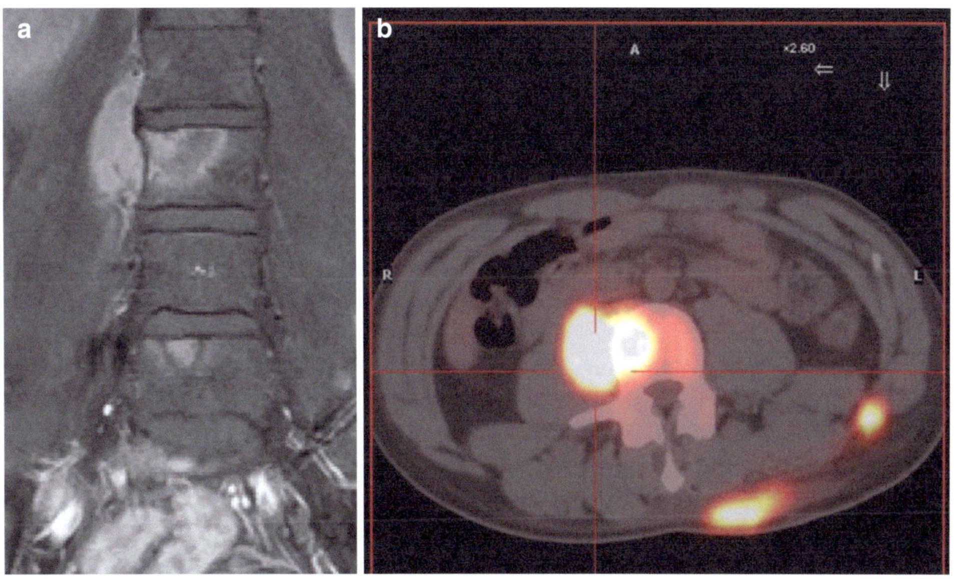

Fig. 4.33 Fungal infection of lumbar. (**a**) Superior anterior margins of L_3 and L_5 vertebral bodies show hyperintense shadows and swelling of adjacent right psoas major shows patchy hyperintense shadow on MRI T_2WI fat-suppressed sequence; (**b**) ^{18}F-FDG PET/CT shows that the destruction focus in lumbar vertebra has hypermetabolism and there are two hypermetabolism areas in subcutaneous soft tissues of the left lower back

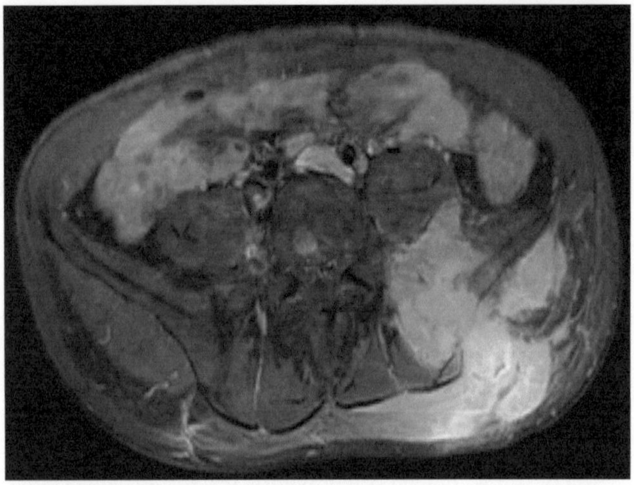

Fig. 4.34 Left iliac bone fungal infection accompanied by peripheral soft tissue abscess and formation of subcutaneous sinus. Male, 25-year-old, positive for coccidioides in pus culture. MRI T_2WI fat-suppressed sequence shows bone destruction in left iliac bone, local defects, large, patchy hyperintense shadow of peripheral soft tissue, and involvement of subcutaneous tissues (Special thanks to Tang Yonghua of Ruijin Hospital, Shanghai Jiao Tong University School of Medicine, who provides Figs. 4.32, 4.33, and 4.34)

sis of peripheral irregular bones (especially on bearing surfaces), joint space stenosis, and bony ankylosis in the advanced stage, mostly concurrent with joint dislocation, which may occur earlier than bone destruction. Fungous arthritis progresses slowly and insidiously. It is common in patients with immune deficiency and those who are long treated with steroids and have received joint replacement. Imaging findings show that the margins of bone destruction is clear and sclerosis is uncommon.

2. **Rheumatoid arthritis (RA).** The disease often affects multiple joints in a symmetric way, among which the facet joints of hands and feet are most susceptible. Imaging findings include symmetric, universal osteoporosis of facet joints of limbs, fusiform-shaped swelling of joint peripheral soft tissues, joint space stenosis, and utricular bone destruction inferior to bony articular surface (commonly occurring on the edges of joints adjacent to articular capsule). The serological test for rheumatoid factor is positive. Fungous arthritis usually involves unilateral large joints. However, sporotrichosis is also common in the facet joints of hands and feet, thus it is difficult to be distinguished from rheumatoid arthritis through imaging alone.
3. **Tuberculosis of bone and joint**. According to imaging findings, fungal infections of the bones and joints and osteoarticular tuberculosis are both manifested as osteolytic bone destruction (usually with no sclerosis margins), joint effusion, synovial thickening, accompanied by swelling of peripheral soft tissues and formation of sinus. It is difficult to distinguish the two diseases, which requires combination of clinical symptoms, clinical signs, and results of laboratory tests. The positive tuberculin test and T-SPOT test are helpful for the auxiliary diagnosis of tuberculosis; In tuberculosis bone destruction area, sequestrum is common, and fungal infection is relatively rare.
4. **Ewing sarcoma.** It occurs more often in long bone metaphysis, wherein invasive damage can be observed on the inner margin of the bone cortex, the bone cortex is intact, surrounded by obvious periosteal proliferation with onion-peel pattern and soft tissue mass. As the disease progresses, the edge of the bone destruction area becomes blurred. Fungal osteomyelitis bone destruction area usually has clear margins, with a periosteal reaction milder than that of Ewing sarcoma.

Status Quo and Progress of Research

^{18}F-FDG PET/CT is a recognized imaging method that can reflect the function and metabolism of lesions. It is widely used in the oncology field and has been increasingly introduced into diagnosis of inflammatory diseases in recent years. In the early stage, ^{18}F-FDG PET/CT can detect functional changes that occur prior to morphologic changes. In addition, since fungal infections of the bones and joints are usually a part of systemic infection, PET/CT can display the involved systems throughout the body. For example, it can identify whether there is occult involvement of the lungs, liver, spleen, or other organs. Research on the value of ^{18}F-FDG PET/CT application in the diagnosis and treatment of invasive fungal infections in immunocompromised patients conducted by Leroy-Freschini et al. [68] indicates that ^{18}F-FDG PET/CT can deliver high sensitivity (93%) and accuracy (90%) in the diagnosis and treatment of opportunistic invasive fungal infections. That said, as for the fungemia without obvious involvement of substantial organs, ^{18}F-FDG PET/CT's diagnostic value is limited. The research further indicates that changes in ^{18}F-FDG intake intensity are associated with the clinical course of the infection, which can be used for treatment monitoring and efficacy assessment of fungal infection, thus helping clinicians provide therapeutic optimization during treatment. A research on in-vivo detection of aspergillus fumigatus pulmonary infection with PET/MRI carried out by Davies et al. [69] demonstrates the great potential of antibody-guided PET/MRI in accurate diagnosis of invasive pulmonary aspergillosis.

4.5 Brucella Infection

Overview

Brucellosis, an animal-derived infectious disease caused by Brucella infection, is a pandemic zoonosis. It was first diagnosed in the Mediterranean region, and was initially named "Malta fever," also known as Mediterranean remittent fever, abortus fever, or undulant fever. It is widely distributed around the globe, in particular the Middle East and the Mediterranean region. In China, it mainly affects Inner Mongolia, and Northwest & Northeast China. The disease can involve multiple organs and tissues throughout the body, among which bones and joints are the most susceptible, accounting for 10%–85% of the body organs suffering from brucellosis [70]. The involvement of the bones and joints mainly includes spondylitis, sacroiliitis, osteomyelitis, peripheral arthritis, bursitis, and tenosynovitis. The involved site of bones and joints depends on the patient's age. As for children and young people, the disease is most common in sacroiliac joint and knee joint; as for senior patients, vertebral columns, especially lumbar vertebra, are the most susceptible.

Brucella is a Gram-negative micrococcus or curtobacterium without flagellum or spore. It is a smooth strain and has microcapsule. Based on hosts, biochemical characteristics, metabolic ways, and immunology gaps, WHO Brucellosis Expert Committee divides brucella into 6 species and 19 biotypes, among which the Brucella abortus, Brucella melitensis, Brucella suis, and Brucella canis are pathogenic to human [9]. Thanks to its strong resistance, the bacterium can survive for several weeks to even several months in soil, fur, organs, secretions, meat, milk, and dairy products of sick animals. It can be killed at a hot & humid condition above 60 °C or direct sun exposure for 20 min. It is sensitive to general disinfectants and broad-spectrum antibiotics. Brucella becomes pathogenic mainly by endotoxins, capsules, and invasive enzymes. It is believed that human are the occasional host of brucella. Usually, the pathogen first spreads among the same species of the infected animals, making animals carrying the pathogen and infected, thus involving human. Brucellosis spreads by: ① Occupational exposure (such as veterinarian, butcher, or stockman), wherein the brucella mainly spreads via direct contacting of sick animals or their secretions, excreta from vaginal delivery and feces; or via skin or conjunctiva infection during processing of skin, wool, and meat products. ② Digestive tract, wherein the brucella mainly spreads via drinking or eating water, raw milk or uncooked meat contaminated by the bacterium. ③ Respiratory tract, wherein the disease is caused by inhalation of droplets and dust contaminated by the pathogen [9, 71]. ④ Other ways, such as fly carrying, tick bites, breastfeeding, sexual behavior, blood transfusion, bone marrow transplantation.

The clinical manifestation of brucellosis usually lacks specificity, thus easy to be misdiagnosed and resulting in insufficient treatment. The disease has an incubation period of 1–6 weeks, up to several months. The average incubation period is 2 weeks. According to the length of the course, the disease can be divided into: ① Acute phase, which refers to disease course less than 8 weeks; ② Subacute phase, which refers to disease course within 8–52 weeks; ③ Chronic phase, which refers to disease course above 52 weeks [72]. Brucellosis of bones and joints is manifested as inflammation in bones and/or joints (such as swelling, pain, dysfunction, fever, tenderness, and redness); The disease typically involves knee, shoulder, hip, and other large joints. Spondylitis can occur if the bacterium invades vertebral column, among which the lumbar vertebra is the most susceptible. Fever, sweating, and backache are known as triad of brucellar spondylitis [73]. Brucellosis in joints of limbs has less specific clinical symptoms and signs in acute and subacute phases. Ninety-five percent of patients have slow onset manifested as fever, and mostly suffer from intermittent fever (undulant fever) with hidrosis. More than 70% of patients are accompanied by large joints migrating pain, which is a fierce pricking. Physical examination shows enlargement of liver, spleen, and lymph nodes; The disease generally has atypical, diverse symptoms in chronic phase, mainly manifested as fatigue, weakness, general malaise, and even melancholia. Fixed or recurrent pain may occur in joints and muscles, and a small number of patients may suffer from organic lesions in bones and joints.

Brucellosis laboratory test mainly includes pathogen culture and serological examination, in which the patient's blood, cerebrospinal fluid, bone marrow, and synovial membrane fluids can all be used for pathogen culture. The golden standard for diagnosing the disease is to separate and cultivate brucella. That said, blood culture, which has a low positive rate, is of greater significance to synovial membrane fluid culture of brucellosis of bones and joints [74]. However, the blood culture is time-consuming, so currently the laboratory diagnosis of brucellosis mainly relies on serological tests, including serum agglutination test (SAT), and ELISA, Coombs test, and complement fixation test (CFT), all of which can be used for definite diagnosis. SAT is the most common test among them. Coombs test can be used to supplement SAT. ELISA, another serological test with high sensitivity and specificity, can target at and detect different antibodies, including non-agglutinative antibodies. CFT mainly aims at IgG, which appears late but lasts long. In China, titer 1:10++ and above is used as the positive standard, which is highly specific to chronic patients [75, 76].

Pathophysiology

After entering human body via skin, mucous membrane, digestive tract, and respiratory tract, brucella is phagocytized by neutrophil or macrophage, and then enters lymph nodes via endolymph circulation. It grows and multiplies in the lymph nodes, to form a primary infection focus. When the pathogen proliferates to a certain number, breaking through the barrier formed by lymph nodes, a large number of bacteria enter the blood, thus causing bacteremia and raising the body temperature. Via blood circulation, the bacteria diffuse into cells of solid organs (such as liver, spleen, and bone) throughout the whole body, and then reproduce in the phagocytes of corresponding tissues and organs after the fever subsides, thus resulting in deformation and necrosis of cells therein. Bacteria can re-enter the blood circulation after they multiply to a certain extent, and when the thallus is destroyed, multiple virulence factors are released, raising the body temperature again. Such a recurrent bacteremia makes the fever type of patient undulant, clinically known as undulant fever. The lesion is prone to evolve into a chronic infection. It is generally believed that the onset and progress of brucellosis is driven by the synthetic effect of bacteria, toxin, and allergic reaction.

Microscope shows that the disease is mainly caused by damage to mononuclear phagocyte system. In the early stage, the lesion is typically manifested as serous exudative inflammation. As fibroblasts proliferate, granulomas composed of epithelial cells, macrophages, plasma cells, and lymphocytes appear in the focus, making the granulomas further fibrotic and finally forming deformed bones and joints.

Imaging Findings

1. **X-ray.** Generally, it cannot be used to make definitive diagnosis, since the positive rate is only between 35% and 42%. Main manifestations in the early stage include peripheral soft tissue swelling and osteoporosis of large joints of limbs. Three months later since onset, bone structure destruction can be found in X-ray plain film, wherein the low-density utricular bone destruction appears inferior to bony articular surface, most of which are 2–5 mm low-density shadows [77], edged with hyperostosis and osteosclerosis. Bone destruction areas can be honeycomb-shaped in severe cases, fusing with each other to form the larger irregular bone destruction area, in which the sequestrum can be found.

   Main manifestations in the advanced stage include periosteum ossification, sclerotic and uneven articular surfaces, and formation of osteophytes around the articular surface. Small bone destruction areas may reappear in the osteophytes, further worsening the reactive hyperplasia of peripheral bones, forming the larger osteophytes and resulting in a higher density of joint bone. When the joint synovium and bursa are involved, chronic brucellosis can form articular capsule, calcification of bursa, and osseous loose body in the articular capsule. The joint space can be narrowed, widened, or has uneven width. The degree of stenosis is related to the degeneration of the secondary arthrosis.
2. **CT.** Compared with X-ray, CT can provide multidirectional display for the subtle changes in bones through 3D reconstruction, thus better identifying changes in small bone destruction area, small sequestrum, joint effusion as well as peripheral soft tissue.
   (a) It is a typical manifestation of the disease that the focal bone destruction area inferior to bony articular surface often invades the bone by which the articular capsule is attached and the cystic change inferior to articular cartilage. CT can best display the lesion involving sacroiliac joints in transverse plane. More than 80% of patients are unilaterally affected [78], manifests as moth-eaten, utricular bone density reduction area inferior to bony articular surface of sacroiliac joint, surrounding by sclerosis margins. Large bearing joints, such as the knee joint and hip joint, are the most susceptible among peripheral joints.
   (b) Reactive new bones and periosteal proliferation can be obviously seen around the bone destruction area, and new bone destruction area may form in regenerated bones.
   (c) The joint space can be widened, narrowed, coarsened, or blurred. Lesions involving synovial membrane, bursa, and tendinous sheath can result in joint effusion, synovial membrane cyst, ossification of articular cartilage, and calcification of joint bursa, thus eventually causing joint bony ankylosis [79] (Fig. 4.35).
   (d) Peripheral soft tissues are swollen. Lesions occurring in the lumbar vertebra may be accompanied by paravertebral and psoas abscesses. The abscesses are localized, not beyond the scope of two vertebral bodies, with thin, heterogeneous cyst walls, which may be distinguished from psychrapostema of tuberculosis.
3. **MRI.** It is the preferred method for diagnosing intra-articular effusion, bone marrow edema and involvement of peripheral soft tissue of joint, in particular in the early stage of the disease (Fig. 4.36). The lesion shows non-specific signal intensity on MRI and typically shows homogeneous hypointense on T_1WI, heterogeneous intensity on T_2WI, and hyperintense on fat-suppressed sequence. The lesion can be homogeneously enhanced in enhanced scan (Fig. 4.37).

Key Points of Diagnosis

1. Epidemiological history.
2. Brucella separated from blood culture in laboratory test; Positive serum agglutination test.
3. The disease progresses slowly, involving multiple parts, joints, and tissues.
4. According to X-ray and CT, focal bone destruction appears inferior to bony articular surface of large bearing joints; obvious reactive hyperostosis and periosteal pro-

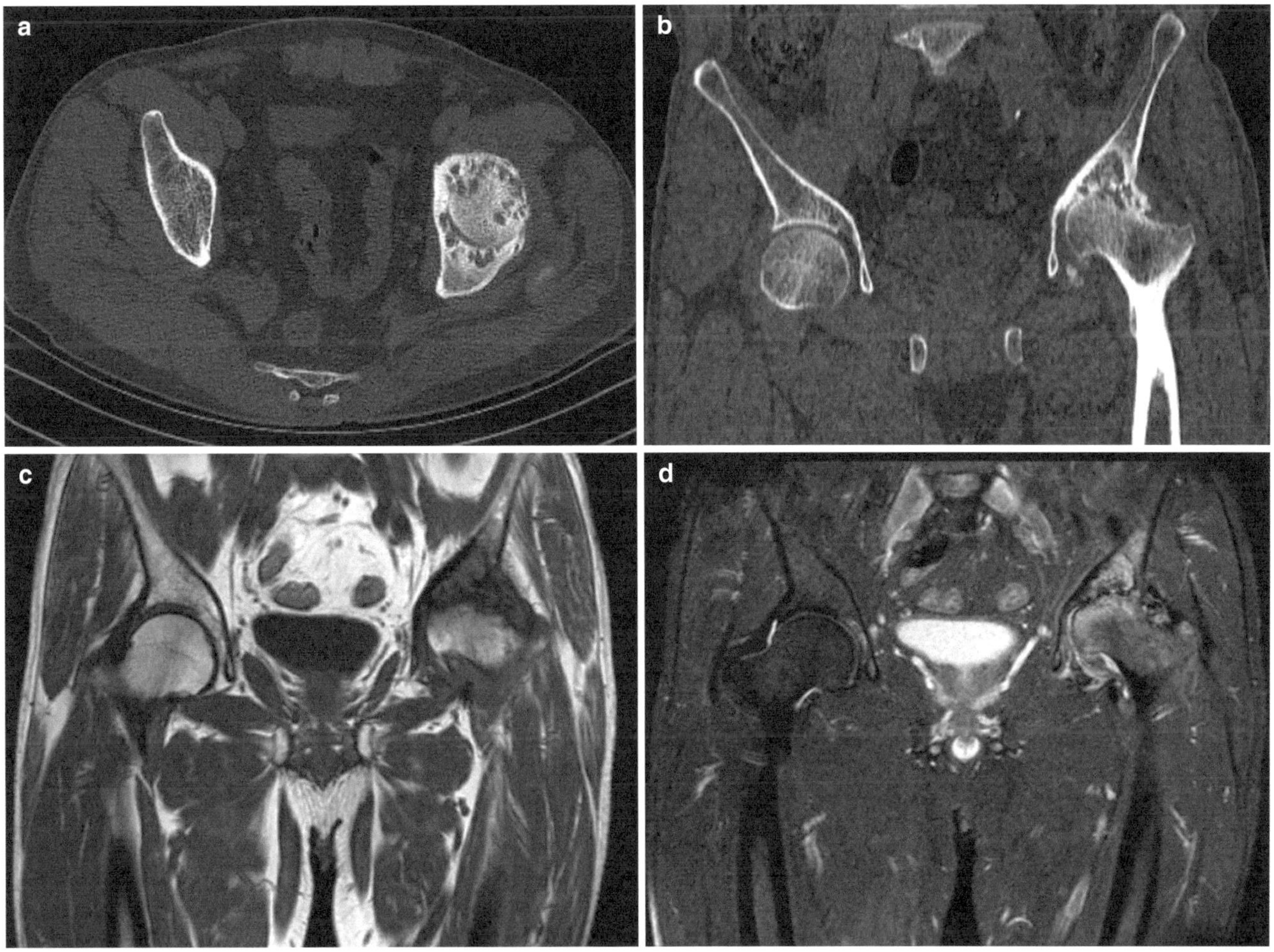

Fig. 4.35 Brucellosis in left hip joint. (**a**) CT shows that there are multiple utricular low-density shadows in subarticular left hip joint (including the surface of acetabulum and femoral head), with sclerosis margins, joint space stenosis, bone trabecula passing through the joint, and bony ankylosis; (**b**) CT coronal plane better displays hyperostosis at the edge of acetabulum and formation of osteophyte, in which utricular destruction area can be seen; (**c**, **d**) According to MRI, left hip subarticular bone destruction area mainly shows hypointense on T_1WI and heterogeneous hyperintense on T_2WI fat-suppressed sequence, with joint space stenosis and roughness

liferation can be seen at the edge; new destruction area may form in the new bones, wherein the new and old focuses coexist.

5. MRI plain scan can detect the lesion in the early stage, manifested as bone marrow edema and joint effusion showing hypointense on T_1WI and hyperintense on T_2WI.

Differential Diagnosis

1. **Tuberculosis of bone and joint.** Most patients have a clinical history of tuberculosis infection. More than 95% of osteoarticular tuberculosis cases are secondary to pulmonary tuberculosis, mainly manifested as fatigue, night sweat, and weight loss, with much longer course than brucellosis. According to imaging findings, bones and joints are severely destroyed; hyperostosis and osteosclerosis of peripheral bones and periosteal reaction are relatively mild; sand-like sequestrum is common in destruction area; cold abscesses form in peripheral soft tissues, typically involving a more extensive area than brucellosis and accompanied by calcification; in the advanced stage, fibrous ankylosis may occur and bony ankylosis is rare.
2. **Rheumatoid arthritis.** Clinical manifestations typically include swelling, pain, and morning stiffness of joints. The disease has a long course and occurs repeatedly. Serum antistreptolysin "O" test is positive and brucella serology test is negative; The disease mainly occurs in facet joints of limbs, common in proximal interphalangeal joints, metacarpophalangeal joints, and wrist joints. The lesion rarely bypasses proximal articular surface to affect distal articular surface, and is manifested as bilateral, symmetric arthritis. MRI shows formation of characteristic synovitis and pannus, and in the earlier stage, MRI shows cartilage destruction and involvement of joint soft tissues. Generally, the disease does not cause joint deformity.

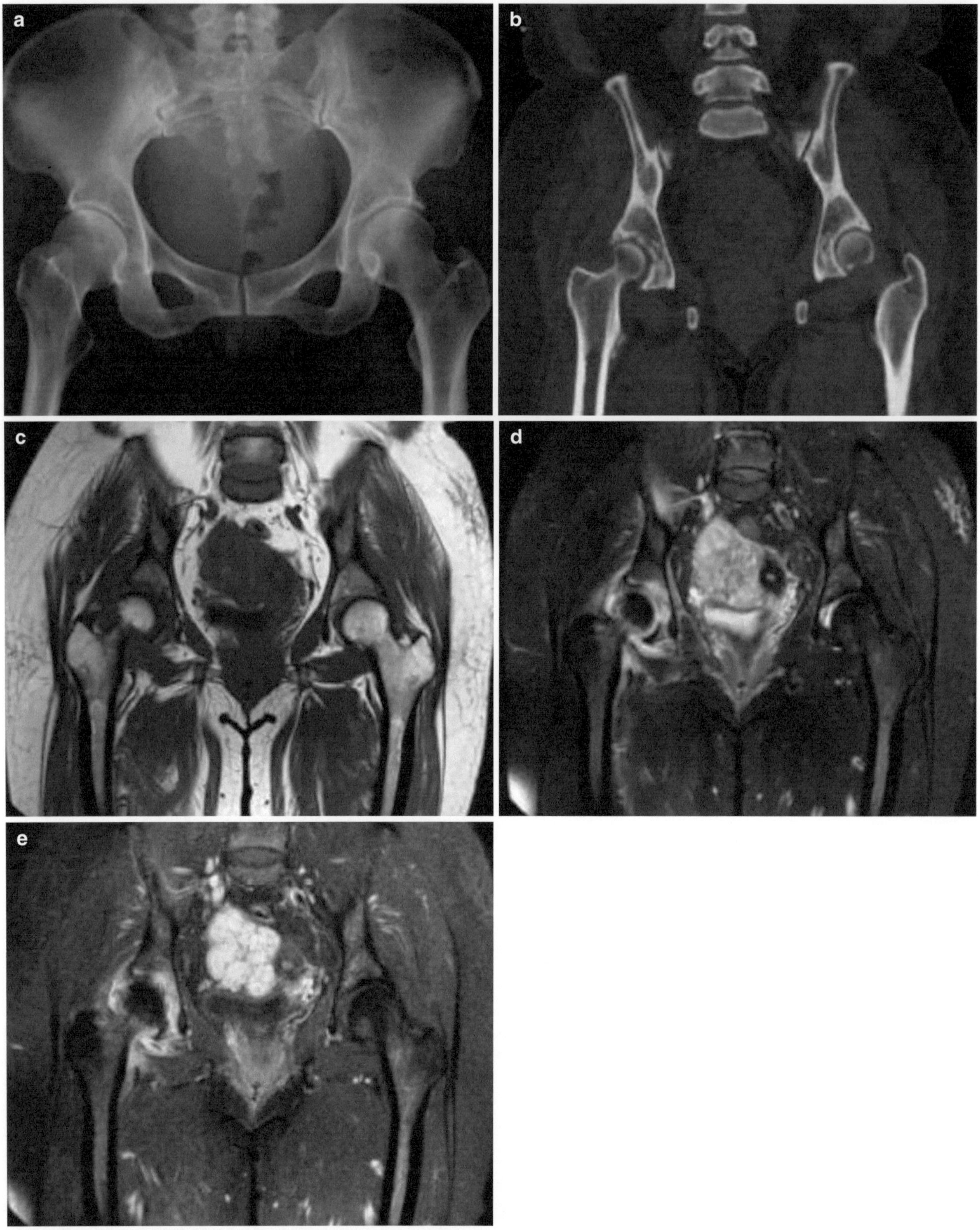

Fig. 4.36 Early brucellosis in right hip joint. (**a**) There is no obvious abnormality in bilateral hip joint DR. (**b**) CT plain film shows negative coarseness on right hip articular surface, wherein subarticular micro-utricular low-density area can be seen, and morphological density of femoral head has no obvious abnormality. (**c**, **d**) According to MRI, right hip subarticular lesion shows hypointense on T_1WI and hyperintense on T_2WI fat-suppressed sequence, with coarse margins. The lesion not only involves the acetabulum, and plain film and CT fail to detect the abnormal signal intensity of femoral head. (**e**) T_1WI enhanced scan shows that the lesion in right hip joint is remarkably enhanced

3. **Degeneration of bones and joints.** It is common in the middle-aged and elderly and occurs frequently in hip joints, knee joints, spine, and other large bearing joints. The clinical symptoms mainly include inflexibility and pain of joints, free from migratory pain, with normal erythrocyte sedimentation rate and negative brucella agglutination test. Imaging findings show lip-shaped hyperostosis or osteophyte formed at the edge of joints, heterogeneous stenosis of joint space, especially at the bearing side. Joint instability, deformity, joint mouse, and subarticular cystic degeneration may occur in the later stage.
4. **Pyogenic arthritis.** Main symptoms include joint swelling and limitation of motion. Acute infection symptoms including redness, swelling, fever, and pain in local soft tissues may occur. In addition, symptoms of systemic poisoning may also appear. In the early stage, image findings mainly show swollen soft tissues around joints and effusions, accompanied by widened joint space and local osteoporosis. In the progressive stage, joint space becomes narrow, and subchondral bone destruction occurs, especially at the bearing side. In the advanced stage, the disease is mainly manifested as hyperostosis and osteosclerosis, accompanied by large sequestrum and bony ankylosis. Due to the high content of protein in exudate, MRI plain scan shows hyperintense.
5. **Ischemic osteonecrosis.** Brucellosis occurring in the hip joint shall be distinguished from aseptic necrosis of femoral head. Patient with ischemic osteonecrosis has no infection history and is clinically manifested as progressive local pain and dysfunction. Imaging findings include moth-eaten bone destruction on the surface of the femoral head, subarticular cystic change, articular surface collapse in the advanced stage, femoral head deformation, and joint space stenosis, all of which may affect the heterolateral articular surface. Typical double-line signs can be found in MRI.

Status Quo and Progress of Research

1. Compared with X-ray plain film and CT, MRI boasts a higher resolution to soft tissue, capable of detecting the bone marrow edema and changes in peripheral soft tissues that cannot be detected by X-ray and CT in the early stage. For this reason, MRI has incomparable superiorities over the other two imaging examination methods. Having said that, MRI is not as good as X-ray plain film and CT in terms of displaying subtle bone destruction. The latter can realize thin-slice reconstruction and curved multi-planar reconstruction not greater than 1 mm, thus better observing the subtle changes in bones from multi-dimensions and multi-directions. It is necessary to combine the three imaging examination methods in a reasonable manner to achieve the best diagnostic performance in clinical practices.
2. DWI, a method for detecting the diffuse movement of water molecules in living tissues, can perform quantitative analysis based on apparent diffusion coefficient (ADC) value, to reflect movement of intercellular water molecules in tissues. During acute phase, brucellosis is mainly manifested as bone marrow edema inferior to articular surface. DWI is highly sensitive to the manifestations during this phase, and thus can detect those tiny bone marrow edema focuses. Besides, researches on brucellar spondylitis have found that [80] DWI sequence can help distinguish the acute and chronic phases of the lesion, with an accuracy as high as 100%. However, it cannot distinguish the acute and subacute phases. The infected vertebral bodies and the paravertebral infected soft tissues of patients with spondylitis show hyperintense in the acute phase and hypointense in the chronic phase on DWI. It is generally believed that the increased accumulation of inflammatory cells during acute spondylitis makes extracellular spaces smaller, thus resulting in limited diffusion of water molecules and increased signal intensity on DWI; By contrast, lesion in chronic spondylitis contains more bone matrixes, while there is no enough mobile protons to measure the diffusion coefficient, thereby the chronic spondylitis showing hypointense on DWI.
3. DTI, a functional magnetic resonance imaging technology based on DWI, has been widely used in central nervous system. The fast development of MRI scanning technology in recent years has effectively reduced the motion artifact. In addition, DTI technology has been increasingly applied in skeletal muscle system, such as articular cartilage and intervertebral disc. The fast scanning speed enables DTI to detect the subtle structural changes in tissue and generate ADC and fractional anisotropy (FA) values for quantification, thereby reflecting the structural integrity of tissue cells and functional changes. ADC value reflects the diffusion capacity of water molecules regardless of directions. The stronger the diffusion, the higher the signal, and the larger the ADC value; FA value reflects the integrity of collagen fibrous tissue, and the complete rules by which the fibrous structure is arranged. The stronger the anisotropy, the higher the FA value. During the acute and subacute phases of brucellosis, chondrocytes are degenerated and necrotic, accompanied by cellular edema and limited water molecule diffusion of collagen fibrous tissue in the parallel direction, thereby decreasing the FA value and increasing the ADC value during the period. It should be noted that the FA value changes earlier than the ADC value. In the chronic phase, thanks to the repair effect of body's immune system, cartilage and collagen matrix are

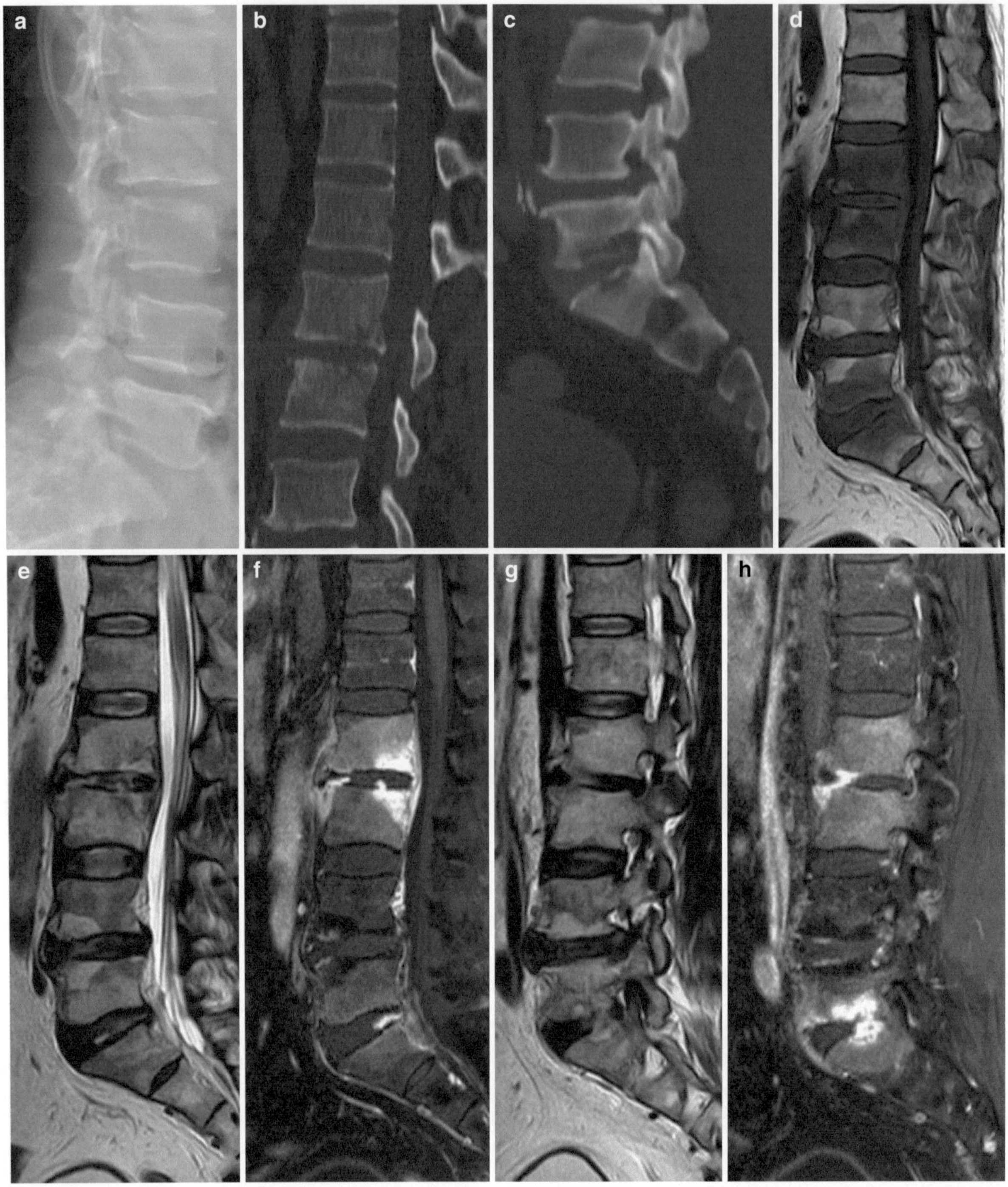

Fig. 4.37 Brucellosis involving multiple lumbar vertebras and right hip joint. Male, 56-year-old, suffering from progressive lumbago, accompanied by discomfort of lower limbs for more than 2 months. (**a**) DR shows that cystic density reduction area can be seen on the inferior margin of L_2 vertebral body, relative margins of L_2–L_3 vertebral bodies have increased local bone density, lip-shaped hyperostosis can be seen at the edge of some lumbar vertebral bodies (especially the L_4–L_5 vertebral bodies), no obvious stenosis is observed in the lumbar intervertebral space; (**b**, **c**) CT sagittal plane shows that relative margins of L_2–L_3 and L_5–S_1 vertebral bodies have utricular, irregular bone destruction areas, characterized by low density, indistinct margins and non-obvious peripheral osteosclerosis. (**d**, **e**, and **g**) According to MRI plain film, posterior relative margins of L_2–L_3 and L_5–S_1 vertebral bodies show small triangular, irregular hypointense on T_1WI and hyperintense on T_2WI; the lesion involves intervertebral disc; patchy, slightly hyperintense area on T_2WI can be seen around the lesion in corresponding vertebral bodies; (**f**, **h**, and **i**) According to MRI enhanced scan, focuses in L_2–L_3 and L_5–S_1 vertebral bodies show marked enhancement; the involved part of intervertebral disc also shows marked enhancement; the area of slightly hyperintense on T_2WI around the lesion shows mild enhancement, which is considered as an inflammatory edema region; there is no obvious swelling and abscess formed in soft tissues around the affected vertebral bodies in the coronal plane; (**j**) The patient reports occasional pain and discomfort in right hip 1 month after the discovery of lumbar vertebra disease. MRI for bilateral hip joint indicates that right acetabulum and subarticular femoral head show small-patchy, hyperintense on T_2WI, which is considered as the early manifestations of brucellosis involving hip joint

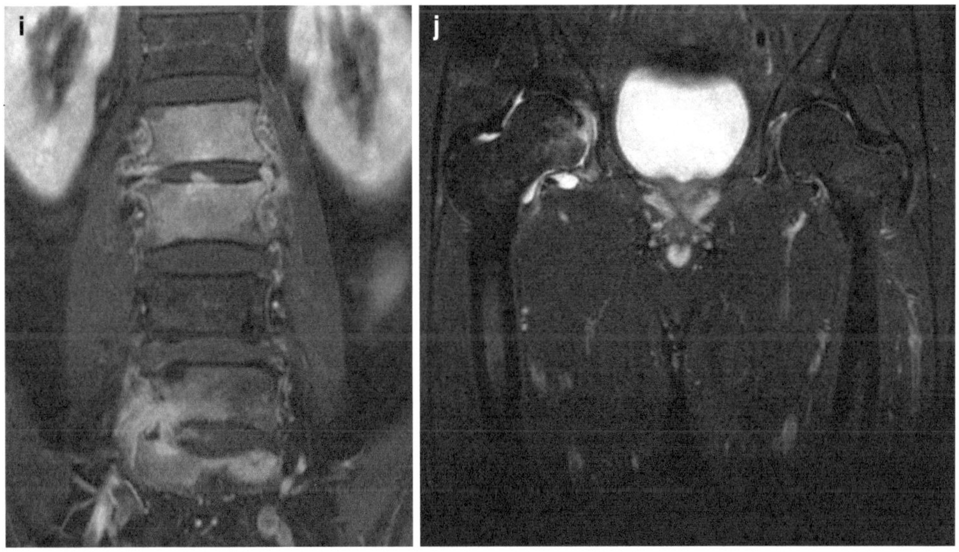

Fig. 4.37 (continued)

restored, generating new tissue cells and small vessels, with less inflammatory exudate than acute and subacute phases. This makes the ADC and FA values closer to the normal, but ADC value is still higher than that of normal structure because of the high water content caused by new tissues. Furthermore, the new tissues enable water molecules to move toward them, thus decreasing the FA value. Therefore, through the quantitative analysis of ADC and FA values, DTI can detect early lesions that have not yet seen morphological changes on the conventional MRI sequence, providing a basis for early clinical diagnosis.

4. At first, suspicious clinical cases may receive screening tests, which mainly include rose bengal plate agglutination test (RBPT) and plate agglutination test (PAT) in China, and then patients with positive results receive confirmation test for definite diagnosis.
5. Polymerase chain reaction (PCR) is a rapid and sensitive molecular method, with a sensitivity of 94.9% and a specificity of 96.5%. It can be applied for identification of the cultured strains and clinical specimens [75]. PCR, however, is yet to be normalized, and its clinical application still requires verification, so it is not suitable for routine inspection currently.

In a word, brucellosis of bones and joints needs to be diagnosed based on epidemiological contact history, clinical manifestations, culture and serological tests, and imaging findings. X-ray plain film is the first choice among all the imaging methods, but MRI also plays an irreplaceable role in early identification and diagnosis of the disease.

4.6 Mycobacterium Tuberculosis Infection

Overview

Tuberculosis of bone and joint is a chronic infectious disease caused by Mycobacterium tuberculosis encroaching on bones and joints. More than 95% cases are secondary to pulmonary tuberculosis, mostly caused by hematogenous spread, wherein Mycobacterium tuberculosis enters bones and joints via blood circulation, remaining in the spongy bone and joint synovium where the blood supply is abundant, thus causing the disease. The incidence of tuberculosis of bone and joint accounts for 2%–5% of the total tuberculosis cases, and 10%–20% of total extrapulmonary tuberculosis cases, which is remarkably higher in developing world than in developed world [81, 82]. The incidence of tuberculosis of bone and joint is second only to lymph node tuberculosis and tuberculosis of urogenital system, ranking third among all the extra pulmonary tuberculosis. Tuberculosis of spine has the highest incidence among tuberculosis of bone and joint, accounting for around 50%, followed by joint tuberculosis. Bone tuberculosis is relatively rare. Peripheral tuberculosis of bone and joint typically affects unilaterally and occurs in large bearing joints of lower limbs, among which hip joint has the highest incidence (12% – 15%), followed by knee joint (10%), ribs (10%), shoulder joint (7%), ankle joint (7%), elbow joint (2%), and wrist joint (2%). According to recent researches, tuberculosis of bone and joint has occurred more in facet joints than in large bearing joints of limbs. Tuberculosis occurring in hands, feet, and other parts is not uncommon especially in children, the elderly, and people with compromised immunity [83]. The incidence of tuberculosis of bone and joint does not vary a lot in gender and race. As far as age is concerned, the disease can occur in all age groups, and incidence among children remains the highest, while the elderly are prone to suffer from bone and joint lesion reactivated after long incubation. In addition, the disease has a higher incidence in poor, densely populated regions with malnutrition. People with underlying diseases (such as combined diabetes), people who long use hormones and immunosuppressive agents, as well as people who are overwrought and HIV-positive are highly susceptible to the disease. In addition, trauma is one of typical causes of tuberculosis of bone and joint.

Mycobacterium tuberculosis, a threadlike, slightly curved aerobe with two slightly blunt ends, has no spore or flagellum. It is motionless and cannot produce endotoxin or exotoxin. It can be divided into human Mycobacterium tuberculosis, Mycobacterium bovis, Mycobacterium murine and the like, among which the human Mycobacterium tuberculosis and the Mycobacterium bovis are, respectively, the most and the least pathogenic to human. Mycobacterium tuberculosis grows slowly and usually forms colonies after 4–6 weeks of cultivation. The thallus contains lipoids, proteins, and polyoses, wherein the lipoids account for 50%–60% of the total weight, thus making the bacterium resistant to dryness, strong acid, alkali and coldness, with strong tolerance, capable of long surviving in external environment. In addition, the bacterium is prone to make drug-fast variation and generate L-type bacterium. The main source of tuberculosis infection is patients with open pulmonary tuberculosis who excrete bacteria. The disease is typically transmitted via respiratory tract. When a patient excreting bacteria coughs or sneezes, aerosol particles contained in droplets are dispersed, and when a healthy person inhales the Mycobacterium tuberculosis carried in the aerosol particles, he/she becomes sick. Besides, dried sputum allows Mycobacterium tuberculosis to float in the air along with the dust, thus resulting in long-distance transmission. In a few cases, the disease can spread via digestive tracts and wounds. Human are generally susceptible to Mycobacterium tuberculosis, among which infants, postpubertal young people, and the elderly have a higher incidence. Normally, 90% of people infected with Mycobacterium tuberculosis do not develop the disease. Some people develop the disease in case of low immunity. Sometimes, the infected person can be self-healed or become a carrier of Mycobacterium tuberculosis for a long time. Tuberculosis of bone and joint is typically secondary to other parts of the body, most common in pulmonary tuberculosis. Via hematogenous dissemination, Mycobacterium tuberculosis is prone to remain in spongy bone and red marrow with rich blood supply, heavily bearing and highly active joints, such as vertebral bodies and long bone metaphysis, and synovium of knee joints, hip joints, and other large joints.

The occurrence, development, and turnover of tuberculosis mainly depend on the quantity and virulence of Mycobacterium tuberculosis and the immune function of the body. Koch's phenomenon has always been used to explain the different pathogenesis of primary tuberculosis and secondary tuberculosis. When the body has allergic reaction, it indicates that the body has acquired immunity to the pathogen. In addition, the allergic reaction is accompanied by caseous necrosis, which attempts to destroy and kill Mycobacterium tuberculosis. The susceptibility of tuberculosis of bone and joint is associated with environmental factors and polymorphism of related genes, which mainly include vitamin D receptor (VDR) gene, interferon-γ (IFN-γ) and its receptor gene, monocyte chemotactic protein-1 (MCP-1) gene, TNF-α gene, and human leukocyte antigen (HLA) gene [84].

Laboratory tests for tuberculosis include: ① Bacteriology test, including smear and culture. Since the specimen of extra pulmonary tuberculosis has a low bacteria count, the smear and culture are not sensitive enough. Besides, the culture is time-consuming, prone to result in delayed diagnosis. ② Molecular biology test. Xpert Mycobacterium tuberculosis/rifampicin (Xpert MTB/RIF), a semi-nested real-time quantitative PCR in vitro diagnosis technique, is very time-effective. It can determine whether a patient is infected with Mycobacterium tuberculosis within 2 hours, and can figure out the patient's resistance to rifampicin. According to studies, Xpert MTB/RIF boasts a sensitivity of 70.9% and a specificity of 100% in the diagnosis of tuberculosis of bone and joint [85, 86]. ③ Pathological test of tuberculosis. ④ Immunologic test, including PPD, interferon gamma release assay (IGRA), and Mycobacterium tuberculosis antibody detection. Among them, PPD is used to detect whether the body has been infected with Mycobacterium tuberculosis. However, it has a low specificity and sensitivity, especially for people with compromised immunity. Furthermore, it can result in false positive in case of nontuberculous mycobacterial infection in the environment and BCG vaccination. IGRA detects T-lymphocytes (i.e., T-SPOT.TB) that release interferon-γ in peripheral blood through enzyme-linked immunospot technique, in which the positive result indicates the presence of effector T cells specific to Mycobacterium tuberculosis in the patient's body, while IGRA can also distinguish the Mycobacterium tuberculosis infection from BCG vaccination and most of nontuberculous mycobacterial infections (except for Mycobacterium kansasii,

Mycobacterium gordonae, Mycobacterium szulgai, or Mycobacterium marinum) in the environment. However, T-SPOT.TB cannot be used alone as a basis for decisive diagnosis of tuberculosis, and clinical symptoms and other test indicators shall be combined to determine whether the tuberculosis is active. Domestic studies show that IGRA has a sensitivity of 53%–98% and a specificity of 60%–90% (or above), both of which are mostly reported to be more than 70%. In 2014, Chinese Society for Tuberculosis, Chinese Medical Association proposed the application of IGRA in China at the present stage based on WHO guidance and our national conditions: Neither PPD nor IGRA can distinguish the latent tuberculosis infection from the active tuberculosis or accurately predict whether the latent tuberculosis infection can develop into active tuberculosis. That said, they can supplement and assist the diagnosis of active tuberculosis that lacks bacteriological diagnosis basis, wherein IGRA negative result can help exclude the Mycobacterium tuberculosis infection. IGRA has a significantly higher sensitive than PPD in AIDS patients. However, since IGRA is not suitable for epidemiological screening, it is not recommended to replace PPD with IGRA as a screening method for healthy people [87–89].

Tuberculosis of bone and joint is a chronic disease, characterized by slow course of development and diverse clinical symptoms and signs. Systemic symptoms include prolonged low fever, night sweats, fatigue, loss of appetite, and weight loss. Swelling, pain, and dysfunction may occur locally in joints of limbs. Cold abscess can form in the peripheral soft tissues in case of lesions in spongy bone breaking through bone cortex. The abscess involves subcutaneous tissues and can form sinus after penetrating skin. Spinal tuberculosis typically causes occult (mostly sore and dull) pain, stiffness, and local tenderness in neck, waist, and back, accompanied by paravertebral, retropharyngeal, and psoas cold abscess. Bone destruction of vertebral bone can form a localized kyphosis. When a paravertebral abscess involves vertebral canal, the spinal cord and nerve roots at the corresponding level can be compressed, resulting in corresponding neurological symptoms, such as sensory and movement dysfunctions in the lower limbs, and even paralysis. As for patients with cervical tuberculosis, abscess can form on their posterior pharyngeal wall, thus compressing the esophagus and trachea, resulting in difficulty in swallowing and breathing. Carpal tunnel syndrome may occasionally appear in patients with tuberculosis of wrist joint.

Pathophysiology

Pathological changes caused by tuberculosis of bone and joint are basically similar to those of tuberculosis in other parts of the body, which include three basic pathological changes, namely exudate, hyperplasia, and caseous necrosis.

1. **Bone tuberculosis.** It is mainly manifested as osteolytic destruction, and rarely forms new bones. The lesion is usually derived from small tuberculosis focuses in spongy bone and then forms tuberculous granuloma, namely tubercle. The lesion is usually localized in this stage and rarely forms sequestrum. It can be seen under the microscope that the tubercle is mainly composed of epithelioid cell, Langhans giant cell, lymphocytes, and a small amount of fibroblast formed by reactive hyperplasia; Caseous necrosis may occur at the center of tubercle. The destroyed bone marrow is gradually replaced by tuberculous granuloma and necrotic tissues. Sequestrum can form in the destruction area. Liquefied necrotic elements form tuberculous abscess around the bone, and the abscess breaks through the skin to form sinus.
2. **Joint tuberculosis.** It can be divided into synovial tuberculosis and osteoarticular tuberculosis, among which the former is caused by Mycobacterium tuberculosis first encroaching on synovial membrane via blood circulation. In the early stage, synovial membrane tuberculosis mainly causes exudative lesion, manifested as hyperemia and swelling of synovial membrane and specific proliferation of granulation tissue. In the advanced stage, the proliferation of fibrous tissue causes synovial thickening, increasing fibrous exudate, eventually resulting in sediment and calcification in the joint, thus forming the white "rice body." As synovial membrane tuberculosis further progresses, it encroaches on articular cartilage first, and then destroys articular surface and subchondral bones at a slow rate. Therefore, the narrowing of joint space in joint tuberculosis happens relatively late and is typically asymmetric. As for osseous joint tuberculosis, lesions mostly penetrate articular cartilage and encroach on the joint based on epiphysis tuberculosis and metaphysis tuberculosis.

Imaging Findings

Imaging examination has always played a key role in the diagnosis of tuberculosis of bone and joint, among which X-ray plain film is the first choice. Having said that, X-ray plain film usually cannot provide positive result until 3 – 4 months after the onset, which is mainly manifested as bone destruction, osteoporosis, and swelling of local soft tissues, wherein sequestrum can be found in bone destruction area, with relatively rare hyperostosis and osteosclerosis and periosteal reaction. In case of bone tuberculosis concurrent with other purulent bacterial infections, obvious hyperostosis and osteosclerosis may appear around the bone destruction area, while CT findings may show small bone destruction area and small sequestrum, abscess, and joint effusion; MRI contributes to the early diagnosis of the lesion and can better display the involvement of vertebral canal, spinal cord, and spinal meninges. Usually, enhanced scan shall be applied after the lesion is identified, thereby better presenting the extent of involvement and pathological changes. The characteristics of different types of bones and joints are introduced below.

4.6.1 Tubular Bone Tuberculosis

Tubular bone tuberculosis refers to tuberculosis that occurs in diaphysis, epiphysis, and metaphysis of limbs and does not encroach on joints. It can be divided into long and short tubular bone tuberculosis. According to patient's age and lesion site, long tubular bone tuberculosis can be further divided into epiphysis and metaphysis tuberculosis and diaphysis tuberculosis, among which the former two are more common, while the latter is relatively rare.

4.6.1.1 Tuberculosis of Epiphysis and Metaphysis

Tuberculosis of epiphysis and metaphysis in long bone occurs frequently in children and teenagers, most of which are under 10 years of age. Clinical symptoms include local swelling, pain, soreness and discomfort, and limitation of motion of affected limbs. It is more common in the superior extremity of femur, proximal ulna, and distal radius, followed by the distal femur and proximal tibia. Without timely treatment, it can gradually affect joints, thus forming osseous joint tuberculosis.

Imaging Findings

1. **X-ray.** Early manifestations include localized osteoporosis in epiphysis and metaphysis and sparse bone trabecula, followed by circular or quasi-circular, eccentric or central area of osteolytic bone destruction. The lesion has sharp and clear margin, without sclerosis margin around it. There may be no or slight periosteal reaction; Small, high-density sand-like sequestrum or calcification can be seen in the bone destruction area. The bone destruction area can extend beyond epiphyseal line, which is a characteristic manifestation of epiphysis and metaphysis tuberculosis for distinguishing the disease from long bone tuberculosis and osteomyelitis lesions in other long bones. Swelling of soft tissue around the joint often indicates that the disease has involved the joint, concurrent with joint tuberculosis.
2. **CT.** Low-density osteolytic bone destruction can be seen in the epiphysis and spongy bone of metaphysis. The destruction area is clearly separated from normal bones, without sclerosis margin at the edge. Compared with plain film, CT can better show the small, high-density sequestrum and punctate calcification in the destruction area. In addition, CT can better display the involvement of joint and peripheral soft tissues.
3. **MRI.** MRI can detect bone marrow edema in the early stage of the disease, which shows hypointense on T_1WI and hyperintense on T_2WI, with blurred margins; As the lesion further progresses, the lesion mainly manifested as tuberculous granuloma shows hypointense on T_1WI and heterogeneous intense on T_2WI, accompanied by edema zone showing hypointense on T_1WI and hyperintense on T_2WI in peripheral area (Fig. 4.38); If caseous necrosis is dominant, it shows hypointense on T_1WI and hyperintense on T_2WI, wherein the small, patchy sequestrum or calcification shadows showing hypointense are scattered. Compared with X-ray, MRI can better display the feature that bone destruction area in epiphysis extends beyond epiphyseal line (Fig. 4.39). According to MR enhanced scan, hyperplastic granulation tissues show marked enhancement, with indistinct boundary and non-enhanced necrotic area at the center; edema in epiphysis shows mild enhancement; peripheral soft tissue forms cold abscess with margin showing rim-like enhancement.

Key Points of Diagnosis

1. It is common in children and teenagers with a history of pulmonary tuberculosis or other tuberculosis.
2. The disease progresses slowly, with mild clinical symptoms.
3. Imaging findings mainly show that osteolytic bone destruction can be found in the epiphysis or metaphysis of long bones of limbs, clearly separated from normal bones, without sclerosis margins; sand-like sequestrum or small calcification can be observed in the destruction area, with osteoporosis around the lesion.
4. The lesion is characterized in that the bone destruction area can extend beyond epiphyseal line.

Differential Diagnosis

1. **Bone cyst.** It is common in diaphysis and metaphysis center of children's long bone, manifested as quasi-circular, expansive and low-density bone destruction area with clear boundary, wherein septa can be seen, and there is no sequestrum; the long radius of the focus is parallel to the long axis of diaphysis, edged with thin, shell-like sclerosis margins; a relatively large lesion may be accompanied by pathologic fracture. MRI shows changes in hypointense on T_1WI and hyperintense on T_2WI. The signals are homogeneous. The lesion cannot be enhanced by enhanced scan.
2. **Giant cell tumor of bone.** It is common in long bone epiphysis of patients aged 20–40 years old, manifested as expansive, eccentric bone destruction on X-ray. It typically shows soap-bubble appearance, with thin bone shell, in which the slender bone ridge can be seen. The

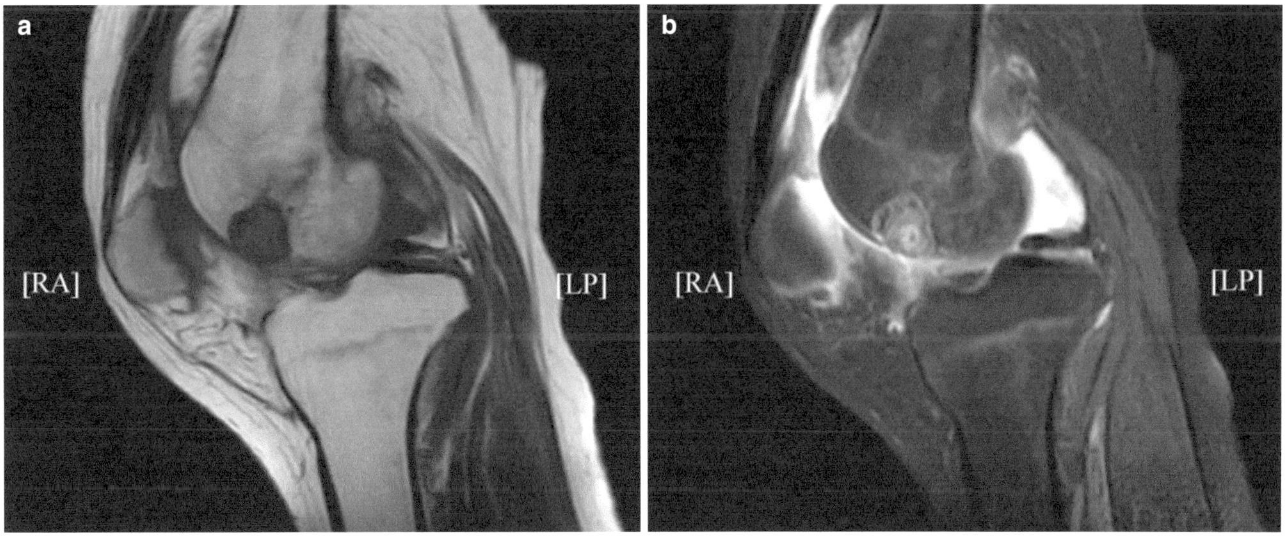

Fig. 4.38 Knee joint epiphysis tuberculosis involving joints. (**a**) MRI indicates that subarticular epiphysis shows quasi-circular hypointense on T_1WI. (**b**) The focus shows heterogeneous, slightly hyperintense on T_2WI fat-suppressed sequence

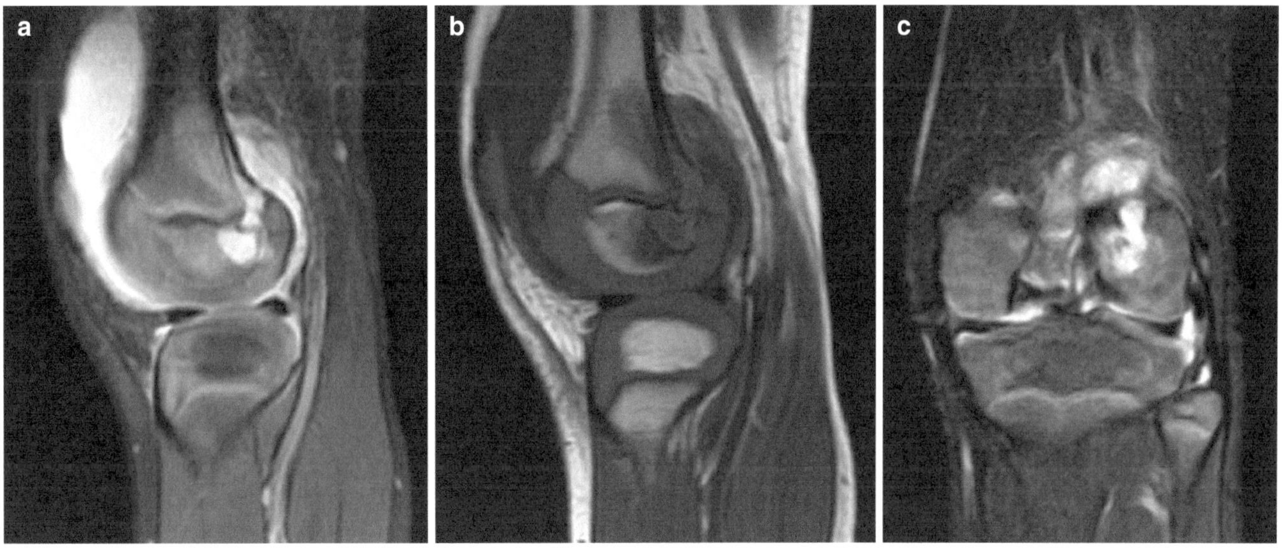

Fig. 4.39 Knee joint epiphysis and metaphysis tuberculosis. (**a**) MRI T2WI fat-suppressed sequence shows that the focus starts from epiphysis and extends beyond the epiphyseal line; (**b**) T_1WI imaging; C. T_2WI coronal plane

tumor tends to expand laterally, and its largest diameter is often perpendicular to diaphysis. Between the bone destruction area and the normal bone there are clear but not sharp boundaries, without sclerosis margin. Besides, there is no calcification or ossification shadows in bone destruction area.

3. **Chondroblastoma.** It is common in teenagers. More than 80% of cases occur in 11–30-year-old patients. The tumor, typically located in the epiphyses of unhealed metaphysis, can break through bone end to enter joints, or extend beyond epiphyseal line to evolve toward metaphysis. However, chondroblastoma that is located solely in metaphysis without involving epiphyseal plate or epiphysis is very rare. According to X-ray, there are quasi-circular bone destruction area with clear boundary, typically surrounded by sclerosis margins; small spot-like and patchy calcification can be noted in the bone destruction area of 20%–50% cases, wherein the soft tissue masses may form around the lesion, accompanied by periosteal reaction.

4.6.1.2 Tuberculosis of Long Tubular Bone Diaphysis

Tuberculosis of long tubular bone diaphysis occurs infrequently, more common in children and extremely rare in people above 30 years old. It typically occurs in long bone diaphysis where there is few muscle attached, such as radius and tibiofibula, with acute or slow onset. Since the focus is far away from epiphyseal plate and joints, the disease generally does not affect bone development and joint functions. Clinical manifestations include chronic, tolerable pain in the affected limb, swelling of local soft tissues, positive tenderness, and touchable subcutaneous fluctuation.

Imaging Findings

1. **X-ray.** When the patient has low immunity, the pathogen is highly virulent, or the disease progresses rapidly, the lesion is mainly characterized by bone destruction. In the early stage, it is manifested as osteoporosis in diaphysis and swollen peripheral soft tissues, followed by moth-eaten, quasi-circular bone destruction area, wherein the lesion has a clear margin; sclerosis margin rarely forms (Fig. 4.40); thin layer of periosteal proliferation whose extent is as same as that of bone destruction can be seen; and soft tissues around the affected bone are swollen in a fusiform shape. As the lesion further progresses, bone cortex becomes thinner, swollen, and thickened in a fusiform shape. The lesion may extend to both ends of diaphysis, but rarely encroaches on joints. In case of slow development, the disease is mainly characterized by proliferation and sclerosis, wherein periosteal proliferation merges with the adjacent bone cortex, to form a large, thick layer of bone cortex. Besides, bone destruction can enlarge marrow cavity, making it difficult to distinguish the disease from sclerosing osteomyelitis. However, the thickening of bone cortex therein is heterogeneous, which can be thinned, ruptured, or interrupted locally. In extremely rare cases, the lesion worsens when the patient's immunity is compromised, resulting in osteolytic destruction in osteosclerosis area or sinus penetrating the skin.
2. **CT.** It can display early osteolytic destruction and osteoporosis from multiple positions via 3D reconstruction, especially good at presenting the internal structure of bone destruction area, such as bone space and small sequestrum. In addition, it also contributes to the display of periosteal reaction and the extent of peripheral soft tissue swelling.
3. **MRI.** Bone destruction area shows hypointense on T_1WI and hyperintense on T_2WI, wherein small sequestrum showing hypointense on both T_1WI and T_2WI can be observed. Some lesions show typical "concentric circles" signs on T_2WI, that is, a caseous necrosis zone with slightly hyperintense at the center, surrounded by a hypointense fibrous capsule at the outer layer and hyperintense granulation tissue and edema zone at the outermost layer. These lesions show rim-like enhancement by enhanced scan. Subperiosteal cold abscess and soft tissue swelling show hypointense on T_1WI and hyperintense on T_2WI, wherein the extent of soft tissue swelling is basically same as that of bone lesion.

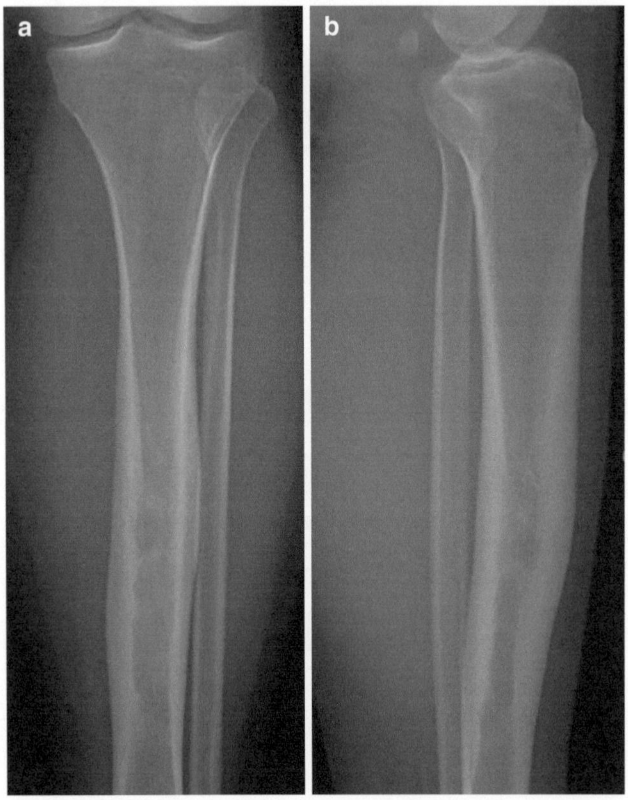

Fig. 4.40 Tuberculosis of left tibia diaphysis. (**a**, **b**) Quasi-circular or quasi-oval bone destruction area with low density can be seen in the middle segment of left tibia, with clear boundary, surrounded by no obvious sclerosis margin

Key Points of Diagnosis

1. The lesion is common in teenagers, frequently occurring in forearm and leg.
2. Main imaging manifestations: Case dominated by bone destruction with compromised immunity is manifested as quasi-circular bone destruction area in diaphysis, rare sclerosis at the edge, and mild, regular, and smooth periosteal reaction. Fusiform swelling can be seen in peripheral soft tissues, with extent in consistent with that of bone destruction; Children or adults with good immunity are manifested as sclerosis, with heterogeneous thickening of the bone cortex, which can be thinned, ruptured, or interrupted locally.

Differential Diagnosis

1. **Sclerosing osteomyelitis.** Hyperostosis and osteosclerosis are obvious; periosteal proliferation occurs; cortex is thickened; marrow cavity is narrow or occluded; exten-

sive or localized osteosclerosis is not obviously separated from normal bones; osteosclerosis zone generally has no bone destruction; usually no sequestrum is formed; peripheral soft tissues are typically not swollen.

2. **Acute suppurative osteomyelitis.** It has acute clinical onset, with obvious systemic and local symptoms of infection. The lesion begins with the metaphysis and then progresses toward the diaphysis. X-ray shows different extent of bone destruction, formation of periosteum new bone and sequestrum without bone expansion, and diffuse swelling of peripheral soft tissues, which is often beyond the extent of bone destruction.
3. **Eosinophilic granuloma of bone.** It is common in children between 5 and 10 years old. As for case occurring in long bone diaphysis, X-ray findings show patchy bone destruction area, which may expand outwards and has no sequestrum or calcification therein. Besides, laminar periosteal proliferation can often be seen around the bone destruction area, and is thick, intact, and larger than the bone destruction area.
4. **Ewing sarcoma.** It is common in long bone diaphysis or metaphysis of 5–15-year-old children, manifested as moth-eaten, large patchy bone destruction area with indistinct boundary, wherein the peripheral bone cortex has lace-like defects, with expansive, lamellar periosteal proliferation, which can be destroyed to form Codman triangle and penetrates cortex to form large soft tissue mass disproportionate to bone destruction in the early stage.

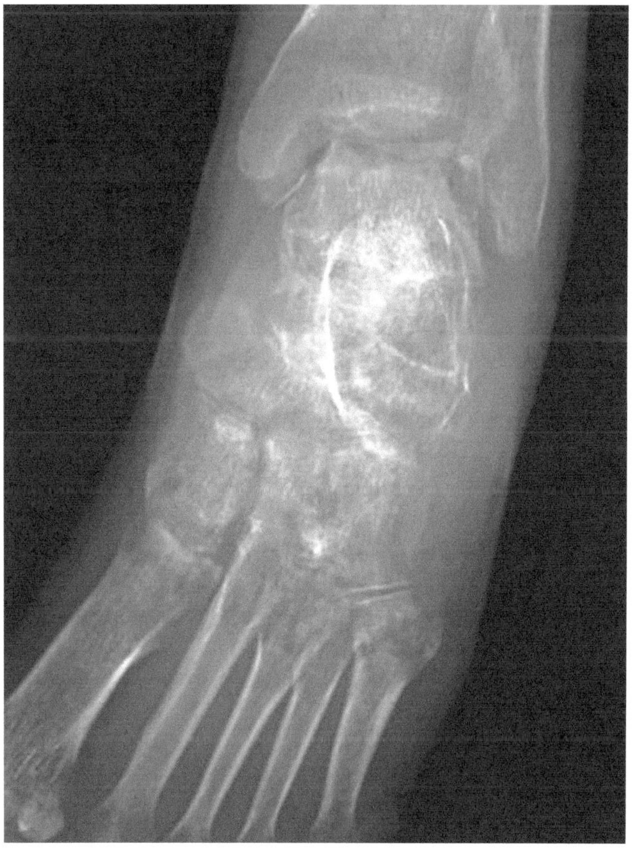

Fig. 4.41 Multiple tarsus tuberculosis involving base of metatarsal. X-ray shows multiple moth-eaten bone destructions, osteoporosis, blurred tarsus space and swollen peripheral soft tissues in the base of tarsus and metatarsus

4.6.1.3 Short Bone Tuberculosis

Tuberculosis of short bone includes tuberculosis in both short tubular bones and block-shaped short bones, such as carpal bones and tarsus, among which tuberculosis of short tubular bone is also known as tuberculous phalanx inflammation or spina ventosa, which refers to tuberculosis in phalanxes of hands and feet, metacarpus, metatarsus, and other short tubular bones. The lesion can be single or multiple, common in proximal phalanges of children below 5 years old, with slow onset. It may cause fusiform swelling of local soft tissues, or be asymptomatic and identified in physical examination. Generally, it causes no tenderness or activity limitation, and sometimes there may be a feeling of slight discomfort. The disease can be self-healed, occasionally forming sinus caused by ulceration.

Imaging Findings

1. X-ray
   (a) This disease typically forms multiple lesions in bilateral hand & feet, involving multiple phalanges (Fig. 4.41), most of which, however, are single lesions. Multiple lesions occurring in the same bone is rare.
   (b) In the early stage, it is manifested as osteoporosis, fusiform thickening of fingers and swelling of soft tissues.
   (c) As disease progresses, circular or quasi-circular bone destruction area appears in the affected bone, manifested as cystic bright area, with clear boundary; bone cortex becomes thinner and expansive; diaphysis is thickened in a fusiform shape, called spina ventosa, mostly located at the center of the bone, with long axis consistent with that of diaphysis. Sometimes, thick, large, and incomplete bone crests can be seen in the lesion. Sequestrum, however, is very rare. Lesions penetrating bone cortex can cause periosteal proliferation but rarely involve joints.
   (d) During repair stage, soft tissues around the lesion become less swollen, destruction area may shrink and osteosclerosis occurs. After healed, short bone tuberculosis may leave no trace or slight bone structural abnormality in children.

(e) Short tubular bone tuberculosis in adults are mostly localized, adjacent to metaphysis, resulting in honeycomb-shaped destruction area and local bone expansion, accompanied by hyperostosis and osteosclerosis around destruction area. In case of severe bone destruction, the entire diaphysis may be involved and pathologic fracture may occur.

(f) Multiple lesions in phalanges of fingers may involve carpal bones and further involve wrist joints, thus forming tuberculosis of wrist joint.

(g) Among all the bones of foot, calcaneus is the most susceptible to tuberculosis. Since there is a large number of tendons and thin, weak soft tissues in the foot, calcaneus is prone to form sinus (Fig. 4.42).

2. **CT and MRI.** The diagnosis of the disease relies mainly on X-ray plain film. However, in case of early stage or atypical X-ray manifestation, CT and MRI can provide highly valuable information, such as mild bone destruction (Fig. 4.43) and changes in peripheral soft tissues. MRI also helps to detect the small caseous necrosis in marrow cavity lesions. Furthermore, CT and MRI can realize enhanced scan, thereby better presenting the extent of involvement and soft tissue abscess enhanced in a rim-like manner.

Key Points of Diagnosis

1. It is common in children below 5 years old, frequently involving multiple phalanges, especially the proximal and middle phalanges of the third finger.
2. Typical X-ray manifestations include quasi-circular bone destruction area at the center of diaphysis, expanded, thinned bone cortex appeared as spina ventosa, peripheral soft tissues swollen in a fusiform shape, and long radius of destruction area in consistent with that of diaphysis, wherein bone ridge can be noted in the destruction area, surrounded by visible periosteal reaction. Joints are rarely involved.

Differential Diagnosis

1. **Multiple enchondroma.** It is common in the short tubular bone metaphysis or diaphysis of hands and feet, among which the lesion occurring in metaphysis and diaphysis mostly grows eccentrically and centrically, respectively. X-ray shows quasi-circular, multilocular bone destruction area, with clear boundary and sclerotic margins. The destruction area is separated from normal bones, wherein bone cortex may become thinned and expansive, and multiple spot-like, irregular calcification can be seen. Generally, there is no periosteal proliferation or soft tissue swelling around the lesion.
2. **Bone cyst.** There is cystic bright area with clear boundary in diaphysis, surrounded by sclerosis margins. Generally, the bright area has no structures and may be accompanied by pathologic fracture, surrounded by no periosteal proliferation or soft tissue swelling.
3. **Gout.** It is common in men between 40 and 60 years old, usually beginning with the first metatarsophalangeal joint, wherein the articular surface has irregular, punched-out bone destruction, surrounded by no sclerosis margins,

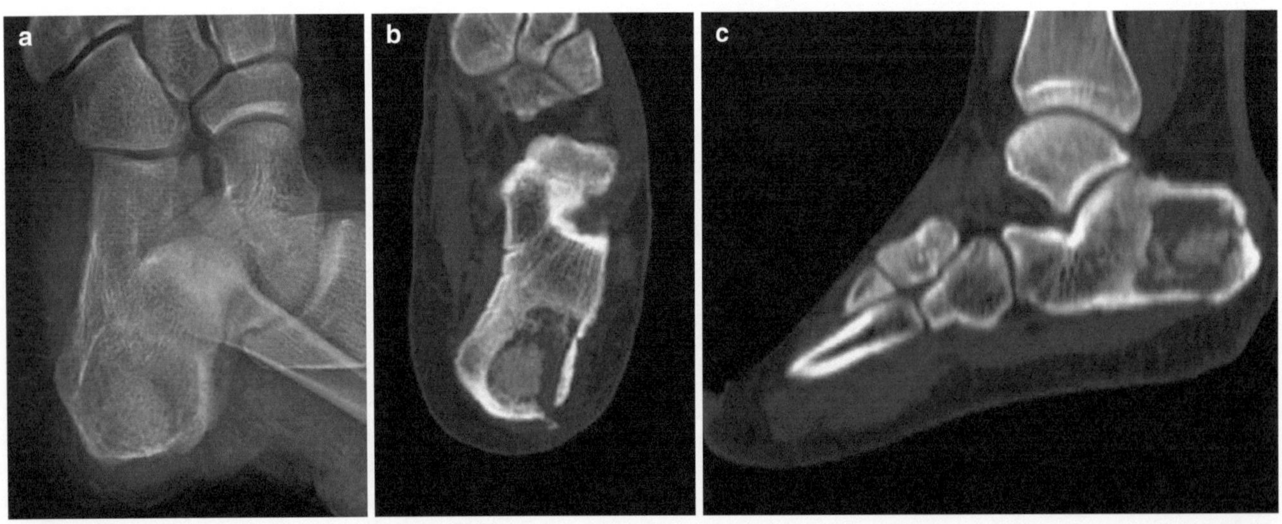

Fig. 4.42 Calcaneus tuberculosis. (**a**) DR indicates that there is quasi-circular bone density reduction area in calcaneus, bone cortex is discontinuous and block-shaped sequestrum can be seen in bone destruction area. (**b**, **c**) CT indicates that bone destruction area has clear boundary, osteosclerosis at the edge of the destruction area is not obvious and local bone cortex is defective, with formation of sinus. (**d**, **e**) According to MRI, bone destruction area in calcaneus shows hypointense on T_1WI and heterogeneous hyperintense on T_2WI fat-suppressed sequence; peripheral soft tissues are swollen; and local sinus extends to subcutaneous tissues

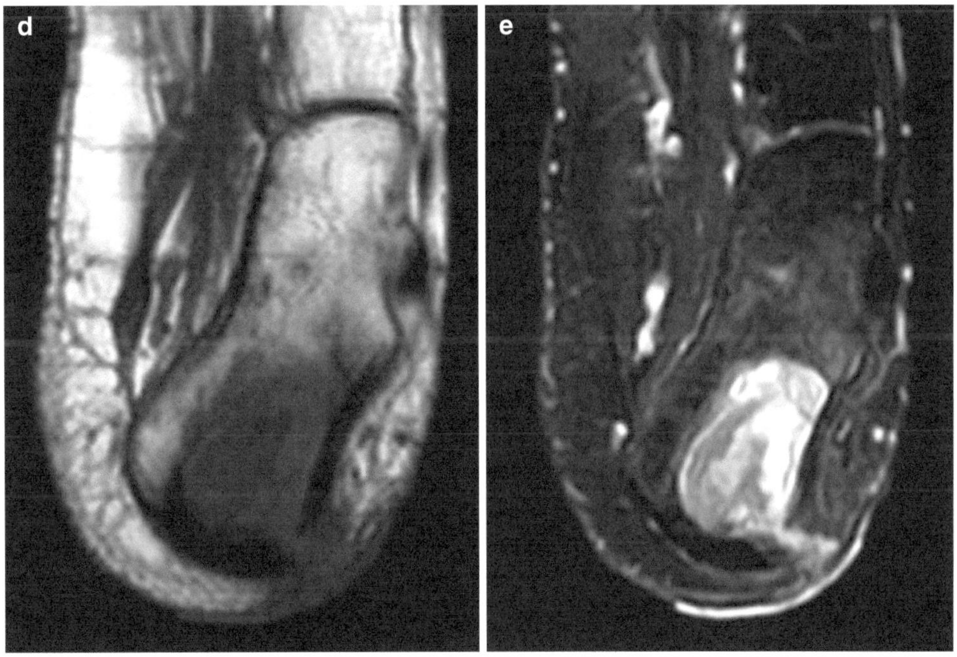

Fig. 4.42 (continued)

and calcific tophus may appear in peripheral soft tissues. Result of clinical laboratory test indicates elevated blood uric acid.

4. **Eosinophilic granuloma of bone.** When occurring in short tubular bone, the lesion mostly involves metaphysis and diaphysis. Osteolytic destruction is located in bone marrow cavity, growing expansively. There are soft tissue dense structures in bone destruction area, with lamellar periosteal proliferation around the lesion and peripheral soft tissue mass.

4.6.2 Flat Bone and Irregular Bone Tuberculosis

Flat bones are mainly distributed in head and chest, including skull, sternum, ribs, and scapula (Fig. 4.44). Irregular bones mainly include vertebra, hip bones, and the like. Tuberculosis rarely occurs in flat bones and irregular bones. Tuberculosis in vertebral body is the most common, followed by tuberculosis of rib, a type of tuberculosis of flat bone.

4.6.2.1 Tuberculosis of Skull

Tuberculosis of skull refers to the specific inflammatory reaction caused by Mycobacterium tuberculosis encroaching on the skull. The disease occurs when tuberculosis focuses in blood circulation, lymphatic system, or adjacent tissues directly spread to skull. Mostly, it is secondary to pulmonary tuberculosis or tuberculosis in other parts of the body. The disease is common in children or adults with compromised immunity. It occurs more frequently in fronto-parietal bone and rarely in skull base bone. With slow onset and long course, the disease is mainly manifested as a lump on head, with no redness or fever in local skin. Severe pain may occur when the lesion encroaches on cerebral dura mater.

Imaging Findings

1. **X-ray.** The lesion can be divided into localized and diffuse types according to the extent of involvement, among which the former is more common, manifested as circular or oval perforated bone destruction and defective areas, with clear but not regular boundary. Tuberculosis of skull usually starts from diploe, wherein the damage to the inner plate is greater than the outer plate, so that double contour sign may sometimes appear at the edge of bony defect. Small sequestrum can be seen in destruction area, with non-obvious peripheral hyperostosis and osteosclerosis, accompanied by local soft tissue swelling. The lesion can extend beyond suturae craniales and encroach on adjacent bones. Diffuse bone destruction area, which is widely distributed with blurred margins, can form sinus.
2. **CT and MRI.** CT manifestations are similar to that of X-ray. CT and MRI can clearly display the extent of involve-

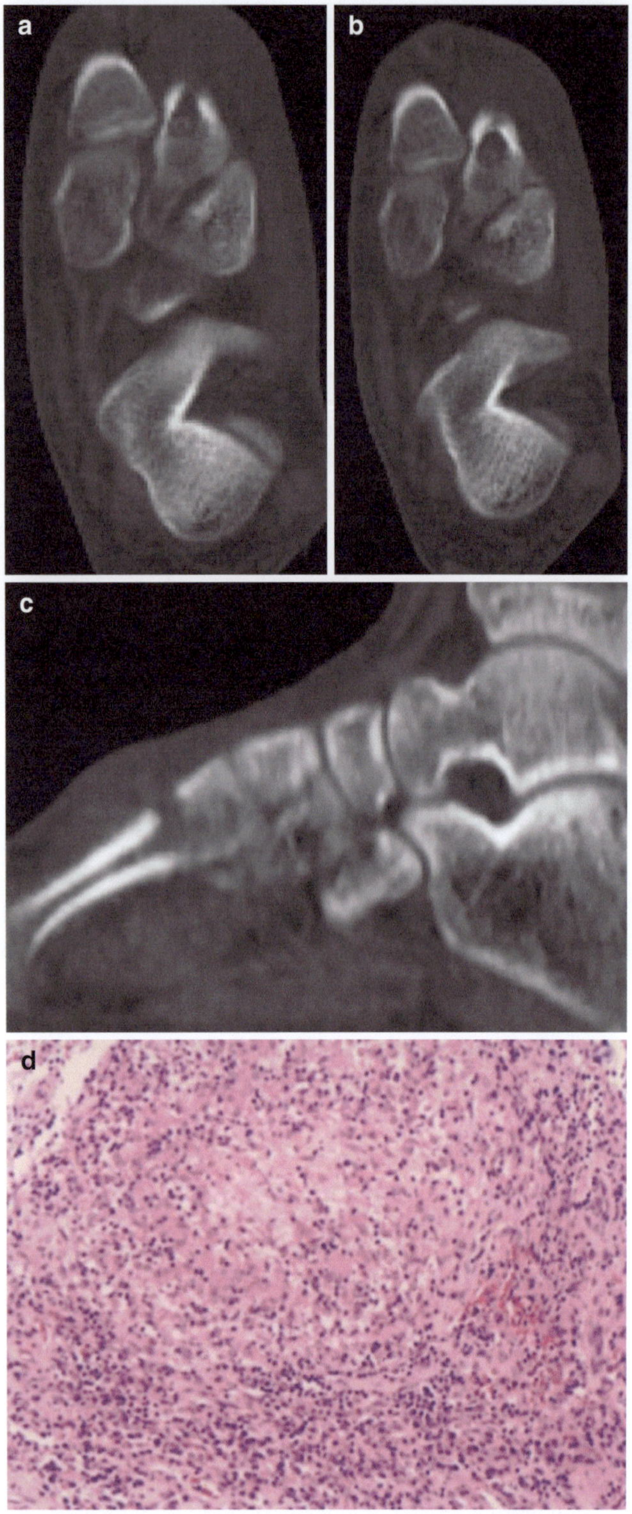

Fig. 4.43 Tuberculosis in the base of the second metatarsus. The patient's left foot is painful, accompanied by subcutaneous abscess formed on dorsum of foot. Local abscess puncture genetics detects MTB and sensitivity to rifampicin with Xpert MTB/RIF technology. (**a**, **b**) CT transverse plane shows there is an utricular bone destruction area in the base of the second metatarsus, wherein small, sand-like sequestrum can be seen; (**c**) CT sagittal plane reconstruction shows cystic bone destruction area in the base of metatarsus. (**d**) Pathology shows granulomatous disease. Nodular focuses formed by epithelioid cells and histiocytes can be seen, with infiltration of lymphocytes and plasma cells in peripheral area

ment in multiple positions. MRI image shows hypointense on T_1WI and hyperintense on T_2WI. Besides, MRI also helps to identify the involvement of subcranial cerebral dura mater, cerebral pia mater, and brain parenchyma.

Key Points of Diagnosis

1. Children or immunocompromised adults often have primary tuberculosis focus, with slowly enlarging lump on head, free from redness or fever in local skin.
2. Typical X-ray findings include single or multiple bone destruction areas with punched-out pattern in skull. The destruction area starts from diploe, wherein the damage to the inner plate is greater than the outer plate. The sclerosis of margin is not obvious, in which small sequestrum can be noted, with swollen peripheral soft tissues. Sinus can be formed.

Differential Diagnosis

1. **Osteomyelitis of skull.** The lesion of osteomyelitis is more extensive than that of tuberculosis, with acute clinical onset and symptoms of acute infection. X-ray shows obvious hyperostosis and osteosclerosis surrounding the destruction area, wherein periosteal reactions can be seen. The lesion usually does not extend beyond suturae craniales, and large sequestrum is common.
2. **Multiple myeloma.** The age of onset is generally older than that of tuberculosis, most of which are above 40 years old, male outnumbers female. It is manifested as different-sized multiple bone destruction areas with punched-out pattern in skull, surrounded by no osteosclerosis, sequestrum or soft tissue swelling. The disease often involves bones of trunk and proximal limb bones except for skull. Bence-Jones protein in urine shows positive result.
3. **Eosinophilic granuloma of skull.** The disease is common in children and teenagers, and also originates from diploe and gradually involves inner & outer plates. Circular or quasi-circular osteolytic destruction area with irregular, sharp boundary is formed, obviously separated from the normal skull. Typical "button sequestrum" can be found in bone destruction area. No swollen soft tissue or abscess is formed in peripheral area.
4. **Skull metastatic carcinoma.** It is common in the middle-aged and elderly people, typically with a history of primary tumor. Imaging findings show multiple osteolytic bone destructions in skull, with indistinct boundaries, free from sclerotic margins, and surrounded by soft tissue density masses.

4.6.2.2 Tuberculosis of Ribs and Sternum

Tuberculosis of ribs and sternum refers to the chronic inflammatory lesion caused by Mycobacterium tuberculosis

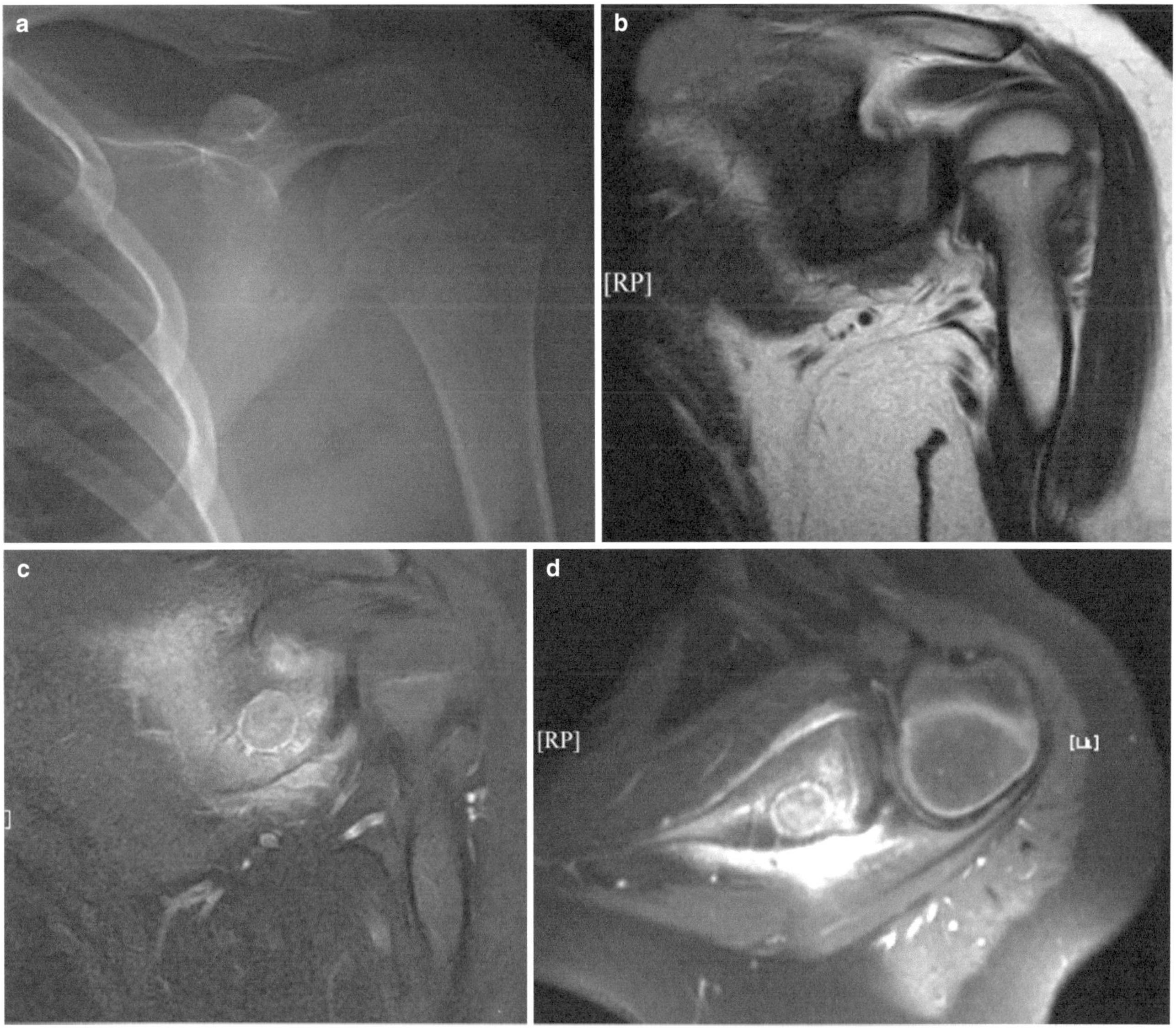

Fig. 4.44 Tuberculosis of scapula. (**a**) DR shows quasi-circular low-density shadows with clear boundary in left scapula, surrounded by no obvious sclerosis margin; (**b**) According to MRI, quasi-circular in scapula shows hypointense shadows on T_1WI; (**c**) Quasi-circular hyperintense shadow is shown on T_2WI fat-suppressed sequence in scapula, with clear boundary. Peripheral bone has patchy bone marrow edema shadows, showing hyperintense on T_2WI. (**d**) T_1WI enhancement shows rim-like enhancement around bone destruction area in scapula, accompanied by swelling of peripheral soft tissues, which shows plaque-like enhancement

directly, or via blood circulation or lymph circulation, spreading to sternum or rib. Clinically, most patients complain of chest wall swelling or dull pain in anterior sternum. In the advanced stage, abscess may appear in chest wall, thus forming sinus. When sinus breaks inwardly through the chest wall, tuberculous empyema can be formed.

Imaging Findings

1. X-ray. Positive manifestations occur much later than clinical manifestations. Tuberculosis of sternum typically occurs in manubrium and gladiolus. In the early stage, chest X-ray examinations of patients are often normal, whereas in the late stage, circular, quasi-circular, irregular-shaped or moth-eaten bone destruction area, in which small sand-like sequestrum is formed, can be seen in the affected bone. Bone destruction often causes heterogeneous density in sternum marrow cavity, raising the density of normal osseous tissues adjacent to the bone destruction area, thus causing hyperostosis and osteosclerosis. Tuberculosis of rib, most of which are single, occurs frequently in the 4th–7th ribs. Spina ventosa may also occur in the affected ribs. When confined to the margin of the ribs, the spina ventosa is mostly manifested as the localized defect formed at the lower ribs. The affected bone is surrounded by swollen soft tissues of chest well and cold abscess, manifested in X-ray plain film as increased density of peripheral soft tissues, in which calcification can be observed. Ulcerated skin may form sinus that cannot be healed for a long time.

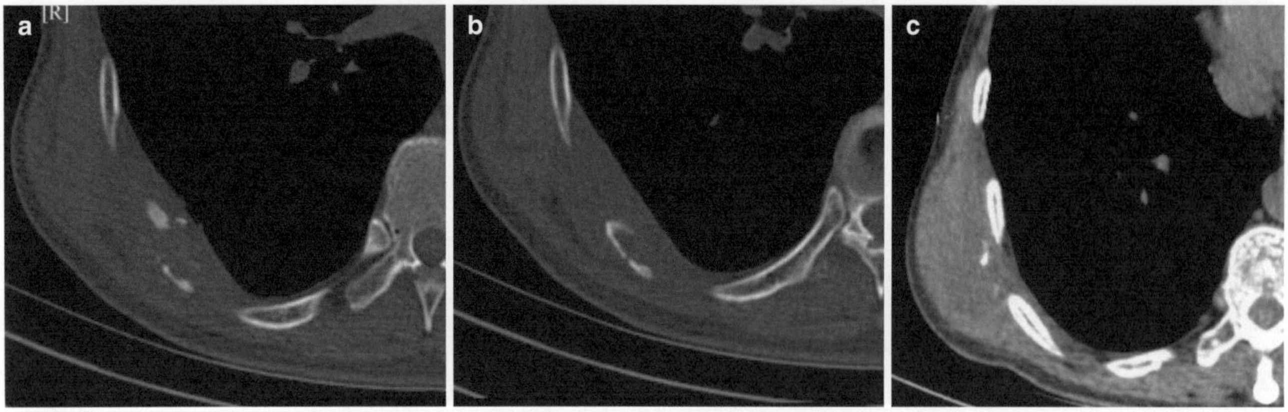

Fig. 4.45 Tuberculosis of right ribs. (**a–c**) According to CT, osteolytic bone destruction with smooth, clear margins can be seen in right ribs, local bone cortex is discontinuous, swollen soft tissues and abscess on right side of the chest wall can be seen in the soft tissue window, wherein calcification is visible (**a**, **b** CT bone window; **c** CT Mediastinum window)

2. CT and MRI. With 3D imaging technology, CT can display small anatomical structures and lesions, showing the extent and range of destruction in sternum and ribs, changes in density of bone marrow cavity, sequestrum, abscess and tiny calcification in a more detailed manner, and better displaying the involvement of sinus and chest wall soft tissues, whether the abscess has broken into the adjacent chest cavity, mediastinum, etc., whether the disease is concurrent with tuberculous pleurisy or pulmonary tuberculosis. Enhanced scan shows rim-like enhancement of abscess in chest wall, with non-enhanced necrotic area at the center (Fig. 4.45). MRI imaging is often applied to detect early tuberculous osteomyelitis and soft tissue changes in sternum and ribs. Compared with CT, MRI can better show the changes in soft tissues and bone marrow edema. However, it is inferior to CT in displaying changes in the fine bone structures and sequestrum.

Key Points of Diagnosis

1. The patient has local chest wall pain, swelling or painless mass on the chest wall.
2. Typical X-ray manifestations include expansive area of osteolytic bone destruction, with smooth, clear margins, in sternum and ribs, wherein small sequestrum can be seen. In case of lesion occurring in sternum, bone surrounding bone destruction area often has a heterogeneously increased density, accompanied by swelling of peripheral chest wall soft tissues and formation of abscess. Ulcerated skin can form sinus, which may progress toward thoracic cage, encroaching on pleura, thus resulting in pleural effusion.

Differential Diagnosis

1. **Metastatic carcinoma of sternum and ribs.** It is common in the middle-aged and elderly people, typically with a history of primary tumor. Imaging findings include osteolytic or osteogenic bone destruction in ribs and sternum, with blurred margins, and non-obvious expansion of ribs. It is usually concurrent with discontinuity of bone cortex, surrounded by localized soft tissue density masses. Through enhanced scan, the soft tissues are enhanced in a holistic manner, instead of rim-like manner in tuberculous abscess.
2. **Fibrous dysplasia of bone.** Fibrous dysplasia of ribs is also manifested as local, expansive bone destruction in rib, wherein ground-glass opacity can be seen, with sclerotic margins, lesion is obviously separated from normal tissues, and peripheral soft tissues are normal.

4.6.2.3 Tuberculosis of Iliac Bone, Pubic Bone, and Ischium

Tuberculosis of iliac bone refers to tuberculosis that is far away from sacroiliac joint and hip articular surface, and simply involves the iliac body. It occurs frequently in ala of ilium and iliac crest. Tuberculosis of pubis and ischium is rare. Tuberculosis of ilium, pubis, and ischium is common in teenagers.

Imaging Findings

Focuses of tuberculosis of iliac bone are mostly single and localized. X-ray plain film shows quasi-circular or irregular bone destruction area. Sequestrum rarely forms, and the surrounding bone shows varying degrees of bone resorption changes, thus blurring margins of the focus. Tuberculosis of iliac bone is prone to form cold abscess, which tends to cause deep multiple abscess in iliacus intermuscular space, most of which are located in leg ends, hypogastric regions and inguinal regions.

Tuberculosis of pubis and ischium are often manifested as osteolytic bone destruction in unilateral pubic bone or ischium, wherein sequestrum can form locally (Fig. 4.46). Periosteal reaction is common when the disease involves

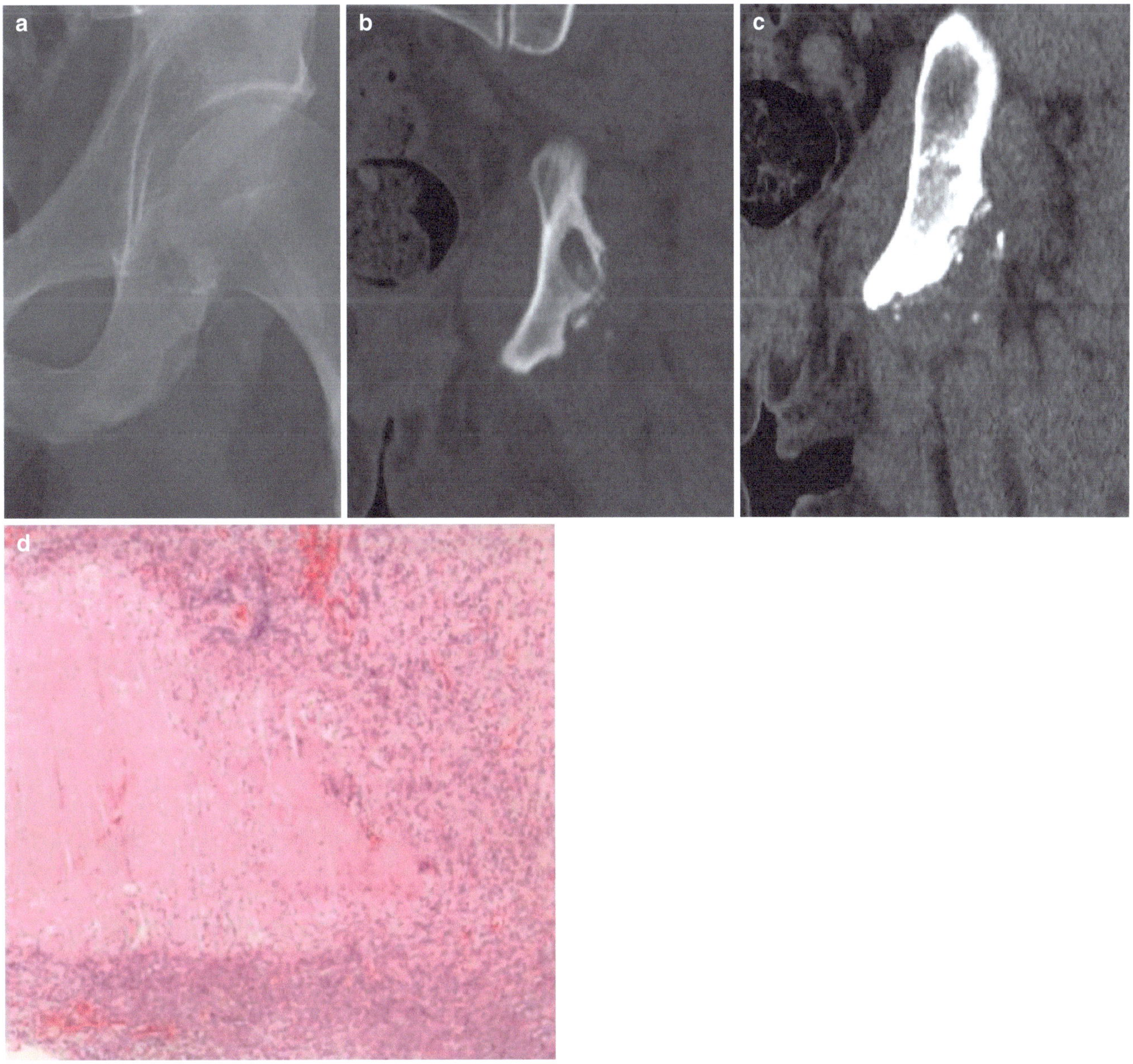

Fig. 4.46 Left tuberculosis of ischium. (**a–c**) In the left ramus of ischium, there is a quasi-oval bone destruction area, which is surrounded by no sclerosis margin, and sand-like sequestrum can be seen therein, with swollen peripheral soft tissues and formation of abscess, in which punctate calcification can be observed; (**d**) It can be seen under the microscope that there is a small amount of inflammatory granulation tissues and focal necroses, scattered multinucleated cells, histiocytes, chronic inflammatory cell infiltration, and formation of focal small abscesses

ramus of pubis and ramus of ischium. The lesion can spread upwards and downwards from body of pubis to pubic branches, crossing the median line, destroying pubic symphysis, and involving the contralateral pubic bone. Tuberculosis of pubic bone forms cold abscess, which can result in deep multiple abscess in inguinal fold or medial thigh along pubic bone and adductor. In severe cases, abscess may appear in scrotum or vagina, forming sinus locally, and discharging light yellow purulent secretions.

Key Points of Diagnosis

Tuberculosis of iliac bone, pubic bone, and ischium is very rare, most common in teenagers, with clinical manifestations of local pain, soreness, and obvious tenderness. Imaging findings mainly show area of osteolytic bone destruction on the iliac bone surface or in unilateral pubic bone and ischium. The lesion is typically localized, with blurred margins, wherein sequestrum can be seen sometimes, which is prone to form swelling of soft tissues, resulting in deep multiple abscess along intermuscular space. Sinus can be formed locally.

Differential Diagnosis

Tuberculosis of iliac bone, pubic bone, and ischium shall be distinguished from osteomyelitis of iliac bone and pubic bone. Osteomyelitis of iliac bone, pubic bone, and ischium is characterized by acute onset, with acute infection symptoms manifested as red, swelling, and heat pain in local area. Despite same manifestation of osteolytic bone destruction in imaging findings, osteomyelitis of iliac bone, pubic bone, and ischium involves more extensively when compared with tuberculosis, and destruction area is often surrounded by obvious hyperostosis and osteosclerosis. Osteomyelitis of pubic bone usually does not extend beyond pubic symphysis, thereby rarely involving contralateral pubic bone.

4.6.3 Joint Tuberculosis

Joint tuberculosis is a common disease. Its incidence is second only to tuberculosis of spine, ranking No. 2 in all the tuberculosis of bone and joint. The disease usually involves a single joint and is divided into two types according to infection routes: (1) Osseous joint tuberculosis. It is caused by tuberculosis of epiphysis and metaphysis adjacent to joint passing through epiphyseal plate to directly encroach on joint, since cartilage cannot block Mycobacterium tuberculosis; (2) Synovial tuberculosis. It is caused by Mycobacterium tuberculosis encroaching on synovial membrane first via blood circulation and then joint; In the advanced stage, obvious destruction appears in both articular tissues and bone ends, manifested as involvement of total joints, which is called total joint involvement. From the perspective of imaging, joint tuberculosis usually develops chronically. In the early stage, imaging finds are mainly characterized in that soft tissues peripheral to joint are swollen, bone destruction first starts from non-bearing parts of joint margins, and joint space stenosis occurs relatively late, wherein the stenosis is typically heterogeneous; affected joint is surrounded by osteoporosis and atrophy of peripheral muscles. In the advanced stage, bony ankylosis does not occur, unless the disease is concurrent with secondary infection.

4.6.3.1 Hip Joint Tuberculosis

The incidence of hip joint tuberculosis ranks first among all the tuberculosis of bone and joint in limbs, among which osseous joint tuberculosis is more common than synovial tuberculosis. The disease occurs frequently in children and teenagers, more common in male than female, and mostly involves unilaterally. No clinical symptom may appear in the early stage. Fall damage and sprain are common predisposing causes. In the later stage, the disease may result in lameness, pain, and limitation of motion. Physical examination shows local percussion pain and swelling in hip joint, accompanied by atrophy of quadriceps femoris sometimes, with positive Thomas signs.

Imaging Findings

1. **X-ray**
   (a) Swelling of soft tissue: X-ray plain film of early hip joint tuberculosis only shows swollen articular capsule, with an increased density and blurred margins. As the disease progresses, soft tissues peripheral to joint become swollen. Besides, atrophy of distal gluteal muscles and upper femur muscles, which is called fusiform swelling, can serve as a valuable sign for reference. In the advanced stage, spot-like calcification may appear in peripheral soft tissue abscess.
   (b) Osteoporosis and bone destruction: Generally, in the early stage (within months or even 1 year) hip joint tuberculosis does not cause bone destruction, only manifested as varying degrees of osteoporosis, mainly characterized in that femoral head, neck and upper third of the femur have gradually worsened osteoporosis. Generally, younger patients may suffer from a more rapid progression and more obvious osteoporosis. As the disease further progresses, localized or diffuse hypointensity bone destruction area starts to appear on the margin of acetabulum, acetabulum is deepened, and bony articular surface of femoral head becomes blurred or has irregular bone destruction area therein (Fig. 4.47).

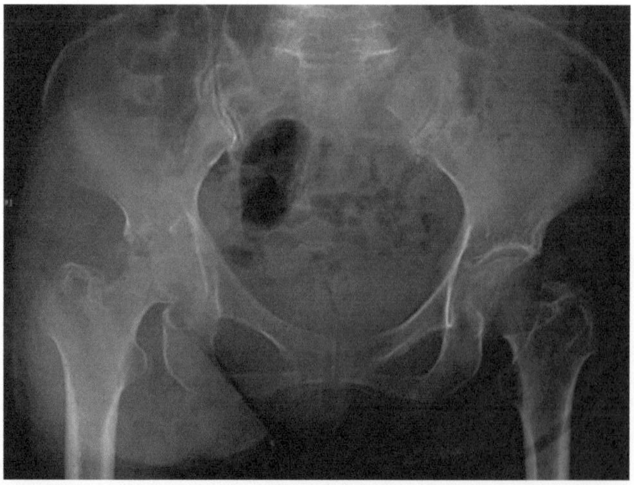

Fig. 4.47 Right hip joint tuberculosis. X-ray shows multiple cystic low-density shadows on margin of right acetabulum and subarticular femoral head, with coarse margins, accompanied by narrowed right hip joint space and obvious swelling of soft tissues peripheral to right hip joint

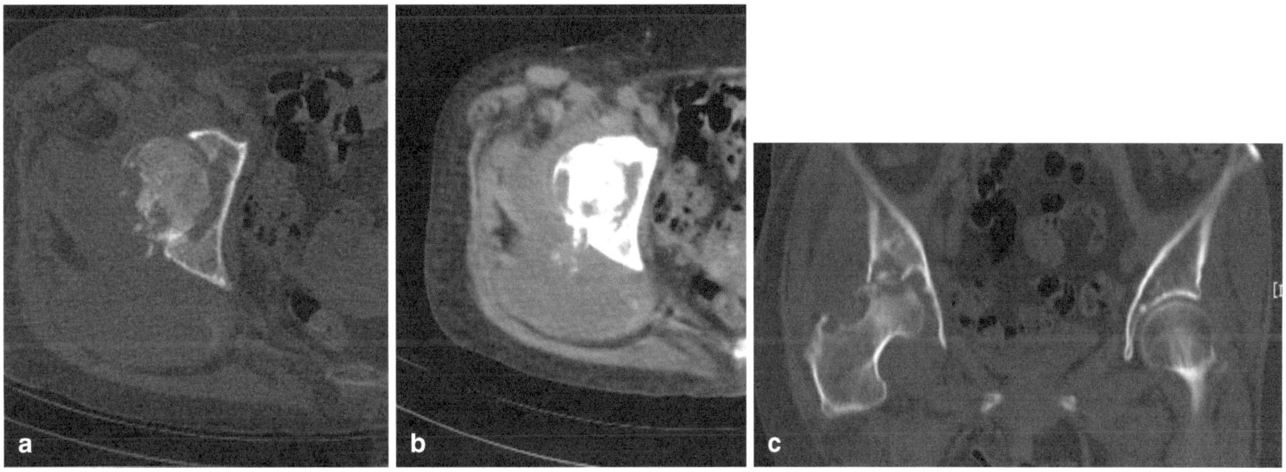

Fig. 4.48 Right hip joint tuberculosis. The same case as Fig. 4.47. (**a**, **b**) CT transverse plane bone window and mediastinum window show cystic bone destruction area in subarticular femoral head and margin of acetabulum, surrounded by no sclerosis margin, wherein sand-like sequestrum can be seen in the destruction area and hip joint spaces appear irregular stenosis; (**c**) CT coronal plane bone window shows right hip joint effusion, and swelling of peripheral soft tissues, in which punctate calcification can be noted

(c) Joint space is widened in the early stage and narrowed in the advanced stage. In the early stage, since X-ray plain film cannot display joint effusion and synovial thickening, the disease is only manifested as widened joint space. As the disease progresses, articular cartilage is destroyed, and heterogeneous narrowing of joint space occurs. In severe cases, articular cartilage, mostly fibrous ankylosis, can happen after the disease is healed.

(d) Joint dislocation or subluxation. In the advanced stage, acetabulum is severely destroyed, margin of acetabulum becomes shallower, and femoral head may shift outward and upward, thus resulting in hip joint dislocation or subluxation.

(e) Hip joint tuberculosis occurring in children can easily cause epiphysis avascular necrosis and epiphysis separation of femoral head, manifested as increased density, irregular shape and dislocation of epiphysis, which may result in joint deformity in the future. Joint deformity caused by hip joint tuberculosis in adults mostly originates from joint tuberculosis occurring in childhood.

2. **CT.** It can clearly display the early articular capsule swelling, joint effusion and pelvic abscess, while is sensitive to sequestrum (Fig. 4.48). Besides, it can provide guidance for puncture treatment and diagnosis of abscess as required.
3. **MRI.** It can show changes in synovial membrane, articular cartilage, articular cartilage, and subchondral bone of the affected joint in a detailed manner. Furthermore, it can analyze pathological components of tissues in articular capsule. In the early stage, MRI of osseous hip joint tuberculosis shows inflammatory infiltrating edema in acetabulum, femoral head epiphysis, and femoral neck bone marrow, with irregular bone destruction focuses, wherein the lesion can spread to joint, resulting in joint effusion and intra-articular and extra-articular abscesses. Synovial hip joint tuberculosis is manifested as remarkably thickened synovial membrane of joints, accompanied by joint effusion, wherein the thickened synovial membrane in articular cavity and granulation tissue show hypointense on T_1WI and heterogeneous intense on T_2WI. Rice-like loose bodies which show heterogeneous hypointense on T_2WI can be noted in joint effusion (Fig. 4.49), pathologically manifested as a mixture of fibrous tissue fragments and caseous necrosis. In case of destroyed articular cartilage, it can be seen that hyperin-

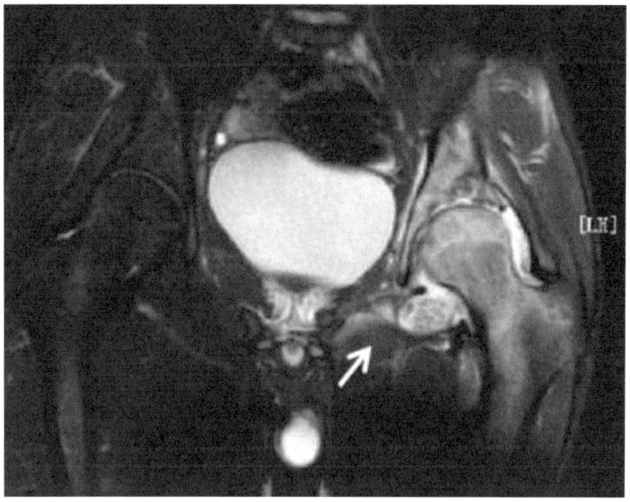

Fig. 4.49 Left hip joint tuberculosis. MRI shows the characteristic "rice body" structure in joint effusion (arrowhead)

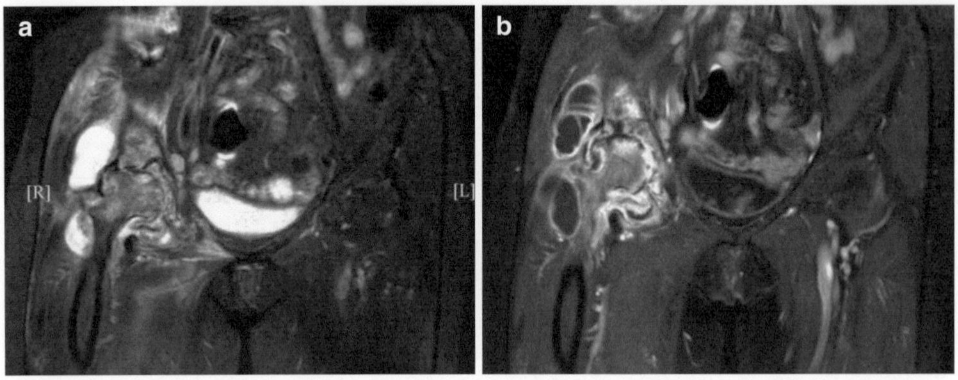

Fig. 4.50 Right hip joint tuberculosis. The same case as Fig. 4.47. (**a**) According to MRI, subarticular right femoral head and margin of acetabulum show multiple, patchy hyperintense shadows on T_2WI fat-suppressed sequence, bone marrow edema appears in adjacent bones, irregular stenosis occurs in right hip joint spaces, with joint effusion and synovial thickening, wherein "rice body" structure can be seen in the effusion, soft tissues peripheral to right hip joint are swollen, and hyperintense abscess area can be observed; (**b**) According to enhanced T_1WI, bones and synovial membrane of right hip show marked enhancement, and peripheral abscess shows rim-like enhancement

tense zone of cartilage becomes thinner and discontinuous, and subchondral bony articular surface is involved, manifested as small, patchy hyperintense shadows inferior to articular surface of affected bones. According to MRI enhanced examination, thickened synovial membrane shows marked enhancement, bursa, and abscess wall peripheral to joint show rim-like enhancement, wherein abscess wall can be both homogeneous and heterogeneous (Fig. 4.50).

Key Points of Diagnosis

1. X-ray shows joint swelling in the early stage. In progressive stage, osteoporosis and bone destruction in acetabulum, femoral head epiphysis, and femoral neck can occur universally. In severe cases, patient may suffer from hip joint dislocation, but sequestrum and hyperostosis and osteosclerosis are rare.
2. MRI shows synovial thickening and joint effusion, wherein the "rice body" structure in articular cavity that shows slightly hypointense on T2WI is characteristic.

Differential Diagnosis

1. **Osteochondrosis of femoral head.** Both are common in children, with similar clinical signs and imaging findings. It is especially difficult to be distinguished from osseous hip joint tuberculosis. Lesions caused by the disease are generally localized in femoral head epiphysis, which may be deformed and defective. Osteoporosis is not obvious. Stenosis usually does not occur in joint spaces, and peripheral soft tissues are not swollen.
2. **Pyogenic coxitis.** It has an acute onset, short course, and large bone destruction area, characterized in that the peripheral hyperostosis and osteosclerosis are obvious, the swelling of peripheral soft tissues is more extensive than tuberculosis, and joint space stenosis can occur in a short time, most of which are homogeneous stenosis. Pyogenic arthritis may cause bony ankylosis in the advanced stage.
3. **Rheumatoid arthritis.** It mostly involves bilateral, symmetric, and multiple joints. In spite of synovial thickening and changes in osteoporosis that are similar to tuberculosis, rheumatoid arthritis causes joint space stenosis earlier, wherein the stenosis is homogeneous, and then encroaches on bony articular surface. A positive rheumatoid factor in laboratory test also contributes to differential diagnosis.

4.6.3.2 Tuberculosis of Knee Joint

Knee joint, the largest and most complicated weight-bearing joint in human body, has the most abundant synovial membranes. Therefore, more than 80% tuberculosis of knee joint are synovial type. The incidence of tuberculosis of knee joint is second only to hip joint, ranking second among tuberculosis of bone and joint in limbs. It is rare in patients below 10 years old, and it has a higher incidence than hip joint tuberculosis in patients above 30 years old. Synovial tuberculosis of knee joint progresses slowly, with a long course and mild clinical symptoms, manifested as painful, swollen joints, and dysfunction. In case of massive joint effusions, ballottement of patella shows positive results. Osseous tuberculosis of knee joint (Fig. 4.51) typically occurs in distal femur and proximal tibia epiphyses and metaphyses. Primary cases in patella are very rare.

Imaging Findings

1. **X-ray and CT.** In the early stage, the disease shows nonspecific manifestations in X-ray and is difficult to be

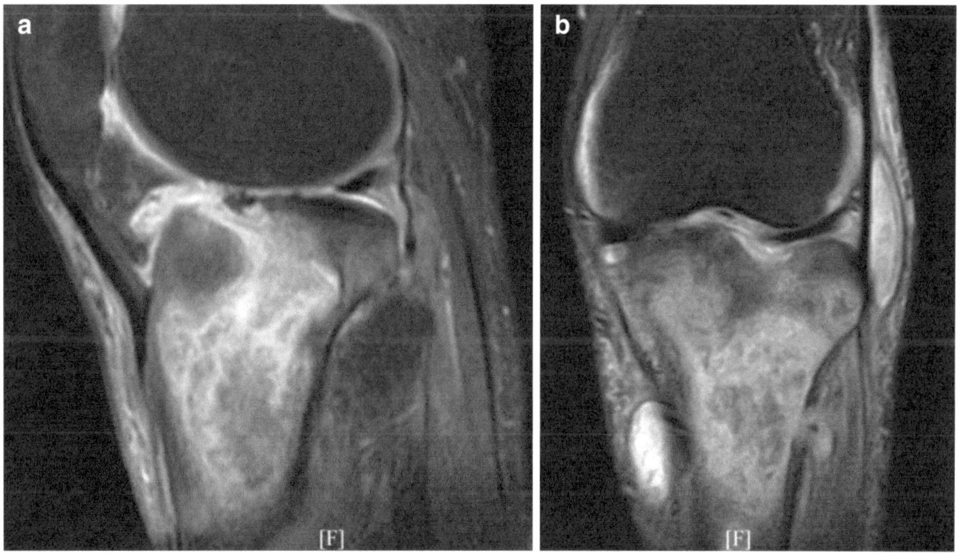

Fig. 4.51 Sinus formed in osseous tuberculosis of knee joint and breaking into joints. According to MRI, proximal tibia shows patchy hyperintense shadows on T_2WI fat-suppressed sequence; sinus forms in local area and breaks into joints; hyperintense shadows appear in knee articular cavity; and soft tissues peripheral to knee joint are swollen

diagnosed. The imaging findings mainly include swelling of articular capsule and joint soft tissues, normal or slightly widened joint space, and osteoporosis in bones which constitute joints. The stage may last long, probably several months and even more than 1 year. As the disease progresses, osteoporosis gradually worsens. Subarticular moth-eaten bone destruction appears, especially in the bones at articular capsule and ligament attachment, resulting in that the non-bearing surface of joint is often involved symmetrically on both upper and lower margins. The lesion area enlarges gradually, forming a quasi-circular bone destruction area, wherein large sequestra can be formed in knee joint and destruction area, most of which are triangular, bottom facing toward articular surface. These sequestra appear symmetrically in both lower and upper articular surfaces, which are called "kissing sequestra" (Fig. 4.52). Swelling of soft tissue becomes worse step by step, accompanied by atrophy in adjacent soft tissues, manifested as the fusiform swelling, a typical sign of joint tuberculosis. Cold abscesses can form around joints and penetrate the skin to form sinus. CT shows effusion in articular cavity. In severe cases, ankylosis may occur in the advanced stage, most of which are fibrous ankylosis. Bony ankylosis may occur when concurrent with pyogenic infection. In childhood, due to synovial hyperemia, epiphysis may be temporarily enlarged or closed in advance.

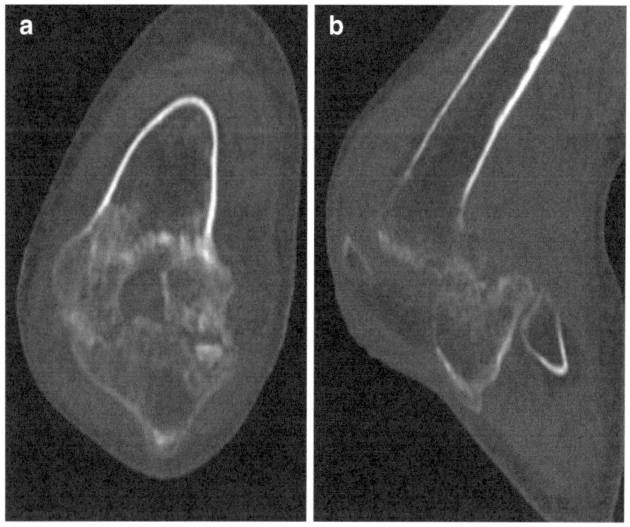

Fig. 4.52 Tuberculosis of knee joint (1). CT shows multiple subarticular quasi-circular bone destruction in distal femur and proximal tibia, wherein block-shaped sequestra can be seen in bone destruction area; upper and lower margins are involved symmetrically, manifested as kissing sequestra; heterogeneous stenosis appears in knee joint spaces and peripheral soft tissues are swollen

2. **MRI.** It especially excels in displaying synovial membrane and subarticular cartilage. Synovial tuberculosis of knee joint is typically manifested as diffuse synovial hyperplasia, wherein the hyperplastic synovial membranes and granulation tissues are mixed together, presenting as twisty strips and blocks, showing hypointense on T_1WI and distinctive slightly hypo/hyper heterogeneous intense on T_2WI (Fig. 4.53). It is generally believed that such a heterogeneous intense may be related to hemorrhage, fibrosis, and caseous necrosis; It can be seen from the sagittal plane that the bursa suprapatellaris is filled with hyperplastic synovial membranes, thus decreasing the normal volume of the bursa suprapatellaris. The hyperplastic synovial tissues show marked enhancement in enhanced scan. Destruction in subarticular cartilage is manifested as coarseness, unevenness, and local thinning and defects on cartilage surface, accompanied by bone marrow edema and bone destruction in sub-

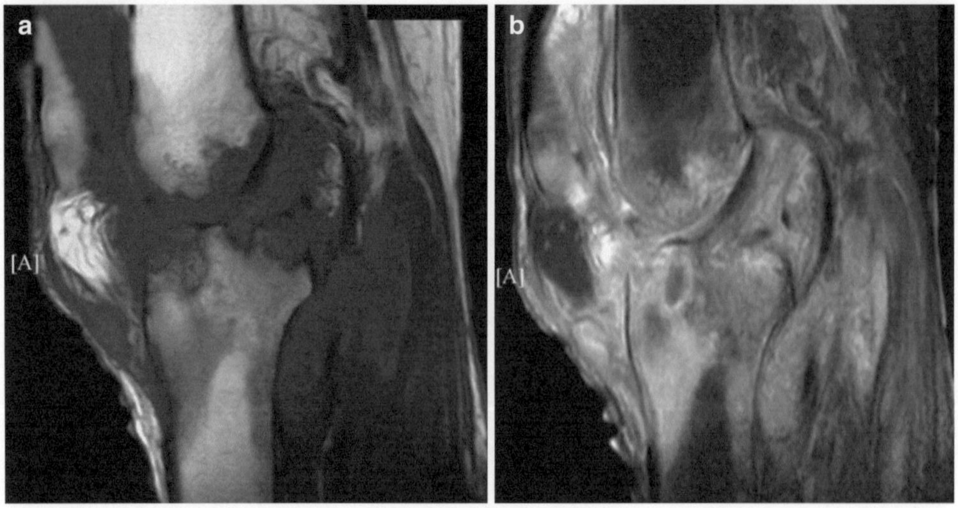

Fig. 4.53 Tuberculosis of knee joint (2). According to MRI, diffuse synovial hyperplasia can be seen in knee joint, showing hypointense on T_1WI and heterogeneous slightly hyperintense shadows on T_2WI fat-suppressed sequence; joint effusion appears and knee joint space is narrowed; subarticular bones are affected

chondral bone, which is best displayed on T_2WI fat-suppressed sequence, showing hyperintense. MRI can also show the damage to cruciate ligament and meniscus by the disease.

Key Points of Diagnosis

1. Early X-ray shows fusiform swelling of joint, osteoporosis peripheral to joint and bone destruction in non-bearing articular surface.

2. According to MRI, synovial thickening shows heterogeneous intense on T_2WI. The hyperplastic synovial membranes and granulation tissues in joints show marked enhancement in enhanced scan, while effusion shows no enhancement, thus forming a sharp contrast.

Differential Diagnosis

1. Pigmented villonodular synovitis occurs frequently in knee joint and ankle joint, mainly involving joint synovium, bursa, and tendinous sheath. Clinical manifestations are mainly pain and swelling of the affected joints, with palpable masses around the joints. Articular puncture fluid shows chocolate color. MRI is the most sensitive to the disease, with certain specificity. MRI findings include extensive synovial hyperplasia, accompanied by massive effusions. Due to repeated bleeding, the hyperplastic synovial membrane shows hypointense hemosiderin deposition on both T_1WI and T_2WI.
2. **Degenerative osteoarthrosis.** It refers to a group of non-inflammatory lesions, which is common in the middle-aged and elderly people, characterized by articular cartilage degeneration in large weight-bearing joints and new bones formed on articular surfaces and their margins. Degenerative osteoarthrosis causes obvious hyperostosis, accompanied by joint effusion and cystic changes at ligament attachment, with non-obvious edema. Peripheral soft tissues are not swollen.
3. **Pyogenic arthritis.** It is difficult to distinguish the disease solely by imaging findings, and medical history shall be combined. Pyogenic arthritis is characterized by acute onset and fast development, which can cause joint space stenosis within a few days. In addition, bone destruction mostly occurs on the weight-bearing articular surface, peripheral soft tissues show diffuse swelling, no muscle atrophy appears in the peripheral area, and bony ankylosis occurs in the advanced stage.

Status Quo and Progress of Research

1. **DWI.** The application of DWI in the diagnosis of tuberculosis of bone and joint has been gradually recognized. As an imaging technology sensitive to the motion of water molecules, it can provide information at molecular level in a quantitative manner for diagnosis. Quantitative analysis can be performed by measuring ADC values. Studies [90] show that ADC values of abscess in spinal tuberculosis vertebral body and paravertebral abscess are higher than that of normal vertebral body, which can help diagnose the atypical spinal tuberculosis. Besides, ADC value can be used as a monitoring indicator during spinal tuberculosis treatment, wherein the ADC value of vertebral body decreases after treatment and approaches normal level during recovery stage.
2. **^{18}F-FDG.** It is a glucose analogue absorbed by inflammatory and tumor cells such as neutrophils, lymphocytes, and macrophages. Inflammation and granulation tissues have enhanced glucose metabolism and permeability, with more glucose transporters, thus increasing the FDG uptaking. For this reason, ^{18}F-FDG PET/CT metabolism imaging can be properly used in the detec-

tion of inflammation in the early stage of the disease. Despite lesions in bones and joints, PET/CT, as a systemic imaging technique, can also detect lesions in other tissues and organs. According to PET/CT imaging, bone tuberculosis focus has heterogeneous glucose uptake, showing ring-like glucose uptake increase in local area. This can be used to distinguish the bone tuberculosis focus from metastasis of malignant bone tumor [91]. In addition, PET/CT can be used to monitor the efficacy of anti-tuberculosis treatment in patients suffering from tuberculosis of bone and joint.

3. **Application of molecular, microbiological, and immunological detection in diagnosis of tuberculosis of bone and joint.** The gold standard for diagnosis of human tuberculosis is to detect Mycobacterium tuberculosis via microbiological ways. However, it may take several weeks to obtain positive results by traditional solid and liquid culture. To this end, fast and sensitive laboratory testing techniques must be developed to assist in clinical diagnosis. Combination of IGRA and Xpert MTB/RIF provides a sensitivity of 91.9% for the diagnosis of tuberculosis of bone and joint, higher than the sensitivity provided by IGRA or Xpert MTB/RIF alone, which is 81.4% and 70.9%, respectively. Furthermore, TNF-α and TGF-β are essential for protective immune responses and anaphylaxis and are closely related to the damage and repair of bone joint tissues. Studies show that patients with tuberculosis of bone and joint have TNF-α and TGF-β levels higher than control groups. In proliferative lesion group, expressions of TNF-α and TGF-β are positively correlated, and expression of TNF-α in this group is significantly higher than that in the caseous necrosis group ($P < 0.01$). In caseous necrosis focus group, expressions of TNF-α and TGF-β are negatively correlated, wherein expression of TGF-β in this group is remarkably higher than that in proliferative lesion group ($P < 0.001$) [86].

4.7 Echinococcosis of Bones and Joints

Hongjun Fu and Ping Wang

Overview

Echinococcosis, also known as hydatid disease, is a zoonosis in which the larva of echinococcus multilocularis parasites on human tissues and organs, thus resulting in damage therein. Echinococcosis is widespread around the world, existing on all continents except Antarctica and can spread across the Arctic, temperate, and tropical regions. It exists in northern and northwestern China, certain regions of South America, East Africa, Australia, Central Asia, the Mediterranean coast, Russia, and Western Europe [92]. Echinococcosis can occur in almost all parts of the body, among which liver (50%–77%) and lung (8.5%–43%) have the highest incidence. The incidence of bone hydatid disease is low, accounting for 0.5%–4% of the total reported cases. The bone hydatid disease is most common in spine (35–50%), pelvis (21%) and long bones, including femur (16%) and tibia (10%). Besides, it is uncommon in distal rib, skull, scapula, humerus, and fibula (2%–6%) [93–95]. Bone hydatid disease progresses slowly, with a long incubation period, typically lacking clinical symptoms during a very long time. Many patients who have been infected since childhood have no symptoms until 10–20 years later. The average age at diagnosis is 50–60 years old, and men are slightly more susceptible than women [96]. Missed diagnosis and misdiagnosis are quite common for bone hydatid disease, especially in non-epidemic region. Early diagnosis is difficult, and the disease usually cannot be detected until pathologic fracture or secondary infection occurs.

Hydatid cyst can be divided into different species, among which Echinococcus granulosus and alveolar echinococcus (Echinococcus multilocularis) parasitize in human body. Echinococcus granulosus is the most common pathogen that causes human echinococcosis [13]. Throughout the life cycle of Echinococcus granulosus, human are occasional hosts, and carnivores such as dog and wolf are definitive hosts. The adult parasite lives in the proximal small bowel of definitive host and is attached to the intestinal mucosa by hooks. It is 2–7 mm long small and thin body consists of scolex, neck, immature proglottid, mature proglottid, and gravid proglottid, where the gravid proglottid takes up about 1/2 of the body. The uterus in gravid proglottid is full of slightly round eggs, with each egg containing an oncosphere. Eggs are released to the host's intestinal tract and passed out in the feces, polluting the land. Sheep are the most common intermediate hosts. They ingest the eggs together with the grass on the polluted lands, then these eggs hatch into oncospheres under the action of digestive juice in the stomach or duodenum, and finally these oncospheres enter the portal circulation via the intestinal wall and then the liver before developing into saccate hydatids. Once the definitive host (such as a domestic dog) eats the internal organs of an intermediate host, the scolex inside the cyst will develop into an adult in the domestic dog's small intestine 3–10 weeks later, completing the cycle [14]. Human beings are possible to become intermediate hosts by touching a definitive host or ingesting polluted water or vegetables.

Hydatids grow slowly. They could grow up to about 1 cm after 5 weeks since entering the human body and then at an annual rate of 1–5 cm. Hydatids can live in the human body for years or tens of years. The cyst wall of hydatid consists of inner and outer layers. The inner layer, as the germinal layer and also known as germ layer, has the multiplication capacity. The outer layer, as the cuticle layer, can protect the germinal layer and absorb nutrients. Cells at germinal layer can bud inwards and form numerous bulges, which gradually develop into brood capsules. After shedding, the germinal cysts become daughter cysts, in which several scoleces can be generated, called protoscolex. Protoscolex breaks the cyst wall and enters into the cyst fluid, which is called cyst sand. Having the same structure as the hydatid (mother cyst), the daughter cyst can develop into a brood capsule again and then a granddaughter cyst after shedding [97]. An old echinococcus cyst can contain hundreds of daughter cysts. Cyst fluid, derived from the host's blood, has antigenicity and can cause the allergic reaction of peripheral tissues after the rupture of echinococcus cyst.

The specific antibody against echinococcosis can be tested by methods such as intracutaneous test for hydatid (Casoni test), indirect hemagglutination (IHA) test, counter immunoelectrophoresis (CIEP), ELISA and gold-labeled antibody (GAB). The Casoni test, IHA, and CIEP are called the three indexes of hydatid test. The relatively accurate and common method is eight indexes of hydatid test, which combines the gold-labeled antibody detection method and ELISA to measure the EgCF, EgP, cystic fluid semi-purified antigen B(EgB) in patients, 4 alveolar hydatid antibodies (Ėm2) suggesting the alveolar hydatid infection, as well as specific antigens and antibodies to the hydatid, showing good sensitivity and specificity [98].

The bone hydatid disease develops slowly and shows insidious clinical symptoms at the early stage. The patient usually goes to the doctor for local limb swelling, ache, or pathologic fracture. The bone hydatid disease involving the spine may show the symptoms of nervous system damage, such as severe backache, hypesthesia, weak lower limbs, paraplegia, and gatism, which may be worsened by fatigue or trauma. The bone hydatid disease involving tubular bones of arms and legs may show symptoms such as mass and sinus at the early stage as well as limp, limb deformity, and limb shortening at the advanced stage.

Pathophysiology

Different from the bone hydatid disease involving soft tissues pathologically, the bone hydatid disease involving bone features exogeneity due to the echinococcus cyst in the bone lacking a reactive fibrous capsule barrier, able to invade and damage the tissue as the tumor does. The Echinococcus granulosus initially lives in the spongy bone. Hard and dense osseous tissues constrain and impede the growth of cyst, preventing it from developing into a big cyst-like hepatic echinococcosis and pulmonary echinococcosis. The lesion extends in the direction of small resistance by spreading along the weak point of Haversian canal, bone marrow cavity, or osseous substance to form a multilocular follicular encapsulation. As time goes on, the cyst keeps growing and its internal pressure rises, resulting that the endocyst ruptures automatically. The leaked cyst fluid invades the osseous substance, resulting in bone destruction. The cyst develops from a spongiform hollow skeleton to a botryoid one and then a fishnet-like one. The parasite reaches and destroys the bone cortex, which may be complicated by the pathologic fracture or dislocation. Subsequently, the lesion spreads toward surrounding soft tissues to form secondary echinococcus cyst of soft tissues. Compared with extraosseous cyst that can be calcified, intraosseous cyst is seldom calcified.

Imaging Findings

1. **X-ray and CT.** It's difficult to use X-ray for diagnosis at the early stage due to lack of specificity (Fig. 4.54). The lesion is mild and occurs within a limited scope at the early stage. It develops from the spongy bone to surrounding areas and then to the bone cortex. The lesion is manifested as osteoporosis and irregular bone absorption. Then it destroys the bone trabecula, forming small round

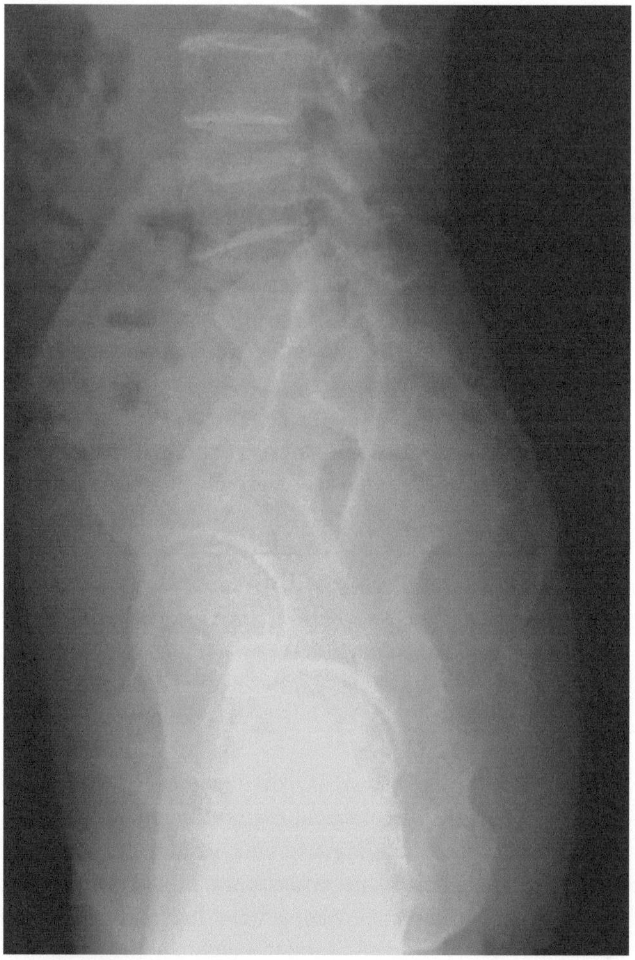

Fig. 4.54 Sacral echinococcosis (1). The X-ray image shows uneven density of sacral osseous substance, multiple utricular low-density shadows and slight expansive changes

cystic low-density areas as well as sharp margins of destruction areas. The cyst walls of some patients may show arc calcification, multiple cysts connected, and botryoid shape. The lesion develops in an increasingly big scope at middle and advanced stages, with foci growing and increasing. It's manifested as multiple cystic bone destruction areas of different sizes, with some foci containing visible ridges. The lesion can expand to compress and thin the bone cortex. There is no reactive hyperostosis, sequestrum, or periosteal reaction around. The lesion expands more significantly if occurring at the flat bone. Once becoming severe, such lesion may break through the bone cortex, invade soft tissues and cause pathologic fracture, but doesn't invade joints. The lesion occurring to the spine doesn't tend to invade the intervertebral disc either. CT can show details better than X-ray (Fig. 4.55). In addition to cystic lesions, the arc calcification of daughter cyst and cyst wall can also be displayed by CT. Some scholars believe that bilayer arc calcification is one of typical CT findings of echinococcus cyst [99].

2. **MRI.** In all imaging examination methods, MRI has the highest diagnosis value due to its characteristics. The multilocular cyst with hypointense on T_1WI and hyperintense on T_2WI is one of the features of bone hydatid disease, and the destruction area has smooth and sharp margins. The intensity of mother cyst signal is higher than that of the daughter cyst signal on T_1WI but lower than that of the daughter cyst signal on T_2WI, which is another feature (Fig. 4.56). In reference to the intensity of muscle signal, the mother cyst signal is close to the muscle signal on T_1WI, while the intensity of daughter cyst signal is similar to that of water signal. Daughter cysts are distributed surrounding the mother cyst or fill up the mother cyst. A false interval is formed between mother and daughter cysts so that the entire focus can be in the shape of a wheel [92, 100]. The cyst wall shows an even and continuous hypointense ring with smooth margins, which is especially clear on T_2WI and enhanced scan image. After rupturing and collapsing, the echinococcus cyst may deform, and has irregular margins as well as separate endocyst and ectocyst. Once co-infection, signals generally become stronger and cyst margins blur.

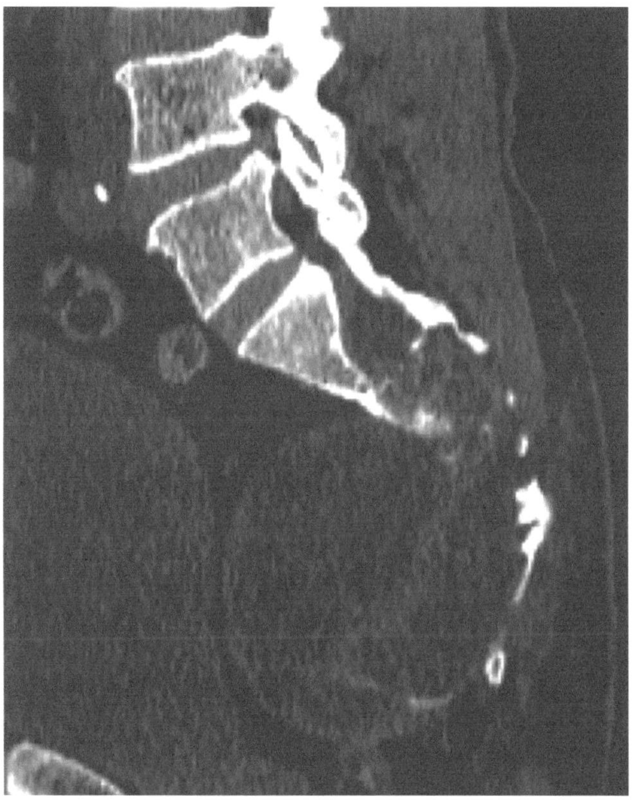

Fig. 4.55 Sacral echinococcosis (2). From the same case as Fig. 4.54. Compared with X-ray image, the CT image can clearly show multiple utricular bone destruction areas, cystic lesions developing toward surrounding soft tissues, as well as mother and daughter cysts

Key Points of Diagnosis

1. The disease mostly occurs in pastoral areas. The patients with the disease have a clear history of close contact with dogs, cows, and sheep or eating raw meat.
2. The disease has a long course that is calculated in years. Most confirmed cases of such disease have been infected as early as in their childhoods.
3. According to X-ray and CT scan images, the multisaccular and expansive bone destruction area originated in the spongy bone can be botryoid. The bone cortex is compressed and becomes thinner. There is no reactive hyperostosis, periosteal reaction, or sequestrum, but possibly complicated by pathologic fracture. It can invade surrounding soft tissues and form echinococcus cysts in them, but usually doesn't invade joints. The cyst wall can be calcified.
4. MRI findings are characteristics to some extent. For multilocular cyst with hypointense on T_1WI and hyperintense on T_2WI, the intensity of mother cyst signal is higher than that of daughter cyst signal as shown on T_1WI but lower than that of daughter cyst signal as shown on T_2WI. Daughter cysts fill up the mother cyst or are distributed surrounding the mother cyst to form the shape of a wheel. It's surrounded by continuous linear hypointense ectocysts.
5. The positive results of Casoni test, IHA, and CIEP as well as EgCF, EgP, B (EgB) and Em2 tests of hydatid by GAB and ELISA can be used to help diagnosis of the disease.
6. In human body, the echinococcosis is the most likely to involve the liver followed by lungs, while the bone hydatid disease is rare. Therefore, in case of any multisaccular focus found in the body of a patient with hepatic bone

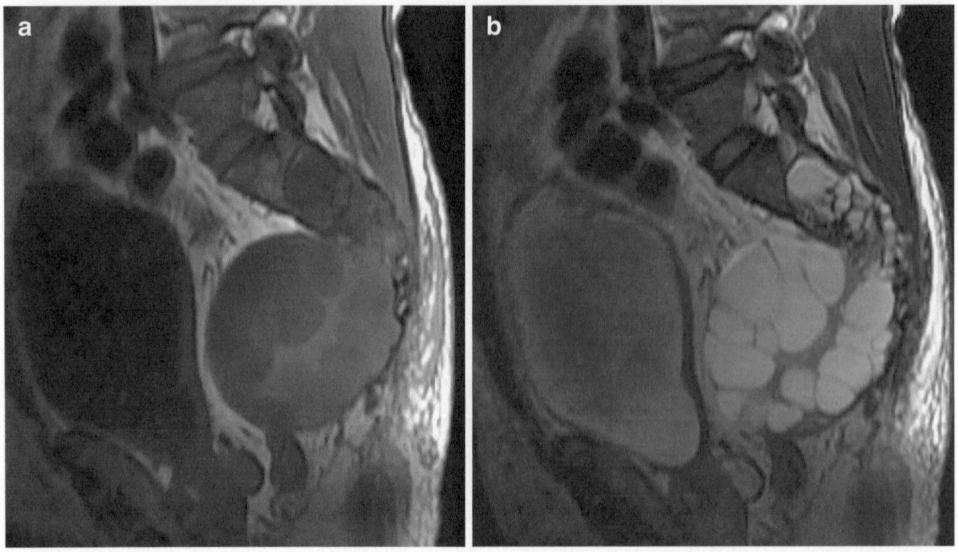

Fig. 4.56 Sacral echinococcosis (3). From the same case as Fig. 4.54. (**a**) As an MRI T_1WI, shows that daughter cysts are distributed around the mother cyst in echinococcus cyst, and that the intensity of daughter cyst signal is lower than that of mother cyst signal. (**b**) As a T_2WI, shows that the intensity of daughter cyst signal is higher than that of mother cyst signal, and that a false interval is formed between daughter and mother cysts so that the entire focus can be in the shape of a wheel.

hydatid disease and pulmonary bone hydatid disease, the possibility of bone hydatid disease shall be highly suspected.

Differential Diagnosis

1. **Bone cyst.** Most confirmed cases of bone cyst are teenagers below 20 years old. The disease usually shows no clinical symptom. It's discovered in PE or when pathologic fracture occurs. As shown in the X-ray image, bone cyst is a quasi-circular bright area with clear border, and the long diameter is consistent with the long axis of diaphysis. However, bone cyst is usually a single cyst without any daughter cyst. It shows isointense on MRI T_1WI and hyperintense on T_2WI, with no hypointense ectocyst at the margin.
2. **Giant cell tumor of bone.** Most confirmed cases of giant cell tumor of bone are young and middle-aged people of 20–40 years old. The giant cell tumor of bone is mostly found at the epiphysis of long bone. It features eccentric and expansive bone destruction as well as typical "soap-bubble" changes in fibrous bone space. The boundary between bone destruction area and normal bone area is clear, with rare sclerotic edge. The long diameter of the focus is vertical to the long axis of the diaphysis. The osseous echinococcus cyst develops in the direction of minimum resistance in the bone. It usually extends from metaphysis to diaphysis. The cystic destruction area is irregular in shape. The giant cell tumor of bone shows isointense on MRI T_1WI, while isointense or hyperintense on T_2WI.
3. **Bone tuberculosis.** The disease is mostly found among teenagers. Patients may have tuberculosis poisoning symptoms such as low fever, night sweats, and weakness. Bones in the lesion area may show quasi-circular moth-eaten bone destruction. Areas surrounding the destruction area are free of sclerosis. Sequestrum is usually found in the destruction area, with possible periosteal reaction. The osseous tuberculosis usually breaks through bone end to affect joints, forming joint tuberculosis. The joint space becomes narrower and it's easy to form cold abscess in surrounding soft tissues.
4. **Aneurysmal bone cyst.** The disease usually occurs before the age of 20. Most aneurysmal bone cysts feature longitudinal growth. It's dominated by eccentric and highly expansive bone destruction of long bone. The boundary between destruction area and normal bone is clear, with sclerosis edges of even thickness visible. Osseous intervals of different thicknesses can be seen in it, and there is usually no surrounding soft tissues affected. CT or MRI examination results usually show many fluid–fluid levels of different sizes as well as diverticulum-like swelling.

Status Quo and Progress of Research

1. **Magnetic resonance hydrography (MRH)**. MRH takes advantage of long water relaxation value, the heavy T_2WI sequence with a long TE, nearly all transverse magnetization vector of other tissues attenuating to show hypointense or no signal, and only tissues containing water able to develop images. MRH features a slice thickness of 0.75–1.50 mm, making it easier to find small focuses than conventional MR sequence. According to the research on alveolar echinococcosis conducted by Wang Jian et al. [101] by MRH, the examination sensitivity of MRH to alveolar echinococcosis focus is 84.38% ± 0.03%, higher than 53.13% ± 0.04% of the conventional MR sequence.

However, the specificity of MRH is lower than that of the conventional MR sequence. Therefore, it's recommended to diagnose alveolar echinococcosis by combining the conventional MR sequence and the MRH sequence so as to ensure both specificity and sensitivity, improving the diagnosis rate.

2. **PCR.** The occurrence of DNA technology, especially PCR technology, provides another method for the definitive diagnosis of Echinococcus granulosus. There are many antigenic substances in the body of Echinococcus granulosus, resulting in complex antigens and that cross reaction is easy to occur. In addition, different periods of the life cycle feature different specific antigens, influencing the sensitivity and specificity of immunologic test results to some extent. The PCR technology can be used to quickly and effectively determine the genotype of Echinococcus granulosus at the gene level, important for diagnosis, treatment, prevention, control, and vaccine research of echinococcosis.

4.8 Pyogenic Arthritis

Hongjun Fu and Liwei Xie

Overview

Pyogenic arthritis refers to the pyogenic inflammation of joints caused by pyogenic bacterium infecting the synovial membrane. It usually presents with acute destructive arthritis. The pathogens can also be fungi or mycobacteria. The disease can occur at any age, but is mostly found among children and babies. It's extremely easy to cause pyemia. The lesion may involve any joint, especially large bearing joints. It's usually accompanied by joint dislocation. It's most common for knee joint and hip joint to be affected by the disease. The disease occurs mostly at simple joints, occasionally also at many joints simultaneously. The multi-joint pyogenic arthritis is most often found in patients with rheumatoid arthritis (RA) or other systematic connective tissue diseases as well as extremely severe sepsis. Early diagnosis and early treatment are essential for the recovery of patients and to keep joint functions.

The same as osteomyelitis, the disease also has three routes of infection: blood infection, direct infection after trauma or puncture, and adjacent soft tissue infection or direct extension of osteomyelitis. The latter isn't unusual in clinical diagnosis. The primary suppurative osteomyelitis focus at the metaphysis runs through the epiphyseal plate, able to involve the subchondral bone of joint and the articular cavity, or the inflammation directly affects joints (such as shoulder joint and hip joint) via the anatomical neck. Its manifestations include acute suppurative osteomyelitis and pyogenic arthritis, both of which occur simultaneously. The extremely destructive pus can destruct affected bones, cartilages, and other accessory tissues at the early stage. Therefore, the pyogenic focus and pus shall be eliminated at the early stage once being found to prevent spreading and relapse. The pyogenic arthritis is usually caused by infection by a single kind of pathogens, but rarely by mixed infection by multiple kinds of pathogens. The disease is usually found in open wound or penetration of joints, direct invasion of enterogenous bacteria, or hematogenous dissemination of the bacteremia caused by multiple kinds of bacteria. Main pathogens include Staphylococcus aureus, streptococcus, Pseudomonas aeruginosa, and meningococcus [3, 102].

Clinical symptoms mainly depend on the lesion location and range as well as especially the type of pathogen. The disease usually occurs acutely. The joint with the disease swells. Surrounding soft tissues show acute inflammation manifestations such as redness, swelling, heat, and pain, as well as systematic toxic symptoms such as chill, fever, and leukocytosis, limiting the joint mobility. For patient with immunodeficiency, the pathogens usually spread to special parts of the body via blood, such as facet joint, sacroiliac joint, acromioclavicular joint, and pubic symphysis [103]. Susceptible factors: old age, diabetes, RA, artificial joint, recent joint operation history, skin infection, drug injection via vein, intemperance, and history of previous corticosteroid injection into the articular cavity. It's reported that about 40% of cases have basic arthropathy. In case of any pyogenic arthritis caused by Staphylococcus aureus, enterococcus or streptococcus without obvious inducement, the possibility of complicated endocarditis shall also be eliminated.

Pathophysiology

The soft tissue swelling caused by pyogenic arthritis is different from general inflammatory reaction and edema. The pus in the articular cavity spreads into adjacent soft tissues, forming abscess in the soft tissues and damaging structures such as ligament, articular capsule, and blood vessel.

1. **Early stage.** At the early stage, which is also called as serous exudate stage, the pathogens enter the joint to cause hyperemia and edema of synovial membrane, leukocyte infiltration, and serous fluid leakage from the articular cavity first. Synovial tissues have no basement membranes serving as their barriers so the pathogens can quickly enter the synovial fluid, causing acute pyogenic arthritis.
2. **Progressive stage.** The disease enters the progressive stage about 1 week after infection. The fluid leaked from the articular cavity is pyogenic. Synovial cell proliferation is obvious. The articular cartilage nearby the lesion is usually normal at the moment, and then the pannus of synovial membrane grows toward the cartilage. Inflammatory cell infiltration can be seen at the surface

layer. Leukocytes decomposition releases a lot of protease and cytokines, able to degrade the cartilage, dissolve, and destruct subchondral bone substances, suppress the chondrogenesis and cause different degrees of articular cartilage injuries. The cartilage usually changes from the attachment point of articular capsule. As the time passes, the change scope expands gradually, chondrocytes degenerate and die, some cartilages fall off, chondrocytes at surface and middle layers gradually die but most of those at the deep layer are still alive. Tissue necrosis can be found in joints. Sometimes neutrophil infiltration can be seen in subarticular bone, some of which can develop to endosseous abscess. The pus destructs the articular cartilage, causing subchondral bone infections and necrosis, erosion and damage of bony articular surface, as well as different degrees of hyperostosis and osteosclerosis.

3. **Healing stage.** The articular capsule becomes fibrosis gradually. Scars form. Granulation tissues form in the articular cavity to cause fibrosis and ossification, resulting in the joint having fibrous ankylosis or bony ankylosis.

The surface components of some germs may play an important role in the occurrence and development of pyogenic arthritis. The adherin of microbial surface components recognizing adhesive matrix molecule (MSCRAMM) can mediate the staphylococci to adhere to the surfaces of intra-articular proteins (such as fibronectin, laminin, elastin, and collagen), hyaluronic acid and artificial joint materials. More and more experiments and clinical evidences show that the Staphylococcus aureus with encoding MSCRAMM gene can cause pyogenic arthritis. The TSST-1 and enterotoxin generated by Staphylococcus aureus can cause strong inflammatory reaction, destruct the articular cartilage, and lead to pyogenic arthritis. For example, animals will have severe arthritis once being infected with the Staphylococcus aureus expressing TSST-1 and enterotoxin, but will have no or just mild arthritis once being infected with the bacterial strain not expressing such toxins. In addition, mice can be inoculated with recombined vaccine against enterotoxin of Staphylococcus aureus to prevent severe arthritis caused by the Staphylococcus containing enterotoxin [104].

The pyogenic arthritis caused by Gram-negative bacillus is mostly found in people with trauma, drug users by intravenous injection, newborns, old people, and patients with immunosuppression. The number of adult cases of the pyogenic arthritis caused by Streptococcus pneumoniae is small but cannot be ignored.

Imaging Findings

1. **X-ray**
   (a) Early stage: There is usually no obvious abnormal change. The articular cavity may be filled with pus 2–3 days after infection, and the articular capsule will be destructed quickly. The pus spill can also invade adjacent bones. The soft tissue swelling surrounding the joint with lesion is similar to the manifestation of acute suppurative osteomyelitis, and diffuse. Its manifestations include unclear boundary, higher density, thick and large strip and reticular interval shadow occurring at the subcutaneous fat layer, as well as intra-muscular fat reposition and blurring. The joint effusion is manifested as enlarged articular capsule. The external fat of articular capsule distends toward both sides, pushing surrounding fat pad to change its position. The joint space becomes wider due to effusion, and joint subluxation may occur in some severe cases (Fig. 4.57a, b).
   (b) Progressive stage: Once the articular cartilage was destructed, joint space stenosis could occur at the early stage. Then blurred, interrupted, eroded, and destructed bony articular surface could be seen. The bearing area of joint was affected first and changed the most significantly (Fig. 4.58). Epiphysitis, periostitis, and metaphysis osteomyelitis may occur in case of severe infection. One to two weeks later, the joint space becomes narrower, and usually an utricular bright area can be seen below the cartilage of the bearing surface of joint, which is the bone destruction focus. As the disease develops, the focus expands, massive bone destruction and sequestrum may occur, and secondary pathological dislocation may be caused. Epiphyseal separation may also occur in case of children. Besides, hyperostosis starts occurring along with the bone destruction. It's manifested as different degrees of hyperostosis and osteosclerosis occurring to surrounding bones of the destruction area. The pus in the joints of some patients may run through the synovial membrane, articular capsule, and skin to form sinus, resulting that it cannot heal for a long time.
   (c) Recovery stage: Local osteoporosis, irregular margins of bone destruction area, and more significant hyperostosis and osteosclerosis can be seen. Various sequel deformities of bones and joints may occur at the advanced stage if the disease isn't cured. Such deformities are manifested as different degrees of abnormal appearances, uneven ossification, structural disorder, epiphysis defect or intamescentia, loss of normal structure of epiphysis, and possible calcification of surrounding soft tissues. Bony ankylosis may occur in case of severe lesion, i.e. joint space and bony articular surface may disappear and the bone trabecula may connect two epiphyses.
2. **CT.** CT examination is better than X-ray examination. It's suitable for examination of some complex joints such

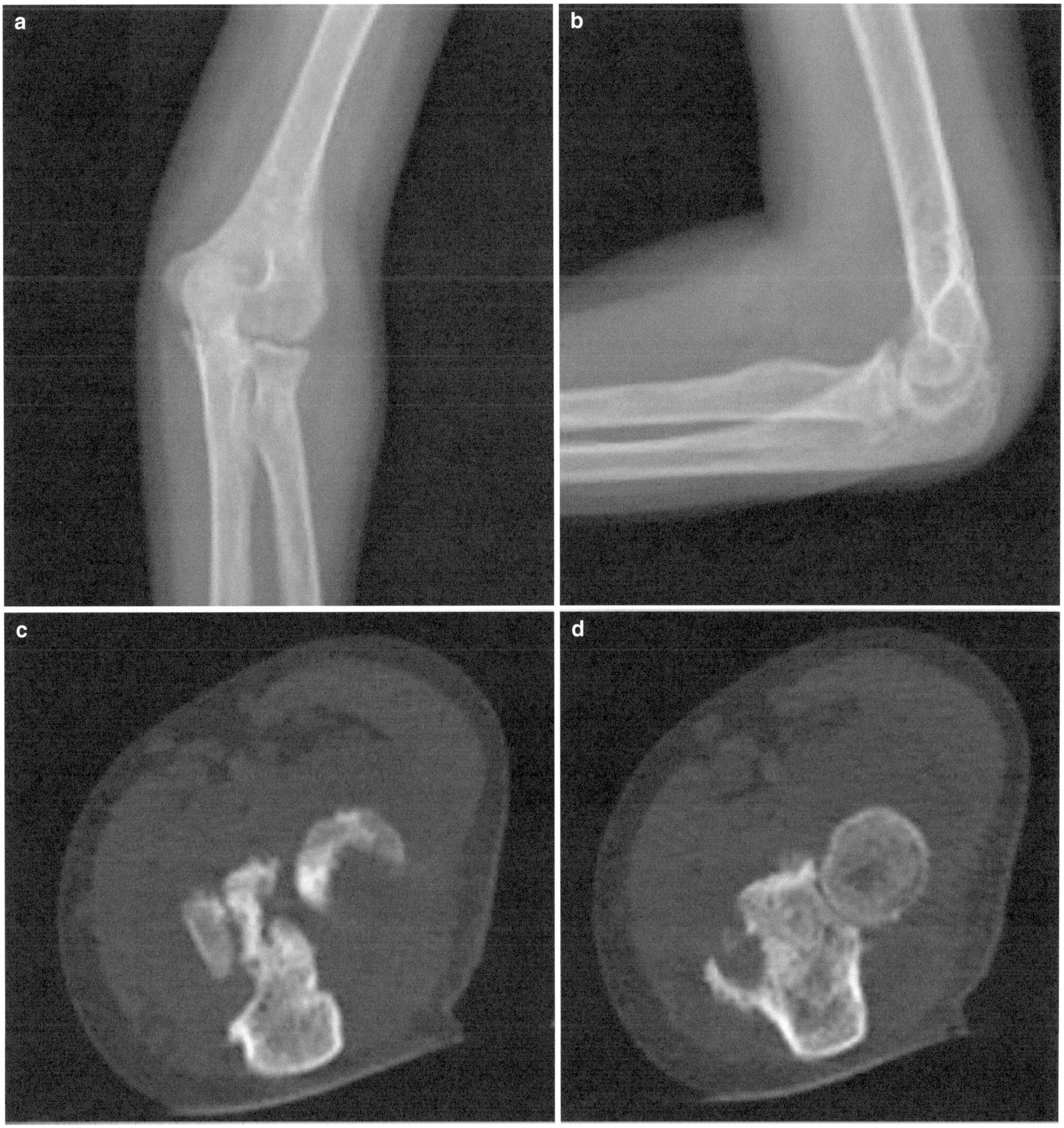

Fig. 4.57 Pyogenic arthritis of left elbow joint. The left elbow joint of a 46-year-old woman ached, swelled, suffered activity limitation and couldn't be stretched after being injured accidentally about 2 years ago. The postoperative pathological diagnosis results showed synovial hyperplasia, interstitial fibrogenesis, vascular proliferation as well as many lymphocyte and plasma cell infiltration, meeting the standard of severe inflammatory changes of synovial membrane. (**a**–**h**) X-ray and CT images show swelling soft tissues surrounding the elbow joint, uneven density, higher subcutaneous fat density, strip shadows, irregular bone destruction areas at the superior extremity of ulna and the head of adjacent radius, many areas of osteolytic bone destruction at the superior extremity of ulna and the inferior extremity of humerus, surrounding hyperostosis and osteosclerosis, soft tissue swelling, and narrower joint space

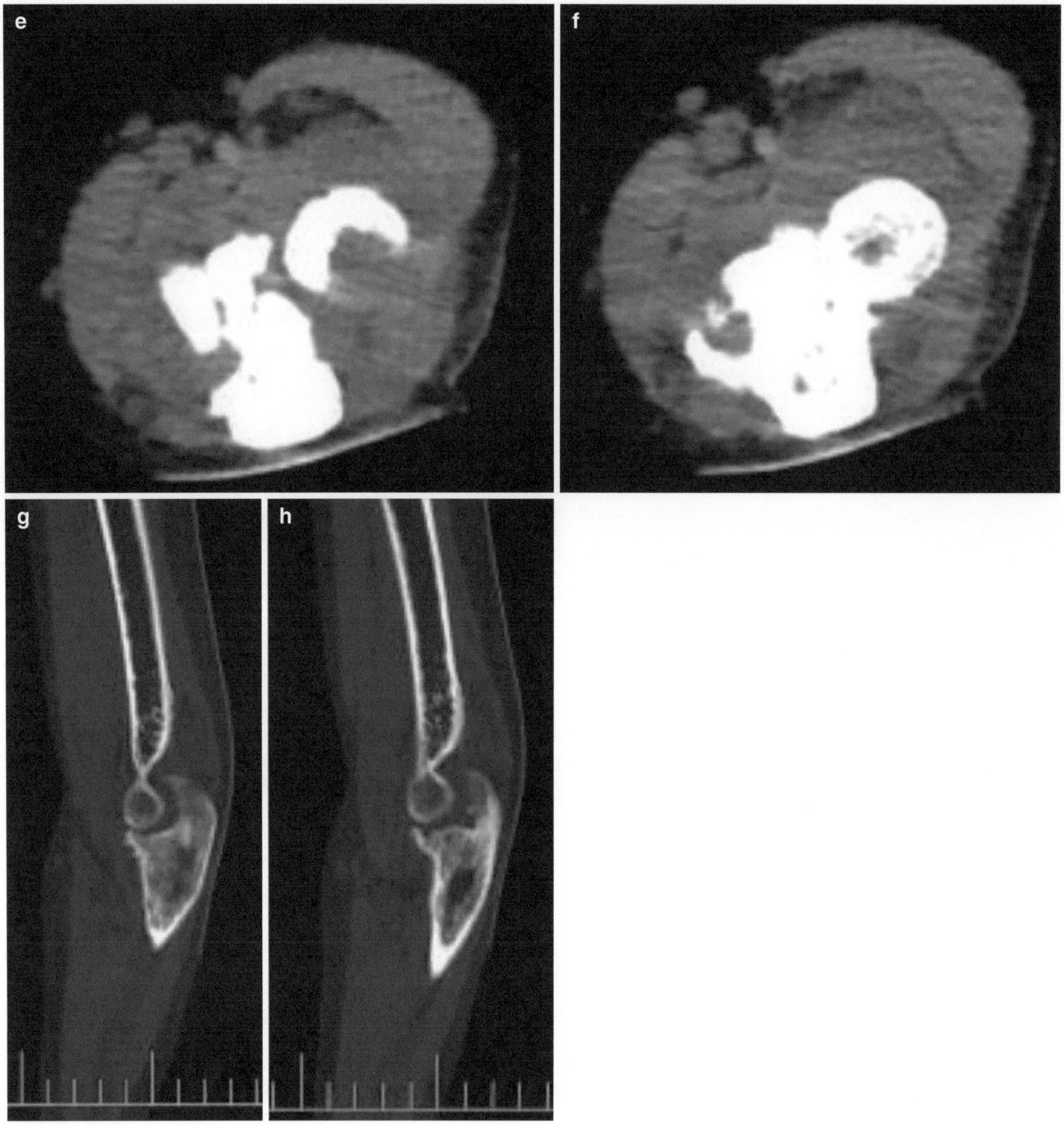

Fig. 4.57 (continued)

as hip joint, shoulder joint, and sacroiliac joint. Abscesses both in and outside joints can be displayed at the acute stage. Its display range of bone destruction and sequestrum, soft tissue swelling and abscess invasion are usually more sensitive than that of X-ray plain film. The soft tissue swelling is manifested as fat and thick muscle surrounding the focus; lower muscle density in the lesion area; higher density, blurring or disappearing of intermuscular fat space; and strip-shaped or grid high-density shadow in subcutaneous fat. Joint space stenosis and joint dislocation and subluxation are clearly displayed on the 3D reconstruction image of coronal plane (Fig. 4.59). The joint effusion is manifested as limited liquid low-density focus in articular cavity and surrounding soft tissues. In addition, it can also be manifested as wider joint space due to joint empyema and joint subluxation. The bone destruction is manifested as rough joint surface, thinner bone cortex, blurred margins, erosive defect, cystic and

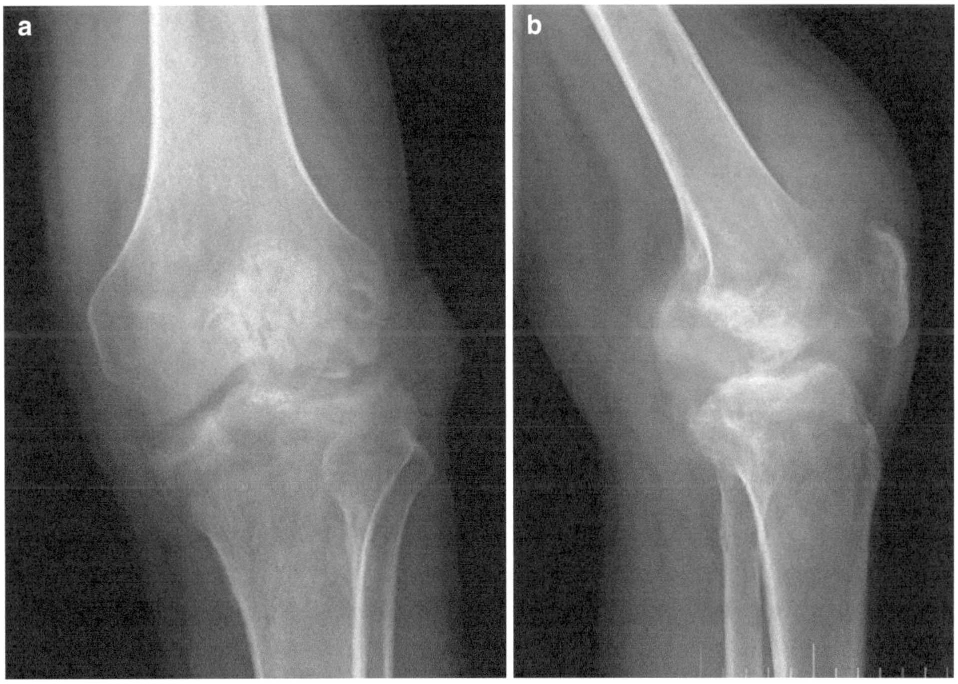

Fig. 4.58 Pyogenic arthritis of left knee joint. X-ray images show many irregular bone destruction areas on the knee joint surface and in adjacent bones, marginal hyperostosis and osteosclerosis, higher density of joint space, swelling surrounding soft tissues, and slightly high density

patchy low-density focus in the subarticular bone, interrupted and disappearing bone trabecula, marginal hyperostosis and osteosclerosis, and osteoporosis surrounding the joint (Figs. 4.57c–h and 4.60a–f). The small sequestrum is manifested as the free high-density shadow located in the vomica, and the large sequestrum contains no bone trabecula structure. The proliferation of synovial membrane and granulation tissue is manifested as visible density shadow of soft tissue in the low-density joint effusion. Especially, contrast-enhanced CT images show the thicker synovial membrane more clearly, and marked enhancement. Occasionally, pneumatosis can be seen in articular capsules or soft tissues.

3. **MRI.** Its soft tissue resolution is obviously higher than that of X-ray and CT. Especially, the enhanced examination by MRI can show the pathologic details of pyogenic arthritis more clearly so as to discover the lesion early. MRI has a high diagnosis value and is the preferred examination method of such disease. However, it's not as clear as CT for observation of the hyperostosis and osteosclerosis at the healing stage. Soft tissues surrounding the lesion joint become thicker. The normal intra-muscular fat space disappears. Normal muscle layers are unclear and have a wide scope. Hypointense is shown on T_1WI, hyperintense on T_2WI, and the fat-suppressed sequence is shown more clearly. The positive rate of effusion in articular cavity can reach up to 100%. It's manifested as hyperintense on T_2WI in the articular cavity. The synovial membrane and proliferous granulation tissues are manifested as mixed signal shadows in the articular cavity as well as marked enhancement after enhancement. The bone destruction area shows that speckle or patchy abnormal signals or those across the bone cortex occur in the bone cortex of extreme hypointense. The surrounding soft tissue abscess is an encapsulated area of hyperintense on T_2WI. The cyst wall is enhanced but the pus is not after Gd-DTPA enhancement (Fig. 4.60g–i). The Charcot's arthritis caused by brain, spinal cord, and peripheral nerve diseases can also cause secondary pyogenic infection of joints. It's usually found among patients with syringomyelia clinically (Fig. 4.60j, k).

In addition, MRI can show the inflammatory reaction of bone marrow. The pathogens have strong invasion ability due to its strong virulence, usually involving adjacent bone marrows. It's manifested as hypointense on T_1WI and hyperintense on T_2WI. However, it's impossible to determine bone marrow edema or osteomyelitis at the moment, requiring regular follow-up. The articular cartilage at the lesion is manifested as diffuse hyperintense on T_2WI first. With the disease develops, the articular cartilage becomes thinner, and the signal becomes heterogeneous gradually. It's manifested as a focal hyperintense on T_2WI, especially the bearing parts.

Key Points of Diagnosis

1. Acute onset, systematic poisoning symptoms, local acute inflammation symptoms, large joints as predilection sites, and obvious swelling and pressing pain at affected parts.
2. Count of leukocytes, neutrophil, and C-reactive protein increase, with a higher erythrocyte sedimentation rate.

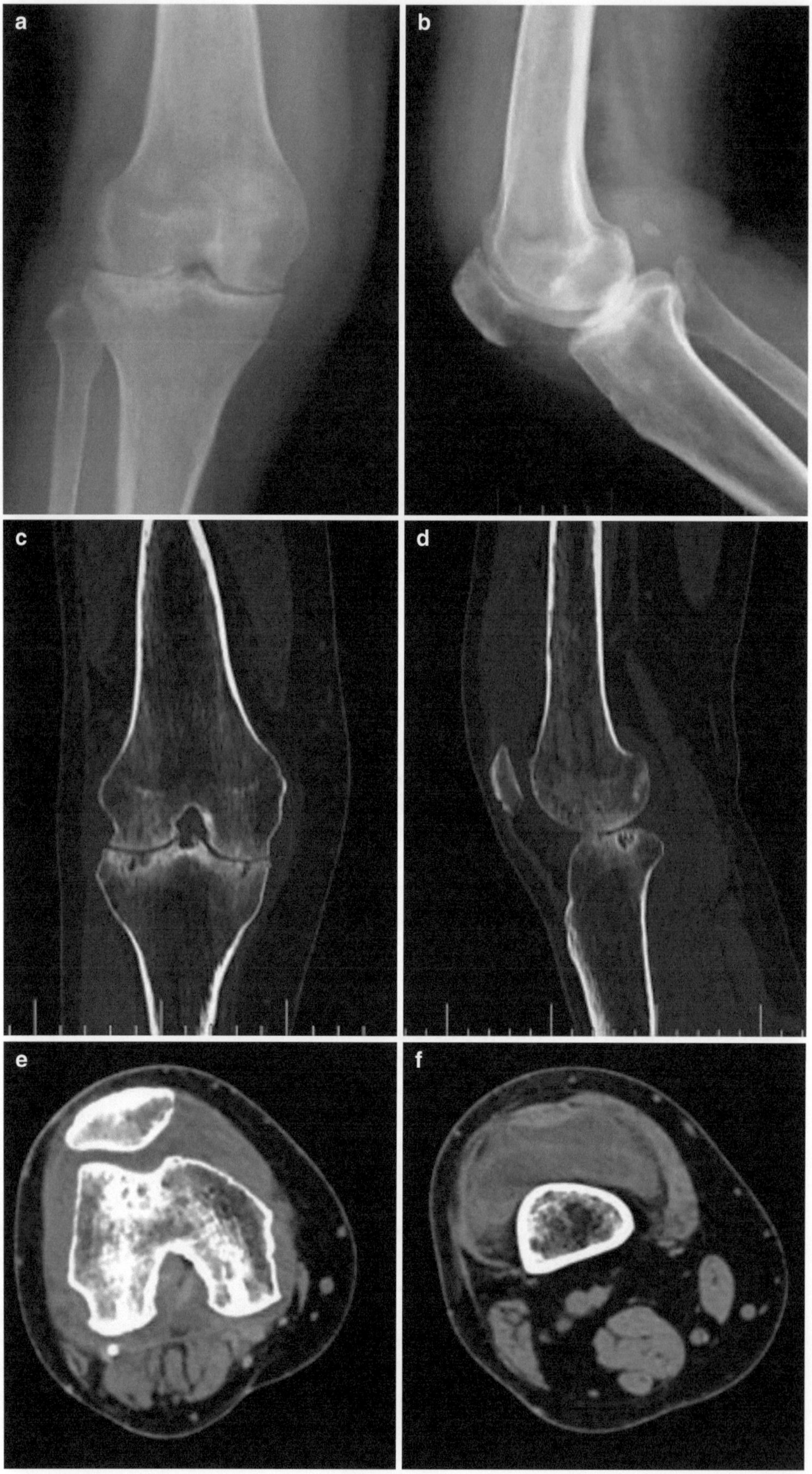

Fig. 4.59 Pyogenic arthritis of right knee joint. (**a**, **b**) As frontal and lateral DR images of right knee, show narrower joint spaces, rough articular surfaces and visible utricular bone destruction areas. (**c**, **d**) As 3D CT reconstruction images of right knee joint, show clearer details, multiple subarticular utricular low-density areas, and visible marginal osteosclerosis ring. (**e**, **f**) Show the effusion in articular capsules

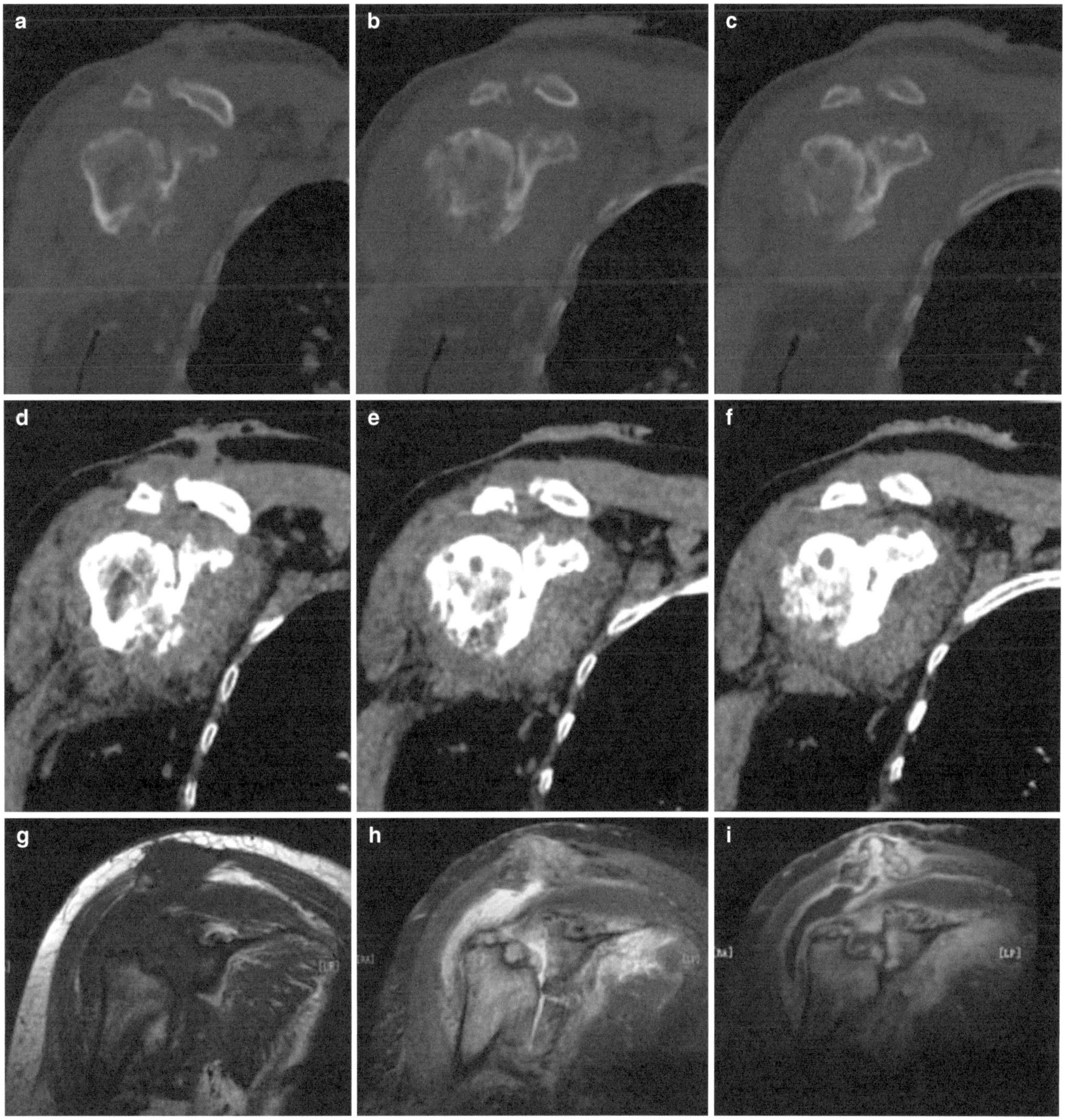

Fig. 4.60 Pyogenic arthritis of right shoulder joint. This case is the secondary pyogenic arthritis of syringomyelia, Charcot's arthritis and joint operation. The blood culture result is Staphylococcus aureus. (**a–c**) As coronal plane reconstruction images of CT bone window, show the glenoid cavity losing its normal form; narrower joint space; slightly flat right humerus head shifting downward; obvious bone destruction, hyperostosis and osteosclerosis; and visible small sequestra. (**d–f**) As coronal plane reconstruction images of CT soft tissue window, show obvious soft tissue swelling around the joint as well as higher density. (**g**, **h**) As MRI images, show a patchy hypointense on T_1WI of humerus head, hyperintense of T_2WI fat-suppressed sequence, articular cartilage injury and destruction, liquid signal shadow visible in the articular cavity, synovial thickening as well as swelling and abscess formation of articular capsule and surrounding soft tissues. (**i**) Shows marked enhancement of right humerus head, its surrounding soft tissues and synovial membrane after MRI enhancement as well as margin enhancement of abscess. (**j**, **k**) As MRI images of cervical vertebra, show visible down movement of tonsil of cerebellum as well as syringomyelia. It's manifested as a bar-type hypointense on T_1WI and hyperintense on T_2WI in the middle of spinal cord

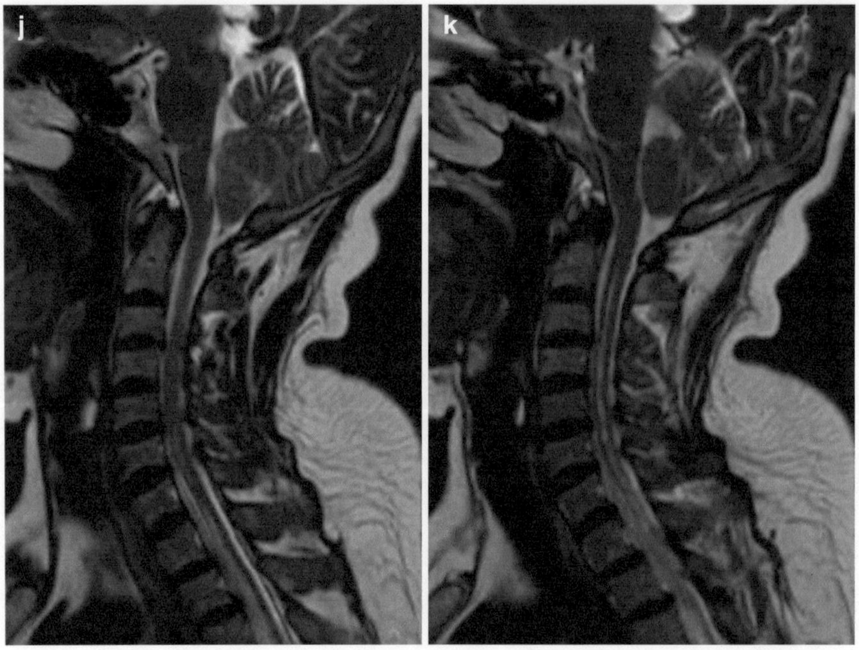

Fig. 4.60 (continued)

3. The X-ray plain film only shows soft tissue swelling surrounding the joint at the early stage. With the disease develops, the joint space becomes wider, the articular surface becomes blurred and interrupted, a subarticular radiolucent area forms, different degrees of proliferation and sclerosis occur in surrounding areas, and symptoms such as joint form change and bony ankylosis can be seen at the later stage.
4. The non-enhanced CT scan image shows the sequestrum in small destruction area and articular cavity well, better than MRI and radionuclide scan ones. In addition, it also shows joint effusion, synovial hyperplasia, and soft tissue swelling clearly.
5. MRI has a diagnosis value at the early stage. It's the preferred examination method of the disease. In terms of display of synovial membrane and exudate, MRI is more sensitive than X-ray plain film and CT. It can define the range of empyema and also show the destruction of joint structures such as articular capsule, ligament, tendon, and cartilage. Especially, it can show the T_2WI fat-suppressed sequence more clearly.
6. The pus is drawn from the joint for microscopic examination, Gram staining, and bacterial culture so as to establish the diagnosis.

Differential Diagnosis

1. **Synovial joint tuberculosis.** Both can have synovitis changes pathologically. However, joint tuberculosis features slow onset, long course of disease, and tuberculosis poisoning symptoms such as low fever and night sweats. Some patients may have a medical history of pulmonary tuberculosis. The disease usually occurs to a single joint and sometimes also to many joints. The synovial joint tuberculosis is manifested as chronic joint swelling, more lymphocytes, fusiform swelling surrounding the joint, and atrophy of adjacent muscle. It can keep normal for a long time before osteoporosis, narrower joint space and bone destruction of non-bearing surface occur several months later. Fibrous ankylosis usually occurs after the disease is cured. The pyogenic arthritis starts acutely and progresses quickly. It features high fever, diffuse swelling, higher level of leukocytes and reactive proteins, and osteoporosis occurring within days. Due to the short course of disease, muscle atrophy isn't obvious, the joint space becomes narrower within a short period, and bone destruction occurs on the bearing surface. Bony ankylosis usually happens after the disease is cured. T_2WI hyperintense change is rare nearby the tuberculous arthritis focus, i.e. there is no obvious bone marrow edema or osteomyelitis change. However, the pyogenic arthritis is on the contrary.
2. **Pigmented villonodular synovitis (PVNS).** The cause to the disease remains unclear. PVNS is mostly found in 20- to 50-year-old people. It usually involves knee joint and hip joint. The disease mainly features synovial nodular or lump-like hyperplasia, bloody effusion in the articular cavity, and hemosiderin deposition. It's complicated by bone destruction and cyst formation. The X-ray image can show many cystic focuses in non-bearing area below

the articular cartilage or beside the joint, clear margin, and thin sclerosis margin. The CT image can show soft tissue masses in the joint and surrounding areas. The hemosiderin is manifested as hypointense on T_2WI, and the MRI signal change of bloody effusion may be different at different blooding times. Joint swelling and bone erosion destruction may also occur. However, due to being chronic diseases, it can be discovered that the involved joint can keep the joint space relatively through long-term observation. Therefore, the disease is different from pyogenic arthritis, and the osteoporosis caused by it isn't obvious.

3. **RA.** RA is a systematic connective tissue disease. The disease starts slowly, most in years. It usually invades small joints such as hands and ankles symmetrically. The disease is usually found in more than one joint. The lesion also begins in synovial membrane. The pannus is formed on the surface of articular cartilage to gradually undermine and absorb the articular cartilage. There is bone erosion or cystic bone defect at joint margins, but the margin is usually sharp and clear. As the disease keeps developing, osteoporosis, subarticular cartilage cystic change, and joint space stenosis may occur; the bone cortex margin of bony articular surface is irregular; and small cystic bone destruction area may occur below the bony articular surface. At the advanced stage, universal osteoporosis and joint subluxation may occur, and fingers may incline toward the ulnar. The pannus and granulation tissue show marked enhancement after Gd-DTPA enhancement. The amount of joint effusion is usually less than that of pyogenic arthritis.
4. **Charcot's arthritis**. Described and named by Charcot in as early as 1868, the disease is mostly found at shoulder joint and usually complicated by syringomyelia or other diseases such as alcohol intoxication, diabetes, and postoperative neuropathy. It's the secondary destructive joint disease of neurosensory disorder and dystrophia, resulting that patients lose their deep sensation of joints, respond slowly to pain, or feel no pain. In this case, patients cannot take protective positions in time, making the joints keep movement and fraction and then causing serious injury. Most common symptoms include swelling, pain, and stiffness as well as joint dislocation. However, the pain isn't severe, and the motion isn't limited usually, not meeting the severity found by imaging examination. Image manifestations include bone destruction, fragmentation, absorption, hyperplasia and bony joint flattening. Some patients may mainly have the pyogenic arthritis clinically. In this case, the disease shall be diagnosed based on the medical history, bone destruction severity of joint and MRI of cervical vertebra comprehensively.
5. **Transient synovitis.** The disease may be relevant with factors such as allergic reaction and trauma. It's self-limited without recurrence. At the early stage, X-ray images show no obvious abnormal change, and CT images only show visible effusion in the articular cavity. MRI manifestations include slight soft tissue swelling surrounding the joint, effusion in the articular cavity, and sometimes effusion in the articular cavity at the normal side.

Status Quo and Progress of Research

MRI has significant diagnosis values and clinical meanings in inflammatory diseases of bone and joint and is usually used as the preferred examination method. It can clearly show the cartilage changes, bone marrow changes, ligament changes, and soft tissue changes that cannot be shown or clearly shown by X-ray plain film and CT. Gd-DTPA is a negatively charged ionic contrast agent. It can change the local magnetic environment of target area and shorten the T_1 relaxation time of tissue within the target area. The granulation tissue and synovial membrane proliferated after enhancement feature marked enhancement [105, 106]. Therefore, MRI, especially contrast-enhanced MRI` examination, can be used to diagnose and evaluate the pyogenic arthritis early so that preventive and treatment measures can be taken at the early stage clinically.

1. The X-ray plain film usually shows no specific sign at the early stage of pyogenic arthritis, with soft tissue swelling surrounding the joint and widened joint space visible sometimes. It shows joint deformity as well as fibrous ankylosis and bony ankylosis clearly at the later stage.
2. Plain CT scan and enhanced CT scan are mainly used to observe the bone structure of joint, soft tissues, and synovial membrane, or for patients with MRI scan contraindication.
3. Plain MRI scan and enhanced MRI examination, as preferred examination methods of pyogenic arthritis, can clearly show not only joint effusion, cartilage and bone destruction but also synovial membrane and granulation tissue. However, the conventional MRI sequence isn't effective in showing the cartilage. The cartilage structure consists of 4 layers histologically, i.e. surface layer, transition layer, radiatum layer, and calcification layer from shallow to deep [107]. Some research results show that T_1-se-cor-water-fil, T_1-flash-3d-water-cor, T_2-me3d-cor, and T_2-me2d-cor are better than the conventional MRI sequence in terms of articular cartilage display, degree of defect, and internal signal [108]. The normal articular cartilage is manifested as band hyperintense relative to the peripheral tissues in 3D-FS-SPGR (a scan technology for continuous thin-slice image scan and MPR, which is free of information loss. The application of fat suppression increases the signal contrast between the cartilage and its adjacent bone marrow, effusion in the articular cavity, fat, and muscle). Therefore, it's easier to observe

the abnormality of cartilage due to the significant contrast with surrounding structures [109, 110].

4.9 Chronic Non-bacterial Osteomyelitis

Liwei Xie and Hongjun Fu

Overview

Chronic non-bacterial osteomyelitis (CNO) is a non-infectious autoimmune inflammatory bone disease. It's manifested as osteodynia caused by recurrent non-bacterial osteomyelitis. The disease broadly refers to the inflammatory disease of bone and joint the pathogen of which cannot be cultured in the blood, bone, and joint. There are three clinical types: ① a single course of disease featuring remission within 6 months; ② persistent course of disease; ③ it's chronic recurrent multifocal osteomyelitis (CRMO) when the disease is recurrent and multiple [111].

CNO/CRMO may be related to multiple autoimmune diseases, which was brought up with by Gideon in 1972 for the first time. The disease can occur at any age and is mostly found in children and teenagers. However, it can last until adulthood. The patient with single symptom and single invasion site is usually misdiagnosed to have bacterial osteomyelitis or bone tumor. Mild cases feature a pain similar to the growing one. It's usually complicated by psoriasis and (or) Crohn's disease. Skin change is not an essential condition of CRMO because ① the typical osteoarthritis change is the same regardless of skin change; ② skin change may occur several years before the occurrence of bone destruction or keep development several years after the occurrence of osteoarthritis.

SAPHO syndrome is a group of skin-related non-bacterial osteoarthritis. The disease is brought up with by Chamot in 1987 for the first time. It includes synovitis, acne, pustulosis, hyperostosis, and osteitis. The disease is mostly found in teenagers and adults, regardless of men or women.

The pathogenesis of CNO/CRMO and SAPHO syndrome remains unclear, neither signs nor symptoms are specific, osteoarticular lesions are extensive, and there is no unified classification or diagnosis standards, resulting in a big dispute. CRMO as a subtype of pediatric SAPHO syndrome or an independent disease is still controversial.

CNO/CRMO, mostly found in children, is usually found at the metaphysis of long tubular bone, while SAPHO syndrome mostly involves the axial bone, especially the anterior chest wall, such as sternum and clavicle areas. The SAPHO syndrome is usually manifested as hyperostosis and osteosclerosis at the medial end of clavicle. Different from adults, the lesion at the clavicle of child patients usually doesn't involve the sternoclavicular joint, and their skin involvement isn't as common as that of adults either [112]. Therefore, CRMO and SAPHO syndrome are introduced separately in the book.

Due to the low incidence of non-bacterial osteomyelitis, there is still no unified clinical therapeutic schedule up to now. NSAID, as the most widely used drug at present, is mainly used to relieve the symptoms and maintain the treatment as a first-line drug. It's usually more effective for patients with a single focus that those with more than one focus. Some researches show that NSAID is effective for most patients within the first 1–2 years. However, the disease may recur to over 50% of patients 2 years later [113].

For patients who cannot be cured with NSAID and pain killers, second-line drugs such as corticosteroid hormone, disease-modifying anti-rheumatic drug (DMARD), diphosphonate and tumor necrosis factor-α antagonist are usually used to help treatment clinically. The corticosteroid hormone can be used to quickly and effectively control the inflammatory activity, relieving symptoms. Especially, it's more effective by the intra-articular administration. However, the drug rarely provides long-term relief, and there is recurrence risk after withdrawal of the hormone [114]. Bisphosphonates can be used to inhibit bone absorption, effective in anti-inflammation to some extent and significantly and continuously relieving the pain. DMARDs include methotrexate, sulfadiazine, and azathioprine.

Some patients also receive surgical treatment such as saucerization, decortication, and partial or total excision of osseous tissues with the lesion, which, however, isn't widely used.

Pathophysiology

It's widely believed that both CNO/CRMO and SAPHO syndrome are autoimmune diseases and have a genetic tendency at present. Their exact pathogenesis remains unclear. There are mainly two opinions: According to one opinion, such diseases are special seronegative spondyloarthropathies (SPAs), usually found at the axial bone and complicated by typical skin changes or inflammatory bowel disease [115]. According to another opinion, in the context of genetic factors, the Propionibacterium acnes infection induces the non-specific T cell immunoreaction of itself [116], increasing inflammatory cytokines (such as TNF-α and IL-6), reducing anti-inflammatory cytokines (especially IL-10) and improving the osteoclast activity. By this way, the bone decomposition can be accelerated at the early stage of the disease to cause the inflammation of bone, which is complicated by other tissue changes such as skin, joint, and intestinal tract sometimes. A research by a German scholar has demonstrated that IL-6 and chemokine CCL11/chemotactic factor for eosinophils can be used to accurately distinguish CNO patients, healthy children, and patients with other inflammatory diseases [117]. It has been proposed to use the serum cytokine profile as a CNO marker.

Most rheumatologists believe that bone biopsy shall be conducted when confirmed diagnosis cannot be made due to non-typical clinical and image manifestations of patients or single focus without other system diseases. On the contrary, patients with the following characteristics may not need receiving bone biopsy: bone defects of typical parts (such as clavicle, metaphysis of long bone, and vertebral body), no symptoms, normal laboratory test results, multiple bone defects, and relevant diseases (such as psoriasis or Crohn's disease).

The histological characteristics of destruction area will change with the development of the disease. At the early stage, it's manifested as the acute inflammation dominated by neutrophil infiltration, with visible bone absorption and significant periosteal proliferation. Subsequently, scattered infiltration of lymphocytes, plasma cells, histiocytes, and a small amount of polymorphonuclear cells can be seen in the focus. The memory T-lymphocytes of $CD8^+$ subpopulation is the main cell type. At the advanced stage, there is no or only slight inflammatory infiltration, sclerosing thickening and myelofibrosis of bone trabecula are visible, the number of osteoblasts increases, and the bone mass increases occasionally. Multinucleated giant cells, granuloma focuses, and necrotic bone chips can be observed in the biopsy specimens of child CNO patients. The histological examination results show no obvious characteristics but can exclude other diagnosis results such as tumor.

Imaging Findings

1. **Chronic non-bacterial osteomyelitis.** The disease usually starts at the metaphysis of long bone but rarely in the diaphysis area for children. For adults, it usually starts at the clavicle, vertebral body, and mandible rich in bone trabecula and with a high bone turnover rate [118]. As the time passes, the disease will develop to a multifocal lesion and keep unchanged throughout the disease process for most patients. Asymptomatic bone focuses are also common.

   The most common complication of CNO is the deformity caused by fracture, slow growth, or growth arrest of affected bones (especially the vertebral body). Kyphosis can be found in patients with multiple vertebral compression fracture. As bone absorption accelerates, the long bone may have pathologic fracture or even damaged epiphyseal plate, leading to asymmetric growth and development of extremities on both sides as well as visible angulation deformity in the joint. Surgical treatment is required in most cases at this point. Two years are needed from the occurrence of initial symptoms to the confirmed diagnosis of CNO averagely. For patients with intermittent or continuous focal bone or arthralgia in lower extremities, clavicle, spine, and (or) mandible, their conditions will deteriorate at night, influencing their sleep. The possibility of CNO shall be considered when the soft tissue at the disease part has fever and swelling. Due to non-typical pain symptoms, no specific laboratory examination and lack of correct comprehensive recognition, the diagnosis of the disease is usually delayed, and exclusive diagnosis is adopted in most cases. Coexisting diseases including psoriasis vulgaris, palmoplantar pustulosis and inflammatory bowel disease may occur before and after CNO, and up to 50% of patients have a family medical history of psoriasis, palmoplantar pustulosis, Crohn's disease or ulcerative colitis, providing a basis for diagnosis of CNO. Tables 4.2 and 4.3 list the scoring standard and diagnosis standard of CNO, respectively [118, 119], providing a reference for the diagnosis of suspected CNO cases.

   The complete blood count of most patients with CNO is normal. The erythrocyte sedimentation rate slightly accelerates and the level of C-reactive protein is elevated. The levels of lactic acid, uric acid, serum calcium, P, alkaline phosphatase, and so on are normal, and the laboratory test is helpful to exclude other diseases.

   (a) X-ray: No abnormal conditions can be found on the images of most patients at the early stage. Its manifestations at the tubular bone include area of osteolytic bone destruction at the metaphysis of adjacent epiphyseal plates, which is separated from the normal osseous tissues by a thin sclerotic margin. Different from the suppurative osteomyelitis, the disease is complicated by periosteal proliferation or sequestrum formation in most cases. However, periosteal proliferation can be observed at the focal margin of clavicle. At the later stage, the disease mainly features hyperostosis and osteosclerosis as well as osseous expansion. The surrounding soft tis-

Table 4.2 Scoring system for diagnosis of Jansson chronic non-bacterial osteomyelitis

Clinical, laboratory, and imaging results	Scores
Normal blood cell count	13
Symmetric injury	10
Marginal sclerosis lesion	10
Normal body temperature	9
The bone destruction area is located in the vertebral column, clavicle,or sternum.	8
Focuses confirmed by radiology: ≥2	7
C-reactive protein: ≥1 mg/dl	6

Note: The total scores are 63. It's mainly used to distinguish non-bacterial osteomyelitis from infectious osteomyelitis as well as benign tumors from malignant tumors of adults and children. The negative predictive value of patients with totally 28 or less scores to CNO is 97%, while the positive predictive value of patients with totally 39 or above scores can reach up to 97% or above

Table 4.3 Primary and secondary diagnosis criteria of NBO/CNO

Primary diagnosis criteria	Secondary diagnosis criteria
1. Lytic bone disease or sclerosing lesion confirmed by radiology	1. Healthy physical conditions and normal hemogram
2. Multiple bone destruction	2 The level of C-reactive protein is slightly elevated, and the erythrocyte sedimentation rate accelerates.
3. Palmoplantar pustulosis or psoriasis	3. Monitoring duration: over 6 months
4. Inflammation as well as (or) fibrosis and sclerosis confirmed by sterile bone biopsy	4. Hyperostosis
	5. Other relevant autoimmune diseases except palmoplantar pustulosis or psoriasis
	6. First or second degree relatives with autoimmune diseases, autoinflammatory diseases, or NBO

Note: Two primary criteria or one primary criterion and three secondary criteria must be met to diagnose NBO/CNO. Prompt: CRMO is a subtype of NBO. It requires multifocal bone injury or focus relevant with palmoplantar pustulosis or psoriasis as well as a chronic (over 6 months) recurrence–remission course of disease. However, the diagnosis criteria of SAPHO syndrome don't include multifocal and chronic requirements. In addition, the recommended diagnosis criteria of NBO only include pure palmoplantar pustulosis or psoriasis, although severe acne, gangrenous pyoderma, and other skin manifestations have also been found in child patients with CRMO. The recommended diagnosis criteria of SAPHO syndrome include severe acne, hidradenitis suppurativa, and palmoplantar pustulosis. The psoriasis vulgaris case in SAPHO syndrome is still controversial. The patients with other autoimmune diseases or their first and second degree relatives are only included in the recommended diagnosis criteria of NBO but not in the diagnosis criteria of SAPHO syndrome

sue swelling isn't obvious. Pathologic fracture (rare) and vertebral body compression fracture (which may cause kyphosis or flat Vertebral body) can be observed at the acute dissolution stage. X-ray has advantages such as quick imaging and low cost, but also disadvantages such as low false negative rate, low sensitivity, and radioactivity.

(b) CT: It's clearer than X-ray in display, especially suitable to display irregular bones (such as mandible). Osteolytic destruction area or mixed density focus, marginal proliferation and sclerosis as well as fusiform enlargement of bone appearance can be observed on the X-ray plain film and in the sternoclavicular joint area with overlapping spine. The involved bone is subject to 3D reconstruction for processing so as to guide the biopsy. However, CT isn't as sensitive as MRI. It's hard to discover the inflammation at the early stage and distinguish the part with inflammation from physiological part by CT. In addition, CT has a high radiation level.

(c) Whole-body radionuclide bone scan: Active and static focuses as well as detailed location of the part with inflammation are found based on the abnormal concentration of tracer. The enhancement of metabolism is relevant with the activity level of the disease. However, it has certain radiation level, unsuitable for daily follow-up.

(d) MRI: It features high sensitivity, accurate location, wider bone marrow focus display scope than X-ray and CT, and no radiation. The focus may also involve the diaphysis, usually without bone abscess or inflammation of soft tissues. The destruction area shows hypointense on T_1WI and hyperintense on T_2WI, and the sclerosis shows hypointense on both T_1WI and T_2WI. Intramedullary hyperintense can be observed in the short time inversion recovery (STIR). Especially at the early stage of the disease, bone marrow edema, and surrounding soft tissue inflammation changes can be found before bone destruction. Diaphysis enlargement, osteoporosis, partial or complete ossification of epiphysis as well as compression vertebral fracture can be observed at the later stage. At the repair stage of the disease, the bone destruction area gradually scleroses and heals. As the time passes, the bone is remodeled and usually can have normal images within 2 years. However, MRI cannot display hyperostosis changes and periosteal reaction clearly, making it hard to distinguish it from osteoblastic metastasis or osclerotic myeloma.

(e) Whole-body MRI: Whole-body MRI is mostly regarded as a golden diagnosis criterion of CNO. The whole-body scanning is helpful to recognize clinical asymptomatic lesions, especially spinal lesions. It is highly sensitive to inflammatory foci, and can be used to accurately evaluate the activity of foci and the level of skeletal injury. Examination plan: Whole-body coronal STIR imaging (4–5 segments), STIR imaging of full spine sagittal view, STIR imaging of sagittal view of feet, as well as STIR imaging of pelvic cavity and the surrounding area of knee joints.

(f) Image monitoring: No consensus has been reached on the imaging examination interval for condition monitoring. More frequent radiationless imaging may be required to accurately evaluate the disease activity so as to guide the treatment. In North America, about 50% of pediatric rheumatologists regularly use the imaging approach, 54% of patients receive repeated imaging examination every 6 months and 25% of patients every 12 months [120]. At the early stage of the disease, it's recommended that patients receive repeated MRI examinations within 3–6 months since starting receiving treatment. It's recommended that patients still taking drugs or having stopped taking drugs receive a repeated MRI examination every 6 to 12 months.

2. **CRMO.** It's more common in western countries, especially Central Europe and North Europe. As mentioned above, CRMO is a subtype of NBO. It requires multifo-

cal bone injury, or focus relevant with palmoplantar pustulosis or psoriasis as well as a chronic (over 6 months) recurrence–remission course of disease. CRMO is mostly found in children, with a boy to girl ratio of about 1:4. It usually occurs at the age of 7–25, with an average onset age of 10. The most common site involved by CRMO is the metaphysis of long bone followed by clavicle and spine. Predilection sites in the long tubular bone include distal femur, proximal tibia, distal tibia, and distal fibula, successively. The focus located in sternum, clavicle, and mandible provides a high specificity for the diagnosis of CRMO. Since CRMO can be complicated by peripheral arthritis, inflammatory bowel disease, psoriasis, and (or) sacroiliitis, most of such patients usually have negative HLA-B27. Therefore, some scholars believe that CRMO may belong to juvenile seronegative spondyloarthropathy [114].

Clinical manifestations, severity levels, and courses of the disease significantly vary with different individual patients. Its main clinical manifestation includes local osteodynia and swelling, possibly complicated by general symptoms such as low fever and weakness. As a benign lesion and with self-limitation, the course of CRMO usually lasts years. The disease has a wide scope, ranging from single asymptomatic or slight bone inflammatory changes to chronic recurrent multifocal bone destruction. It may recur at the original site or any other site and sometimes may also cause osteomyelitis and osteonecrosis. Some patients may have sequelae such as premature closure of epiphysis, bone deformity, and ithyokyphosis deformity. Some CRMO patients may develop to sacroiliitis or spondylitis, and up to 30% of patients may have non-infectious arthritis [113]. Limp may be caused if the long bone is involved. Trauma may be one of its inducement factors since quite a lot of CRMO cases are caused by trauma.

Imaging findings of the involved bone are approximately the same as those of CNO. Please refer to preceding part of the book. The imaging findings at active and repair stages of the disease still have a suggestive effect on the disease to some extent. However, with more knowledge of the disease and a longer clinical observation period, CRMO is likely to be more common than we thought before. The disease is diagnosed based on exclusion of other diseases, including lack of pathogen, no abscess, sinus and sequestrum formation, not predilection site of non-infectious osteomyelitis, frequent involvement of clavicle, incidence at multiple sites, imaging findings of subacute or chronic osteomyelitis, histopathology, non-laboratory test results, longer course of the disease, fluctuation, recurrent pain in many years and other features.

3. **SAPHO syndrome.** As a group of skin-related hyperostosis and osteosclerosis lesions in the bone destruction area, the disease is a group of changes mainly featuring damages such as palmoplantar pustulosis, hidradenitis suppurativa, or severe acne complicated by sternocostoclavicular hyperostosis, CRMO, and sacroiliitis. The SAPHO syndrome has some common features with spondyloarthropathy and other autoimmune diseases. However, it tends more to be part of the spontaneous disease in the autoimmune disease spectrum. It's found that the SAPHO syndrome is very important to avoid unnecessary invasive procedures and treat the osteoarthritis with antibiotics for a long time. Most courses are benign, and good long-term functional prognosis can be achieved if diagnosis and treatment are given in time.

The involved site of an adult is the anterior chest wall followed by the spine in most cases. The thoracic vertebra is the easiest to be involved. Up to 13% to 52% of patients with SAPHO syndrome have sacroiliitis. The disease rarely occurs to bones of the extremities of adult patients with SAPHO syndrome, with only 5% to 10% of patients having their long bones involved and 1% to 10% of patients having bone destruction of mandible [121]. The joints of adjacent involved bones may have arthritis, including sternoclavicular costal joints of anterior chest walls and sacroiliac joints of adults as well as ankle and knee joints of children. Skin changes may be obvious at the early stage of osteoarticular symptoms or occur several years before or after the occurrence of osteoarticular symptoms. Compared with adults, skin involvement is rare in children, with at least 15% of adults and over 70% of children possibly never having any skin change. Skin lesion is a neuropathic skin disease. The most common palmoplantar pustulosis takes up 50% to 70% of all skin diseases, and nearly 60% of patients have extended follow-up times [112]. Hidradenitis suppurativa (also called as acne inversa) is regarded as a type of severe acne and predominantly occurs to men. Other rare skin manifestations include pyoderma gangrenosum and Sweet's syndrome [112].

Nguyen et al. brought up with the diagnosis criteria of SAPHO syndrome in *Semin Arthritis Rheum*: ① osteoarticular manifestations + acne conglobata and acne fulminans or hidradenitis suppurativa; ② osteoarticular manifestations + palmoplantar pustulosis; ③ hyperostosis and hypertrophy, with or without skin change (anterior chest wall, arms, and legs as well as spine); ④ CRMO involving axial bone and appendicular bone, with or without skin change. Diagnosis can be made as long as any of above four criteria is met [122]. SAPHO syndrome can also be considered if the following conditions are combined: possibly relevant with psoriasis vulgaris or inflammatory bowel disease, characteristic change with ankylosing spondylitis (AS) and low toxic bacterial infection. Exclusion criteria: suppurative osteomyelitis, infectious chest wall arthritis, infectious palmoplantar pustulosis, palmoplantar keratoderma, exclusion of incidental diffuse idiopathic skeletal hyperostosis, and osteoarticular changes after treatment with retinol.

Two osteoarticular manifestations of SAPHO syndrome are osteitis as well as hyperostosis and hypertrophy. Both are chronic inflammatory response, chronic periosteal reaction, and cortical hyperplasia of bone cortex and bone marrow cortex. At the early stage of the disease, X-ray and CT images of the lesion area show no abnormal conditions; the focus is only the area of osteolytic bone destruction, with or without sclerotic margin; and typical change is that the disease is complicated by proliferative reaction, bone expansion, and ligament ossification of endosteum and periosteum. As the disease progresses, such focus becomes a mixture of destruction and hyperplasia or complete proliferation and sclerosis. The chronic focus is mainly proliferation and sclerosis, which is complicated by cortical thickening of bone cortex, narrowing of marrow cavity and thickening of bone trabecula. CT, especially multi-slice CT and late 3D reconstruction, is the most suitable to show details of osteoarticular lesions and also an optional examination method of the lesions in sternum and clavicle areas. It's difficult to show such details by X-ray clearly due to the superimposed effects of ribs, vertebral column, and mediastinum.

(a) The anterior upper chest wall is the most susceptible, and the disease is a typical change of SAPHO. Bone destruction can occur at the sternum, clavicle, and any site nearby ribs. The course usually consists of 3 stages: At the first stage, the disease is limited to the ligament area of costoclavicular joint and is possible to be manifested as higher bone mineral density at the attachment point of primary ligament as well as adjacent soft tissue swelling. At the second stage, the lesion of costoclavicular joint is complicated by osteolytic destruction and osteosclerosis changes of structures such as medial clavicle, sternum, the first rib, and costal cartilage. At stage 3, the above structures and their surrounding structures are characterized by hyperostosis, hypertrophy, thickening, and fusion of adjacent joints, which can develop into arthritis or ankylosis (Figs. 4.61 and 4.62a–c).

(b) Axial bone: Its incidence is second only to that of the osseous tissue of the anterior chest wall, which is usually limited to one vertebral level. Generally, the focus does not cross the intervertebral space and is not accompanied by paravertebral abscess. This is another characteristic of CRMO from infection. It occurs frequently in thoracic vertebrae, followed by lumbar vertebrae and cervical vertebrae. Occasionally, 4 adjacent vertebral bodies are seen to be involved, and 5 adjacent focuses may be present in individual patients. The early manifestations were progressive non-specific discitis, and X-ray and CT showed erosive destruction of the endplates with subchondral hyperostosis and osteosclerosis, narrowing of the intervertebral space and ossification of the paravertebral ligaments. MRI shows that the affected intervertebral disc in the acute stage shows hyperintense on both T_1WI enhancement and T_2WI, and the intervertebral disc degenerated in the late stage of the lesion and shows hypointense on T_2WI. In the later stage of the disease, local collapse of the vertebral body, stress fracture, ossification of the paravertebral ligaments, formation of bone bridges across 1 or more intervertebral spaces, and even kyphotic deformity occur. The article by Minhchau et al. mentioned that sacroiliitis in SAPHO syndrome is more common unilaterally, hyperostosis and osteosclerosis are mainly located on the iliac articular surface, while sacroiliitis in ankylosing spondylitis is more com-

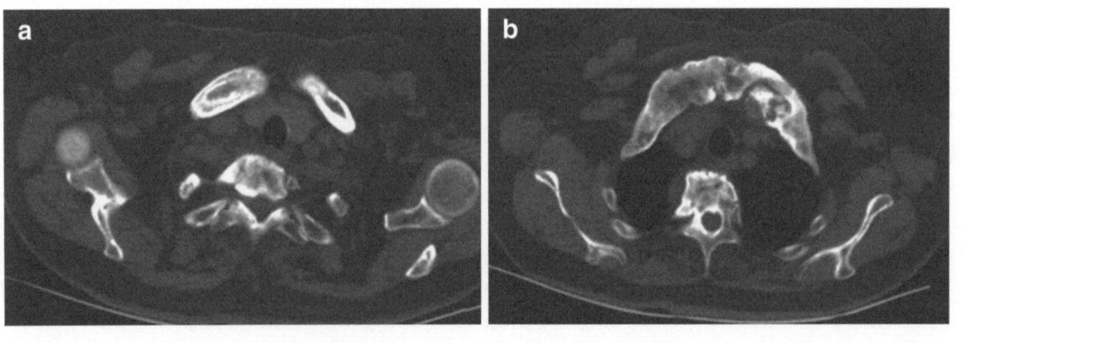

Fig. 4.61 SAPHO syndrome. The manubrium, adjacent bilateral clavicles, part of thoracic vertebrae and adjacent ribs show significant proliferation and sclerosis, with thickening of right clavicle, periosteal proliferation, and thickening of bone cortex. The left sternoclavicular joint showed irregular bone destruction area, without obvious swelling of surrounding soft tissues

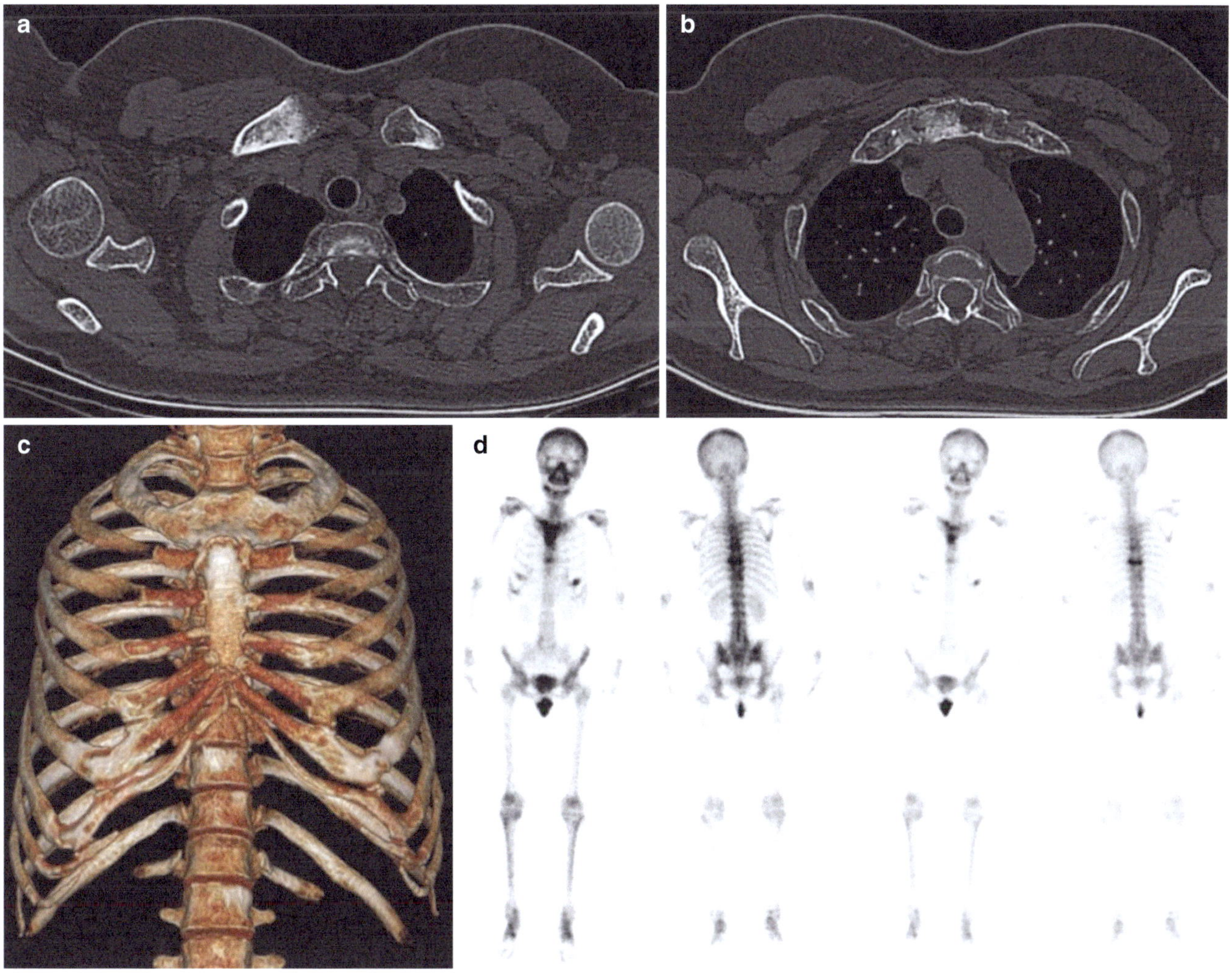

Fig. 4.62 Anterior chest wall SAPHO syndrome. (**a**–**c**) The right sternoclavicular costal joint shows hyperostosis and osteosclerosis, utricular bone destruction area, thin sclerotic margin at the edge, bone fusion of the sternoclavicular costal joint space; (**d**) Bone scan showed "bull-head sign" change of the sternoclavicular costal joint, local tracer concentration in the left clavicle, and thoracic vertebra

mon bilaterally [122]. As for the results of Xu Wenrui et al., in contrast, most of them show bilateral sacroiliac joint involvement, more obvious on the sacral side, and a higher proportion of bone marrow edema, fat deposition, bone destruction, and osteosclerosis in the bone adjacent to the joint, indicating the coexistence of old and new focuses, but the worm-like changes and space changes on the articular surface are not obvious and occur frequently in women [123].

Chronic diffuse sclerosing osteomyelitis of the mandible may be caused by overuse of masticatory muscles and is divided into localized and diffuse types, usually affecting the mandibular body and branches, while the temporal-mandibular joint is usually unaffected, and is often accompanied by pain and swelling of the overlying soft tissues. Now it is generally considered as a form of SAPHO symptoms, whether it is an independent disease or a disease associated with other sites is still controversial. Imaging findings are mainly unilateral or diffuse hyperostosis and osteosclerosis, low-density focuses are seen in some sclerotic areas, and the degree of periosteal reaction depends on the extent of the affected bone focus, which is usually more pronounced in small diameter bones and heals in a way of progressive hyperostosis and osteosclerosis [121, 124].

(c) Appendicular bone is the most common site in pediatric patients, and long bone involvement is less common in adult patients. In the early stages, the typical presentation is the presence of areas of osteolytic bone destruction in the metaphysis close to the epiphyseal plate.
(d) Whole-body scintigraphy is highly sensitive because it can not only show focuses with abnormal bone metabolism, but also show the clinically silent

focuses. The so-called "bullhead sign" is produced by high tracer uptake in the sternal-clavicular region, with the manubrium constituting the "bull's head" and the infected sternoclavicular joint and the adjacent clavicles constituting the "bull's horn" (Fig. 4.62d).

(e) Whole-body magnetic resonance imaging: MRI has no radiation and can be repeatedly applied during follow-up, especially for children. MRI is more sensitive than X-ray and CT and can also show bone marrow edema and adjacent soft tissue inflammation. It is especially suitable for vertebral examination and can be used to monitor the progression of the disease because chronic sclerosing bone destruction foci shows hypointense on both T_1WI and T_2WI; while active focuses showed hypointense on T_1WI and hyperintense on T_2WI.

Key Points of Diagnosis

1. SAPHO syndrome can be diagnosed as long as 1 of the 4 inclusion criteria is met.
2. Whole-body radionuclide bone scan or MRI can show osteoarticular involvement focuses and clinically silent focuses.
3. Corresponding histological results and negative bacterial culture results can be obtained by biopsy, and then infectious osteomyelitis or bone tumors can be ruled out.
4. For patients with both typical pain sites (such as the anterior chest wall), corresponding imaging findings and characteristic skin lesions, the diagnosis is relatively simple. The diagnosis is relatively difficult when the lesion site is single, atypical, or without skin change. A detailed medical history, especially enquiry about whether the skin and bones were previously involved, may provide a basis for diagnosis.

Differential Diagnosis

Due to the lack of recognized diagnostic criteria and specific laboratory tests and markers, SAPHO syndrome belongs to the exclusion diagnosis, mainly due to its non-specific imaging findings in the early stages, and the differential diagnosis mainly includes tumors and infections.

1. **Chronic hypotoxic osteoarthritis.** It mostly occurs singly, occasionally collectively, with asymmetric distribution, and mostly not accompanied by characteristic skin changes. Pathogens can be cultured by biopsy of bone and soft tissue.
2. **Infectious osteoarthritis** mostly occurs singly, and the surface soft tissue of the affected area is presented with obvious redness, swelling, heat, and pain. Sequestrum was observed in the bone destruction area, abscess formation was observed in the bone and surrounding soft tissues, laboratory tests showed high inflammatory indicators, and pathogens could be cultured.
3. **Eosinophilic granuloma of bone.** It is more common in children under 10 years of age and may occur singly or collectively. Single eosinophilic granuloma occurs frequently in skull and femur, multiple eosinophilic granulomas occur frequently in vertebral body, with pathological features of granuloma formed by reticular cell proliferation and eosinophilic granulocyte infiltration. Long bone lesions mostly involve metaphysis and diaphysis, manifested as a single irregular bone destruction area, which is usually located in the marrow cavity, growing in an expansive way with clear edges. Small, patchy dense osteosclerosis may be observed in the destruction area, accompanied by lamellar periosteal reaction and hyperostosis and osteosclerosis, and surrounded by soft tissue masses. The symptoms of the affected bone are similar to those of aseptic osteomyelitis and can be differentiated in combination with the site of disease, laboratory tests of eosinophilia and pathological characteristics.
4. **Paget's disease** is characterized by an older age of onset and a familial predisposition and may occur singly or collectively. Osteoporosis is followed by rapid hyperostosis, resulting in limb enlargement and deformity. On imaging, not only cystic low-density areas but also hyperostosis and osteosclerosis areas could be seen, without obvious periosteal reaction or soft tissue mass shadow. There is no characteristic skin change compared with SAPHO syndrome, and the blood alkaline phosphatase is elevated.
5. **Diffuse idiopathic skeletal hyperostosis (DISH).** It is characterized by unexplained hyperostosis and osteosclerosis, thickened bone cortex and no obvious areas of bone destruction. However, it generally does not involve adjacent joints, there is no characteristic skin change, and the sternoclavicular costal joint is rarely affected.
6. **Primary bone tumors or metastases.** Primary bone tumors have fewer areas of bone destruction with significant hyperostosis and osteosclerosis, while evident soft tissue masses. For sclerotic bone tumors, osteogenic bone metastases show intrabony patchy or conglomerate high-density shadows with uniform density, mostly intact bone cortex, and no change in the shape of the bone, and the osseous tissue of the anterior upper chest wall is less affected compared with SAPHO syndrome.
7. **Other seronegative spondyloarthropathy (SPA)** rarely involves the anterior upper chest wall, without characteristic skin change, and occurs frequently in male patients, mostly HLA-B27 positive, and frequently in sacroiliac joint and spinal fusion.

Status Quo and Progress of Research

1. Plain X-ray is the most basic screening method. When the above 3 diseases are highly suspected in clinical

practice, whole-body MRI and radionuclide scan are preferred. In the monitoring stage after the diagnosis of diseases, MRI is the best examination method due to the absence of radiation.

2. The CRMO may be related to gene mutations, i.e., the 166pb allele on human chromosome 18. Majeed syndrome is also related to this gene, which belongs to autosomal recessive disorders and is a group of syndromes characterized by early onset MO, dyserythropoietic anemia, and joint contracture, mainly caused by defects in its function due to mutations in the LPIN2 gene encoding lipoprotein 2 [125].
3. The study results of Li Chen et al. confirmed that for patients with refractory SAPHO syndrome (those whose disease was not controlled after treatment with NSAIDs and glucocorticoid (GC) and anti-rheumatic drugs), the response rate was 100% after treatment with TNF-α antagonists [126]. At present, the short-term efficacy of such drugs has been generally recognized. Therefore, experimental treatment can be adopted when this disease is highly suspected in clinical practice, but the long-term efficacy, course of treatment, and potential risks need to be debated.
4. The sequences strongly T_2-weighted and Gd-DTPA enhancement are helpful to show inflammatory bone injury and/or periosseous reactions, and varying degrees of enhancement are observed in the affected bones in the acute stage. The surrounding soft tissues in STIR show hyperintense; new areas of osteolytic bone destruction indicate progression and deterioration of CRMO, which eventually resolves in a sclerotic fashion. This repeated process of inflammation leads to progressive hyperostosis and osteosclerosis of the bone, which may persist for years and gradually expand circumferentially. For long-term CRMO focuses, the affected bone is rarely able to return to normal shape. In the repair stage of CRMO, the resolution of bone marrow edema is the most representative imaging feature, and the bone marrow signal is not as high or with no hyperintense change as in the acute stage on T_2WI and STIR sequences.

References

1. Renju B, Xuelin Z. Medical imaging diagnostics. 3rd ed. Beijing: People's Health Publishing House; 2010.
2. Shuling B, Dajun Y. Systematic anatomy. 9th ed. Beijing: People's Medical Publishing House; 2018.
3. Guo Q. Applied radiology. 3rd ed. Beijing: The People's Medical Publishing House; 2007.
4. Pugmire BS, Shailam R, Gee MS. Role of MRI in the diagnosis and treatment of osteomyelitis in pediatric patients. World J Radiol. 2014;6(8):530–7.
5. Hui Q, Wu W, Rongjie B. Orthopedic imaging: a practical approach. 5th ed. Beijing: Science Press; 2012.
6. Lattar SM, Tuchscherr LP, Centron D, et al. Molecular fingerprinting of Staphylococcus aureus isolated from patients with osteomyelitis in Argentina and clonal distribution of the cap5(8)genes and of other selected virulence genes. Eur J Clin Microbiol Infect Dis. 2012;31(10):2559–66.
7. Mc Carthy AJ, Lindsay JA. Genetic variation in Staphylococcus aureus surface and immune evasion genes is lineage associated: implications for vaccine design and host-pathogen interactions. BMC Microbiol. 2010;10(173):2–15.
8. Nelson GE, Pondo T, Toews KA, et al. Epidemiology of invasive group A streptococcal infections in the United States, 2005-2012. Clin Infect Dis. 2016;63(4):478–86.
9. Adetunji SA, Ramirez G, Foster MJ, et al. A systematic review and meta-analysis of the prevalence of osteoarticular brucellosis. PLoS Negl Trop Dis. 2019;13(1):e0007112.
10. Zheng R, Xie S, Lu X, et al. A systematic review and meta-analysis of epidemiology and clinical manifestations of human brucellosis in China. Biomed Res Int. 2018;2018:5712920.
11. Rando MM, De Matteis G, Gessi M, et al. Tuberculous arthritis of the ankle. Eur J Case Rep Intern Med. 2018;5(6):000870.
12. Vanhoenacker F, Sanghvi D, De Backer A. Imaging features of extraaxial musculoskeletal tuberculosis. Indian J Radiol Imaging. 2009;19(3):176–86.
13. Babitha F, Priya PV, Poothiode U. Hydatid cyst of bone. Indian J Med Microbiol. 2015;33(3):442–4.
14. Nouroallahian M, Bakhshaee M, Afzalzadeh MR, et al. A hydatid cyst in an unusual location-the infratemporal fossa. Laryngoscope. 2013;123(2):407–9.
15. Gurzu S, Beleaua MA, Egyed-Zsigmond E, et al. Unusual location of hydatid cysts: report of two cases in the heart and hip joint of Romanian patients. Korean J Parasitol. 2017;55(4):429–31.
16. Melissa DJ, John RP. Fungal infections of the bones and joints. Curr Infect Dis Rep. 2001;3(5):450–60.
17. Anagnostakos K, Kelm J, Schmitt E, et al. Fungal periprosthetic hip and knee joint infections clinical experience with a 2-stage treatment protocol. J Arthroplast. 2012;27(2):293–8.
18. Chen S, Chen Y, Zhou YQ, et al. Candida glabrata-induced refractory infectious arthritis: a case report and literature review. Mycopathologia. 2019;184(2):283–93.
19. Elias JA, Michael RM, Michael AP. Clinical mycology. 2nd ed. Amsterdam: Elsevier; 2009. p. 525–45.
20. Hung CY, Hsu AP, Holland SM, et al. A review of innate and adaptive immunity to coccidioidomycosis. Med Mycol. 2019;57(Suppl 1):S85–92.
21. Xu K, Qiyong G, Ping H. Medical imaging. 8th ed. Beijing: People's Health Publishing House; 2018.
22. Lima AL, Oliveira PR, Carvalho VC, et al. Recommendations for the treatment of osteomyelitis. Braz J Infect Dis. 2014;18(5):526–34.
23. Zhi Y, Jian L, Hu Y, et al. The application of anti-infective active bone in the treatment of adult traumatic osteomyelitis. Chin J Trauma. 2009;4(25):333–7.
24. Kan JH, Young RS, Yu C. Clinical impact of gadolinium in the MRI diagnosis of musculoskeletal infection in children. Pediatr Radiol. 2010;40(7):1197–205.
25. Gotthardt M, Bleeker-Rovers CP, Boerman OC, et al. Imaging of inflammation by PET, conventional scintigraphy, and other imaging techniques. J Nucl Med. 2010;51(12):1937–49.
26. Averill LW, Hernandez A, Gonzalez L, et al. Diagnosis of osteomyelitis in children: utility of fat-suppressed contrast-enhanced MRI. AJR Am J Roentgenol. 2009;192(5):1232–8.
27. Jaramillo D. Infection: musculoskeletal. Pediatr Radiol. 2011;41(1):S127–34.
28. Browne LP, Guillerman RP, Orth RC, et al. Community-acquired staphylococcal musculoskeletal infection in infants and young children: necessity of contrast-enhanced MRI for the diagnosis of growth cartilage involvement. AJR Am J Roentgenol. 2012;198(1):194–9.

29. Guillerman RP. Osteomyelitis and beyond. Pediatr Radiol. 2013;43(Suppl 1):S193–203.
30. Meiwen Z. MRI features and diagnostic utility of chronic osteomyelitis. Chin J CT MRI. 2013;11(1):105–10.
31. Prieto-Perez L, Perez-Tanoira R, Petkova-Saiz E, et al. Osteomyelitis: a descriptive study. Clin Orthop Surg. 2014;6(1):20–5.
32. Acikgoz G, Averill LW. Chronic recurrent multifocal osteomyelitis: typical patterns of bone involvement in whole-body bone scintigraphy. Nucl Med Commun. 2014;35(8):797–807.
33. Song C, Xingyu C, Wang G, et al. MRI features of atypical chronic osteomyelitis. Diag Imaging Interven Radiol. 2013;6:471–4.
34. Yan Z, Zhu Y, Zitao Z, et al. Progress in imaging research on the diagnosis of chronic osteomyelitis. Chin J Orthop Trauma. 2016;1(18):89–92.
35. Bires AM, Kerr B, George L. Osteomyelitis: an overview of imaging modalities. Crit Care Nurs Q. 2015;38(2):154–64.
36. Hedrich CM, Hahn G, Girschick HJ, et al. A clinical and pathomechanistic profile of chronic nonbacterial osteomyelitis/chronic recurrent multifocal osteomyelitis and challenges facing the field. Expert Rev Clin Immunol. 2013;9(9):845–54.
37. Kudva A, Kamath AT, Dhara V, et al. Chronic recurrent osteomyelitis: a surgeon's enigma. J Oral Pathol Med. 2019;48(2):180–4.
38. Harmer JL, Pickard J, Stinchcombe SJ. The role of diagnostic imaging in the evaluation of suspected osteomyelitis in the foot: a critical review. Foot (Edinb). 2011;21(3):149–53.
39. Wang GL, Zhao K, Liu ZF, et al. A meta-analysis of fluorodeoxyglucose-positron emission tomography versus scintigraphy in the evaluation of suspected osteomyelitis. Nucl Med Commun. 2011;32(12):1134–42.
40. Nag HL, Kancherla R, Malpura A. Brodie's abscess of medial distal femoral condyle after a thorn prick: rare clinical presentation. Chin J Traumatol. 2012;15(2):126–8.
41. Agrawal P, Sobti A. A Brodie's abscess of femoral neck mimicking osteoid osteoma: diagnostic approach and management strategy. Ethiop J Health Sci. 2016;26(1):81–4.
42. Kanoun ML, Khorbi A, Khmiri C, et al. Diagnosis and treatment of Brodie's abscess in adults: about twenty cases. Tunis Med. 2007;85(10):857–61.
43. Olasinde AA, Oluwadiya KS, Adegbehingbe OO. Treatment of Brodie's abscess: excellent results from curettage, bone grafting and antibiotics. Singap Med J. 2011;52(6):436–9.
44. Heng Z, Fei C, Yi L, et al. A case of Brodie abscess involving epiphyseal plate. Chin Med J. 2018;98(17):1366–7.
45. Qi R, Colmegna I. Brodie abscess. CMAJ. 2017;189(3):e117.
46. Foster CE, Taylor M, Schallert EK, et al. Brodie abscess in children: a 10-year single institution retrospective review. Pediatr Infect Dis J. 2019;38(2):32–4.
47. Hao J. Bone and joint MRI. 2nd ed. Shanghai: Shanghai Science and Technology Press; 2011.
48. Min Z, Yaling C, Yuke L, et al. Application of image fusion technology to diagnose bone inflammation. J Traditional Chin Orthop Traumatol. 2010;22(11):22–6.
49. Strobel K, Hany TF, Exner GU. PET/CT of a Brodie abscess. Clin Nucl Med. 2006;31(4):210.
50. Segev E, Hayek S, Lokiec F, et al. Primary chronic sclerosing (Garré's) osteomyelitis in children. J Pediatr Orthop B. 2001;10(4):360–4.
51. Akgül HM, Çağlayan F, Günen Yılmaz S, et al. Garre's osteomyelitis of the mandible caused by infected tooth. Case Rep Dent. 2018;8:1409539.
52. Wang G, Xu H, Xie J, et al. Sequential sclerosing osteomyelitis in bilateral tibia:1 case report. J Clin Orthop. 2014;17(1):116.
53. Ogawa A, Miyate H, Nakamura Y, et al. Treating chronic diffuse sclerosing osteomyelitis of the mandible with saucerization and autogenous bone grafting. Oral Surg Oral Med Oral Pathol Oral Radiol Endod. 2001;91(4):390.
54. Bai S, Zhang H, Li Z, et al. A 53-year-old man with a sclerosing rib lesion: a case report. Medicine (Baltimore). 2017;96(47):e8692.
55. Shen S, Guozhi Z. Status quo of researches on etiology and treatment of diffuse Sclerosing osteomyelitis in mandible. J Jinan Univ. 2003;24(2):88–92.
56. Hayati MA, Fatma C, Sevcihan GY, et al. Garre's osteomyelitis of the mandible caused by infected tooth. Case Rep Dent. 2018;2018:1409539.
57. Rongjie B, Cheng X, Xiang G, et al. Comparison of radiography, CT and MR imaging in detection of atypical osteomyelitis. J China Clin Med Imaging. 2008;19(7):488–92.
58. Van de Meent MM, Pichardo SEC, Rodrigues MF, et al. Radiographic characteristics of chronic diffuse sclerosing osteomyelitis/tendoperiostitis of the mandible: a comparison with chronic suppurative osteomyelitis and osteoradionecrosis. J Craniomaxillofac Surg. 2018;46(9):1631–6.
59. Singh S, Graham ME, Bullock M, et al. Chronic sclerosing osteomyelitis of the mandible treated with hemimandibulectomy and fibular free flap reconstruction. Plast Reconstr Surg Glob Open. 2016;3(12):e580.
60. Goff TAJ, Rambani R, Ng AB. Current concepts in the management of periprosthetic fungal joint infection using antifungal bone cement. Curr Orthop Pract. 2014;25(2):169–74.
61. Melissa DJ, John RP. Fungal infections of the bones and joints. Curr Infect Dis Rep. 2007;3(5):450–60.
62. Giles JT, Bathon JM. Serious infections associated with anticytokine therapies in the rheumatic diseases. J Intensive Care Med. 2004;19(6):320–34.
63. Vechi HT, Theodoro RC, Oliveira ALD, et al. Invasive fungal infection by Cryptococcus neoformans var. grubii with bone marrow and meningeal involvement in a HIV-infected patient: a case report. BMC Infect Dis. 2019;19(1):220.
64. Henry MW, Miller AO, Walsh TJ, et al. Fungal musculoskeletal infections. Infect Dis Clin N Am. 2017;31(2):353–68.
65. Alvarenga JA, Martins DE, Kanas M, et al. Paracoccidioidomycosis in the spine: case report and review of the literature. Sao Paulo Med J. 2016;134(3):263–7.
66. Ferreira LC, Barroso PF, Tonomura E, et al. Osteomyelitis caused by Sporothrix schenckii in an immunocompetent patient. Rev Soc Bras Med Trop. 2016;49(4):527–9.
67. Belthur MV, Blair JE, Shrader MW, et al. Musculoskeletal coccidioidomycosis. Curr Orthop Pract. 2018;29(4):400–6.
68. Leroy-Freschini B, Treglia G, Argemi X, et al. 18F-FDG PET/CT for invasive fungal infection in immunocompetent patients. QJM. 2018;111(9):613–22.
69. Davies G, Rolle AM, Maurer A, et al. Toward translational ImmunoPET/MR imaging of invasive pulmonary aspergillosis: the humanised monoclonal antibody jf5 detects aspergillus lung infections in vivo. Theranostics. 2017;7(14):3398–414.
70. Esmaeilnejad-Ganji SM, Esmaeilnejad-Ganji SMR. Osteoarticular manifestations of human brucellosis: a review. World J Orthop. 2019;10(2):54–62.
71. Zheng R, Xie S, Lu X, et al. A systematic review and meta-analysis of epidemiology and clinical manifestations of human brucellosis in China. Biomed Res Int. 2018;2018:1–10.
72. Ulu KA, Metan G, Alp E. Clinical presentations and diagnosis of brucellosis. Recent Pat Antiinfect Drug Discov. 2013;8(1):34–41.
73. Mehanic S, Baljic R, Mulabdic V, et al. Osteoarticular manifestations of brucellosis. Med Arh. 2012;66(3 Suppl 1):24–6.
74. Elnour EF, Nisreen S. Brucella septic arthritis: case reports and review of the literature. Case Rep Infect Dis. 2016;2016:4687840.
75. Avijgan M, Rostamnezhad M, Jahanbani-Ardakani H. Clinical and serological approach to patients with brucellosis: a common

diagnostic dilemma and a worldwide perspective. Microb Pathog. 2019;129:125–30.
76. Editorial Board of Chinese Journal of Infectious Diseases. Expert consensus on diagnosis & treatment of brucellosis. Chin J Infect Dis. 2017;35(12):705.
77. Wang Y. Chinese medical imaging·musculoskeletal system. 2nd ed. Beijing: People's Medical Publishing House; 2012.
78. Bozgeyik Z, Aglamis S, Bozdag PG, et al. Magnetic resonance imaging findings of musculoskeletal brucellosis. Clin Imaging. 2014;38(5):719–23.
79. Remide A, Berna DM. Musculoskeletal brucellosis. Semin Musculoskelet Radiol. 2011;15(5):470–9.
80. Oztekin O, Calli C, Adibelli Z, et al. Brucellar spondylodiscitis: magnetic resonance imaging features with conventional sequences and diffusion-weighted imaging. Radiol Med. 2010;115(5):794–803.
81. Held M, Bruins MF, Castelein S, et al. A neglected infection in literature: childhood musculoskeletal tuberculosis: a bibliometric analysis of the most influential papers. Int J Mycobacteriol. 2017;6(3):229–38.
82. Qian Y, Han Q, Liu W, et al. Characteristics and management of bone and joint tuberculosis in native and migrant population in Shanghai during 2011 to 2015. BMC Infect Dis. 2018;18(1):543.
83. Moore SL, Rafii M. Advanced imaging of tuberculosis arthritis. Semin Musculoskelet Radiol. 2003;7(2):143–54.
84. Feng N, Qiuye W. Research progress on the susceptibility of tuberculosis of bone and joint and polymorphisms of related genes. J Chin Pract Diagn Therapy. 2017;31(4):391–3.
85. Broderick C, Hopkins S, Mack DJF, et al. Delays in the diagnosis and treatment of bone and joint tuberculosis in the United Kingdom. Bone Joint J. 2018;100-B(1):119–24.
86. Tang Y, Yin L, Tang S, et al. Application of molecular, microbiological, and immunological tests for the diagnosis of bone and joint tuberculosis. J Clin Lab Anal. 2018;32(2):e22260.
87. Auguste P, Tsertsvadze A, Pink J, et al. Comparing interferon- gamma release assays with tuberculin skin test for identifying latent tuberculosis infection that progresses to active tuberculosis: systematic review and meta-analysis. BMC Infect Dis. 2017;17(1):200.
88. Chinese Society for Tuberculosis, Chinese Medical Association and Editorial Board of Chinese Journal of Tuberculosis and Respiratory Diseases. Recommendations for the application of interferon-γ release assays in China. Chin J Tuberculosis Respirat Dis. 2014;37(10):744–7.
89. Wang T, Tan YJ, Wu SJ, et al. The ratio of tuberculosis-specific antigen to phytohemagglutinin in T-SPOT assay in the diagnosis of active tuberculosis. Zhonghua Jie He Hu Xi Za Zhi. 2019;42(4):262–7.
90. Madhok R. Evaluation of apparent diffusion coefficient values in spinal tuberculosis by MRI. J Clin Diagn Res. 2016;10(8):TC19–23.
91. Albano D, Treglia G, Desenzani P, et al. Incidental unilateral tuberculous sacroiliitis detected by 18F-FDG PET/CT in a patient with abdominal tuberculosis. Asia Oceania J Nucl Med Biol. 2017;5(2):152–6.
92. Song XH, Ding LW, Wen H. Bone hydatid disease. Postgrad Med J. 2007;83(982):536–42.
93. Manciulli T, Mustapayeva A, Juszkiewicz K, et al. Cystic echinococcosis of the bone in Kazakhstan. Case Rep Infect Dis. 2018;2018:9682508.
94. Agudelo HN, Brunetti E, McCloskey C. Cystic echinococcosis. Clin Microbiol. 2016;54(3):518–23.
95. Cattaneo L, Manciulli T, Cretu CM, et al. Cystic echinococcosis of the bone: a European multicenter study. Am J Trop Med Hyg. 2019;100(3):617–21.
96. Meinel TR, Gottstein B, Geib V, et al. Vertebral alveolar echinococcosis-a case report, systematic analysis, and review of the literature. Lancet Infect Dis. 2018;18(3):e87–98.
97. Gurzu S, Beleaua MA, Egyedzsigmond E, et al. Unusual location of hydatid cysts: report of two cases in the heart and hip joint of Romanian patients. Korean J Parasitol. 2017;55(4):429–31.
98. Dapeng L, Xiaohui F, Jingping Z, et al. Application of EgCF, EgP, B (EgB) and Em2 tests of hydatid by GAB and ELISA in diagnosis of bone hydatid disease. Chin J Orthop. 2010;30(2):198–202.
99. Thapa S, Ghosh A, Ghartimagar D, et al. Hydatidosis of infratemporal fossa with proptosis-an unusual presentation: a case report and review of the literature. J Med Case Rep. 2018;12(1):309.
100. Salamone G, Licari L, Randisi B, et al. Uncommon localizations of hydatid cyst. Review of the literature. G Chir. 2016;37(4): 180–5.
101. Wang J, Wenxiao J, Hong C, et al. Value of MRH in diagnosis of alveolar echinococcosis. Chin J Radiol. 2009;43(4):402–5.
102. Willegger M, Kolb A, Windhager R, et al. Acute haematogenous osteomyelitis in children: diagnostic algorithm and treatment strategies. Orthopade. 2017;46(6):541–56.
103. Alaya Z, Zaghouani H, Osman W, et al. Septic arthritis of the pubis symphysis: clinical and therapeutic features. Pan Afr Med J. 2017;26:215.
104. Kehl-Fie TE, Porsch EA, Yagupsky P, et al. Examination of type IV pilus expression and pilus-associated phenotypes in Kingella kingae clinical isolates. Infect Immun. 2010;78:1692.
105. Boesen M, Kubassova O, Sudot-Szopińska I, et al. MR imaging of joint infection and inflammation with emphasis on dynamic contrast-enhanced MR imaging. PET Clin. 2018;13(4):523–50.
106. Montgomery NI, Epps HR. Pediatric septic arthritis. Orthop Clin North Am. 2017;48(2):209–16.
107. Wu K, Wang T, Liang H, et al. Comparison and analysis of display of articular cartilage of knee by different 3.0T MRI technologies. J Pract Radiol. 2013;8(22):1010–3.
108. Crema MD, Roemer FW, Marra MD, et al. Articular cartilage in the knee: current MR imaging techniques and applications in clinical practice and research. Radiographics. 2011;31(1): 37–61.
109. Li X, Cheng J, Lin K, et al. Quantitative MRI using T1ρ and T2 in human osteoarthritic cartilage specimens: correlation with biochemical measurements and histology. Magn Reson Imaging. 2011;29(3):324–34.
110. Theologis AA, Schairer WW, Carballido-Gamio J, et al. Longitudinal analysis of T1ρ and T2 quantitative MRI of knee cartilage laminar organization following microfracture surgery. Knee. 2012;19(5):652–7.
111. Yu K, Shen M. Autoinflammatory bone disease. Chin Med J. 2016;96(15):1230–2.
112. Colina M, Govoni M, Orzincolo C, et al. Clinical and radiologic evolution of synovitis, acne, pustulosis, hyperostosis, and osteosis syndrome: a single center study of a cohort of 71 subjects. Arthritis Rheum. 2009;61:813–21.
113. Schnable A, Range U, Hahn G, et al. Unexpectedly high incidences of chronic non-bacterial as compared to bacterial osteomyelitis in children. Rheumatol Int. 2016;36:1737–45.
114. Wolber C, David-Jelinek K, Udvardi A, et al. Successful therapy of sacroiliitis in SAPHO syndrome by etanercept. Wien Med Wochenschr. 2011;161(7–8):204–8.
115. Jurik AG. Chronic regional multifocal osteomyelitis. Semin Musculoskelet Radiol. 2004;8:243–53.
116. Govoni M, Colina M. SAPHO syndrome and infections. Autoimmun Rev. 2009;81(8):256–9.
117. Hofmann SR, Bottger F, Range U, et al. Serum interleukin-6 and CCL11/eotaxin may be suitable biomarkers for the diagnosis of chronic nonbacterial osteomyelitis. Front Pediatr. 2017;5:1–11.

118. Jansson A, Renner ED. Classification of non-bacterial osteitis: retrospective study of clinical, immunological and genetic aspects in 89 patients. Rheumatology. 2007;46(1):154–60.
119. Jansson AF, Muller TH, Gliera L, et al. Clinical score for nonbacterial osteitis in children and adults. Arthritis Rheum. 2009;60(4):1152–9.
120. Zhao Y, Dedeoglu F, Ferguson PJ, et al. Physicians' perspectives on the diagnosis and treatment of chronic nonbacterial osteomyelitis. Int J Rheumatol. 2017;2017:7694942.
121. Depasquale R, Kumar N, Lalam RK, et al. SAPHO: what radiologists should know. Radiol Med. 2014;119(3):156–63.
122. Nguyen MT, Borchers A, Selmi C, et al. The SAPHO syndrome. Semin Arthritis Rheum. 2012;42(3):254–65.
123. Xu W, Chen L, Xiali S, et al. Sacroiliac joint MRI findings in SAPHO syndrome. Chin J Magn Reson Imaging. 2017;8(6):441–5.
124. Zemann W, Pau M, Feichtinger M, et al. SAPHO syndrome with affection of the mandible: diagnosis, treatment, and review of literature. Oral Surg Oral Med Oral Pathol Oral Radiol Endod. 2011;111(2):190–5.
125. Beck C, Girschick HJ, Morbach H, et al. Mutation screening of the IL-1 receptor antagonist gene in chronic non-bacterial osteomyelitis of childhood and adolescence. Clin Exp Rheumatol. 2011;29:1040–3.
126. Chen L, Jing L, Dong Z, et al. Tumor necrosis factor-alpha blockers in SAPHO syndrome. J Med Res. 2013;42(4):91–5.

Spinal Infection

5

Rongjie Bai, Zhanhua Qian, and Huili Zhan

5.1 Anatomy of Spine and Imaging Anatomy

5.1.1 Anatomy of Spine

The spine is located in the middle of the posterior wall of the trunk, which is the central axis of the trunk and is involved in constituting the thoracic cage, abdominal cavity, and pelvic cavity, with support, protection, and motor functions. The spine is composed of vertebrae, intervertebral discs, ligaments between vertebral bodies, spinal cord in the vertebral canal, and rete vasculosum around the spine, whose anatomy is more complex.

1. **Vertebra.** At an early age, the human body has a total of 32 or 33 vertebrae, including 7 cervical vertebrae, 12 thoracic vertebrae, 5 lumbar vertebrae, 5 sacral vertebrae, and 3 or 4 caudal vertebrae; in adulthood, 5 sacral vertebrae are fused into the sacrum, and 3 or 4 caudal vertebrae synthesize into the coccyx, so the adult spine includes 24 vertebrae, 1 sacrum and 1 coccyx [1]. Except for the first and second cervical vertebrae, the shape of the vertebrae is similar and they consist of an anteriorly cylindrical vertebral body and a posteriorly plate-like vertebral arch. The vertebral body and vertebral arch form a vertebral foramen, and all vertebral foramina are connected superiorly and inferiorly to form a vertebral canal that accommodates the spinal cord. The vertebral arch consists of 1 pair of pedicles of vertebral arch and 1 pair of lamina of vertebral arch. The pedicle of vertebral arch is located in the lateral rear of the vertebral body, with 1 notch superiorly and inferiorly, and the notches of the superior and inferior pedicles of vertebral arch form a vertebral foramen, where the spinal nerves and blood vessels pass through; 7 processes emanate from the vertebral arch, including 1 spinous process, 2 transverse processes, 2 superior and 2 inferior articular processes, respectively, and the superior and inferior articular processes of the adjacent vertebral bodies constitute the facet joints. Due to the increase in weight bearing, the vertebral body increases in size gradually from the cervical vertebra downward and reaches its maximum at the fourth and fifth lumbar vertebrae and sacrum, and then decreases in size gradually from the sacral auricular surface downward. In the sagittal plane, there are four physiological curvatures of the spine, which are the cervical, thoracic, lumbar, and sacral curvatures, with the cervical and lumbar curvatures anteriorly and the thoracic and sacral curvatures protruding posteriorly [1].

   The first cervical vertebra, also known as the atlas, is composed of an anterior and posterior arch and bilateral masses, with the superior articular surface articulating with the occipital condyle of the skull base and the inferior articular surface articulating with the superior articular surface of the second cervical vertebra. The second cervical vertebra, also known as the axis, is composed of the vertebral body and vertebral arch, and the vertebral body forms a protrusion superiorly, called the odontoid process, which constitutes a joint with the posterior border of the anterior arch of the atlas [2].
2. **Connection between vertebrae.** The vertebral bodies are connected by intervertebral discs, ligaments, and joints.

   The intervertebral disc is located between two adjacent vertebral bodies and acts as a connection and cushion. Except between the first and second vertebral bodies, there were intervertebral discs between other vertebral bodies. The centre of the intervertebral disc is a jelly-like nucleus pulposus; it is surrounded by an annulus fibrosus composed of multiple layers of fibrocartilage arranged in a concentric circle; the upper and lower surfaces of the intervertebral disc are covered by a thin layer of hyaline cartilage, known as the hyaline cartilage plate [1].

R. Bai (✉) · Z. Qian · H. Zhan
Department of Radiology, Beijing Jishuitan Hospital, Beijing, China
e-mail: bairongjie@126.com

H. Li et al. (eds.), *Radiology of Infectious and Inflammatory Diseases - Volume 5*,
https://doi.org/10.1007/978-981-16-5003-1_5

The main ligaments connecting the spine include the anterior longitudinal ligament, posterior longitudinal ligament, ligamentum flavum, supraspinal ligament, and interspinal ligament. The anterior longitudinal ligament is attached to the anterior margin of the vertebral body and intervertebral disc, arises superiorly from the skull base, and extends inferiorly to the sacrum. The posterior longitudinal ligament binds tightly to the posterior border of the vertebral end-plate and intervertebral disc, while it binds loosely to the middle of the vertebral body. It starts from the axis and ends at the sacrum. The cervical segment of the posterior longitudinal ligament is thicker while the thoracolumbar segment is thinner. The ligamentum flavum is connected to adjacent lamina of vertebral arch. The interspinal ligaments are connected to adjacent spinous processes. The ligamentum flavum is composed of elastic fibres with a thin neck that gradually thickens inferiorly. The supraspinal ligament is a longitudinal ligament connecting all spinous processes [2].

The joints of the spine include the zygapophysial joints, atlanto-occipital joints, and atlanto-axial joints. The zygapophysial joint is articulated by the inferior articular process of the upper vertebral body and the superior articular process of the lower vertebral body, that is, the facet joint [2].

3. **Intraspinal contents.** Intraspinal contents mainly include the spinal cord and cauda equina, spinal nerve roots, spinal dura mater, epidural space and the vertebral venous plexus and connective tissue located in it, arachnoid, spinal pia mater, and subarachnoid space [1].

   The medulla oblongata extends inferiorly at the level of the foramen magnum to form the spinal cord. The conus medullaris is the end of the spinal cord and is located approximately at the level of the L_1 vertebral body in adults. The conus medullaris continues inferiorly as the filum terminale, ending at the first caudal vertebra. The spinal cord is thickest at the level of C_6 to C_7, known as cervical enlargement, thinnest at the level of T_5 to T_9, and thickened at the level of T_{10} to the conus medullaris [1].

   The spinal nerve is composed of the ventral anterior root and the dorsal posterior root, including 8 pairs of cervical spinal cord, 12 pairs of thoracic spinal cord, and 5 pairs of lumbar spinal cord. The first 7 cervical spinal nerves perforated the vertebral canal from the upper border of the pedicle of vertebral arch of the corresponding vertebral body and the eighth pair from the lower border of the C_7 pedicle of vertebral arch. From the T_1 spinal nerve, all of them perforate the vertebral canal by the vertebral foramen below the same ordinal vertebra [1].

   The spinal dura mater in the vertebral canal continues with the cerebral dura mater in the cranial cavity; the arachnoid is closely apposed to the spinal dura mater; and the spinal pia mater is closely apposed to the surface of the spinal cord and nerve roots and is not easily separated. The space formed between the spinal pia mater and the arachnoid is called the subarachnoid space, which is filled with cerebrospinal fluid and communicates with the cerebral subarachnoid space [2].

5.1.2 Imaging Anatomy of Spine

In clinical practice, the most commonly used examinations to determine spinal lesions include X-ray anteroposterior/lateral, CT, and MRI. X-ray opening position can also be used to determine the alignment of atlanto-axial vertebra, dual oblique position can be used to determine the intervertebral foramen and vertebral arch isthmus, hyperextension and hyperflexion position can be used to determine the stability of spine, and CT myelography (CTM) can be used to determine the intramedullary lesion and intraspinal brachial plexus root injury.

1. **X-ray anatomy.** On the PA X-ray, the vertebral body showed a slightly wider quadrangle at the bottom edge, a dense fine line shadow in the bone cortex, and slightly thicker superior and inferior end-plates of the vertebral body. The intervertebral space shows a certain thickness of radiolucent area between adjacent vertebral bodies, and the radiolucent shadow between adjacent vertebral laminas is the intervertebral foramen. The pedicle of vertebral arch is projected on both sides of the vertebral body and is symmetrically round or oval, and the distance between the two pedicles of vertebral arch is called the interpediculate distance, which represents the width of the vertebral canal. The superior and inferior articular processes are projected to the superior and inferior borders of the pedicle of vertebral arch, the superior articular process is located outwards superiorly, the inferior articular process is located inwards inferiorly, and the adjacent superior and inferior articular processes constitute the facet joints. The portion between the superior and inferior articular processes is called the isthmus of vertebral arch. The transverse process was projected on both sides of the vertebral body, except for C_7, where the transverse process of the cervical spine was not obvious, rib pits and costal bones were observed on both sides of the thoracic vertebral body, and the transverse process of L_3 was the most obvious. Part of the paravertebral soft tissues can be displayed beside the spine, such as the psoas major, quadratus lumborum, and parathoracic vertebral lines. In children, annular epiphyses are seen above and below the vertebral body, and epiphyseal ossification may present as a thin layer of ossification shadow at the superior and inferior borders of the vertebral body [3].

The vertebral body is rectangular on the lateral X-ray. The superior and inferior borders of the adjacent vertebral arches constitute the intervertebral foramen. The intervertebral space is clearer in the lateral view than in the PA view, 2–6 mm tall, and gradually widened from the cervical to the lumbar segments. The superior and inferior articular processes and spinous processes are observed in the posterior part of the vertebral arch, the spinous processes are obliquely downward, and the C_7 spinous process is the longest. In childhood, there is a deep notch in the middle of the anterior and posterior borders of the vertebral body, and a thin layer of ossification shadow appears at the superior and inferior borders of the vertebral body [3].

The C_1 and C_2 vertebral bodies, that is, the atlas and axis, cannot be displayed in ordinary PA views due to mandibular occlusion, and an opening position needs to be taken. In the opening position, the atlanto-occipital joint is formed by the two lateral masses of the atlas and the occipital condyle, and the pivot odontoid process is located between the two lateral masses, with symmetrical left and right spaces. The atlanto-odontoid joint is formed by the odontoid process of the axis and the anterior arch of the atlas, and its anteroposterior space is observed in the lateral view, which is normally about 2 mm. The inward triangular protrusion of the bevel is seen on both sides of the superior border of the cervical vertebral body, which is called the uncinate process, and the blunt bevel on both sides of the interior border of the vertebral body is called the clivus, which of the above two form the unique uncovertebral joint of the cervical vertebra and is most clearly displayed on the PA view. When the uncovertebral joint proliferates and degenerates, it is easy to compress the nerve root in the intervertebral foramen and the vertebral artery in the transverse foramen. The anteriorly arcuate physiological curvature of the cervical process can be observed in the lateral view, with the apex approximately at the posterosuperior border of the fifth vertebral body. The articular surface of the facet joints is obliquely downward by about 45°. The oblique film is mainly used to show the intervertebral foramen and its relationship with the uncovertebral joint, the left anterior oblique view shows the right intervertebral foramen, and the right anterior oblique view shows the left intervertebral foramen [4] (Fig. 5.1).

On the PA view of the thoracic vertebra, the capitulum costae of the 12 pairs of ribs beside the thoracic vertebra and the rib pits of the thoracic vertebral body constitute the joint thoracic vertebra, while the costal tubercles and the transverse rib pits form the costotransverse joint, while there is no costotransverse joint in the 11th and 12th ribs. Lateral views may show thoracic curvature, vertebral body, intervertebral foramen, zygapophysial joints, and ribs [4] (Fig. 5.2).

PA view of the lumbar vertebra may show the shape of the lumbar vertebra, the facet joint space, and the paravertebral soft tissues. Lateral views show the shape and

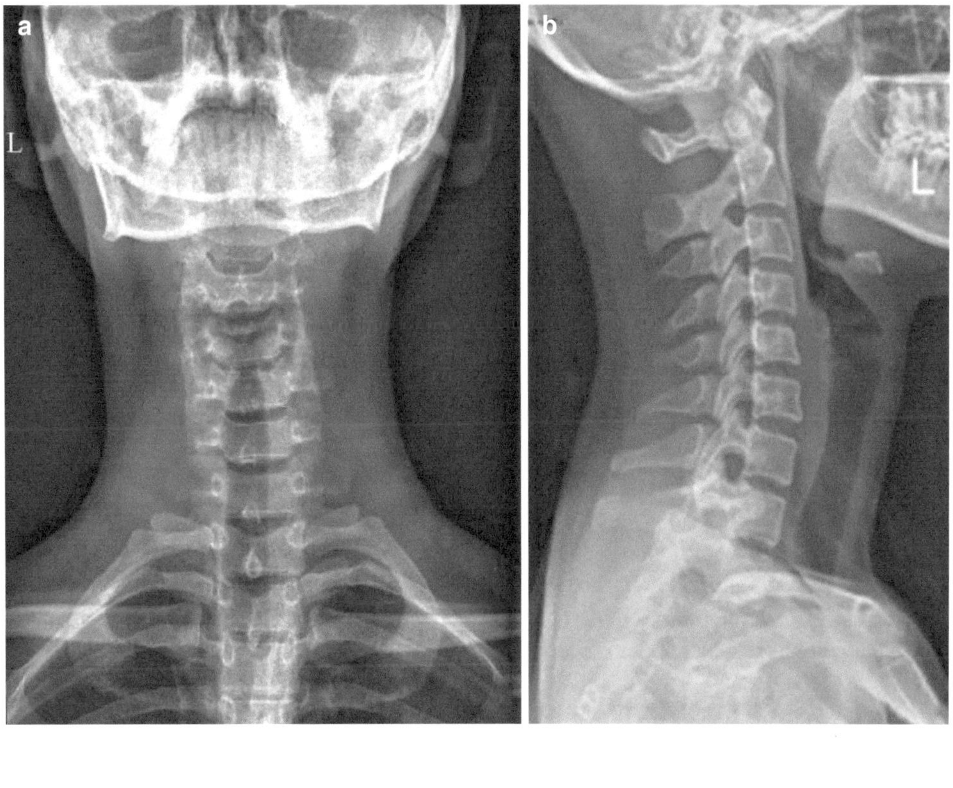

Fig. 5.1 Anteroposterior and lateral X-ray of cervical vertebra. (**a**) Anteroposterior X-ray of cervical vertebra; (**b**) Lateral X-ray of cervical vertebra

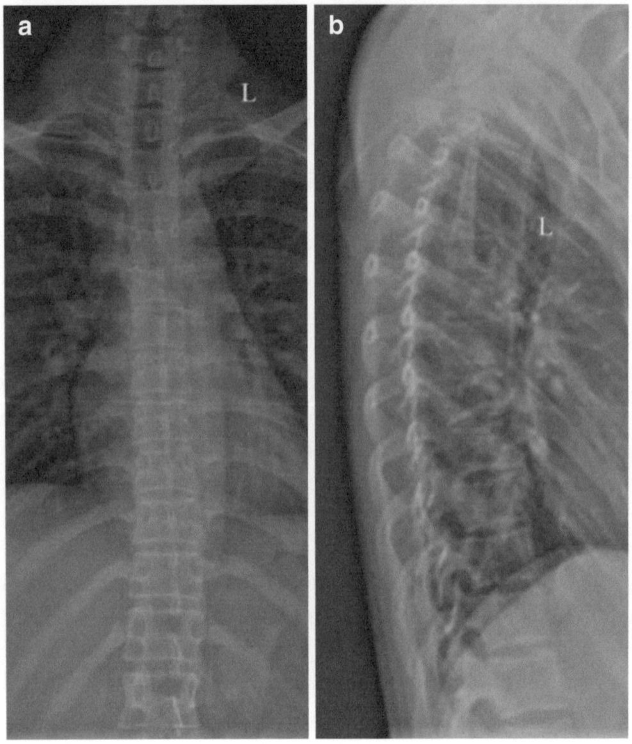

Fig. 5.2 Anteroposterior and lateral X-ray of thoracic vertebra. (**a**) Anteroposterior X-ray of thoracic vertebra; (**b**) Lateral X-ray of thoracic vertebra

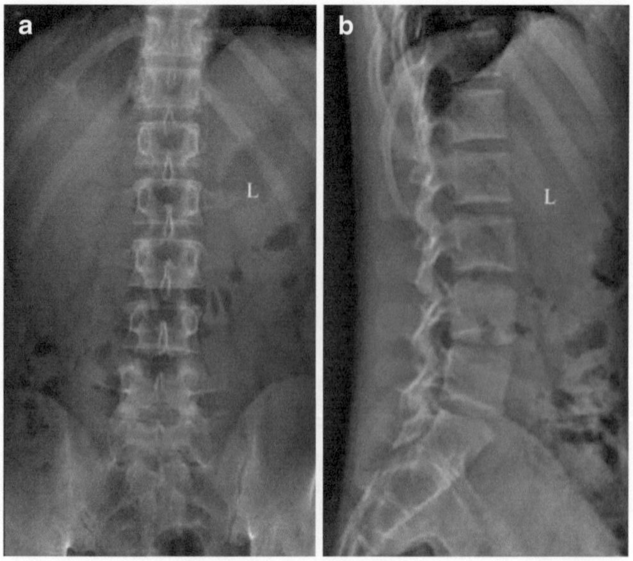

Fig. 5.3 Anteroposterior and lateral X-ray of lumbar vertebra. (**a**) Anteroposterior X-ray of lumbar vertebra; (**b**) Lateral X-ray of lumbar vertebra

structure of the vertebral body, intervertebral space, intervertebral foramen, spinous process, and zygapophysial joints (Fig. 5.3). Oblique film may show the isthmus of vertebral arch. The superior and inferior joints of the pedicles of vertebral arch and the isthmus of vertebral arch on both sides resembled canines on oblique films, with the proximal transverse process equivalent to the canine mouth, the pedicle of vertebral arch as the canine eye, the superior articular process as the canine ear, the inferior articular process as the canine anterior leg, the vertebral lamina as the canine abdomen, the isthmus as the canine neck, the distal transverse process as the canine tail, and the inferior articular process as the canine posterior leg. Isthmus spondyloschisis of vertebral arch occurs frequently at L_5 [3].

2. **CT anatomy.** CT can be used to observe structures including vertebral body, vertebral arch, facet joint, intervertebral space, intervertebral disc, dural sac, ligament, vertebral canal, spinal cord, and nerve root. In the transverse plane, except for the C_1 and C_2 vertebral bodies, the remaining cervical vertebral bodies are generally oval in shape with a slightly straight posterior border (Fig. 5.4); the thoracic vertebra is roughly cordate with approximately equal transverse and anteroposterior diameters and an procoelous posterior border; the lumbar vertebra is kidney-shaped with a Y-shaped low-density shadow extending into the spongy bone in the anterior and posterior middle of the vertebral body, which is the vertebral venous foramen and is only observed in the transverse plane and is often misdiagnosed as a fracture (Fig. 5.5).

The vertebral bodies were rectangular in sagittal and coronal planes. The atlas is approximately round in the transverse plane, with anterior and posterior nodules in the midline of the anterior and posterior arches, short transverse processes on both sides, and transverse foramen in it. The odontoid process of axis is articulated with the atlas, anterior to the posterior wall of the anterior arch of the atlas, posterior to the transverse ligament of the atlas, with transverse processes and transverse foramina on both sides. The atlanto-axial joints space can be visualized in the sagittal and coronal planes. The facet joints of the cervical vertebra are approximately located in the transverse plane, the thoracic vertebra is approximately located in the coronal plane, and the lumbar vertebra is approximately located in the sagittal plane, including the articular cartilage and the articular surface of the superior and inferior articular processes. The vertebral canal is about 12 mm in anteroposterior diameter in the cervical vertebra, 14–15 mm in the thoracic vertebra, and 20 mm in the lumbar vertebra. The intervertebral foramen is located between the superior and inferior pedicles of vertebral arch. The anteromedial wall of the cervical intervertebral foramen is the posterior aspect of the uncinate process, the intervertebral disc and the inferior part of the vertebral body, and the posterolateral wall is the medial part of the zygapophysial joint. The anterior wall of the thoracic and lumbar vertebrae is the vertebral body and intervertebral disc, and the posterior wall is the zygapophysial joint. In the sagittal plane, the intervertebral

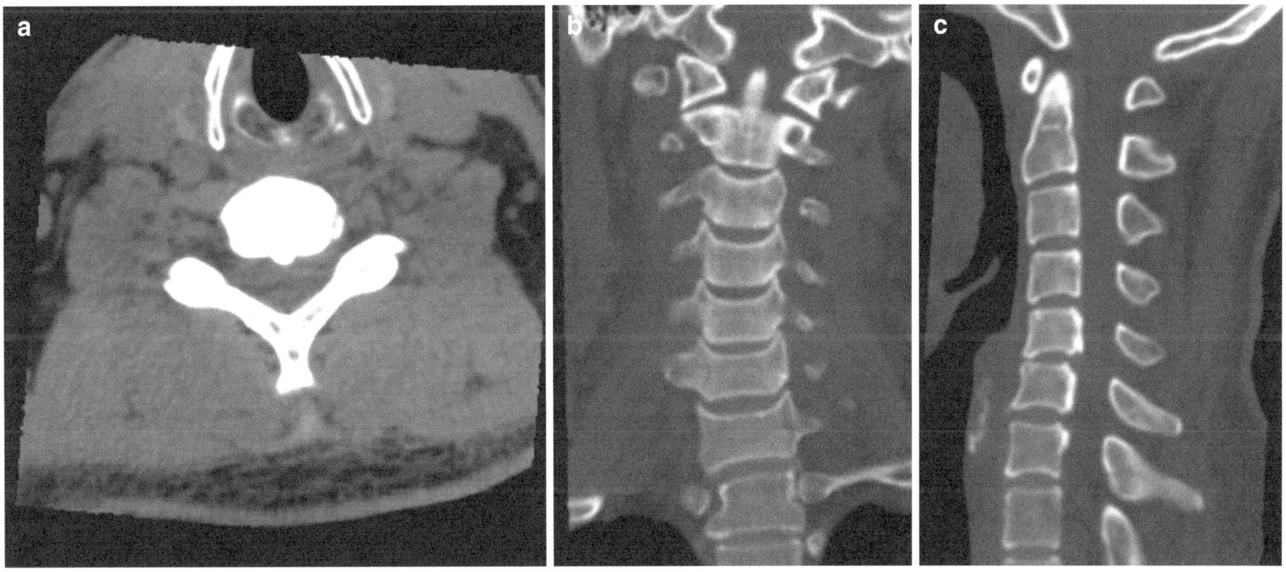

Fig. 5.4 Cervical CT. (**a**) In the transverse plane of cervical CT, the cervical body is approximately oval, and the punctate protrusion in the posterior part of the vertebral body is a calcified posterior longitudinal ligament; (**b**) In the coronal plane of cervical CT, the vertebral body is close to the rectangle, and attention should be paid to the uncovertebral joints on both sides of the vertebral body; (**c**) In the sagittal plane of cervical CT, the vertebral body is approximately rectangular in the sagittal plane

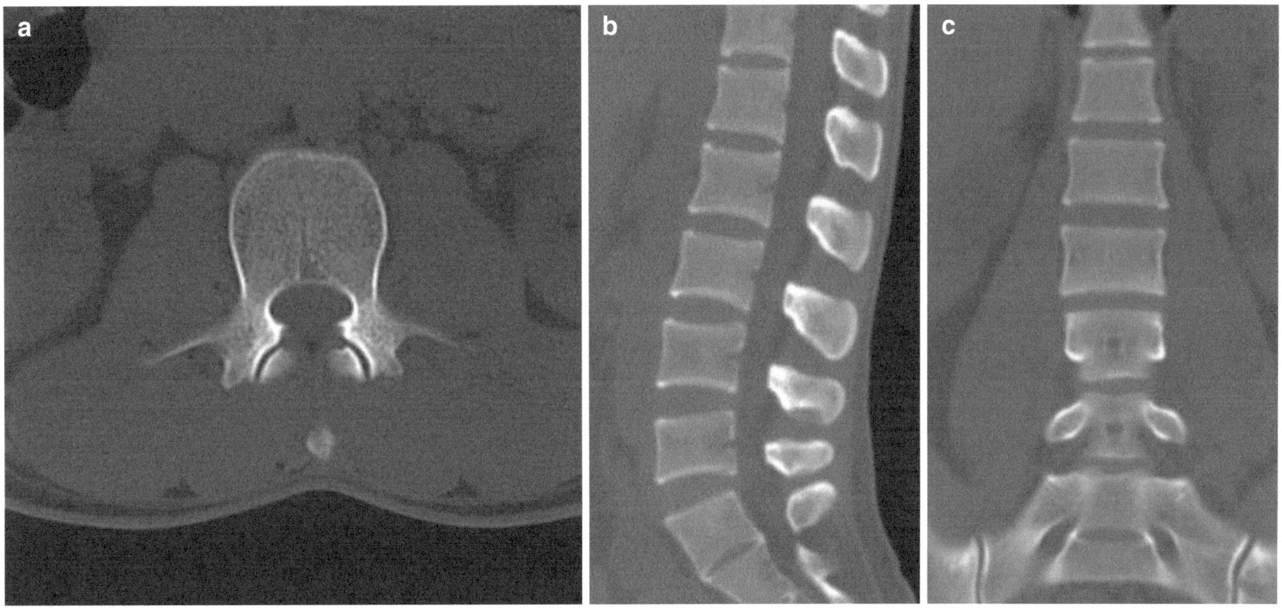

Fig. 5.5 Lumbar CT. (**a**) In the transverse plane of lumbar CT, the lumbar vertebra is approximately reniform, and the low-density line shadow in the middle of the vertebral body is the vertebral venous foramen; (**b**) In the sagittal plane of lumbar CT, the vertebral body is close to the rectangle in the sagittal plane; (**c**) In the coronal plane of lumbar CT, the vertebral body is close to the rectangle

foramen is round or oval, and nerve roots can be seen passing through it [3].

There are intervertebral discs from $C_2 \sim C_3$ to $L_5 \sim S_1$. In the transverse plane, the cervical intervertebral disc is round, the thoracic intervertebral disc is cordiform, and the lumbar intervertebral disc is reniform. They are coiled in the sagittal and coronal planes, and the borders are flush with those of the superior and inferior vertebral bodies. The intervertebral discs of $L_5 \sim S_1$ can be straight or slightly herniated, with a CT value of 50 ~ 100 HU, and the thickness is gradually thickened from top to bottom. The anterior and posterior borders of the vertebral body are covered with the anterior and posterior longitudinal ligaments, which are not normally visualized. Except for C_1 and C_2, the rest of the epidural space is filled with fat and connective tissues, which could contrast out the smooth, round, or oval borders of the dural sac. The normal dural sac contains arachnoid, cerebrospinal fluid, spinal pia mater, and spinal cord, with a CT value of 30 ~ 50 HU. The intraspinal venous plexus is distributed between the periosteum and spinal dura mater of the vertebral canal and cannot be distinguished from the peripheral tissues during plain scanning, and marked enhancement of the epidural space is observed after enhancement. Spinal nerve roots are round or cord-like soft tissue density shadows that penetrate out of the vertebral canal through the intervertebral foramen. The ligamentum flavum is located in the medial aspect of the zygapophysial joints and vertebral laminas and is in a "V" shape with a CT value of 40 ~ 60 HU, which gradually thickens from top to bottom, 2 ~ 3 mm [4].

3. **MRI anatomy.** The intensity of the vertebral signal depends on the type of bone marrow and the ratio of red and yellow bone marrow. The proportion of yellow bone marrow in the vertebral body of ordinary adults is higher than that of red bone marrow, so it shows hyperintense on both T_1WI and T_2WI. The end-plates show hypointense on both T_1WI and T_2WI due to mixed effects and chemical shift artefacts in different tissues. The cartilage of the facet joints shows hypointense on both T_1WI and T_2WI and is not easily distinguished from the bone cortex [3].

   The signal of the intervertebral disc is determined by its water content, and the water content in the nucleus pulposus of the normal intervertebral disc is high, so it shows hypointense on T_1WI and hyperintense on T_2WI. The annulus fibrosus on the lateral side of the nucleus pulposus has a low water content and shows hypointense on both T_1WI and T_2WI and is not easily distinguished from the anterior longitudinal ligament, posterior longitudinal ligament, and vertebral end-plate (Fig. 5.6) [5].

   The anterior longitudinal ligament, posterior longitudinal ligament, supraspinous ligament, and interspinous ligament contain a large amount of collagen components and thus show similar hypointense of bone cortex on all sequences of MRI. The ligamentum flavum shows isointense on both T_1WI and T_2WI due to its 80% content of the elastin component [5].

   The spinal cord shows isointense on T_1WI and hypointense on T_2WI. In the case of small FOV imaging, nerve roots can be visualized by the background of water or contrast agent [5].

5.2 Characteristics and Pathophysiological Changes in Common Pathogen Infection

Spinal infections are a collective term for a range of infectious diseases, including spondylitis, spondylodiscitis, zygapophysial joint arthritis, epidural infection, radiculitis, and myelitis, accounting for 2% ~ 7% of systemic musculoskeletal infections [6]. Spinal infection can be divided into three categories: pyogenic infection, granulomatous infection, and parasitic infection. It can be divided by pathogenic species into bacterial infection, fungal infection, virus infection, and parasitic infection. Pyogenic spondylitis and spinal tuberculosis are the two most common types of spinal infections [7]. Both pyogenic spondylitis and spinal tuberculosis are frequently seen in patients over 50 years of age. Spinal infections are relatively rare seen in children and adolescents.

Staphylococcus aureus is the most common pathogens in pyogenic spondylitis, accounting for about 60%, and other pathogens include Escherichia coli, pseudomonas aeruginosa, streptococcus pneumoniae, and salmonella. The annual incidence of pyogenic spondylitis is (0.2–2.4)/100,000 and the male to female ratio is (1.5–3):1. Spinal tuberculosis accounts for 1.5% ~ 3% of systemic tuberculosis [6, 8].

Pyogenic spondylitis is generally infected by haematogenous dissemination of bacteria in distant sites, frequently seen in lumbar vertebra, with the main symptoms of fever and back pain, most patients with unexplained acute, subacute fever. It can be infected via the arterial and venous routes, with pathogens from the urinary system, respiratory system, pelvis, or subcutaneous [9]. The terminal branches of arterial vessels in the end-plate area of spinal vertebral body-intervertebral disc are widely distributed, especially in the anterior region of vertebral body. Therefore, haematogenous infection in adults first and most commonly involves the sub-end-plate area of anterior vertebral body, and then the inflammation invades beyond the bone cortex, and towards the subligamentous region, intervertebral disc, adjacent vertebral body and even the spinal canal; The intravenous route is through the Batson venous plexus without valves and is the main haematogenous spread route of the infected spine in the urinary system and pelvic organs; Non-haematogenous routes include penetrating trauma, direct exposure to skin or open wounds, direct spread such as interventional procedures, and adjacent infections from head and neck, chest and abdominal viscera [6, 10].

Spinal tuberculosis is mostly haematogenous infection. Patients develop lung, lymph nodes, digestive tract, and other organs of tuberculosis, and then mycobacterium tuberculosis through haematogenous dissemination. Tuberculosis of spine is frequently seen in the thoracic/thoracolumbar segment. Patients may have fatigue, discomfort, weight loss, night sweats, and other symptoms. Patients at the chronic healing stage may have back stiffness, deformity, and neurological symptoms. Most patients do not have fever.

Spinal infection in children first involves the intervertebral disc, while spinal infection in adults over 20 years of age first infects the end-plate and then the intervertebral disc. It can spread directly from adjacent spinal-discitis or facet arthritis, or can be infected after haematogenous spread or interventional procedures, which are more frequently seen in the thoracic vertebra, and more than 70% are located dorsal to the vertebral canal. Primary facet arthritis is mostly trans-

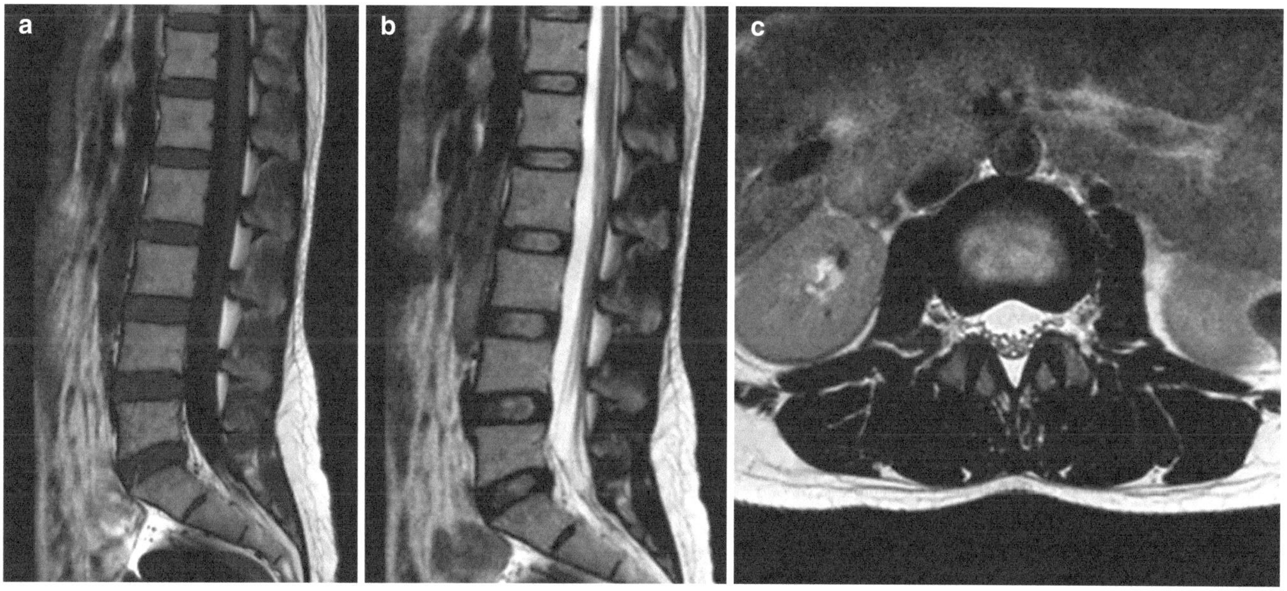

Fig. 5.6 Lumbar MRI. (**a**) MRI lumbar T_1WI sagittal plane; (**b**) MRI lumbar T_2WI sagittal plane; (**c**) MRI lumbar T_2WI transverse plane. The vertebral body shows hyperintense on both T_1WI and T_2WI, the nucleus pulposus of the intervertebral disc shows hypointense on T_1WI and hyperintense on T_2WI, and the fibres lateral to the nucleus pulposus show hypointense on both T_1WI and T_2WI

mitted by non-haematogenous routes [6, 11]. Complications such as diabetes, end-stage renal disease, and cirrhosis are high risk factors for spinal infection [12].

5.3 Bacterial Infection

Rongjie Bai, Zhanhua Qian, and Huili Zhan

Overview

Spinal bacterial infection is the most common type of spinal infection, and the most common diseases include vertebral osteomyelitis, discitis, and epidural abscess. The routes of infection include haematogenous transmission from other sites of infection, direct spread and spread of infection from other adjacent sites [13]. The most common route of infection in discitis is lumbar puncture, or infection after discography and discectomy, with onset 2 to 3 days after surgery, severe local pain, elevated body temperature, and activity limitation of lumbar vertebra. Spinal infections are less common than joint infections of the extremities, and the vulnerable population for spinal bacterial infections can be divided into three age groups. (1) Neonates within 6 months of age, especially those with toxaemia; (2) Children aged 2 ~ 8 years, with a relatively low incidence in this age group, frequently involved with spondylodiscitis; (3) The elderly over 50 years of age, accounting for about 60% of all patients with spinal bacterial infections [9].

Most of the pathogens are staphylococcus aureus or Escherichia coli, and cervical vertebra or thoracolumbar spine may be infected. Staphylococcus aureus infections account for more than 50% of all patients with spinal bacterial infections. Urinary tract infection is often associated with Escherichia coli and proteus infection; Pseudomonas aeruginosa infections often have a history of intravenous drug abuse or immune system defects; Salmonella infections generally occur in patients with sickle cell anaemia; anaerobic infections can occur secondary to patients with open spinal injuries and are also more frequently seen in diabetic patients; Chronic low-toxicity infections are usually caused by low-toxicity bacteria, such as alpha-hemolytic streptococcus and staphylococcus epidermidis [13].

Low back pain and muscle spasm are the earliest and most important clinical symptoms in patients with spinal bacterial infection, with sudden onset, persistent high fever, spinal pain, activity limitation, aggravated during exercise and relieved after rest. In patients with thoracic vertebra infection, pleural irritation may occur; in patients with lumbar vertebra infection, peritoneal irritation may occur. Acute pyogenic spondylitis can also form abscesses in the paravertebral region and can enter the vertebral canal to compress the spinal cord and produce spinal cord compression symptoms. Patients with slow onset, mild symptoms have hyperostosis and even ligament ossification after examination of the vertebral body. According to the different location of the lesion and the progression of the disease, it is still often accompanied by symptoms such as physical discomfort, weight loss, and anorexia. Infection of intervertebral disc may present with posterior peritoneal irritation sign, flatulence of the small intestine, paralytic intestinal depression, and vertebral destruction at 2–3 weeks later, and may invade the facet joints. Pyogenesis of intervertebral disc can easily enter the vertebral canal, compress the spinal cord, and cause spinal cord compression symptoms. Peripheral bone destruction, hyperplasia, and sclerosis occur in the late stage.

Laboratory tests show increased or unchanged leukocyte, increased erythrocyte sedimentation rate, and elevated C-reactive protein. Etiological isolation of pathogens is one of the diagnostic criteria, but only 1/2 ~ 2/3 of patients have positive culture results [13].

MRI is the preferred choice of examination for the diagnosis of spinal infection, and its sensitivity, specificity, and accuracy can reach 96%, 92%, and 94%, respectively. Enhanced MRI enables early diagnosis of spinal infection. CT has high sensitivity for spinal infection, but low specificity, and easily misses epidural abscess [7].

Pathophysiology

The routes of spinal bacterial infection include haematogenous transmission from other sites of infection, direct spread and spread of infection from other adjacent sites. The Batson paravertebral venous plexus of the vertebral body is a valve-free venous system in which reverse blood flow can occur during increased thoracic or intra-abdominal pressure. This venous plexus is associated with central vertebral infections, skip vertebral infections, and disseminated infections such as infective endocarditis. The sub-end-plate region of vertebral cartilage is supplied by the anterior and posterior vertebral arterial plexus and is associated with haematogenous infection in this region [10].

Many factors predispose patients to pyogenic spinal infections, including advanced age, malnutrition, immunocompromise, diabetes, intravenous drug abuse, AIDS, malignancy, chronic steroid use, renal failure, septicaemia, spinal surgery, and the presence of intravascular devices and foreign bodies. Bacterial endocarditis is the most common risk factor for this disease, and nearly 30% of haematogenous spinal infections are associated with bacterial endocarditis [13].

Imaging Findings

1. Typical radiographic findings include osteolysis, end-plate destruction, and vertebral collapse. The role of plain X-ray in the diagnosis of early spinal bacterial infection is limited, and abscesses in the paravertebral soft tissues are seen within 2 weeks of onset. Cervical infection forms an abscess in the posterior wall of the throat. Swelling and thickening of fusiform soft tissue is observed beside the vertebrae during thoracic vertebra infection. Lumbar infection shows swelling of the psoas major. Vertebral bone destruction can be seen at 2 ~ 4 weeks after onset, and signs of blurred end-plate bone and narrowing of the intervertebral space may occur in the affected vertebral body, which are not easily observed. In severe cases, vertebral compression fractures occur, or the adnexa and facet joints of the vertebral body are destroyed, which may be accompanied by periosteal new bone beside the vertebral cortex. In the late stage of the disease, hyperostosis and osteosclerosis around the vertebral destruction area, ossification of paravertebral ligaments, formation of intervertebral bone bridges, or bone fusion of the vertebral body occur (Fig. 5.7a, b). Pyogenic discitis, within 10 days of onset, can show destruction of the superior and inferior end-plates of the vertebral body of the infected intervertebral disc. Osteolytic destruction can occur 2 weeks later, the intervertebral space narrows, and the paravertebral soft tissue swells. Bone fusion of vertebral body occurs in the late stage. The diagnostic sensitivity and specificity of X-ray are lower than those of CT. However, X-ray can still provide very useful information for the evaluation of the overall sequence and stability of the spine and can also play a very important role in the late follow-up of patients [12].
2. **CT.** Compared with plain X-ray films, CT can detect early bone destruction of the vertebral body in patients with spinal bacterial infection, and can show abscesses and calcifications around the affected vertebral body, and can better assess vertebral destruction and local spinal stability (Fig. 5.7c ~ e). Paravertebral abscesses are frequently seen in pyogenic bacterial infections, and paravertebral calcifications and involvement of pedicle of vertebral arch are more frequently seen in granulomatous inflammation. Vertebral bone destruction is a characteristic feature of this disease, but it is not specific and can be seen in any vertebral tumour or infectious lesion. CTM can be used to observe epidural involvement in spinal bacterial infections, but in the cervicothoracic part, it is easy to cause missed diagnosis due to artefacts. CT-guided puncture is commonly used for lesion biopsy [10].
3. **MRI.** It is the preferred choice of examination for the diagnosis of spinal bacterial infections. It shows that the effect of pathological changes in each stage of pyogenic spondylitis is the best. Contrast-enhanced MRI should be performed in patients with suspected spinal bacterial infection unless there are clear contraindications.

   Bone marrow oedema is the earliest imaging findings of this disease, but the specificity is low, and narrowing of the intervertebral space is also an earlier manifestation of this disease. With intravertebral osteomyelitis infiltration, oedema and congestion to pus production, vertebral bone marrow shows hypointense on T_1WI and hyperintense on T_2WI or proton-weighted images. Narrowing of the intervertebral space, irregular shape of the intervertebral disc, and rupture of the nucleus pulposus are common MRI findings of this disease (Fig. 5.7f, g), and the affected intervertebral disc shows hyperintense on T_2WI (Fig. 5.7g), which is a very important feature of this disease. It shows hypointense on T_1WI, and the demarcation from the vertebral end-plate is blurred on T_1WI. When end-plate bone destruction occurs, a hypointense band on T_1WI may appear under the vertebral end-plate, which is significantly enhanced after enhancement (Fig. 5.7h),

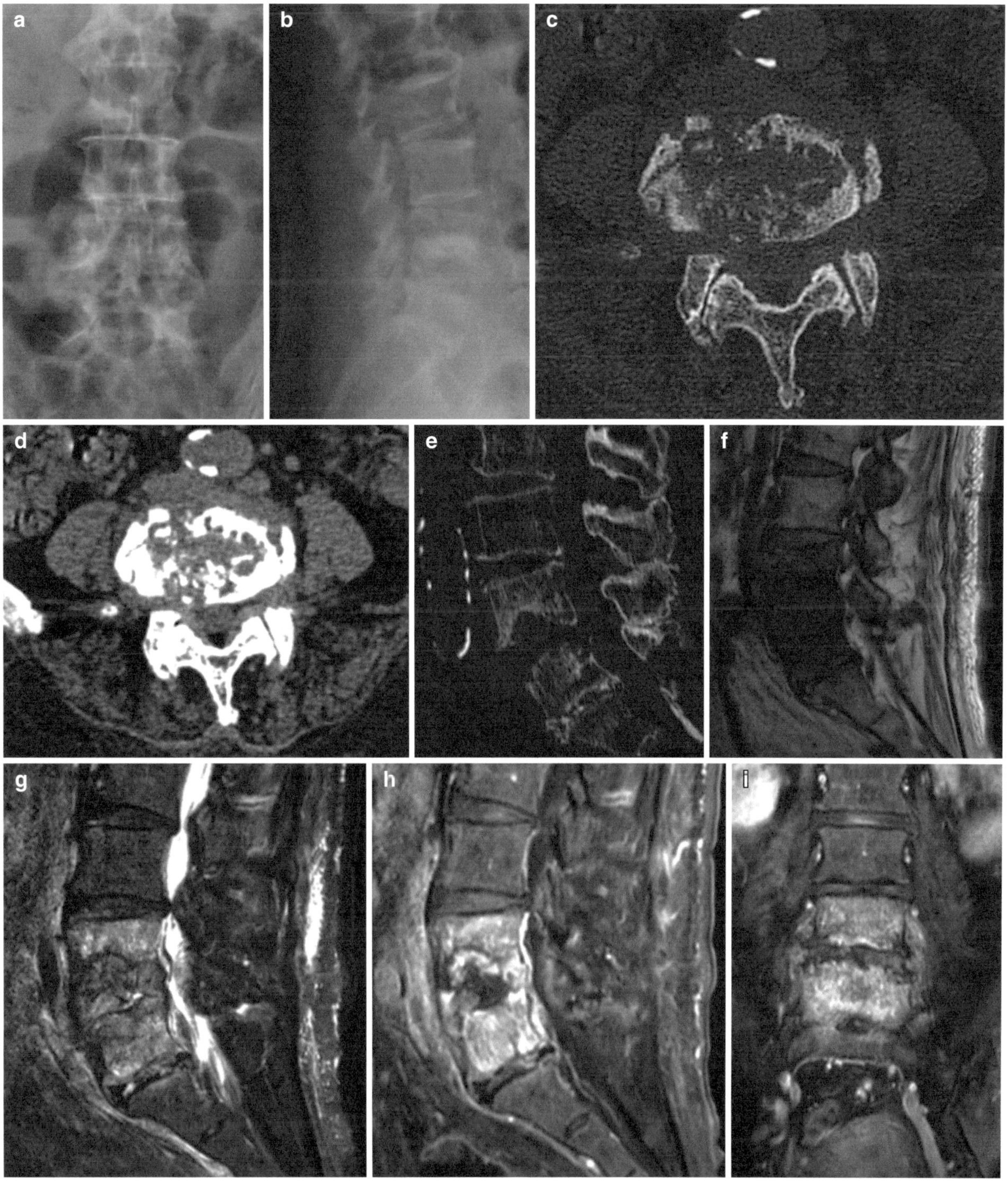

Fig. 5.7 Lumbar bacterial infection. (**a**) PA X-ray of lumbar vertebra shows blurred space from L_4 to L_5, and unclear display of adjacent cortex border of vertebral bodies $L_4 \sim L_5$; (**b**) Lateral X-ray of lumbar vertebra shows blurred space from L_4 to L_5, depression of lower border of vertebral body L_4, visible bone defect, rough articular surface, local osteosclerosis, and blurred bone at superior border of vertebral body L_5; (**c**) CT transverse plane bone window shows bone erosion and destruction of vertebral body L_4, multiple fragmentation, with osteosclerosis; (**d**) CT transverse plane soft tissue window shows soft tissue density in the destruction area of vertebral body, and the boundary is still clear; (**e**) CT sagittal plane bone window reconstruction shows bone erosion and destruction of vertebral bodies $L_4 \sim L_5$, with uneven density, mainly low density, with osteosclerosis and multiple fragmentation, and the vertebral body has not slipped; (**f**) MRI lumbar T_1WI sagittal plane shows bone destruction at the inferior border of vertebral body L_4 and the superior border of vertebral body L_5, showing hypointense on T_1WI, involving the intervertebral disc; (**g**) MRI lumbar T_2WI fat-suppressed sequence sagittal plane shows uneven signal intensity in the bone destruction area of vertebral bodies $L_4 \sim L_5$, showing slightly hyperintense, hyperintense in the vertebral body of non-destruction area, loss of normal shape of lumbar intervertebral disc, local hyperintense and exudation shadow in the subcutaneous area of lower back; (**h**) T_1WI fat-suppressed enhanced sequence of lumbar vertebra shows significant heterogeneous enhancement in the destruction area of vertebral bodies $L_4 \sim L_5$, marked enhancement zone in the sub-end-plate area of vertebral body L_4, local nodular enhancement of intervertebral disc and quasi-circular non-enhanced area in the intervertebral space; (**i**) Coronal plane shows localized enhancement of paravertebral soft tissues

with no enhancement of paravertebral abscesses and necrotic tissue and sequestrum, while marked enhancement of the affected bone marrow and periabscess tissue (Fig. 5.7i). Epidural abscess is common in this disease, but it is not a specific manifestation of this disease, and it is easily missed on T_2WI sagittal plane images when the abscess involves multiple sites [6]. In the subacute and chronic stages, due to vertebral destruction with surrounding hyperostosis and pus formation in residual lesions, it shows hypointense on T_1WI and hypointense or mixed hyperintense-hypointense on T_2WI. If spinal cord compression occurs, MRI can comprehensively assess the degree of compression and spinal cord injury.

Key Points of Diagnosis

1. Most of them have a definite history of pyogenic bacterial infection.
2. Bacterial endocarditis is the most common risk factor for this disease.
3. Typical imaging findings include osteolysis, end-plate destruction, and vertebral collapse.
4. CT can detect vertebral bone destruction early in patients with spinal bacterial infection.
5. MRI is the preferred choice of examination for this disease with an accuracy of 94%.
6. Bone marrow oedema shows hypointense on T_1WI and hyperintense on T_2WI; the affected intervertebral disc shows hyperintense on T_2WI, with blurred demarcation from the vertebral end-plate on T_1WI; the paravertebral abscess and necrotic tissue are not enhanced on contrast-enhanced scan, and the affected bone marrow and periabscess tissues show marked enhancement.
7. Laboratory tests show accelerated erythrocyte sedimentation rate and elevated C-reactive protein.

Differential Diagnosis

1. **End-plate osteochondritis.** MRI findings include: irregular and thickened outline of two adjacent vertebral bodies, hypointense on T_1WI, and hyperintense on T_2WI for bone marrow, intervertebral disc with possible vacuum sign, and end-plate cortex generally continuous without destruction. Heterogeneous enhancement is observed through enhanced scan, and linear hyperintense shadow with clear boundary is observed at the junction between the focus of abnormal end-plate osteochondritis and adjacent bone marrow and the normal bone marrow on the DWI image [6], and the intervertebral space can be narrowed; the paravertebral soft tissues and epidural space are generally not affected.
2. **Ankylosing spondylitis.** The findings include: mostly blurred outline of facet joints and subchondral osteosclerosis in the early stage, straightening of lumbar curvature in the middle stage, and calcification of articular capsule between the articular processes with two parallel longitudinal dense bands in the late stage, forming bamboo vertebrae, extensive ligament calcification and facet joint fusion, but no stenosis is observed in the intervertebral space.

Status Quo and Progress of Research

Bacterial spinal infections in adults can have significant adverse consequences, including pain, neurological impairment, spinal instability, deformity, or death. Many factors predispose people to spinal infections, many of which can affect the immune status of patients. The routes of spinal bacterial infection include haematogenous transmission from other sites of infection, direct spread and spread of infection from adjacent sites. Infections are usually classified into several categories based on anatomical location and are broadly classified as vertebral osteomyelitis, discitis, and epidural abscess [8].

5.4 Fungal Infection

Overview

Spinal fungal infections are uncommon, frequently seen in immunocompromised patients, and rare in immunocompetent patients with chronic obstructive pulmonary disease. The pathogens causing fungal spinal infection can be divided into two categories: opportunistic pathogens and pathogenic fungi. Opportunistic pathogens (including Aspergillus, Candida, and Mucor) rarely cause diseases in healthy people, but are frequently seen in immunocompromised people; Pathogenic fungi (including Blastomyces, Coccidioides, Histoplasma capsulatum) can cause disease in healthy people, accounting for 5% ~ 10% of all spinal fungal infections. Due to the widespread use of immunosuppressive drugs and broad-spectrum antibiotics, the increase in the use of venous indwelling needles and the increase in the number of patients with AIDS in recent years, the incidence of this disease has increased. The disease is mostly caused by haematogenous transmission at other sites (mainly in the lungs) or direct transplant during invasive procedures [14].

Because the clinical manifestations of spinal fungal infections lack specificity and there is also a lack of specific laboratory tests, spinal fungal infections are difficult to be diagnosed in early stage.

Pathophysiology

Cryptococcus, Candida, and Aspergillus are the most common pathogens of this disease. These fungi are usually endophytic fungi of the human body, but in some cases, such fungi can spread along the vasculature to organs or spine.

Cryptococcus is present in soil and pigeon faeces. This fungal infection is the fourth most common infection in HIV-infected individuals, with an incidence of 1% ~ 5% in organ transplant recipients. Normally, Candida is part of human commensal bacteria, commonly found in the skin, gastrointestinal tract, but also in the female genital tract and in the urine of patients with indwelling catheters. Most of them are endogenous infections and can also be seen in human-to-human transmission. Aspergillus is a ubiquitous saprophytic fungus that can produce many microspores (2 ~ 4 μm in diameter). Spores are frequently seen in water, soil, decaying vegetation, hay, and cereals. The spores are very small in size and can diffuse into the airflow of a contaminated air-handling system at any time and deposit into the human alveoli [14].

Fungal infection can cause a series of inflammatory reactions such as chronic inflammatory reactions and pyogenic granuloma formation, leading to local calcification, infarction, or causing allergic reactions.

Imaging Findings

1. **X-ray.** The plain X-ray of spinal fungal infection is similar to that of tuberculosis, which is characterized by involvement of the anterior margin of vertebral body, relatively mild destruction of intervertebral disc, and paravertebral abscess formation [9]. It invades the adjacent ribs and posterior part of the vertebral body, and sinus formation is rare. Certain specific types of fungal infections may show specific signs, for example, in patients with coccidioidomycosis, swelling of the soft tissues around the vertebral body, especially the soft tissues behind the spine. Vertebral collapse and kyphotic deformity are more common in patients with Blastomyces infection [7]. Osteolytic lesions in the vertebral bodies of cryptococcus-infected individuals are similar to cystic lesions of coccidioidomycosis or spinal tuberculosis, with discontinuous margins and surrounding abscess formation. Spinal fungal infections may also be characterized by separate vertebral collapse with infiltrative bone destruction. Patients tend to have more severe bone lesions than clinical symptoms [14].
2. **CT.** In spinal fungal infections, CT and MRI are effective means of determining the extent of the disease. The affected vertebral body with spinal fungal infection is characterized by small fragments and irregular residual bone in the osteolytic destruction on CT [10]. Unlike suppurative osteomyelitis of the spine, fungal infections often do not involve the intervertebral disc. These are not specific imaging findings of spinal fungal infections and can also appear in other spinal non-pyogenic infections, such as tuberculosis of spine [12].
3. **MRI.** In immunocompromised patients, T_2WI signals may not change, or appear slightly increased, in vertebral lesions due to the lack of inflammatory response. The intervertebral disc shows significant signal increase on T_2WI, the structure of the nucleus pulposus is intact, and its pathological mechanism remained unclear [8].

   Aspergillus spinal infection can cause necrotizing arteritis and further lead to thrombosis, vessel rupture, or infarction. Aspergillus infection may lead to multiple vertebral body involvement, and its vertebral body destruction is similar to that of tuberculosis of spine; anterior/posterior bulging of the intervertebral disc with annulus fibrosus destruction, no or mild enhancement of the intervertebral disc after enhancement, marked enhancement of the anterior/posterior longitudinal ligaments and subligamentous space, occasional vertebral collapse, backward protrusion into the vertebral canal, and spinal instability. Infection may be characterized by an epidural abscess or myelitis.

   Candida spinal infections may be accompanied by or secondary to haematogenous disseminated candidiasis. Candida albicans infection may cause vertebral and intraspinal abscesses and large paravertebral abscesses and granulomas without intervertebral disc involvement.

   Blastogenic spinal infection is clinically and radiologically similar to tuberculosis and is characterized by osteolytic lesions with mild reactive sclerosis, jumping lesions, vertebral collapse, spinal abscess or granuloma, spinal meningitis with spinal cord compression, paravertebral abscess, and occasional adjacent rib involvement, which can be used for differentiation from tuberculosis.

   Cryptococcal spinal infection is usually characterized by an intraspinal granulomatous mass with compression of the spinal cord. Cryptococcal meningitis is frequently seen in AIDS patients, where the inflammatory response is mild and meningeal enhancement is rare. Vertebral body and adnexal lesions are frequently seen in the lumbar vertebrae, well-defined osteolytic lesions are observed, and periosteal reactions are mild or absent.

   Coccidioidal spinal infection is characterized by osteolytic bone destruction with sclerotic edges, lesions not involving the intervertebral space and vertebral lamina, common adnexal involvement, and extensive paravertebral soft tissue swelling and thickening.

Key Points of Diagnosis

1. The pathogens of spinal fungal infections are generally conditional pathogen, found in immunocompromised people.
2. Cryptococcus, Candida, and Aspergillus are the most common pathogens of this disease.
3. The plain X-ray of spinal fungal infection is similar to that of tuberculosis, which is characterized by involvement of the anterior margin of vertebral body, relatively

mild destruction of intervertebral disc, and paravertebral abscess formation.
4. In spinal fungal infections, CT and MRI are effective means of determining the extent of the disease.
5. MRI findings of spinal fungal infections are not specific, and in immunocompromised patients, T_2WI signals may not change, or appear slightly increased due to the lack of inflammatory response.

Differential Diagnosis

1. **Spinal tuberculosis.** Spinal fungal infection and tuberculosis of spine are difficult to differentiate. Spinal fungal infection may be accompanied by necrotizing arteritis and adjacent rib involvement, and T_2WI signal changes may be mild. A thorough physical examination and history may be helpful in differentiating.
2. **Pyogenic spondylitis.** Intervertebral space and intervertebral disc are commonly involved, but rare in this disease.
3. **Primary tumour/metastatic tumour.** There is no paravertebral abscess; mild signal change in vertebral body, and high degree of enhancement after enhancement.

Status Quo and Progress of Research

Spinal fungal infections are rare diseases that are sometimes difficult to be diagnosed. Early diagnosis of the disease requires knowledge of the patient's history and detailed physical examination. Prompt and appropriate medical treatment is the preferred choice of treatment for this disease and requires close monitoring of the clinical course. Ineffective medical treatment, spinal instability, and neurological dysfunction are indications for debridement treatment of spinal fusion. The prognosis depends on the premorbid state of the patient, the type of fungus, and the timing of treatment [14].

5.5 Brucella Infection

Overview

Brucellosis, also known as Malta fever and undulant fever, is a zoonotic systemic infectious and allergic disease caused by various types of Brucella [15], which occurs around the world and is more frequently seen in the Mediterranean and Arab regions [16]. In China, the disease is mainly concentrated in pastoral areas in Inner Mongolia, Northeast China, and Northwest China. Sick sheep, cattle, canines, and other animals are the main source of brucellosis infection. People who have direct contact with sick animals and other occupational groups or who eat undercooked beef or mutton are at high risk of infection with the disease. In recent years, due to the increasing consumption of fresh dairy products and beef and mutton year by year, the incidence of brucellosis has also increased, with 500,000–1,000,000 new patients with brucellar spondylitis each year [9]. The disease occurs frequently in young and middle-aged, but rare in elderly and infants. With a long course of the disease, it is easy to invade the bone and joints, causing spondylitis, sacroiliitis, osteomyelitis, peripheral arthritis, bursitis, and tenosynovitis. Spondylitis occurs most frequently in adults, and the lumbar vertebra is the most vulnerable. The sacroiliac joints and knee joints are most commonly affected in young adults. The location of bone and joint damage is fixed, mainly in weight-bearing joints, which are more common in large joints such as the hip joint and knee joints, characterized by joint enlargement, pain, arthritis, dysfunction, and persistent soreness or dull pain in the skeletal muscles. Fever, hyperhidrosis, and low back pain are known as the triad of brucellar spondylitis, and orchitis is also one of the characteristic symptoms of brucellosis.

Brucella can involve tissues and organs such as liver, spleen, lymph nodes, and bone marrow after dissemination with blood [17]. Brucellosis laboratory test mainly includes pathogen culture and serological examination, in which the patient's blood, cerebrospinal fluid, bone marrow, and synovial membrane fluids can all be used for pathogen culture. Isolation and culture of Brucella is the gold standard for the diagnosis of the disease, but the positive rate of blood culture is low. Tube agglutination test is a common serological diagnostic method for brucellosis and helps to diagnose brucellar spondylitis [18].

Pathophysiology

Brucella enters the human body through the skin, mucous, digestive tract, and respiratory tract, is phagocytosed by neutrophils and macrophages, reaches nearby lymph nodes with the endolymphatic circulation in the body, and then enters the blood circulation, and thus invading the liver, spleen, bone marrow, joints, and other tissues. The main change of this disease is serous exudative inflammation, and then with the proliferation of fibrocytes, granulomas composed of epithelioid cells, macrophages, plasma cells and lymphocytes appear in the lesion. Bacteria multiply to a certain extent and can enter the blood circulation again. After bacterial destruction, a variety of virulence factors are released, and the body temperature increases again. The lesions are prone to protracted chronic infection and can eventually form bone and joint deformation. Granulation tissue proliferation in the bone destruction area is observed, in which neutrophils, monocytes, eosinophils, and lymphocytes are infiltrated.

Imaging Findings

1. **X-ray.** It can display the whole picture of spine, and the flattening of vertebral body, stenosis of intervertebral

space, and physiological curvature of spine can be visually observed in lateral position. Adnexa such as vertebral arches and articular processes may also have bone destruction changes. Typical presentations are described below.

(a) Inflammation of vertebral body: The lesions are multiple and mostly invade the superior and inferior borders of 1 ~ 2 vertebral bodies. In the early stage, it is characterized by small focal bone mineral density reduction and bone defects a few weeks later, which are quasi-circular hypodense lesions of 2 ~ 5 mm in diameter (Fig. 5.8a) surrounded by a significant sclerosis strap, and larger lesions are "insular". The destruction area shows soft tissue density, sharp margin, irregular knife-saw appearance, later edge sclerosis and hyperplasia to form bone spurs, and adjacent vertebral bodies can form bone bridges. The centre of the vertebral body can also be invaded. Usually, the lesion in the centre of the vertebral body is presented with rapid sclerosis without the formation of deep bone destruction and is gradually replaced by new bone later [9, 16].

(b) Zygapophysial joint arthritis: It occurs frequently in the adjacent vertebral body. The joint space gradually narrows, or even disappears. The articular surface is irregularly destroyed, and multiple joints can also be invaded at the same time, resulting in bony ankylosis.

(c) Ligament calcification: It occurs frequently in the lower lumbar vertebra and can gradually progress from bottom to top, with cord-like calcified ground-glass opacity in the anterior and posterior longitudinal ligaments.

(d) Spondylodiscitis: In the early stage, it is characterized by narrowing and increased density of the intervertebral space, but no destruction of the vertebral end-plates [9, 16].

2. **CT.** The bone destruction foci are multiple, quasi-circular low-density lesions with the diameter of no more than 5 mm, with varying degrees of obvious proliferation and proliferation and sclerosis zone at the edge, mostly distributed at the edge of vertebral body, a few were found in the centre of vertebral body. The bone trabecula is thick and disordered, the structure is unclear, and there is no sequestrum or destruction of pedicle of vertebral arch (Fig. 5.8b). Vertebral body destruction is accompanied by adjacent intervertebral disc destruction, intervertebral space stenosis, generally increased density of adjacent vertebral bodies, and proliferation and sclerosis of articular surface. The periosteum of the vertebral body is hypertrophic and bulges from the middle to both sides, so that the vertebral body shows mottled heterogeneous density increase, shuttle deformation, coracoid protrusion, and armor involucrum at the edge of the affected vertebral body, forming new osteophytes, which constitute the characteristic features of "lacelike vertebrae" with the destruction foci in between. Ligament calcification or ossification also appears on one or all sides of 2 ~ 3 vertebral bodies, showing fine strip high ground-glass opacity. Intervertebral osteochondritis is characterized by narrowing of the intervertebral space and rare formation of paravertebral abscesses. Similar changes are also observed in the zygapophysial joints, mostly limited to 1 ~ 2 facet joints, with irregular or narrowed joint spaces. The above findings may coexist or appear alone. Soft tissue ground-glass opacity connected to the destruction area of the vertebral body is observed beside the vertebra, with irregular shape and clear boundary, pushing the adjacent psoas major.
3. **MRI.** It can detect early abnormal signals of vertebral body and surrounding involved soft tissues, with heterogeneous signals. The disrupted intervertebral disc or inflammatory granulation tissue protruding into the vertebral canal, spinal cord compression, and intervertebral space stenosis can also be found [12]. Epidural abscesses in brucellar spondylitis are extremely rare and are characterized by the absence of significant local tissue reaction. Brucellar spondylitis MRI is characterized by thick and irregularly enhanced abscess walls and ill-defined paraspinal abnormal signals, hypointense on T_1WI and hyperintense on T_2WI, hyperintense on T_2WI until bone destruction is evident, and heterogeneous hyperintense in the vertebral body, intervertebral disc, adnexa and in vertebral canal on T_2WI fat-suppressed sequence [9] (Fig. 5.8c ~ e).

Key Points of Diagnosis

1. The disease shows some regional clustering and is mainly concentrated in pastoral areas.
2. RBPT and SAT are commonly used serological diagnostic methods.
3. The X-ray findings include inflammation of vertebral body, zygapophysial joint arthritis, ligament calcification, and spondylodiscitis.
4. The "lacelike vertebrae" formed by new osteophytes and destruction focuses therein is a characteristic CT finding of the disease.
5. MRI features include thick and irregular abscess wall, and ambiguous abnormal intensity observed in paravertebral region.

Differential Diagnosis

1. **Tuberculosis of spine.** Thoracolumbar segment is the most common site of focuses, and vertebral bodies concerned are mainly destroyed by osteolysis. These focuses can be observed in multiple spinal segments, leading to

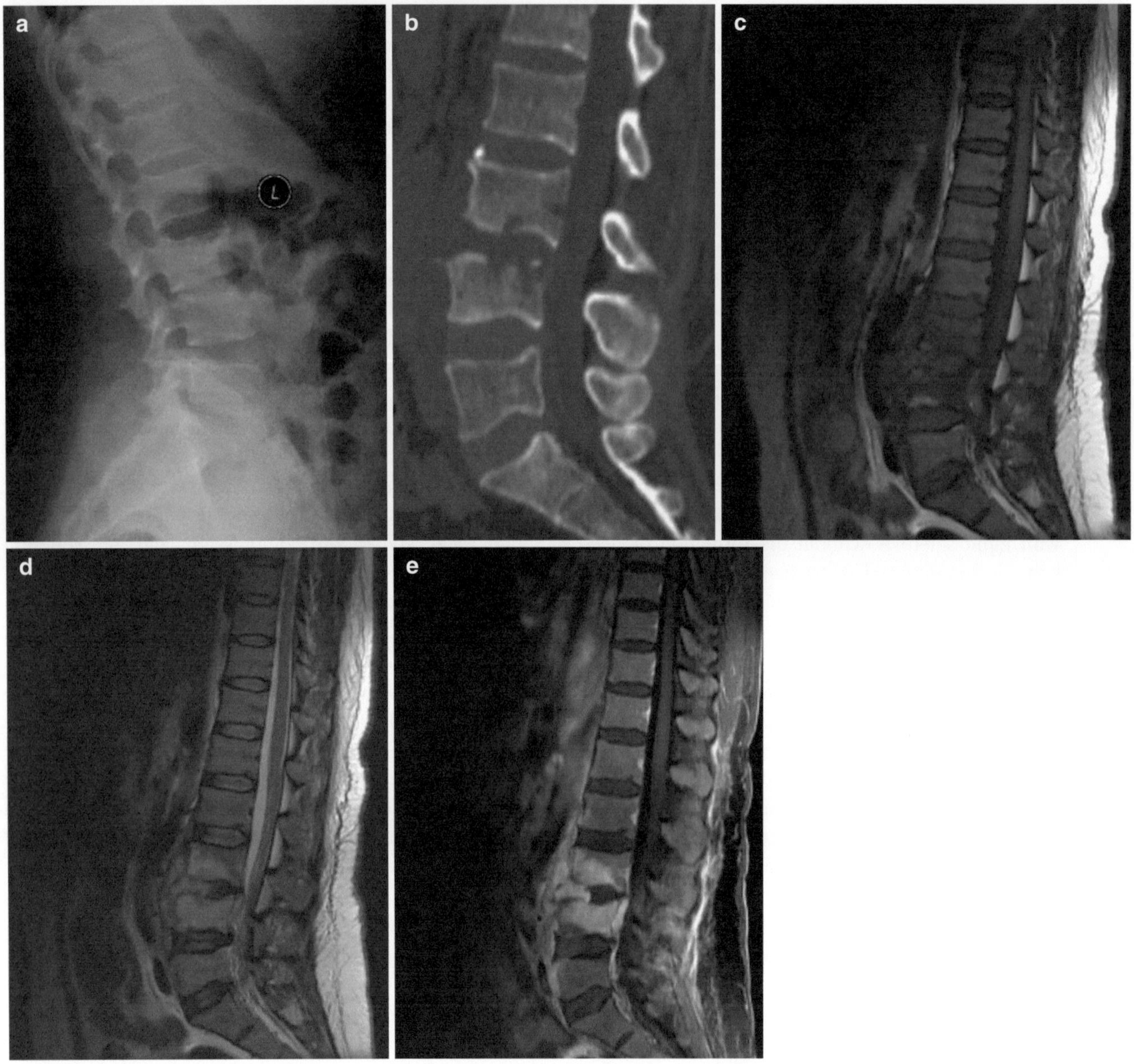

Fig. 5.8 Brucella infection of spine. (**a**) Lateral X-ray of lumbar vertebra, narrowing of L_3 ~ L_4 space, osteoporotic changes of vertebral bodies L_3 and L_4, worm-eaten bone destruction at the anterosuperior border of vertebral body L_4, clear margin, no sclerosis, no calcification in the lesion area; (**b**) CT sagittal plane of lumbar vertebra, blurred bone trabecula of vertebral bodies L_3 and L_4, multiple worm-eaten bone destruction, clear boundary, no sclerosis, no calcification in the lesion; (**c**) MRI lumbar T_1WI; (**d**) MRI lumbar T_2WI; (**e**) MRI lumbar T_1WI enhanced sequence, oedema of vertebral bodies L_3 and L_4, showing hypointense on T_1WI and hyperintense on T2WI, irregular conglomerate isointense on T_1WI and hyperintense on T_2WI in the intervertebral disc, enhancement after enhancement, suggesting abscess wall, irregular soft tissue thickening at the anterior margin of vertebral body, showing hypointense on T_1WI and heterogeneous hyperintense on T_2WI, unclear boundary, enhancement after enhancement (thanks to Junlin Li from Inner Mongolia People's Hospital who provided the picture)

sequestrum in the destruction area of vertebral body, narrowed adjacent intervertebral space, incarceration of two adjacent and destroyed vertebral bodies, and kyphosis. In most cases, the disease occurs with osteoporosis involving the pedicle of vertebral arch, and the focuses can affect the paravertebral soft tissue and lead to psychrapostema formation. After enhanced scan, a ring enhancement in abscess wall uniform in thickness is observed, with well-defined abnormal intensity in the paravertebral region.

2. **Pyogenic spondylitis.** The main symptoms are spinal pain, limitation of motion, and possibly acute infectious manifestations of local soft tissues (e.g. redness, swelling, fever, and pain). With persistent high fever, the rapid-onset spondylitis has severe symptoms of systemic poisoning and mainly targets the spongy bone; and leads

to subchondral bone destruction beginning from the bearing surface, and the intervertebral disc is ill-defined and presented as diffuse hyperintense on T_2WI. At advanced stage, hyperostosis and osteosclerosis are mainly observed with large sequestrum and extensive fusion between the intervertebral discs and adjacent vertebral bodies, and bony ankylosis is demonstrated in most cases. Through the enhanced scan, marked enhancement is noticed in vertebral bodies and intervertebral disc concerned, and plaque-like enhancement is observed in focus-centred diffuse soft tissue swelling, with ill-defined margins.

3. **End-plate osteochondritis**. MRI findings include: irregular and thickened outline of two adjacent vertebral bodies, hypointense on T_1WI and hyperintense on T_2WI, intervertebral disc with possible vacuum sign, and end-plate cortex generally continuous without destruction. Heterogeneous enhancement is observed through enhanced scan, and linear hyperintense shadow with clear boundary is observed at the junction between the focus of abnormal end-plate osteochondritis and adjacent bone marrow and the normal bone marrow on the DWI image.

Status Quo and Progress of Research

Dynamic enhanced magnetic resonance imaging (MRI) has been widely used in diagnosis of tumour-like and inflammatory focuses in various systems of the human body. The cases at acute stage of brucellosis primarily manifest as subarticular bone marrow oedema. Micro focuses of bone marrow oedema can be located by DWI hypersensitive to manifestation at the stage. IVIM-DWI is the only noninvasive imaging examination technique available for detecting the diffuse movement of water molecules in vivo tissues. It measures the intensities of focuses at different *b* values based on multiple focus images with different *b* values, and provides additional and accurate information for clinically judging the benign and malignant focuses via analysis of the time-signal intensity curve with respect to these focuses. In addition, it shows the diffuse movement and blood perfusion of tissues in focus regions with quantitative parameters, and evaluates the microstructure of the focus by using the specific apparent diffusion coefficient [17].

5.6 Mycobacterium Tuberculosis Infection

Overview

Patients with tuberculosis of bone and joint account for 1% ~ 2% of all tubercular patients. The disease is normally secondary to tuberculosis developing in other parts of the body, especially in lung. The primary focus of tuberculosis cannot be located in most (about 80%) patients with tuberculosis of bone and joint. The tuberculosis of bone and joint is a local manifestation of a systemic disease. Mycobacterium tuberculosis is trapped in bones and joints (including spine) through blood circulation [11]. Patients with tuberculosis of spine, also known as Pott disease, account for approx. 10% of all cases with extra-pulmonary tuberculosis and 50% with the tuberculosis of bone and joint. Patients with vertebral body tuberculosis account for 90% ~ 95% while patients with adnexa tuberculosis account for 5% ~ 10% of all cases with the tuberculosis of spine. Tuberculosis of spine mostly occurs in lumbar vertebra, secondly in thoracolumbar segment and rarely in cervical vertebra. Children are susceptible to the tuberculosis of thoracic vertebra and adults are susceptible to the tuberculosis of lumbar vertebra [19].

The vertebral body tuberculosis can be distinguished from the adnexa tuberculosis depending on the first focus of bone destruction, and the vertebral body tuberculosis can be further divided into central type, marginal type, and subligamentous type [20]. The spinal tuberculosis is normally attributed to haematogenous dissemination of bacteria from distant body sites. There are abundant terminal arteries distributed in the end-plate region of the spine, especially the anterior parts of vertebral bodies. Therefore, in most cases, the adult haematogenous infection affects the sub-end-plate bone in the anterior part of vertebral body, and then invades beyond the cortex and downwards to sites under ligaments, intervertebral discs, adjacent vertebral bodies, adnexa, and vertebral canal. The spinal tuberculosis also spreads via a vein approach, valveless Batson venous plexus. The blood flow of the venous system depends on changes in intrapleural pressure and intra-abdominal pressure. When the tuberculosis is disseminated through the system, the focus may be originated from the centre of vertebral body [11, 21].

The focuses of vertebral body tuberculosis are commonly observed at regions surrounding intervertebral disc, anterior margin of the vertebral body, and the centre of vertebral body. The intervertebral disc of patients suffered from simple central vertebral body tuberculosis is generally unaffected, but the vertebral body is prone to be compressed and deformed into vertebrae plana. As an artery anterior to a vertebral body is divided to nourish a superior and an inferior vertebral body, respectively, the spinal tuberculosis usually affects at least two vertebral bodies. The tuberculosis dissemination inferior to the anterior and posterior longitudinal ligaments of the spine will affect multiple vertebral bodies. The spread of the infection is attributed to absence of proteolytic enzyme in patients with mycobacterial infection [11].

The characteristic findings of spinal tuberculosis include the disappearance of intervertebral space, bone destruction and collapse of adjacent vertebral bodies, and forward angulation deformity of spine. In most cases, more than one vertebral body is affected and the vertebral body is more susceptible than adnexa. The spinal deformity is common [10].

Patients with spinal tuberculosis may have such symptoms as fatigue, discomfort, weight loss, night sweats, and patients at chronic healing stage may have back stiffness, deformity, and neurological symptoms [21]. Most patients are free from fever, with increased or unchanged leukocyte count. Accurate diagnosis partly depends on the isolated pathogens. However, both positive rates obtained by means of direct smear and rapid culture of mycobacterium tuberculosis are less than 50%, and the rapid culture of mycobacterium tuberculosis takes too much time (4 ~ 8 weeks). Tuberculin test is applied to judge whether a patient has ever contracted the tubercle bacillus.

Pathophysiology

Proliferative spinal tuberculosis mainly leads to formation of tuberculous granulation tissues in bone destruction focuses, without prominent caseous necrosis or large sequestrum. Small residual bone trabeculae are familiar in the tuberculous granulation tissues. Caseous exudative spinal tuberculosis mainly leads to bone destruction, with new bone formation in few cases. Extensive caseous necrosis and sequestra can be observed with abscess formation [10]. No redness, swelling, fever, or pain are noted in focus, which is called cold abscess or psychrapostema. The cold abscess is composed of caseous necrosis tissues, plasma, sequestra, and tubercle bacillus, with a few reactive changes in epitheloid cells in peripheral region.

Imaging Findings

1. **X-ray.** It is the preferred examination method for tuberculosis of spine. Typical X-ray findings include osteoporotic and thinning vertebral end-plate, descending vertebral body, bone destruction, narrowed intervertebral space, new bone formation, soft tissue abscess, and angulation deformity of spine. These focuses generally involve multiple vertebral bodies, especially the vertebral fusion and collapse [8].

   Tuberculoses of spine can be divided into four types depending on results from X-ray radiographs.

   (a) Central type: The type occurs most commonly in children. The focus results in centrally bright area with blurred border in one or two adjacent vertebral bodies due to spongy bone destruction at early stage. The destruction area expands with the development of the focus, and further leads to wedged collapse involving the intervertebral disc and adjacent vertebral bodies in case of rapid development of the disease. The collapse of the vertebral body can result in kyphosis deformity, and prominent shadow indicating abscess can be observed in the paravertebral region.

   (b) Marginal type: It is the most common type with focus from the end-plate regions of the superior and inferior margins of the vertebral body. The type manifests as narrowed intervertebral space, blurred or irregular superior and inferior margins of the vertebral body, and incarceration of two adjacent and destroyed vertebral bodies (Fig. 5.9a, b). The paravertebral abscess is helpful diagnostically. Sometimes, the abscess is unilaterally prominent, especially in thoracic vertebra, the paravertebral line shadow bulging is more noticeable than the change in psoas cold abscess [22].

   (c) Subligamentous type: It is mainly observed in thoracic vertebrae, with focuses extending inferior to the anterior longitudinal ligament, bone destruction at the anterior margin of vertebral body, and intact intervertebral disc.

   (d) Adnexa type: It is a rare type manifesting mostly as bone destruction in spinal adnexa and transarticular involvement of articular processes.

   Cold abscess of tuberculosis manifests as shadow of soft tissue surrounding the spine on radiograph. On the lateral view of cervical vertebra, the widened space in prevertebral soft tissue indicates the formation of retropharyngeal abscess. The formation of abscess surrounding the thoracic vertebra is suggested by the widened shadow of mediastinum on the PA view of thoracic vertebra, as well as the increased density of prevertebral soft tissue and protruded shadow of trachea on the lateral view. The formation of abscess surrounding lumbar vertebra is suggested by the increasing density of soft tissues around bilateral and dorsal lumbar vertebra on the anteroposterior and lateral views of the lumbar spine. Punctate calcification in abscess is a characteristic finding of the cold abscess of tuberculosis [10].

   Bone focuses in atlanto-occipital joint and spine at the cervicothoracic junction, involved spinal cord and soft tissues, and abscess area are not clear on X-ray radiograph. Early focuses are not shown clearly on the X-ray radiograph [23].

2. **CT.** CT scan may demonstrate early focuses not apparent in X-ray radiograph, including fragmentary bone destruction, osteolytic focuses, localized sclerosis, subperiosteal focuses, paravertebral soft tissue focuses, and paravertebral cold abscess. CT can clearly show punctate calcification in the cold abscess and epidural focuses containing sequestrum. CT further clearly shows the spinal cord compression in case of invasion to vertebral canal by inflammatory tissues, sequestra, or collapsed vertebral

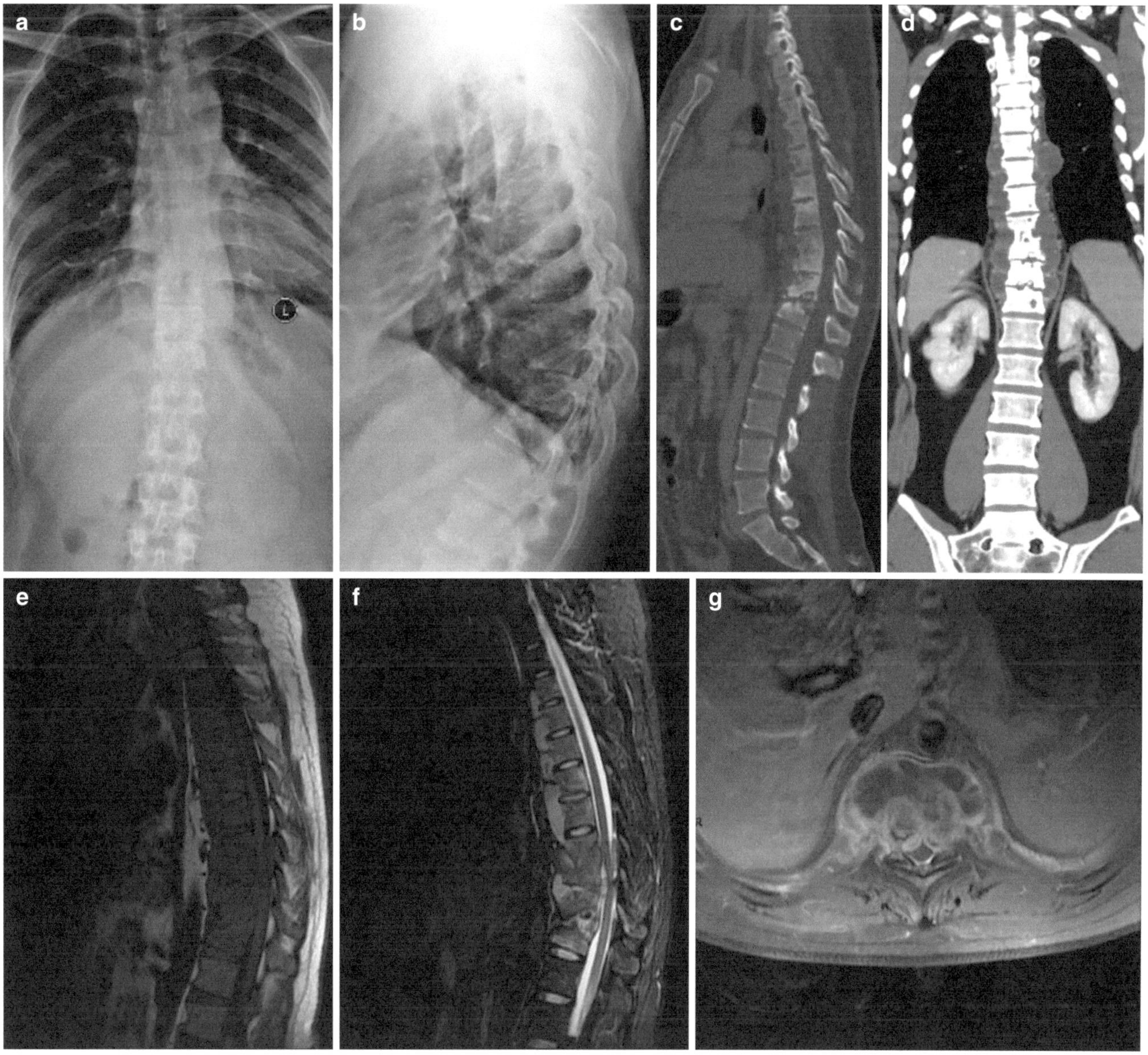

Fig. 5.9 Tuberculosis of spine. (**a**) PA X-ray of thoracic vertebra, showing widened mediastinum surrounding the lower thoracic vertebra with increased density, blurred and disappeared space between T_9 and T_{10}, and increased density of $T_9 \sim T_{12}$ vertebral bodies; (**b**) X-ray lateral view of thoracic vertebra, showing blurred and disappeared space between T_9 and T_{10}, and blurred and destroyed bone on the anterior margins of $T_9 \sim T_{12}$ vertebral bodies; (**c**) CT sagittal plane of total spine, showing destroyed and disappeared space between T_9 and T_{10}, multiple patchy calcification focuses in $T_{10} \sim T_{11}$ vertebral bodies, as well as bone erosion on anterior borders and increased vertebral bone density of $T_4 \sim T_{12}$; (**d**) CT enhanced-coronal plane of total spine, showing localized abscess formed around $T_4 \sim T_{12}$ vertebral bodies, and peripheral enhancement by enhanced scan; (**e**) Sagittal plane of thoracic vertebra by MRI T_1WI; (**f**) Sagittal plane of thoracic vertebra by MRI T_2WI fat-suppressed sequence; (**g**) Transverse plane of thoracic vertebra by MRI T_1WI enhanced sequence, showing destroyed and disappeared space between T_9 and T_{10}, oedema in $T_4 \sim T_{12}$ vertebral bodies, localized hypointense on T_1WI and hyperintense on T_2WI around vertebral bodies, and marked enhancement of margin by enhanced scan

bodies. Abscess manifests as monolocular or multilocular cyst, and further manifests as liquid density shadow with marginal ring enhancement and unremarkable central enhancement by enhanced scan [8] (Fig. 5.9c, d).

3. **MRI**. It demonstrates bone destruction between adjacent vertebral bodies and involvement of intervertebral disc there between; and shows hypointense on T_1WI, as well as mixed intensity, hyperintense and hypointense on T_2WI. The destruction of vertebral body is prominent, and it produces specific, localized, and heterogeneous enhancement by enhanced scan, which is associated with vertebral body compression fracture and angulated kyphosis in multiple cases; The early intervertebral disc failure is less disruptive, with some normal or degenerated nucleus pulposus

intensities observed as a criterion to distinguish the early intervertebral disc failure from early pyogenic spondylitis; In most cases, the segments with focuses were associated with paravertebral abscess, with remarkable hyperintense on T_1WI with respect to muscle tissue, and hyperintense on T_2WI. These focuses manifest as well-defined ring enhancement by enhanced scan. For some severe cases, the abscess cavity communicated with the destruction area of vertebral body and spreading widely in subligamentous region is observed, and multi-level vertebral bodies are involved. Tuberculosis of spine is more likely to involve the spinal membrane and facet joints and leads to formation of epidural abscess. At advanced stage, the hypointense on T_1WI and T_2WI suggests the vertebral lamina collapse with end-plate sclerosis.

Atypical tuberculosis of spine can manifest as abnormal solitary vertebral body, abnormality between solitary vertebral body and adjacent intervertebral disc, abnormal multiple vertebral bodies and normal intervertebral disc, simple adnexal focuses, etc. The type of tuberculosis mostly occurs in adolescents or patients with hypoimmunity, and may be associated with invasion by extraspinal bones. Therefore, the tuberculosis should be distinguished from the metastatic tumour or lymphoma [21] (Fig. 5.9e ~ g).

Key Points of Diagnosis

1. Tuberculosis of spine is normally secondary to tuberculosis developing in other parts of the body, especially in lung.
2. The tuberculosis of spine mostly occurs in lumbar vertebra, secondly in thoracolumbar segment, and rarely in cervical vertebra. Children are susceptible to the tuberculosis of thoracic vertebra and adults are susceptible to the tuberculosis of lumbar vertebra.
3. Typical X-ray findings include osteoporotic and thinning vertebral end-plate, descending vertebral body, bone destruction, narrowed intervertebral space, new bone formation, soft tissue abscess, and angulation deformity of spine. These focuses generally involve multiple vertebral bodies, especially the vertebral fusion and collapse.
4. Early manifestations of focus can be demonstrated by CT scan, including fragmentary bone destruction, osteolytic focuses, localized sclerosis, subperiosteal focuses, paravertebral soft tissue focuses, and paravertebral cold abscess.
5. Bone destruction of two or more adjacent vertebral bodies is observed with hypointense on T_1WI and mixed intensity on T_2WI, involved intervertebral disc and narrowed intervertebral space.

Differential Diagnosis

1. **Pyogenic spondylitis**. The main symptoms are spinal pain and limitation of motion. The spondylitis mainly targets the spongy bone, and leads to subchondral bone destruction beginning from the bearing surface, and the intervertebral disc is ill-defined and presented as diffuse hyperintense on T_2WI. At advanced stage, hyperostosis and osteosclerosis are mainly observed with large sequestrum and extensive fusion between the intervertebral discs and adjacent vertebral bodies, and bony ankylosis is demonstrated in most cases. Through the enhanced scan, marked enhancement is noticed in diseased vertebral bodies and intervertebral disc, and plaque-like enhancement is observed in focus-centred diffuse soft tissue swelling, with ill-defined margins.
2. **Vertebral metastasis.** It mostly occurs in middle-aged and aged patients with known primary cancer. It causes pain confined to an extent and progressively aggravates. The non-continuous destruction can be observed in multi-level vertebral bodies. In most cases, the bone destruction is observed and other adnexa are involved, including pedicle of vertebral arch. The intervertebral space is not involved or narrowed, and the mass in paravertebral tissue is relatively confined and often invades the intraspinal spinal cord.
3. **Chordoma**. It occurs mostly in sacrum and produces osteolytic bone destruction, expansive growth, thinning and intact bone cortex, and giant soft tissue mass in presacral region. It is a slowly progressing disease.

Status Quo and Progress of Research

X-ray radiography is one of the most commonly used methods for diagnosing the tuberculosis of spine. In case of small focus area, CT scanning is significantly superior in showing clear focus range, calcification conditions, bone destruction, osteosclerosis, peripheral abscess morphology, tiny sequestrum, clear paravertebral soft tissue abscess, and involved bony vertebral canal. Multi-plane, multi-position, and multi-sequence MRI is helpful to locate imperceptible changes in vertebral bodies and intervertebral discs and define their extents, thereby being far superior to other means for early diagnosis. MRI is significantly superior to X-ray and CT scanning in showing involved extent of focuses, intraspinal invasion, collapse and deformity of vertebral body, spinal stenosis caused by kyphosis deformity and spinal nerves compression. MRI further visually distinguishes the granuloma from abscess and locates the abscess extent, septa and relationship with adjacent structures. However, MRI is inferior to CT scanning in showing calcification conditions [24].

5.7 Hydatid Disease of Spine

Zhanhua Qian, Rongjie Bai, and Huili Zhan

Overview

Spinal parasitic infections include hydatid disease of spine, onchocerciasis, and toxoplasmosis. The echinococcosis, also known as hydatid disease, is a chronic parasitosis produced by parasitism of echinococcus at larval stage [25]. According to the pathogenic larvae, the echinococcoses can be divided into spinal granulosa echinococcosis and spinal alveolar echinococcosis. Some carnivores and canids in pastoral and forest areas are the definitive hosts of these parasites, and human beings expose to second infection by ingesting food or water contaminated by parasitic eggs [26]. The oncospheres hatched from these eggs in the intestinal tract enter the systemic circulation and reach the bones for parasitism, which causes the bone hydatid disease. The echinococcosis mostly occurs in liver and lung. The patients with hydatid disease of spine account for 50% of cases with bone hydatid disease, which only accounts for 0.5% ~ 4.0% of all echinococcosis cases. For hydatid disease of spine, the most susceptible positions are the vertebral body and pedicle of vertebral arch of thoracic vertebra (about 50%), followed by the lumbar vertebrae, sacrum, and cervical vertebrae. According to the parasitic sites of hydatid, the echinococcosis can be divided into intramedullary, subdural extramedullary, extradural intraspinal, vertebral and paravertebral echinococcoses [27, 28].

The specific antibody detection methods for echinococcosis include Casoni test, IHA, CIEP, ELISA, and gold-labelled antibody detection method, and the first three are collectively known as the three indexes for hydatid. The relatively accurate and common method is eight indexes of hydatid test, which combines the gold-labelled antibody detection method and ELISA to measure the EgCF, EgP, cystic fluid semi-purified antigen B(EgB) in patients, 4 alveolar hydatid antibodies (Em2) suggesting the alveolar echinococcus hydatid infection, as well as specific antigens and antibodies to the hydatid.

The bone hydatid disease develops slowly and shows insidious clinical symptoms at the early stage. The patient usually sees the doctor for local limb swelling, ache, or pathologic fracture. The echinococcosis involving the spine may show the symptoms of nervous system damage, such as severe backache, hypaesthesia, weak lower limbs, paraplegia and gatism, which may get worse by fatigue or trauma.

Pathophysiology

Generally, osseous hydatid invades the spongy bone of vertebral body through portal vein-vertebral vein system. Therefore, the hydatid disease of spine develops from the spongy bone. As the cyst growth is confined by hard and dense osseous tissue, the cyst grows towards the direction of low resistance in the bone trabecula space, and then develops by continuous bone erosion and absorption. Continued growth may affect the vertebral adnexa, and even lead to pathologic fracture, or invade into paravertebral soft tissue and vertebral canal to form secondary echinococcus cyst.

Imaging Findings

1. **X-ray**. Early manifestations include multiple osteolytic bony defect areas in utricular, moth-eaten, and cellular forms in the bones involved, multiple focuses, and clear-cut margins with sclerosis. The wedging of vertebral body is possibly observed with calcification of cyst wall in the focuses. At the progressive stage, prominent expansive and osteolytic bone destruction is noticed in the vertebral body, which may be associated with pathologic fracture or spondylolisthesis. At the advanced stage, the bone destruction area may be affected by infection, hyperostosis, and osteosclerosis, or calcium deposition and bone deformity. These focuses may invade into the pedicle of vertebral arch, vertebral lamina, and other adnexa, and lead to blurred pedicle of vertebral arch. The intervertebral disc is not typically involved. The paravertebral soft tissue may be invaded to form pseudo-paravertebral abscess [29] (Fig. 5.10a).
2. **CT.** CT image reveals multiple cystic bony defects different in size in vertebral bodies, external osseous expansion, bulging, thinning, fracture or defect of bone cortex, and shadow of fluid density in the cyst (including single-cyst type, multi-cyst type, and mother-daughter cyst type). The cyst wall is well-defined and surrounded by sclerotic margin. The sharp and clear margin and soap bubble sign are observed with multiple septa. When the cyst wall is calcified, punctate calcification can be identified in the focus. Most focuses affect the vertebral body, and then invade into the pedicle of vertebral arch, vertebral lamina, spinous process, transverse process, and caput costae, leading to intervertebral foramen enlargement [26]. The invasion into paravertebral soft tissue and vertebral canal produces round mass in the paravertebral soft tissue. If the rupture of cyst causes infection, the air-fluid level in focus can be observed with thickened and sclerotic cyst wall. Consolidation and calcification components can be observed at advanced stage (Fig. 5.10b, c).
3. **MRI.** For diagnosis of echinococcosis, MRI is the most valuable imaging examination technique in accurately locating and identifying the extent and characteristics of the hydatid. The findings on MRI include multiple cystic

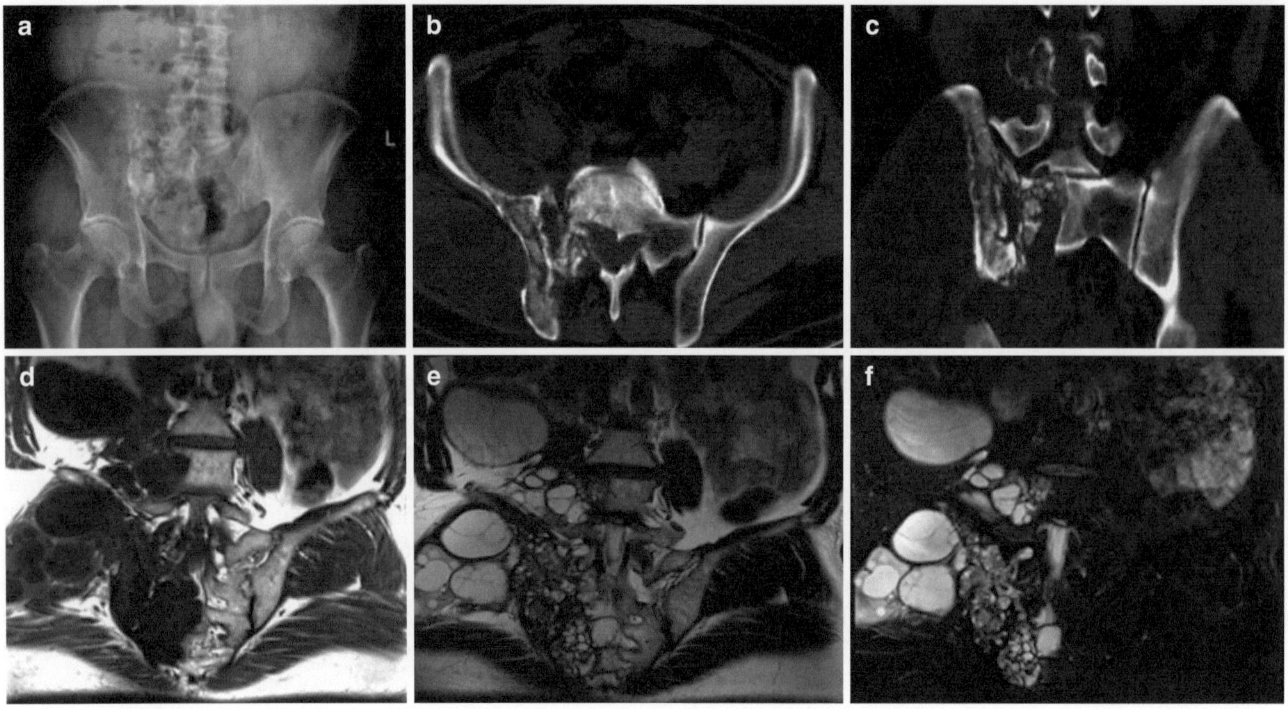

Fig. 5.10 Hydatid infection of spine. (**a**) PA X-ray of pelvic, showing multiple cystic and cellular bone destruction and margin sclerosis of the right sacroiliac joint; (**b**) CT transverse plane of pelvis; (**c**) CT coronal plane of pelvis, showing multiple expansive osteolytic bone destructions in transverse process, sacrum and ilium on the right side of L4, multiple calcification focuses in the sacrum and ilium, and multiple cystic low-density focuses in right gluteus maximus. (**d**) Coronal plane of pelvis on MRI T_1WI; (**e**) Coronal plane of pelvis on MRI T_2WI; (**f**) Coronal plane of pelvis by MRI T_2WI fat-suppressed sequence, showing multiple cystic hypointense on T_1WI and hyperintenses T_2WI in transverse process, sacrum, ilium, and gluteus maximus on the right side of L_4, and daughter cysts in some focuses (hereby thanks Hui Guo of The First Affiliated Hospital of Xinjiang Medical University for providing the image)

or lobulated bone destructions in different sizes in one or more adjacent vertebral bodies. The cyst wall is smooth and sharp-outlined, and the vertebral bodies may be wedge-shaped. The hypointense on T_1WI and heterogeneous hyperintense on T_2WI are shown in destruction areas. Multiple small daughter cysts may be observed in a large cyst. Among the important imaging findings, the mother cyst shows remarkable hyperintense on T_1WI and hypointense on T_2WI with respect to the daughter cyst. A hypointense focus suggesting the hydatid can be observed in almost every large cyst or small cyst in some cases. The onset of echinococcosis in multi-vertebral bodies normally involves adjacent vertebral bodies rather than the intervertebral discs. The hydatid cyst wall shows hypointense on MRI and remarkable hypointense on T_2WI. The vertebral canal, vertebral adnexa, and peripheral soft tissues are susceptible to hydatid disease of spine, which leads to formation of multi-cystic or single-cystic lesions in these tissues, and even deformed cyst in some cases. Especially in the cases with involvement of psoas major, the confined mother cyst containing multiple daughter cysts of different sizes can be observed in the paravertebral region. The polycystic echinococcus cyst can be observed more clearly by means of the T_2WI fat-suppressed sequence. The hydatid in vertebral body is unremarkable in case of no rupture infection. However, the mild enhancement of cyst wall can be identified on MRI when the cyst wall ruptures (Figs. 5.10d ~ f, 5.11, 5.12, and 5.13).

Key Points of Diagnosis

1. The disease is common in pastoral and forest areas in the Northwest and Southwest of China.
2. Casoni test, IHA, and CIEP as well as EgCF, EgP, B (EgB), and Em2 tests of hydatid by GAB and ELISA are commonly used serological diagnostic methods.
3. The intervertebral disc is typically not involved in hydatid disease of spine.
4. On MRI, multiple daughter cysts of different sizes can be observed in the cystic destruction area of vertebral body, with significant hypointense of cyst wall, typically normal intervertebral disc and multiple daughter cysts in the peripheral soft tissues.

Differential Diagnosis

1. **Spinal tuberculosis.** With respect to tuberculosis of spine, the hydatid disease of spine is featured by polycys-

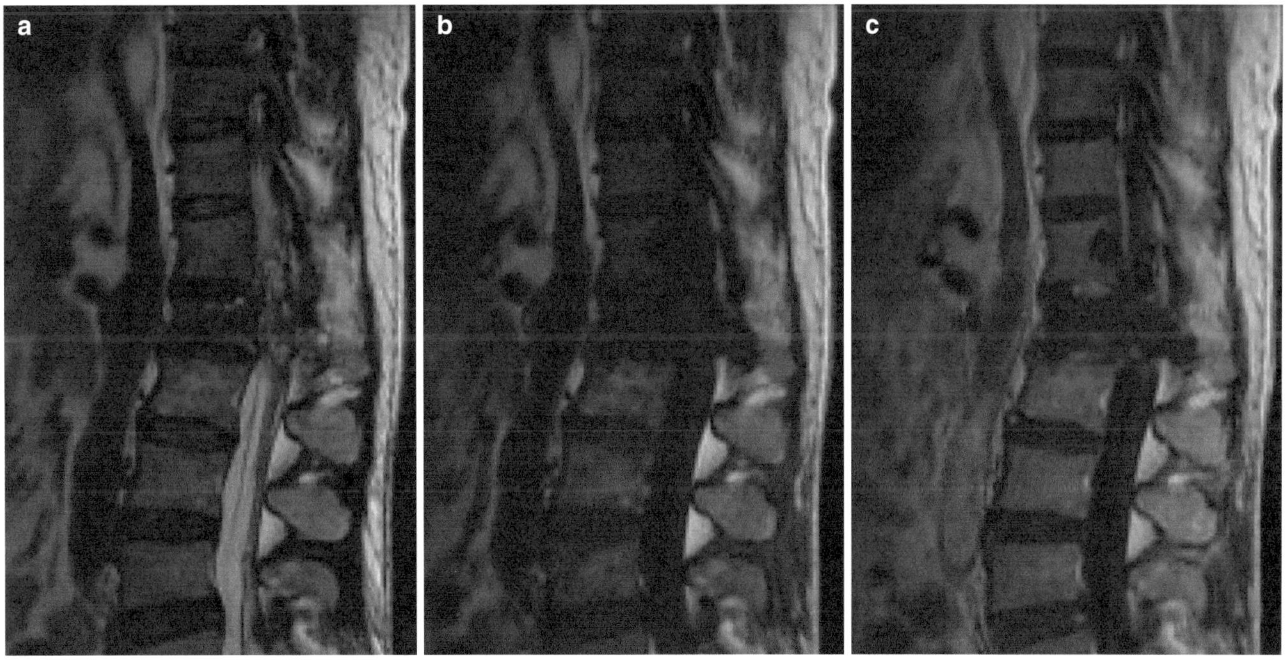

Fig. 5.11 Alveolar hydatid infection of spine. A 48-year-old man with bone destruction in $L_1 \sim L_2$ vertebral bodies, intraspinal protrusion by focus, and normal intensity of intervertebral disc. (**a**) Plaque-like hypointense shadow and multiple hyperintense vesicles are observed in the focuses on MRI T_2WI. (**b**) Hypointense on T_1WI; (**c**) Enhancement in linear and spotty manner is observed at the margin of the focus by enhanced scanning

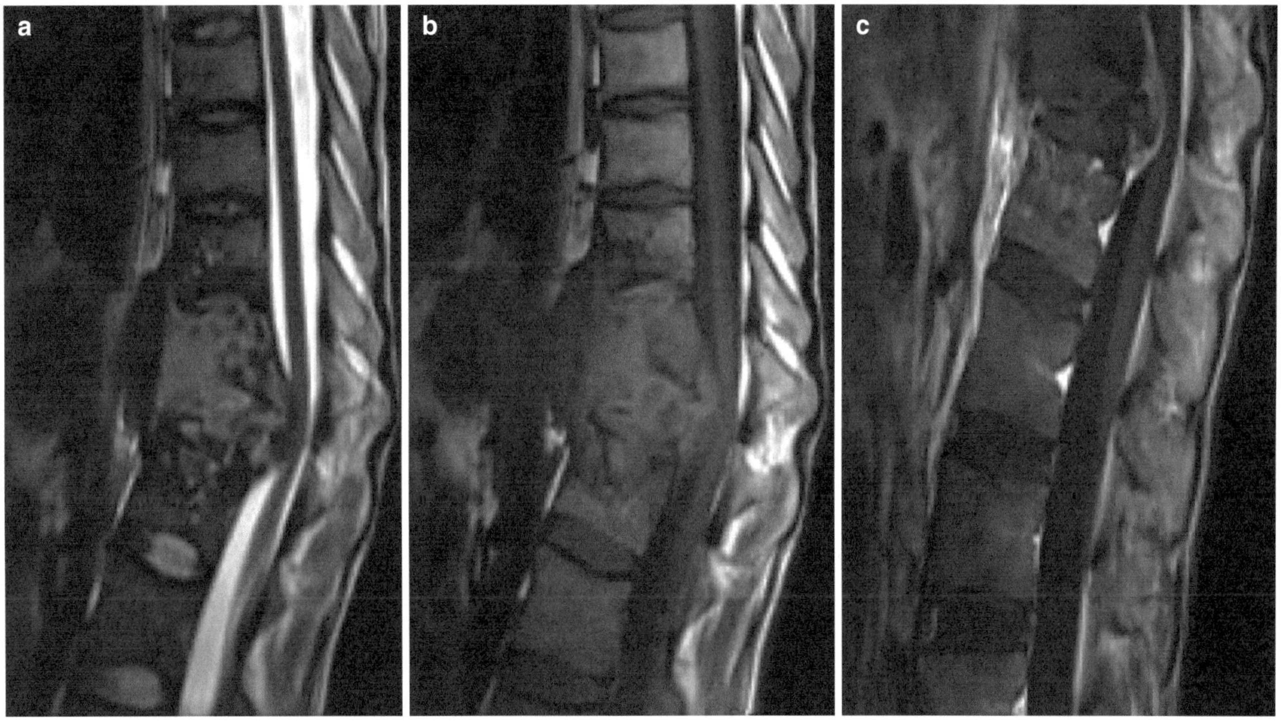

Fig. 5.12 Alveolar hydatid infection of spine. A 35-year-old woman with focus involving $T_{11} \sim L_1$ vertebral bodies, and destroyed and disappeared intervertebral disc between T_{11} and T_{12}. (**a**) On MRI T_2WI, a slight hyperintense is dominantly observed with scattered hyperintense of vesicles and hypointense of soft tissue focuses anterior to the vertebral body. (**b**) Isointense is dominant on T_1WI; (**c**) Spotty enhancement can be observed by enhanced scanning

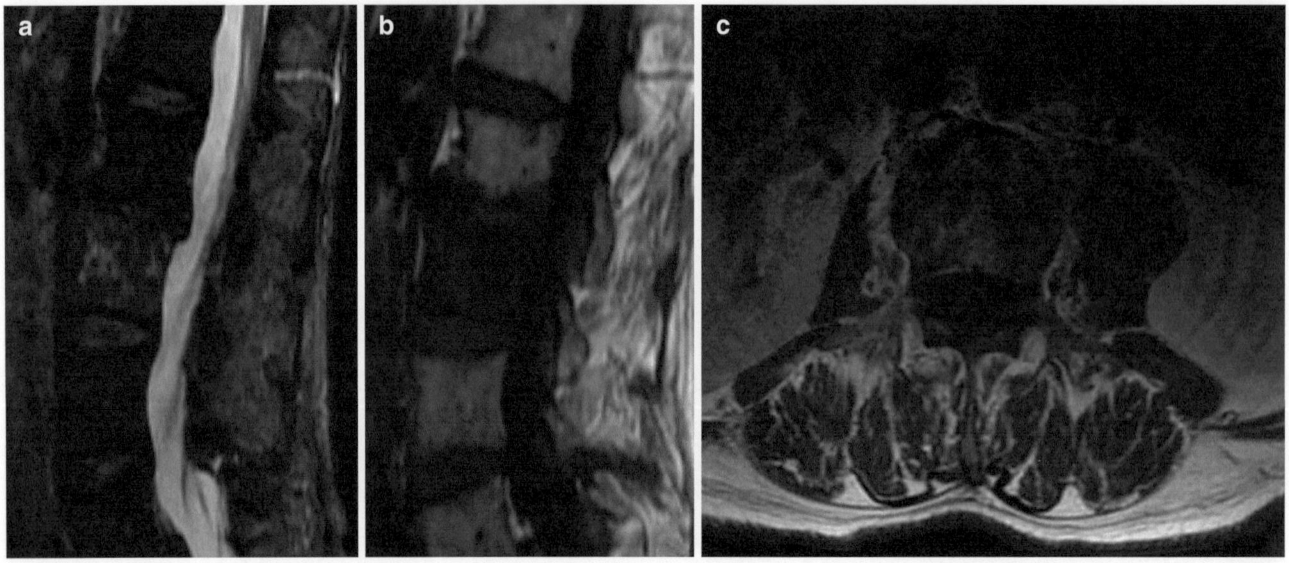

Fig. 5.13 Alveolar hydatid infection of spine. A 26-year-old man. (**a**, **b**) Most of focuses manifest as hypointense by MRI T_2WI fat-suppressed sequence and hypointense by T_1WI sequence, and multiple spotty hyperintense is observed in the vertebrae and intervertebral disc involved. (**c**) No enhancement is observed by enhanced scanning. The psoas major is compressed by focus on the left side of vertebral body, and no focus is observed in the adnexa (hereby thanks Hu Haixia and Xu Hui of Qinghai Provincial People's Hospital for providing Figs. 5.11, 5.12, and 5.13)

tic vertebral body and adnexa involved in echinococcosis; collapse of vertebral body with severe focus; typically unilateral soft tissue mass in paravertebral region; and normally intact intervertebral disc free from narrowing. Tuberculosis of spine affects the adjacent vertebral bodies and the intervertebral disc there between, and leads to narrowing of the intervertebral space. In addition, a fusiform soft tissue density shadow can be observed in bilateral regions of vertebral body, and even spread widely along the vertical axis of the spine.

2. **Aneurysmal bone cyst of vertebral body**. With expansive cystic bone destruction in vertebral bodies and typically involved vertebral arch, the disease is difficult to be distinguished from the bone hydatid disease. However, they can be easily distinguished on MRI as the aneurysmal bone cyst manifests as stepladder-like fluid-fluid level and diverticulum-like processes of different sizes in most cases.
3. **Arachnoid cyst of vertebral canal**. The disease manifests as a single cyst without shadow of daughter cysts, vertebral body free from involvement or deformity under compression, insignificant bone destruction, and non-enhanced cyst wall by enhanced scanning.

Status Quo and Progress of Research

Focuses can be accurately located and extent and morphology of focuses can be shown by means of multi-row spiral CT in combination with three-dimensional reconstruction and spectral imaging, which have been an important imaging technique for screening and diagnosing the echinococcosis. The myelography is helpful to demonstrate the echinococcus cyst clearly, especially superior in showing size and extent of the echinococcus cyst. As a cutting-edge imaging technology, PET is far superior to the other techniques in detecting systemic metastatic echinococcosis depending on wide coverage.

References

1. Shuling B, Dajun Y. Systematic anatomy. 8th ed. Beijing: People's Medical Publishing House; 2015.
2. Zhenyu W, Wenjian X. Human sectional and imaging anatomy. 3rd ed. Beijing: People's Medical Publishing House; 2010.
3. Jincheng C, Li H, Sirun L. Practical clinical anatomy and imaging diagnosis. Beijing: Science Press; 2007.
4. Jiyang J, Gaojun T. Fundamentals of applied anatomy for diagnostic imaging. Beijing: People's Military Medical Press; 2007.
5. Berquist. MRI of the musculoskeletal system. Translated by Cheng Jingliang et al. Zhengzhou: Zhengzhou University Press; 2004.
6. Ning Z, Xianjun Z, Laichang H, et al. Present research situation of the MRI manifestations of spinal infection and its imitations. Chin J Magn Reson Imag. 2019;10(3):73–7.
7. Tins BJ, Cassar-Pullicino VN. MR imaging of spinal infection. Semin Musculoskelet Radiol. 2004;8(3):215–29.
8. Tali ET. Spinal infections. Eur J Radiol. 2004;50(2):120–33.
9. Mukherji SK. Spinal infections. Neuroimaging Clin N Am. 2015;25(2):xiii.
10. Stäbler A, Reiser MF. Imaging of spinal infection. Radiol Clin N Am. 2001;39(1):115–35.
11. Garg RK, Somvanshi DS. Spinal tuberculosis: a review. J Spinal Cord Med. 2011;34(5):440–54.

12. Kourbeti IS, Tsiodras S, Boumpas DT. Spinal infections: evolving concepts. Curr Opin Rheumatol. 2008;20(4):471–9.
13. Cornett CA, Vincent SA, Crow J, et al. Bacterial spine infections in adults: evaluation and management. J Am Acad Orthop Surg. 2016;24(1):11–8.
14. Ganesh D, Gottlieb J, Chan S, et al. Fungal infections of the spine. Spine. 2015;40(12):E719–28.
15. Solera J, Lozano E, Martinez-Alfaro E, et al. Brucellar spondylitis: review of 35 cases and literature survey. Clin Infect Dis. 1999;29(6):1440–9.
16. Xinming Y, Wei S, Yakun D, et al. Clinical imaging findings and pathological findings of brucellosis spondylitis. J Pract Radiol. 2008;24(4):122–7.
17. Shen L, Jiang C, Jiang R, et al. Diagnosis and classification in MRI of brucellar spondylitis. Radiol Infect Dis. 2017;4(3):102–7.
18. Xiaopeng W, Guangming N, Yang G. Research progress of magnetic resonance imaging in brucellosis spondylitis. Chin J Magnet Reson Imag. 2017;8(4):317–20.
19. Kumar K. Spinal tuberculosis, natural history of disease, classifications and principles of management with historical perspective. Eur J Orthop Surg Traumatol. 2016;26(6):551–8.
20. Yu J. Research progress on diagnosis of cervical tuberculosis. Trauma Crit Care Med. 2014;2(4):230–3.
21. Yingang Z, Ning J, Jing L, et al. Imaging analysis of tuberculosis of spine. J Pract Radiol. 2004;20(1):54–6.
22. Ning Z, Xianjun Z, Laichang H, et al. Research status of MRI manifestations and differential diagnosis of spinal infection. Chin J Magnet Reson Imag. 2019;10(3):73–7.
23. Tali ET. Spinal infections. Eur Radiol. 2004;50(2):120–33.
24. Yilian H. Classification of tuberculosis of spine and imaging diagnosis and differential diagnosis thereof. Modern Med Imagel. 2013;2:121–4.
25. Jain A, Prasad G, Rustagi T, et al. Hydatid disease of spine: multiple meticulous surgeries and a long term follow up. Indian J Orthop. 2014;48(5):529–32.
26. Weibin S, Yi L, Xiaoxiong X, et al. Characteristics and diagnosis of spinal hydatid disease. Chin J Orthop. 2006;26(1):7–12.
27. do Amaral LL, Nunes RH, da Rocha AJ. Parasitic and rare spinal infections. Neuroimaging Clin N Am. 2015;25(2):259–79.
28. Sayit M, Wenxiao J. MRI findings of spinal hydatid disease. Chin J Radiol. 2009;43(8):858–61.
29. Ivan P. Hydatid disease: radiologic and pathologic features and complications. Radiographics. 2000;20(3):795–817.

Bone and Joint Infection in Children

6

Wei Li, Qi Li, Heng Zhao, Junlin Li, Wei Zhou, and Xiaohong Lv

6.1 Bone Development in Children and Imaging Anatomy

The motor system is a set of bones, joints, and tissues related, including cartilages and muscles. Bone is one of the important components of the system. For osteogenesis and development of many bones, cartilage serves as the precursor tissue in fetal period. These bones construct a rigid framework to maintain and support most soft tissues of the body as a pillar and lever system.

Human beings grow fastest throughout the pediatric period. Therefore, dysfunction or structural abnormality in any tissues and organs will lead to dysplasia and even pathological changes during the period, including the bone and joint system. In case of congenital malformation, metabolic disorder, trauma, inflammation, tumor and other diseases, the growth and development of children's bone and joint system will be stunted and impaired, leading to abnormal function and structure in some cases. It is necessary to master the characteristics of bone and joint in children during the development process and understand the essence of related diseases, thereby distinguishing normality and abnormality, improving the imaging diagnostic capability of pediatric bone and joint diseases, and realizing accurate diagnosis.

6.1.1 Development of Bone

The growth and development of bone mainly covers three processes: osteogenesis, growth, and maturation.

1. Osteogenesis

   The osteogenesis can be implemented by: (1) intramembranous ossification, including skull and facial bone; and (2) endochondral ossification, including basion, spine, and bones of the extremities.

   (a) **Intramembranous ossification**. The mesenchymal cells evolve into osteoblasts in the differentiated membranous tissues, and then produce osteoid tissues to form an ossification center. The ossification center grows in all directions to form a radial bone trabecula, which is thickened to form a reticular structure and a spongy bone thereon; Meanwhile, the mesenchyme surrounding the membranous connective tissues form the periosteum, and the osteoid tissue secreted by osteoblasts in the inner layer of the periosteum is calcified to form the bone trabecula, which thickens to form compact bone substance.

   (b) **Endochondral ossification**. Most bones in human body are generated by endochondral ossification, including long and short bones of extremities. In this process, the mesenchymal cells form a cartilage model, which is differentiated into the diaphysis and epiphysis covered by perichondrium after developing to a certain extent.

W. Li (✉)
Department of Radiology, Shengjing Hospital of China Medical University, Shenyang, Liaoning, China
e-mail: drliwei@126.com

Q. Li
Department of Radiology, Liaoning Electric Power Central Hospital, Shenyang, Liaoning, China

H. Zhao
Department of Radiology, The First Affiliated Hospital, Hengyang Medical School, University of South China, Hengyang, Hunan, China

J. Li
Department of Radiology, People's Hospital of Inner Mongolia Autonomous Region, Hohhot, The Inner Mongolia, China

W. Zhou
Department of Radiology, The General Hospital of Northern Theater Command, Shenyang, Liaoning, China

X. Lv
Department of Radiology, The First Affiliated Hospital of Jinzhou Medical University, Jinzhou, Liaoning, China

H. Li et al. (eds.), *Radiology of Infectious and Inflammatory Diseases - Volume 5*,
https://doi.org/10.1007/978-981-16-5003-1_6

2. Bone Growth

The growth of long bones includes the growths in vertical and transverse diameters.

(a) **Growth of long bone in vertical diameter**. All long bone diaphyses have been ossified at birth (primary ossification centers), but both ends are still covered by cartilages, i.e., epiphysis. The secondary ossification center is established and enlarged in the epiphysis, until it divides the epiphyseal cartilage into two parts: the cartilage plate proximal to the joint, which develops into articular cartilage; and the epiphyseal plate proximal to the diaphysis, which progressively disappears with age. The epiphysis and the metaphysis of diaphysis merge together on the epiphyseal plate (Fig. 6.1).

For growing children, bones grow vertically in the epiphyseal plate between the epiphysis and metaphysis. The chondrocytes of epiphyseal plate divide continuously and they are arranged in parallel rows or cell columns vertically, which orientate to the diaphysis. Cells and columns are individually separated by matrix. The metaphysis is in a relatively primitive and active state throughout the bone development. When cells divide and grow continuously, the metaphysis undergoes a series of morphological changes and is divided into proliferation zone, maturation zone, and hypertrophy zone of chondrocytes (i.e., provisional calcification zone). The cartilage is consistently calcified until the long bone is completely ossified, and the epiphysis and the metaphysis of diaphysis merge together.

(b) **Growth of long bone in transverse diameter.** It occurs in periosteum. The periosteum mainly consisting of osteoblasts and dense collagen fibers is divided into two layers: an external layer is the collagen fibrous tissues fixing the periosteum on the surface of bone cortex; and an inner layer clinging to the bone cortex, with osteoblasts therein constantly form new bones on the bone cortex to thicken the diaphysis. Meanwhile, with the presence of osteoclasts, spongy bone is gradually formed on the inner surface of the bone cortex due to absorption and destruction of bone substance. As the bone trabecula is gradually absorbed, the bone marrow cavity is gradually widened. The mutual interaction of constant osteogenesis of periosteum and osteoclasis on the inner surface of bone cortex will change the thickness of bone cortex and the width of marrow cavity. In most cases, the marrow cavity is widening throughout the puberty and remains unchanged in adulthood.

3. Bone Maturation

The diaphysis is growing and thickening throughout the growth and development period of long bone. Meanwhile, the long bone is subject to remodeling, including the epiphysis and new bone at metaphysis. The migration of metaphysis to diaphysis produces thickened diaphysis and reamed marrow cavity and diversifies the bone morphology.

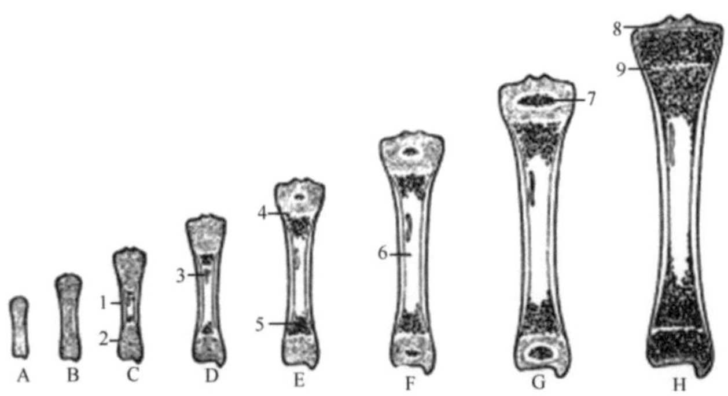

Fig. 6.1 Diagram of all development stages of long bone. (**a**) Primitive cartilage primordia; (**b**) Chondrocyte enlargement and increase of cartilage primordia lead to formation of the precursor of primary ossification center; (**c**) Subperiosteal bone is formed in the central area of the early primary ossification center, and the periosteum invades into the cartilage matrix to form a channel, namely the nutrient canal; (**d**) The ossification extends from the diaphysis to both ends, and marrow cavity is formed by bone absorption in the central area; (**e**) ~ (**g**) Secondary ossification centers are initially formed and continuously ossified; (**h**) Ossification of epiphyseal plate in adulthood and closure at the metaphysis. 1. Bone cortex; 2. Epiphysis and metaphyseal cartilage; 3. Nutrient canal; 4. Provisional calcification zone or epiphyseal plate; 5. Spongy bone; 6. Bone marrow cavity; 7. Secondary ossification center; 8. Articular cartilage; 9. Epiphyseal line remained after epiphyseal plate closure

6.1.2 Anatomy of Bone

1. **Compact bone substance and spongy bone**. The compact bone substance mainly makes up the external layer (i.e., bone cortex) of bones, which is a hard and dense structure composed of multiple closely arranged bone lamella and having strong compressive strength; Spongy bone is the main component of both ends of a bone as well as interior of flat bone and irregular bone (Fig. 6.2). The orientation, number, and thickness of children's bone trabecula depend on load, muscle tension, and special functions, and some bone trabeculae are arranged in the pressure direction, namely pressure curve; Some bone trabeculae are arranged in the tension direction, namely tension curve. In this way, pressure can be dispersed in all directions to allow the bones to work under high pressure.
2. **Periosteum**. It is a connective tissue membrane covering the bone and nourishing it with abundant blood vessels and nerves. During the pubertal development period, there is a periosteum inside and outside the bone cortex, respectively, i.e., the periosteum and endosteum.

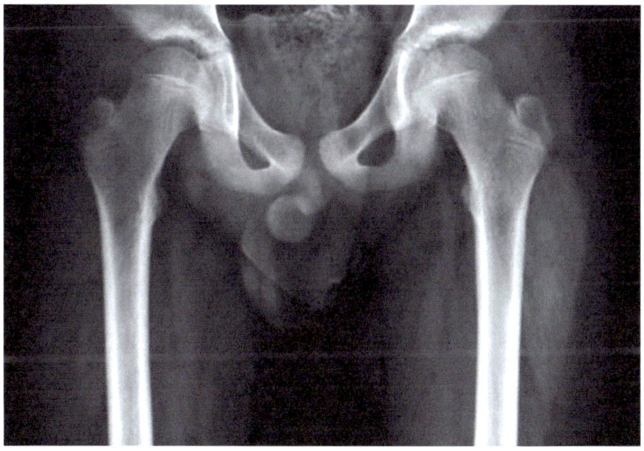

Fig. 6.2 X-ray anatomy of long bone in children. On the X-ray radiograph of bilateral hip joints in children, the thickest and densest area in the middle-superior 1/3 segment of femur and on the external diaphysis indicates the bone cortex. Spongy bone is located in the proximal femur with low density

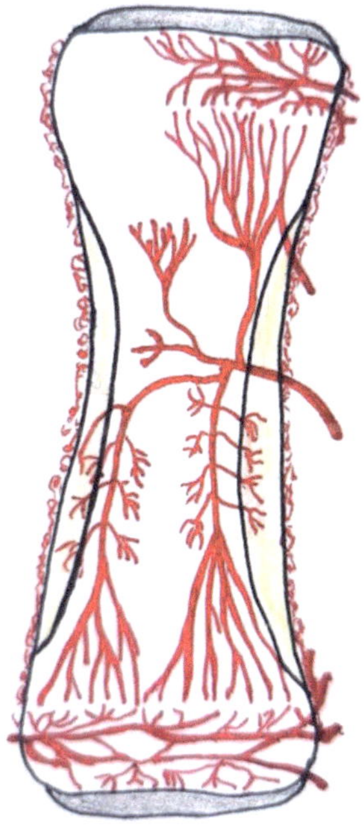

Fig. 6.3 Blood supply to long bones. Attention should be paid to the comparison of the blood supply of diaphysis, metaphysis, and epiphysis as well as their communication with blood vessels in periosteum, endosteum, and periarticular area

3. **Bone marrow cavity**. It occupies the center of bone and is covered with endosteum and filled with bone marrow. The bone marrow of children is red hematopoietic tissue. The red bone marrow is replaced by yellow bone marrow with age and losses the hematopoietic activity. However, the red bone marrow remains in spongy bone at both ends of long bone and within the flat bone for life.

6.1.3 Blood Supply to Bones

There are two typical approaches for supplying blood to bone: a set of blood vessels (namely nutrient arteries) running obliquely from the nutrient foramen into the Haversian canal and bone marrow cavity in the bone; and a set of blood vessels transversely entering the bone through the perforating canal from periosteum, and communicating with the longitudinal blood vessels in the Haversian canal. During the growth period of bone, blood vessels cannot penetrate the epiphyseal plate. Therefore, the blood vessels of diaphysis cannot reach the epiphysis. The nutrient vessels of epiphysis are from the articular capsule, and the metaphysis is supplied by the terminal branches of nutrient arteries. These terminal branches anastomose with the blood vessels entering the bone through perforating canal and that in adjacent soft tissues. After mutual merging between the diaphysis and epiphysis, the vascular branches of the metaphysis anastomose with the vessels of the epiphysis.

Taking tubular bone of growing children for example, there are four kinds of nutrient arteries, namely periosteal artery, nutrient artery, metaphyseal artery, and epiphyseal artery (Fig. 6.3).

1. **Periosteal artery**. The trunk courses along the long axis of bone and gives off multiple branches at different locations on the periosteum to form a periosteal artery network nourishing the periosteum and enter the bone cortex.
2. **Nutrient artery**. It enters the bone through the nutrient foramen and canal in the bone. The branches of nutrient artery enter the bone cortex and anastomose with blood vessels from the periosteal vascular plexus. Therefore, the bone cortex has double blood supply and collateral circulation.
3. **Metaphyseal artery**. There are numerous tiny through-holes in the cortex (vascular foramen) in the metaphyseal region of the bone, which allow the small branches of articular blood vessels to enter the bone through the bone cortex. The metaphyseal artery anastomoses with the terminal branches of ascending and descending branches of the nutrient artery.
4. **Epiphyseal artery**. The nutrient vessels in epiphysis also arise from vascular plexus around joints. Before merging between the epiphysis and metaphysis, the blood supply around the epiphyseal cartilage plate is from: (1) the terminal branches of epiphyseal artery distributed in the germinal layer of chondrocytes; (2) the terminal branches of metaphyseal artery distributed in the cell hypertrophy layer of epiphyseal cartilage plate.

During the development process of bones, the blood supplies to epiphysis and metaphysis are not completely isolated. There are microvascular communicating branches between the periosteal vessels and the epiphysis and metaphysis.

6.1.4 IV Joint

A joint is the connection made between bones. According to the nature and activity of connective tissues, joints can be divided into diarthrosis, amphiarthrosis, and synarthrosis.

1. **Diarthrosis**. It is mainly composed of articular surface, articular capsule, and articular cavity. The differentiation of some special structures (e.g., ligament, articular disc, articular labrum, and fold of synovial membrane) from part of joints aims to meet the functional requirements. These structures are collectively called auxiliary structures of synovial joints.
   (a) Articular surface: Each joint includes at least two smooth articular surfaces, which are covered with articular cartilages for life. The articular cartilage is rubbery and mainly used to reduce friction and absorb the impact and shock during articulated motion. The articular cartilage consists of cells, matrix, and fibers and is divided into three layers: surface layer, intermediate layer, and deep layer. The cartilage fibers in the surface layer are closely arranged and parallel to the surface; the intermediate layer is inclined and arched; and the deep layer is vertical. Calcification zone and bone lamella are located inferior to the deep layer. The nutrition for articular cartilage is supplied by penetration through the cartilage matrix and blood of subchondral bone tissue. Articular cartilage lacks the ability of regeneration after being destroyed or impaired.
   (b) Articular capsule: It is divided into inner and external layers: the external layer is a tough fibrous layer that strengthens the stability of joint with the surrounding ligaments; and the inner layer is a synovial layer that is composed of loose connective tissues and abundant blood vessels, and it can secrete synovial fluid. Synovial fluid can lubricate joints and nourish articular cartilage.
   (c) Articular cavity: It is an airtight space formed by joint epiphysis end and synovium, with a small amount of synovial fluid. Some joints contain ligaments in their articular cavities, such as knee joint and shoulder joint.
2. **Amphiarthrosis**. It is a transitional connection between the diarthrosis and synarthrosis. Its characteristic is that there is no articular capsule, and two bones may be directly connected by cartilage tissue, with a slit-like lacuna in the cartilage to limit the range of motion, including pubic symphysis.

   Two bones may also be connected by connective tissue or osseous tissue without gap there between, namely lacuna-free connection. Such connections include interosseous connection of skull, synostosis among ischium, pubis and ilium, and synostosis between sacral vertebrae.

6.1.5 Imaging Anatomy of Bones in the Extremities of Children

As children are in the period of growth and development, the imaging findings of bones and joints of children vary with age. Familiarity with normal manifestations of bones and joints of children of all ages is helpful to distinguish the normal conditions and pathological conditions and has important implications for the diagnosis of related diseases.

1. X-ray anatomy of bones in the extremities
   (a) **Epiphysis and Metaphysis**
      (i) Epiphysis: The secondary center of ossification in the epiphyseal cartilage is called secondary ossification center. The ossification center enveloped by bone cortex contains the spongy bone. During the growth and development period, the ossification center increases with age.
      (ii) Metaphysis: It is located between the epiphysis and the enlargement parts on both ends of tubular diaphysis, with relatively thin bone cortex in local part. The cartilage between epiphysis and metaphysis manifests as a transparent linear shadow on X-ray image, which is called epiphyseal plate (Fig. 6.4). In childhood, the division, proliferation, and ossification of chondrocytes in epiphyseal plate make the tubular bone grow in the vertical direction and gradually narrow the epiphyseal plate. The dense linear shadow on the metaphysis near the epiphyseal plate is called the provisional calcification zone, and the radiolucent area between the provisional calcification zone and epiphysis gradually narrows to an epiphyseal line with age. Finally, the epiphyseal cartilage is completely ossified and merged with the diaphysis, and the merging can be shown as a transversely dense line, namely connected epiphyseal line or growth line existing for several years or for life.
   (b) **Diaphysis**. It is a tubule composed of a relatively thin 1/3 intermediate part connecting to thick ends.
      (i) Periosteum: It is a membranous structure enveloping the bone. It is similar to the peripheral

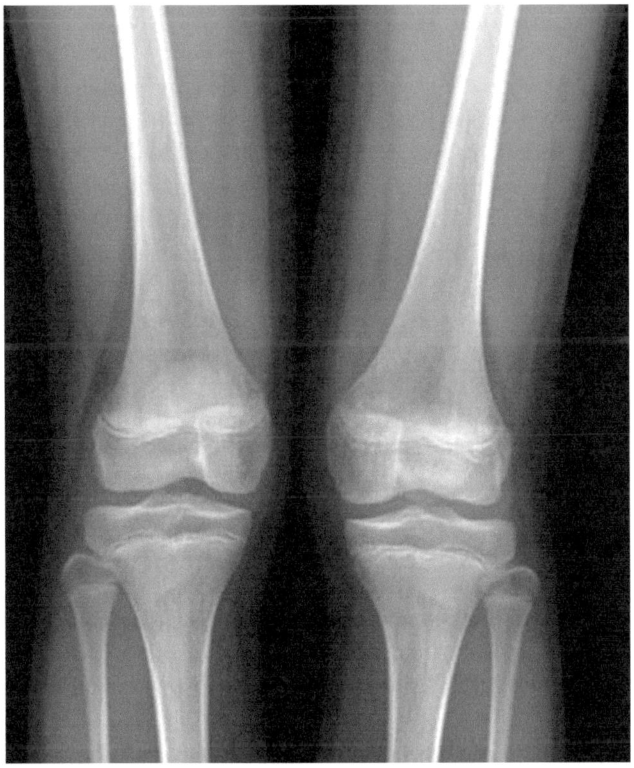

Fig. 6.4 X-ray anatomy of long epiphyseal plate of children. On X-ray image of distal femur and proximal tibia and fibula of children, a bright linear shadow between the epiphysis and metaphysis of long bone suggests a cartilage, namely epiphyseal plate. The dense linear shadow of metaphysis proximal to the epiphyseal plate is called provisional calcification zone. The radiolucent area between the provisional calcification zone and epiphysis gradually narrows to the epiphyseal line with age

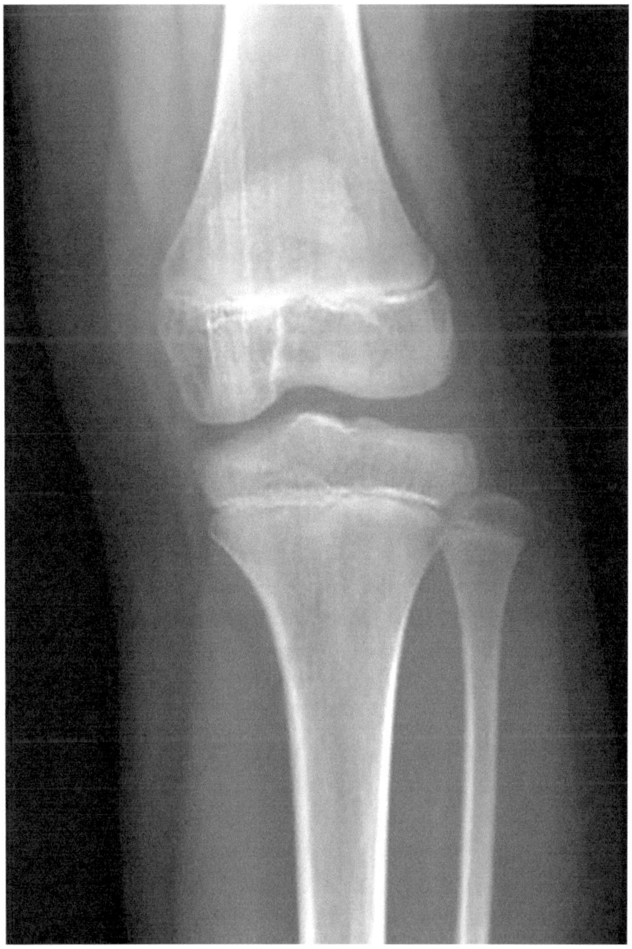

Fig. 6.5 X-ray anatomy of long bone joint space in children. On the X-ray image of knee joint in children, the bright space between the articular surfaces of bilateral metaphyses of long bones (i.e., distal femur and proximal tibia) is the joint space, which is wider than the actual space of knee joint

soft tissues in density and opaque on X-ray image. With less collagen fibers in the external periosteum, the periosteum fixation ability of children is inferior to that of adults, so their periosteal is easy to be peeled off.

(ii) Bone cortex: It is uniform and dense, and thickest and densest in the central diaphysis. The vascular channel formed by nutrient vessels can be occasionally observed, and the cortex is thinning as it extends to both ends. The bone cortex is connected with spongy bone at inner margin, which is ill-defined and less smooth than external margin in most cases. The external margin of bone cortex is mostly neat, but localized prominence or notch can be noticed at the attachment sites of muscle or tendon. Premature newborns possibly have relatively thick bone cortex.

(iii) Spongy bone: It is known as trabecular bone and composed of dense bone trabecular and bright bone marrow gap. The trabeculae intersecting with each other are reticularly connected and arranged in the directions of pressure and tension on the bone.

(iv) Bone marrow cavity: It is filled with bone marrow tissues, which mainly consist of fat, blood vessels, nerves, and body fluids. In contrast to the bone cortex, it is a bright area on X-ray radiograph.

(v) Nutrient foramen of bone: In most cases, it is located in the middle 1/3 segment of the diaphysis. When passing through the bone cortex, the nutrient artery of bone forms a slender channel in an initial direction perpendicular to the bone cortex, and the artery gradually inclines with the growth of bone.

(c) **X-ray anatomy of joint**. The joint consists of articular surface, joint space, and articular capsule [1–4] (Fig. 6.5).

(i) Articular surface: The surfaces of bones in relative positions that make up the joint are cartilages invisible on X-ray image. The articular surface observed is composed of subchondral calcification zone and thin dense bone, manifesting as smooth and sharp linear dense shadow.

(ii) Joint space: It is the transparent space between the articular surfaces of two metaphyses in relative positions. Since the articular cartilage and fibroplate and soft tissues share the similar density and indistinguishable on the X-ray radiograph, the joint space observed is wider than actual space.

(iii) Articular capsule: With same density as that of the peripheral soft tissues, it cannot be noticed in most cases, but sometimes its margin can be observed against the adipose layer outside the articular capsule.

(iv) Joint appendages: The ligaments around some large joints (e.g., knee joint, hip joint and ankle joint) can be observed against the adipose tissue.

2. CT anatomy of bones in the extremities

Depending on tomography, CT images eliminate the overlapped and shielded shadows among anatomical structures, clearly show various bone structures at high-density resolution, and reveal subtle focuses and changes in soft tissue that are difficult to be located by X-ray scan. CT enhanced examination further display the blood supply of focuses to distinguish the normal tissues from pathological tissues.

(a) **Bone.** The bone cortex and trabecula can be clearly observed in CT bone window. The bone cortex manifests as dense linear or strip-shaped shadow, and the bone trabecula manifests as reticular shadow. Bone marrow cavity manifests as low-density area due to fat components in the bone marrow (Fig. 6.6a, b). In the soft tissue window, muscles, tendons, and epiphyseal cartilages at moderate density can also be observed against the adipose tissue at low density.

(b) **Joint.** CT image clearly reveals the metaphysis and bony articular surface, but unavailable for showing the articular cartilage in most cases. The articular capsule, peripheral muscles, and ligaments inside and outside the capsule at moderate density can be observed in the windows of proper widths and positions. A small amount of fluid in normal articular cavity is difficult to be identified by CT, and the joint space manifests as low-density shadow (Fig. 6.6c).

(c) **Soft tissue.** CT can show soft tissue structure and further reveal tissues and organs with similar densities, including fat, muscle, and blood vessels. On the CT image, there are "linear" moderate-density skin, low-density subcutaneous fat, and moderate-density muscle from exterior to interior (Fig. 6.6c). The fat, blood vessels, and nerves can be observed among intermuscular spaces. The blood vessels and nerves manifest as small quasi-circular or strand-like shadow at moderate density, which can be distinguished against the low-density adipose tissue and course continuously at all levels.

3. MRI anatomy of bones in the extremities

MRI findings include cartilage, ligament, articular cavity, and other tissues difficult to be distinguished on X-ray image and reveal focus in the bone marrow cavity and soft tissues surrounding the bones [5–8].

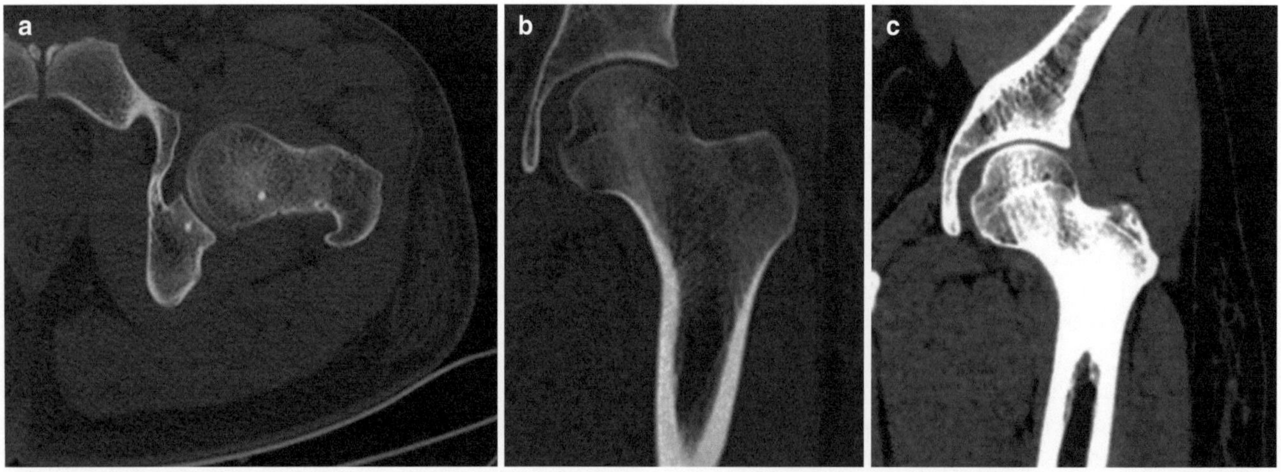

Fig. 6.6 CT anatomy of long bones in children. (**a**, **b**) Transverse plane and coronal plane for proximal femur of children by CT bone window reconstruction, clearly showing bone cortex and trabecula. The bone cortex manifests as dense strip-shaped shadow along the bone margin, and the bone trabecula manifests as reticular shadow in the bone marrow cavity shown as a low-density area. (**c**) Soft tissue window reconstructed, showing moderate-density articular capsule as well as surrounding muscles, fat, skin, and other soft tissues

Epiphyses are located at both ends of the diaphysis. Ossification nucleus manifests as hyperintense and is located in the center of epiphysis. Epiphyseal cartilage manifests as slightly hypointense and surrounds the ossification nucleus. The bone cortex of diaphysis cannot produce magnetic resonance signal as it is rich in calcium salts. Therefore, it manifests as hypointense on T_1WI and T_2WI. The periosteum clinging to the bone cortex cannot be distinguished by conventional scanning. Bone marrow intensity varies with its components: after birth, the intensity increases as the red bone marrow is replaced by adipose yellow bone marrow with age. The heterogeneous intensity is possible depending on the replacement progress. The bone marrow intensities in different sites of a femur are proximal metaphysis, distal metaphysis, and diaphysis in ascending order (Fig. 6.7). The bone marrow intensities of these sites decrease in younger people. That is, the red bone marrow of relevant sites is replaced by yellow bone marrow with age, and the fat components are increasing continuously. The intensities of all sites of femur are homogeneous after the age of 20 [5–8].

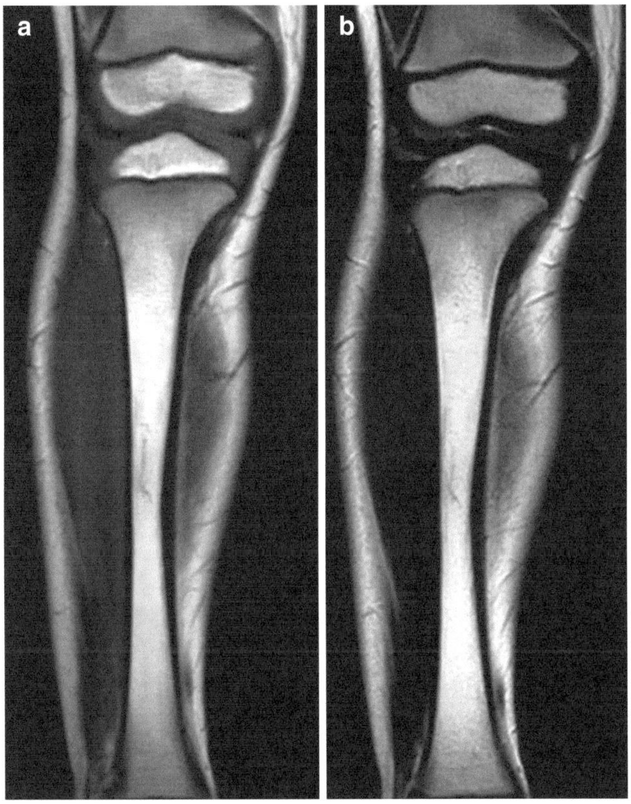

Fig. 6.7 MRI anatomy of long bones in children. On the MRI image, the ossification nucleus manifests as hyperintense, epiphyseal cartilage manifests as slightly hypointense, bone cortex shows hypointense on T_1WI and hypointense on T_2WI, and the bone marrow intensity increases from bilateral metaphyses to diaphysis

MRI is irreplaceable in displaying joint structures with its superiority. Taking knee joint for example, articular cartilage (e.g., meniscus) manifests as homogeneously triangular hypointense shadow as it is mainly composed of elastic fibers. However, linear slightly hyperintense shadow can be observed in the meniscus, and the articular surface is not involved. It is a normal manifestation due to the existence of blood vessels in meniscus in infants; Similarly, the intra-articular ligament structure manifests as homogeneously strip-shaped or linear hypointense shadow. Considering that the tiny ligament structures in children cannot be shown clearly on the MRI image, the impairments should be evaluated and judged according to indirect signs. Refer to femur for the changes in intensity of periarticular bone structures. It should be noted that the bone marrow of infants often manifests as hyperintense on T2WI fat-suppressed sequence, which should be differentiated from bone marrow edema caused by trauma. The components of synovial fluid in articular cavity manifest as hypointense on T_1WI and hyperintense on T_2WI (Fig. 6.8).

6.2 Characteristics and Pathophysiological Changes in Common Pathogen Infection

Qi Li and Wei Li

Common pathogens causing infectious lesions of children's bones and joints mainly include bacteria, fungi, parasites, and spirochetes. The pathogens of suppurative osteomyelitis and pyogenic arthritis are Staphylococcus aureus in most cases, and enterobacter, streptococcus, Pseudomonas aeruginosa, and Typhoid bacillus in some cases, followed by Mycobacterium tuberculosis. For fungal infection and other rare infections, the pathogens include Aspergillus, Candida, and Cryptococcus. The main parasitic infection involving bone and joint is echinococcosis, and spirochete infection is mainly caused by syphilis.

6.2.1 Staphylococcus aureus

Staphylococcus is a group of Gram-positive cocci widespread in nature. However, these cocci often become Gram-negative after aging, death, or phagocytosis by neutrophils. They are generally nonpathogenic and produce no capsule and can live with or without oxygen. The Staphylococcus aureus are the most common clinically pyogenic pathogens. It can cause multiple diseases and is also the most common pathogen leading to bacterial infection of bone and joint system [9].

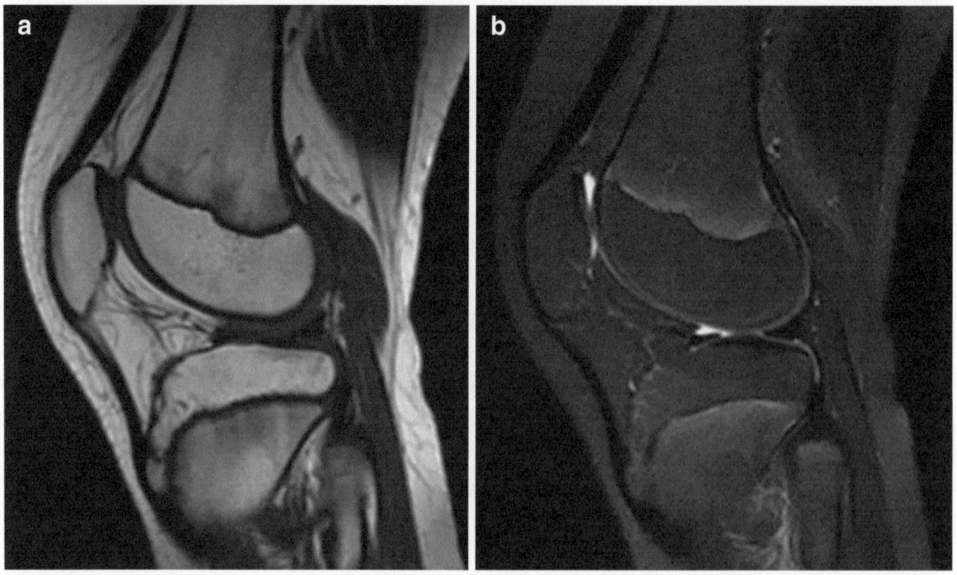

Fig. 6.8 MRI anatomy of knee joint in children. For knee joint of children on MRI T_1WI and T_2WI fat-suppressed sequence, the articular cartilage (e.g., meniscus) manifests as homogeneously hypointense shadow. On T_2WI fat-suppressed sequence, bone marrow manifests as slightly hyperintense

The pathogenicity of Staphylococcus aureus depends on its toxin and invasive enzyme and is related to the formation of biomembrane [10].

The onset of disease mainly depends on the relationship between virulence of the staphylococci and immunity of host. In the skin or other organs invaded, staphylococci multiply quickly and produce various toxins and enzymes in the same time, leading to corresponding pathological lesions. The phagocytosis by neutrophils and macrophages in the body limits the focus and forms suppurative inflammation. Meanwhile, local microthrombosis in the focus causes blood circulatory disorder, leading to tissue necrosis, liquefaction, and formation of vomica [11].

6.2.2 Streptococcus

Streptococcus belonging to Gram-positive bacteria is named because it is in circular or oval shape and arranged in chain-like conformation in the culture medium. The bacterium belongs to body normal flora and widely exists in nature. It can be found in feces of human and animals as well as nasopharynx of healthy people. According to hemolytic ability in relation to erythrocytes, streptococci can be divided into 3 types: (1) α-hemolytic streptococcus; (2) β-hemolytic streptococcus, which is highly pathogenic and accounts for the majority of pathogens; and (3) γ-hemolytic streptococcus with low pathogenicity.

The streptococcus is only second to Staphylococcus aureus in incidence of bone and joint infectious diseases. Pathogenic streptococci mainly include Streptococcus-a and Streptococcus pneumoniae. Streptococcus-a is Gram-positive, in circular or oval shape, with a diameter of 0.6 ~ 1.0 μm, arranged in chain-like conformation, and aerobic or facultative anaerobic, including anaerobe. The streptococcus-a has capsule formed by hyaluronic acid and is free of spores and flagella. It can invade all ages of people, with the highest incidence in children.

Streptococcus-a can cause various suppurative inflammations, toxic diseases, and allergic diseases. After invasion to body and organs, it inhabits locally by anti-phagocytosis and adhesion mechanism of bacteria, and then multiplies significantly to produce various toxins and exoenzymes, kill, lyse and destroy host cells and interstitial tissues, and spread through lymphatic vessels and interstitial spaces, leading to widespread tissue infection. The generated pyrogenic exotoxin enters the blood circulation and possibly leads to systemic toxemia, and even necrosis of important and parenchyma organs in severe cases, including liver, kidney, and heart [11]. Viridans streptococcus and group B streptococcus are opportunistic pathogens, which cause infections in case of compromised immunity.

6.2.3 Meningococcus

Meningococcus belongs to Neisseria and can cause epidemic cerebrospinal meningitis (i.e., meningococcal meningitis). Meningococci belong to Gram-negative diplococcus. They are kidney-shaped or bean-shaped and arranged in pairs with concave surfaces in relative positions, with a diameter of 0.6 ~ 0.8 μm and irregular arrangement. Meningococcus can be found in the nasopharyngeal cavity of healthy people. The morbid substances mainly include capsule, fimbriae, lipooligosaccharide (LOS) antigen, and IgA1 protease. The IgA1 protease is an exoenzyme produced by the meningococcus to initiate specific lysis of human IgA1 and assist the meningococcus in adhering to cell mucosa, thereby destroying immunity.

The disease is most common in infants aged 6 months to 2 years old, and mainly transmitted by close contact, including co-sleeping, breastfeeding, and kissing among these child patients. The early symptom is upper respiratory infection in most cases, which decreases the body resistance. After reproduction to a tremendous number in the nasopharynx, these bacteria enter the blood circulation and cause transient bacteremia, which develops to septicemia in a few cases. These bacteria can stay in the bone and joint system through bloodstream, causing suppurative osteomyelitis or allergic inflammation of bone and joint. In case of autolysis and death of bacteria, lots of endotoxin is released to cause systemic multi-system failure and toxic shock.

6.2.4 Brucella

Brucella is a zoonosis pathogen first isolated by David Bruce, a British military doctor, in 1886. For this reason, it was named brucella. Based on hosts, biochemical characteristics, metabolic ways, and immunology gaps, WHO Brucellosis Expert Committee divides brucella into 6 species and 19 biotypes, among which the Brucella abortus, Brucella melitensis, Brucella suis, and Brucella canis are pathogenic to human [12]. These bacteria vary in pathogenicity, among which the Brucella melitensis can cause severe infection and evolve into caseous granuloma. After directly touching the sick animals or their secretions/feces, or eating/using the products of the animals, humans are thereby infected with the bacteria via their skin and mucous membranes, respiratory tracts as well as digestive tracts [13].

Brucella can cause allergic inflammations of bone and joint system, mainly including arthritis, ankylosis, spondylitis, and osteomyelitis. These diseases can involve one or more joints, including sacroiliac joints, hip joints, knee joints, shoulder joints, and other large joints. Some patients are subject to redness and suppuration of joints, and synovitis, tenosynovitis, and periarthritis are common.

6.2.5 Mycobacterium tuberculosis

Mycobacterium is a kind of slender and slightly curved bacillus with remarkable characteristics: cell wall containing a lot of lipids; without spores and flagella; immobile; and producing no endotoxin or exotoxin.

Mycobacterium tuberculosis can be divided into human Mycobacterium tuberculosis, Mycobacterium bovis, Mycobacterium murine, and the like, among which the human Mycobacterium tuberculosis mainly threatens human health [14]. Mycobacterium tuberculosis is mainly transmitted via respiratory tracts, and a small number of the bacteria enter the body through digestive tracts and infected skin wounds, thus infecting multiple systemic tissues and organs, such as lung, brain, bones, and joints, intestinal tracts and urogenital system, among which tuberculosis is the most common disease. Humans are generally susceptible to Mycobacterium tuberculosis, among which infants have a higher incidence. It can cause systemic disseminated tuberculosis in severe cases. The macrophages phagocytose the tubercle bacillus invading to body and send the processed antigen information to T lymphocytes for sensitization. The T lymphocytes will play a major role in phagocytosis of tubercle bacillus by immune response and form tubercle. In most cases, tuberculosis of bone and joint occurs secondary to tuberculosis. Through hematogenous dissemination, Mycobacterium tuberculosis tends to stay in the spongy bone and red bone marrow, where the blood supply is sufficient, and joints, such as synovial membrane of vertebral body, long bone metaphysis, knee joint, hip joint, and other large joints, which are heavy-loaded and highly active.

6.2.6 Hydatid

There are different species of hydatids, among which the Echinococcus granulosus, Alveolar echinococcus, Echinococcus vogeli, and Echinococcus oligarthrus are parasitized in human body. The Echinococcus granulosus is the most common pathogen of human echinococcosis [15]. Echinococcosis, distributed in vast pastoral areas around the globe, spreads between humans and animals. Hydatid can grow up to 30 ~ 40 cm, and infiltration and hyperplasia of monocytes, acidophilic granulocytes, foreign body giant cells, epithelioid cells, and fibroblasts can be observed around the focuses, which compress the peripheral tissues for a long time and resulting in secondary liver cirrhosis, atelectasis, and other diseases.

6.2.7 Aspergillus

Aspergillus of a great variety exists extensively in nature. Aspergilli can be divided into 18 groups, 132 species, and 18 varieties. Most of them are nonpathogenic, and only about 20 kinds of aspergilli cause human diseases. With extremely low pathogenicity to human beings, aspergillus only threatens individuals with low immunity. The common pathogens are Aspergillus fumigatus and Aspergillus flavus. By invading multiple organs of body, aspergillus can cause diseases including direct infection, hypersensitivity, and aspergillosis poisoning. Aspergillus is an opportunistic pathogen. Lung and paranasal sinus are most susceptible to aspergillus spores by inhalation, and wound infection can be caused by skin lesion, which mainly presenting exudative inflammation, abscess, necrotic ulcer, and granuloma, and leading to visceral congestion and swelling. The pathogen grows slowly and only invades into deep tissues in a few cases. Invasive aspergillosis may occur in case of granulocytopenia and abnormal T lymphocytes for a long time. The skeletal system is mostly infected via direct diffusion from lung to adjacent vertebrae, intervertebral disc spaces, and ribs or via blood. GM, which has been confirmed as a surrogate marker for invasive aspergillosis, is suitable for the specific diagnosis of aspergillus infection [16].

6.2.8 Candida

Candida, belonging to candida species, with circular or oval thin-wall body and a diameter of 4 ~ 6 μm, is Gram-positive and reproduced by budding. It is easy to form blastospores and pseudohyphae in tissues, a few can form chlamydospores and fungal mycelium, but Candida glabrata cannot form mycelium. Candida is an opportunistic pathogen. The most common disease caused by the bacterium is Candida albicans infection, which is more common in the patients with body dysbacteriosis or decreased immunity, hematological malignant tumor, long-term administration of steroid pills, prosthesis implantation, long-term use of broad-spectrum antibiotics, and the like. However, the Candida albicans is among the body normal flora, with the highest carrier rate in digestive tract. Candida can cause infections of skin, mucous membranes, and systemic and local deep tissues [17]. It normally exists in the gastrointestinal tracts of human and animals. Candida infections are mostly caused by endogenous exposure and spread to the whole body through the digesting tract. The iatrogenic factor plays the major role in the infection. The infection by exogenous exposure is relatively rare and normally associated with occupation.

The candida infection in skeletal system mainly occurs in patients using antibiotics for a long term due to open injuries, manifesting as an acute suppurative inflammation with coagulative necrosis in the center as well as cavitation, fibrosis, and granuloma.

6.2.9 Cryptococcus neoformans

Cryptococcus neoformans, one species of cryptococcus, is a circular or oval-shaped bacterium with a diameter of 5 ~ 20 μm. Different from other yeast-like fungi, it reproduces by budding and does not produce pseudohyphae. It is surrounded by a wide, thick polysaccharide capsule, which serves as a main virulence factor to inhibit the phagocytosis of phagocytes and lower the body's immunity. The microscopic examination after negative staining with ink shows that the bacterial body is circular, oval-shaped and transparent against the black background. Cryptococcus neoformans is ubiquitous in the nature. It can be isolated from pigeon feces, fruits, soil, and skin, mucous membranes, and feces of healthy human, especially abundant in pigeon feces. For mankind, Cryptococcus neoformans is opportunistic pathogen that leads to congenital or acquired infection in infants. Like many pathogenic fungi, cryptococcus invades mostly through the respiratory tract. The infection usually starts from the lungs, forming early white jelly-like focuses and granulomas in different sizes at the advanced stage. These focuses contain caseous necrosis, small cavities, rare pyogenesis, no calcification or significant capsule. As the Cryptococcus neoformans has special affinity to the central nervous system, patients concerned often see the doctor due to clinical symptoms of neurological involvement (e.g., chronic meningitis), and 90% of these patients have cerebral injury or spinal cord (membrane) injury. Bone and joint infections are caused by hematogenous dissemination, more common in osteomyelitis. Joint involvements are mostly aroused by spread of adjacent osteomyelitis [18], and the cellulitis can be caused by invasion to skin. The symptoms of synovial tissues include acute and chronic synovitis, with multinucleated giant cells, granulomas, and a large number of budding yeasts stained by special colors found under the microscope.

6.2.10 Coccidioides

Coccidioides, a dimorphic fungus, presents as yeast type and mycelium type, respectively, in a 37 °C tissue and a 28 °C culture medium. It can rupture into arthrospores. Coccidioidomycosis mainly occurs in the arid areas of southwestern America [19], mostly due to inhalation of arthrospores in contaminated soil. The coccidioides in the soil presents as mycelium. Once invading the tissues, it will transform into an ablastemic spherule with a diameter of 2 ~ 200 μm, containing many endospores. The ruptured ablastemic spherule releases endospores, which are transmitted to other parts of the body via lymph or blood. Each spore can become an ablastemic spherule again and start a new lifecycle. Like other fungal diseases, bone infections induced by coccidioidomycosis are mainly observed at joints. Joint infections are mostly caused by the spread of adjacent osseous tissue. Depending on etiology, the definite diagnosis can be made if sporangium is detected under the microscope.

6.2.11 Syphilis

Syphilis is a chronic infectious disease caused by Treponema pallidum. It can invade all organs and tissues of whole body and be transplacentally transmitted to the fetus. The bacterial body is 4 ~ 14 μm long and 0.2 μm wide, consists of 8 ~ 14 regularly arranged helices, and has low survival rate in vitro. Treponema pallidum are abundant on the surface of skin and mucosa membrane, and they can also be found in saliva, milk, semen, and urine. The Treponema pallidum can be transmitted by close contact, such as sexual abuse, kissing, breastfeeding. After entering the human body, the pallidum invade nearby lymph nodes within several hours, and spread to the whole body after 2 ~ 3 days via the blood circulation. Organs could be infected through lymphatic and hematogenous metastasis, including arteries, bones, nerves, and sensory organs, and viscera will be affected at advanced stage, such as liver, kidney, and stomach. At early stage, the pallidum causes endarteritis and endophlebitis and results in vascular endothelial swelling and proliferation. The thickening of vascular wall in the lesion area can be observed microscopically, a large number of pallidus were accumulated in the perivascular and/or endothelial cell areas, and the fibrous connective tissue hyperplasia, neutrophil and lymphocyte infiltration, fewer plasma cells, and single acidophilic granulocyte are observed [20]. The giant cell granuloma with central coagulative necrosis can be observed in advanced nodular syphilis and gumma.

6.3 Bacterial Infection

Heng Zhao and Wei Li

6.3.1 Acute Suppurative Osteomyelitis

Overview

Acute suppurative osteomyelitis is a suppurative inflammation caused by pyogenic bacteria transmitting through blood circulation or directly invading bones, and affecting bone marrow, sclerotin, or periosteum. It mostly occurs in children and adolescents, especially in children under 12 years old. It is common in metaphysis of long tubular bones with abundant blood vessels, especially in lower extremities. The tibia, fibula, and femur are the most susceptible parts [21, 22]. With rapid onset and severe symptoms, it should be diagnosed definitively as soon as possible. Meanwhile, the existence of abscess and its location and extent should be defined, and effective and timely treatment should be provided accordingly for satisfactory efficacy. Delay of treatment will inevitably lead to irreversible bone destruction and osteonecrosis, which affect bone development and even cause bone deformity.

Acute suppurative osteomyelitis can be divided into hematogenous osteomyelitis and non-hematogenous osteomyelitis according to infection mechanism, and hematogenous infections are more common in related patients. For patients with hematogenous infection, the pyogenic bacteria enter the bloodstream from the pyogenic infection focus and infect bones. The disease can be induced by trauma (e.g., sprain), local infections (e.g., furuncle and amygdalitis), and systemic diseases (e.g., upper respiratory tract infection) or produce infection without definitely inducing factors. Pathogens causing the hematogenous osteomyelitis mainly include Staphylococcus aureus (accounting for 72% ~ 85%), which is followed by Staphylococcus haemolyticus, pyogenic streptococcus, Escherichia coli, Diplococcus pneumoniae, etc. Non-hematogenous infection mostly occurs after open injury or spread of soft tissue infection to adjacent bone. Pathogenic factors are associated with type and virulence of the pathogens, and closely related to the sensitivity to infection, natural immunity and locally decreased immunity of body.

Acute pyogenic infections of bone in infants and children are mostly hematogenous infections, which have different characteristics in clinical pathogenetic process, symptoms, signs, imaging findings, and prognosis. The reason for these differences is that the anatomical structures of bone marrow tissues and intraosseous blood supply vary with bone development. In fetal period, there are only a few large veins without venous sinus in the bone marrow. In infancy, the intraosseous blood supply remains the characteristic. The veins are still wide as there are only a few primary venous sinuses formed. These veins are surrounded by hemopoietic tissues and a few adipocytes are produced. Therefore, any pyogenic infection in bone can quickly spread throughout the bone and cause pyemia, thus the osteomyelitis in infants and children is an acute disease with severe systemic symptoms of poisoning and extensive bone destruction, which easily lead to chondronecrosis or massive osteonecrosis, bone growth disorder, early metaphysis closure, and bone developmental deformity, as well as invasion to joints resulting in dysfunction.

The acute suppurative osteomyelitis in children has unique anatomical characteristics and is common in metaphysis. The bacteria pass through the terminal branch of bone nutrient artery and the capillary vessel at metaphysis to enter the venous sinus. A U-shaped vascular loop opening towards diaphysis is formed at the arteriovenous end of the metaphysic. With vortexes of sluggish blood stream in the loop, the environment suitable for bacterial reproduction is provided for inflammatory infiltration of bone marrow within a short term. The inflammatory infiltration further develops to destroy the blood supply in bone and cause purulency and abscess. As the pressure on intraosseous abscess increases, the abscess may directly extend to the marrow cavity of diaphysis or the articular cavity adjacent to the metaphysis, or spread to the inferior periosteum through the Haversian canal of bone cortex to form the subperiosteal abscess, destroying the blood vessels and periosteum in the Haversian canal of bone cortex and leading to osteolytic destruction or massive osteonecrosis. The subperiosteal abscess can subperiosteally invade to the distal bone marrow cavity or penetrate the periosteum and flow to the soft tissue, thereby forming soft tissue abscess or invading adjacent joints [23]. The epiphyseal plate provides a temporary barrier throughout the childhood (from 1 year old) until the metaphysis is closed. During this period, the epiphyseal involvement of osteomyelitis is rare in children as the blood vessels cannot penetrate the epiphyseal plate, and the blood supplies of epiphysis and metaphysic are isolated. For children with severe conditions, it can be observed that the metaphysic focus penetrates the epiphyseal plate and affects the epiphysis, and even further invades epiphyseal cartilage and involves the articular cavity. During the repair period, the granulation tissue absorbs pus, and the new bone hyperostosis leads to myelosclerosis and free sequestrum. After medical or surgical treatment, the pyogenic infection can be cleaned up, or develops into chronic osteomyelitis, or causes a lifelong disability due to extensive bone destruction and failure in absorbing large sequestrum.

The systemic symptoms of acute hematogenous osteomyelitis vary with the infection level. Manifestations of mild infection include low-grade fever, and that of severe infection include acute high fever, bacteremia, septicopyemia, and other poisoning symptoms. The lung abscess and suppurative pericarditis can be additionally observed in a few cases. Some children with infant osteomyelitis may suffer mild general conditions and severe local symptoms and signs; some child patients have high fever, convulsion, subcutaneous bleeding spots, multiple pustules, pneumonia, and other symptoms; and severe cases suffer septic shock and coma. The local symptoms include pain in limb affected, muscle spasm, flexion of adjacent joints. The child patients refuse limb activity or cry after passive activity [24]. The affected part has redness, heat pain, tenderness, and fluctuation. The extensive pyogenic focus will cause severe bone destruction and form sequestra of different sizes. In that case, the disease will develop into the chronic osteomyelitis and even cause permanent deformity after abscess incision and drainage. In addition to blood biochemical test, hemoculture and other routine examinations in laboratory test, the DNA-related molecular detection can be conducted to improve the detection rate of corresponding pathogens [25]. Children with acute osteomyelitis require no surgery in most cases. However, the surgical treatment is required in case of abscess and is urgently needed in case of secondary pyogenic arthritis and other severe complications [26]. In clinical practice, the early treatment of acute suppurative osteomyelitis specially emphasizes the importance of abscess elimination by local aspiration of pus and drainage. With accurate time and location for incision and drainage, a timely diagnosis can be made to detect the species of pathogens, and sensitive antibiotics can be selected accordingly to effectively control the disease.

Pathophysiology

The pathological process of suppurative osteomyelitis consists of bacterial invasion to bone, inflammatory infiltration, purulency, bone destruction, sequestrum formation, and extensive hyperostosis for repair. The process can be basically divided into four stages according to pathological manifestations. (1) Inflammatory infiltration and abscess formation: At early stage, infiltration and exudation of intramedullary inflammatory cells in metaphysis increases the intraosseous pressure and obstructs the venous return, and then gradually develops into abscess and causes bone destruction. Microscopically, the abscess is infiltrated with purulent exudate, gliacytes, numerous neovessels, and neutrophils. It is peripherally surrounded by granulation tissues and fibrous connective tissues. (2) Abscess spreading: The abscess spreads in the bone marrow cavity or penetrates the cortex and reaches inferior periosteum, forming the subperiosteal abscess. (3) Sequestrum formation: The enlarged subperiosteal abscess lifts the periosteum and interrupts the blood supply to the diaphysis. Meanwhile, the impact on blood supply by thromboarteritis causes osteonecrosis and even sequestrum formation. (4) Periosteal proliferation: Bone repair and periosteal new bone formation can be observed with the bone destruction, and involucrum formed by new bone is partially visible. Sinus tract formation observed in some cases: pus erodes and penetrates bone and soft tissue, forming a fistula communicating the intraosseous and ectosteal soft tissues and opening to outside.

Imaging Findings

1. **X-ray**
   (a) X-ray radiograph: During the acute period (7 ~ 10 days), X-ray only detects extensive diffuse swelling of soft tissue surrounding the diseased bone, which increases diameter of affected limbs and leads to abnormal limb appearance, but these abnormalities generally do not cross the joint. The density of soft tissue is relatively increased, and the deep tissue adjacent to the bone is involved firstly. The intermuscular fat can be relocated or disappears, gradually developing thickened and rough edema of subcutaneous fat layer with thick reticular shadow. The boundary between the subcutaneous fat and other soft tissues and the muscle is blurred. In most cases, bone change cannot be observed immediately unless 2 weeks after the onset of disease. In the early stage, the confined osteoporosis occurs in the metaphyseal spongy bone; and after about 2 weeks, multiple scattered and irregular bone destruction focuses are formed in moth-

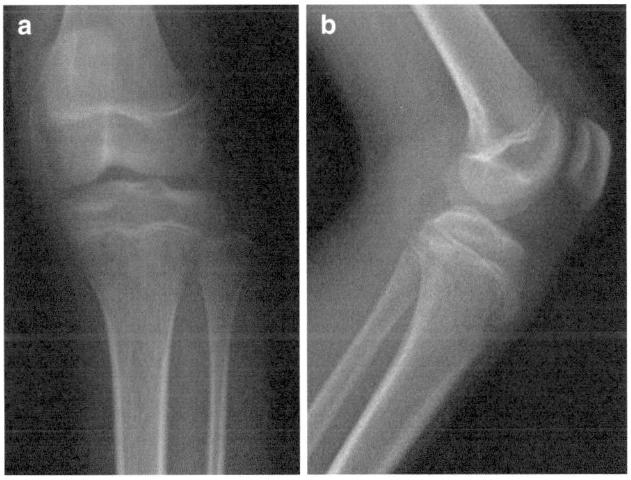

Fig. 6.9 Suppurative osteomyelitis in the proximal left tibia. DR shows metaphyseal osteoporosis of the proximal left tibia, and multiple scattered moth-eaten bone destructions in the spongy bone

eaten and plaque-like pattern. The bone trabecula is discontinuous with ill-defined boundary with the surrounding bone (Fig. 6.9). With rapid progress of the disease, the bone destruction areas are expanded and merged together, manifesting as multiple strip-like low-density shadows. The destruction area may spread to diaphysis and cause pathologic fracture, or cause subperiosteal abscess after destroying the bone cortex, and further stimulate the periosteum to cause periosteal proliferation (Figs. 6.10 and 6.11). The early proliferative response is mild, and then it is enhanced with the progress of the disease, manifesting as linear and laminated dense new bones parallel to the diaphysis. These new bones have irregular margins and relatively high and heterogeneous density. If the proliferative periosteum is penetrated by the inferior abscess and ruptured, the Codman's triangle is formed (Fig. 6.12). Lifted periosteum and thromboarteritis interrupt the blood supply to bone cortex and lead to osteonecrosis, which manifests as well-defined plaque-like and strip high-density bone pieces of different sizes. In severe cases, large plaque-like and long strip sequestra are prominent against the surrounding low-density pus area and osteoporotic bones by bone absorption and destruction. Sequestrum in bone marrow cavity manifests as shadows of small dense bones of different sizes scattered in low-density destruction area. The hyperostosis for repair is carried out with bone destruction, which manifests as hyperplasia and ossification of periosteum as well as heterogeneously increased density of annular shadow around the bone destruction area.

(b) Contrast examination by aspiration of pus: According to findings from X-ray radiograph, sites with suspected abscess and sites with tenderness and fluctuation identified by clinical examination are punctured. The pus is drained out if possible, and water-soluble contrast agent equivalent to or slightly less than the volume of extracted pus is injected. The anteroposterior and lateral views are taken immediately after injection to show the intraosseous and ectosteal abscesses [1].

(i) Subperiosteal abscess: The area developed by contrast agent is a subperiosteal abscess surrounding the diaphysis, clinging to the subperiosteal bone cortex, and free of gap with bone. At

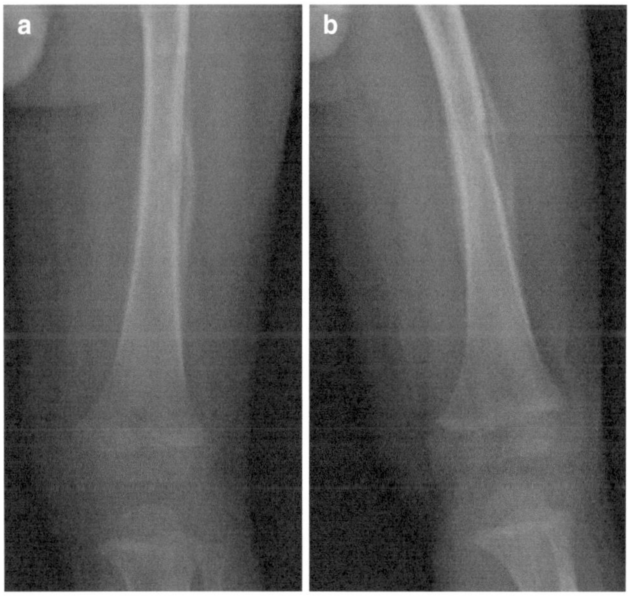

Fig. 6.10 Suppurative osteomyelitis in the middle part of left femur. DR shows confined cortical destruction and periosteal proliferation in the middle part of left femur, with inferior sequestrum

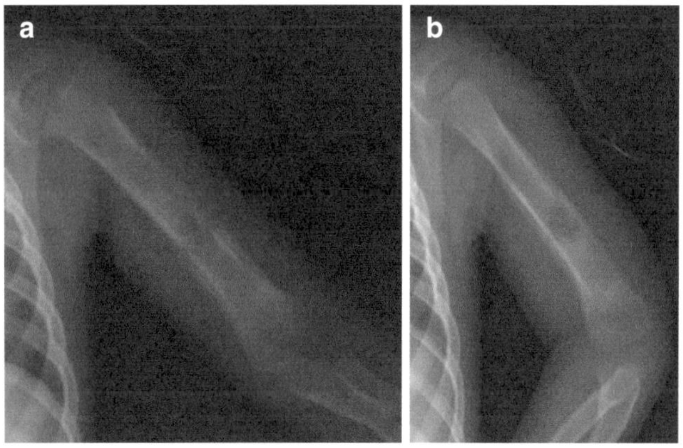

Fig. 6.11 Suppurative osteomyelitis in the proximal left humerus. DR shows osteoporotic diaphysis of left humerus, multiple plaque-like bone destruction, bone cortex involvement, visible periosteal reaction, and peripheral soft tissue swelling

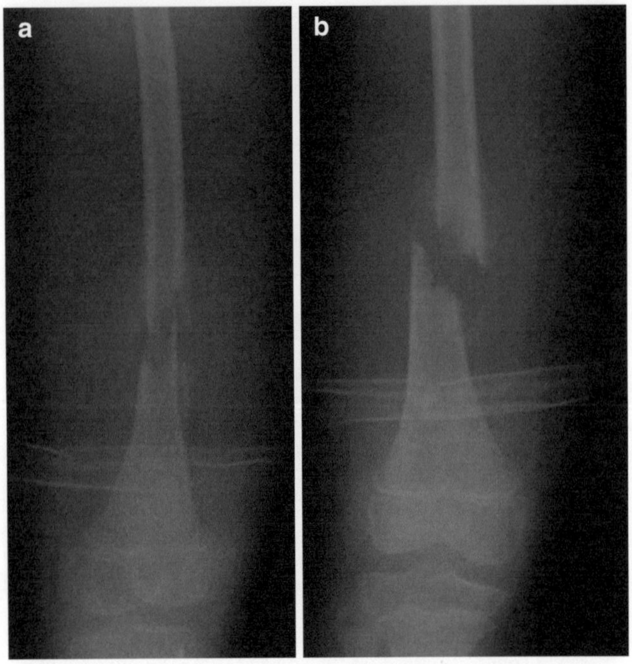

Fig. 6.12 Suppurative osteomyelitis in the distal left femur with pathologic fracture. DR shows bone destruction and fracture in the distal left femur, periosteal proliferation, and formation of Codman's triangle

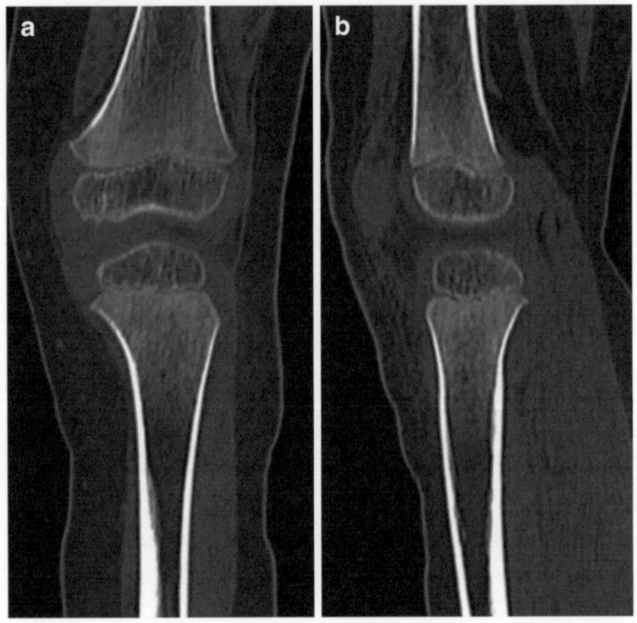

Fig. 6.13 Suppurative osteomyelitis in the proximal left tibia (1). CT coronal and sagittal reconstruction showed a small amount of moth-eaten bone destruction in the metaphysis of the proximal left tibia

the early stage, the abscess has smooth margin and slight bulging and is relatively confined. After 5 ~ 6 days of onset, the subperiosteal abscess spreads extensively and produces irregular margin, which proves that the periosteum has been destroyed. After 7 ~ 8 days of onset, the subperiosteal abscess ruptures, and the contrast agent spreads to the peripheral soft tissues or intermuscular space. In this time, the distribution of contrast agent in the vomica is highly irregular. If the subperiosteal abscesses are adjacent to the joints, the capsular ligament may be invaded to develop the joint space. The subperiosteal abscess may cause the development within the bone at the time of pyography, as the intraosseous pus can spread through the Haversian canal to the subperiosteum and after the subperiosteal pus was extracted, the contrast agent can also enter the bone through the Haversian canal.

(ii) Soft tissue abscess: the results showed that the development of the vomica was irregular, and the contrast agent was distributed in masses with some space with the bone. Even though the development of the deep vomica was close to the bone, there was also a narrow clear gap. If the contrast agent has closed to the bone cortex, it indicates that the periosteum here has been damaged, which will inevitably lead to the erosion of bony substance.

2. **CT.** It is more likely to detect soft tissue swelling than X-ray in the early stage and can determine in a more precise manner the increased soft tissue density and the thickened edema of subcutaneous fat layer and find the thick reticular shadow and that intermuscular fat can be transferred or disappeared. CT is helpful to finding the small lesions in the bone and there is localized osteoporosis in the metaphyseal spongy bone in the early stage, which forms the scattered bone destruction foci about 2 weeks, with the worm-etched shape, small patchy shape, and indistinct boundary from the surrounding normal osseous substance (Fig. 6.13). As the disease worsened, the damage was gradually expanded and spread to the diaphysis (Fig. 6.14), and the subperiosteal abscess (Fig. 6.15) occurred to the bone cortex after cortical destruction, which caused periosteal proliferation by stimulating the periosteum, the result of which showed linear and layered dense new bone with uneven edges, higher density, but not heterogeneous. Significant periosteal proliferation could form changes of bone involucrum (Fig. 6.16). The proliferating periosteum was punctured by the abscess below, forming a Codman triangle. Lifted periosteum and thrombotic arteritis may also cause the disruption of blood supply to the bone cortex, leading to osteonecrosis, the symptoms of which showed patchy and strip high-density bone mass of different sizes, with clear boundaries; in severe cases, large flaky elongated sequestrum can be seen (Fig. 6.16), while the sequestra in the

bone marrow cavity were manifested as small dense bone masses of different sizes scattered in the low-density destruction area.

The hyperostosis for repair is carried out with bone destruction, which manifests as hyperplasia and ossification of periosteum as well as heterogeneously increased density of annular shadow around the bone destruction area. For advanced diseases, CT is clearer and accurate than X-ray in showing bone destruction, small sequestrum, bone fistula, soft tissue sinus, and even foreign substances, intraosseous or soft tissue gas.

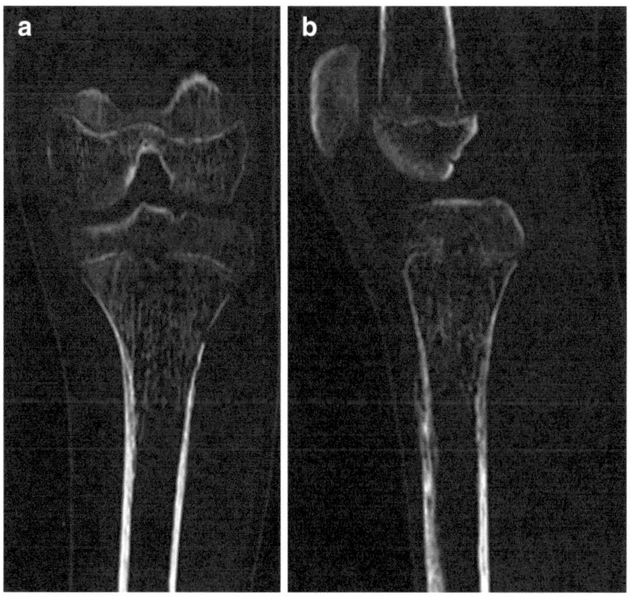

Fig. 6.14 Suppurative osteomyelitis in the proximal left tibia (2). CT coronal and sagittal reconstruction showed osteoporosis in the metaphysis of the proximal left tibia, with multiple moth-eaten bone destruction and local cortical being involved

3. **MRI**. In the early stage of the disease (2 ~ 3 days), MRI examination can detect the lesions as the bone marrow inflammation causes exudation, edema, congestion, and increased water content. Hypointense or isointense can be seen on T_1WI, while hyperintense can be seen on T_2WI and fat-suppressed sequence, with a clearer boundary than that on T_1WI. In the progressive stage, multiple irregular and unequal bone destruction area can be seen, which presented hypointense on T_1WI and heterogeneous hyperintense on T_2WI and STIR sequence (Fig. 6.17), and intraosseous vomica and subperiosteal abscess presented hyperintense on T_2WI (Fig. 6.18). After the appearance of sequestra, hypointense can be seen both on T_1WI and T_2WI and the periosteum showed "linear" hypointense. STIR sequences are clearer in showing abscesses, inflammatory responses, and intramuscular edema, which can provide accurate pathologic anatomic images for surgery. After enhancement, there is marked enhancement in the granulation tissue around the vomica, but without enhancement in the vomica (Fig. 6.18).
4. **Radionuclide bone imaging.** As one of the infectious diseases, the acute suppurative osteomyelitis can cause changes in blood supply in the early stage, which is manifested as high blood supply in the lesion area. Thus, the radionuclide bone imaging is of great significance for the early detection of acute osteomyelitis. The bone imaging should include the three-phase bone imaging, and the local increased blood flow can be seen in the blood flow phase, blood pool phase, and delayed phase, which shows a concentration of radioactivity (Fig. 6.19). Sometimes,

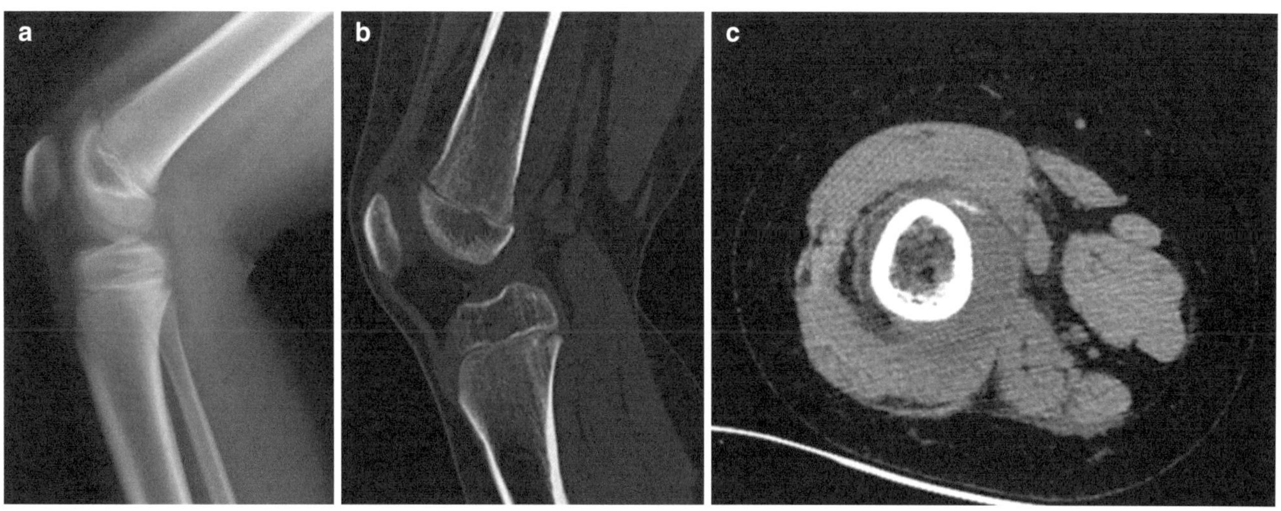

Fig. 6.15 Subperiosteal abscess at the distal end of right femur. (**a**) The shadow of increased soft tissue density in the dorsal arc of the distal end of the right femur is observed on DR lateral views; (**b**) CT sagittal reconstruction shows arc-shaped low-density area with clear margins outside bone cortex; (**c**) CT soft tissue window shows the formation of subperiosteal abscess in the fluid density area outside the bone cortex

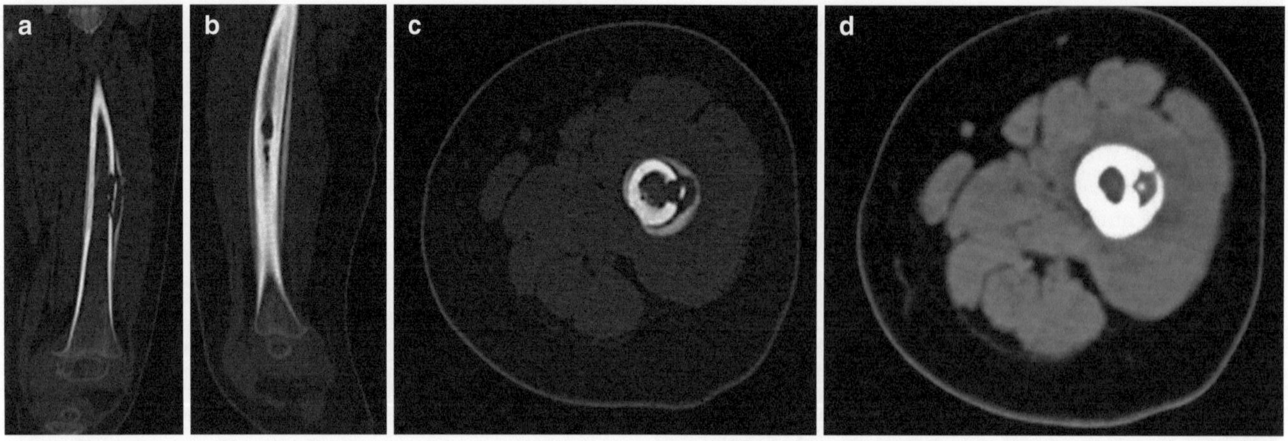

Fig. 6.16 Suppurative osteomyelitis in the middle part of left femur. (**a**, **b**) CT bone window reconstruction shows localized cortical destruction and the formation of sequestrum and periosteal proliferation in the middle part of the left femur; (**c**) CT transverse plane shows localized cortical destruction, the formation of sequestrum, periosteal proliferation, and changes of bone involucrum; (**d**) CT soft tissue window shows that the lesions of femur presents soft tissue density under periosteum, with soft tissue swelling around

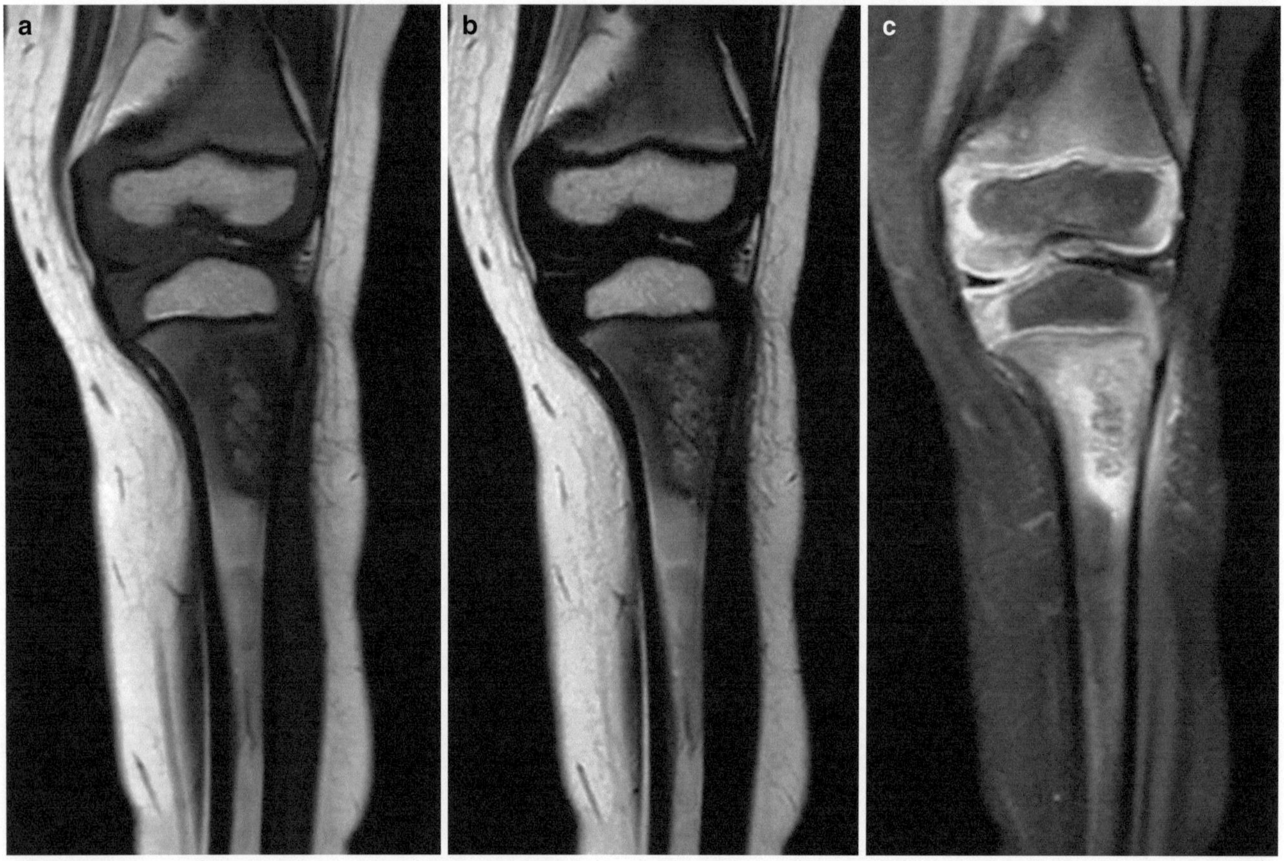

Fig. 6.17 Suppurative osteomyelitis in the proximal left tibia (3). Long-and-round shape destruction area of bone in the metaphysis of the proximal left tibia. (**a**) On MRI, T_1WI showed mixed isointense/hypointense; (**b**) T_2WI showed isointense/slightly hyperintense; (**c**) T_2WI STIR sequences showed that there were heterogeneous slightly hyperintense in the bone destruction area, and patchy slightly hyperintense edema zones can be seen around, with the edema and exudation of periosseous soft tissue

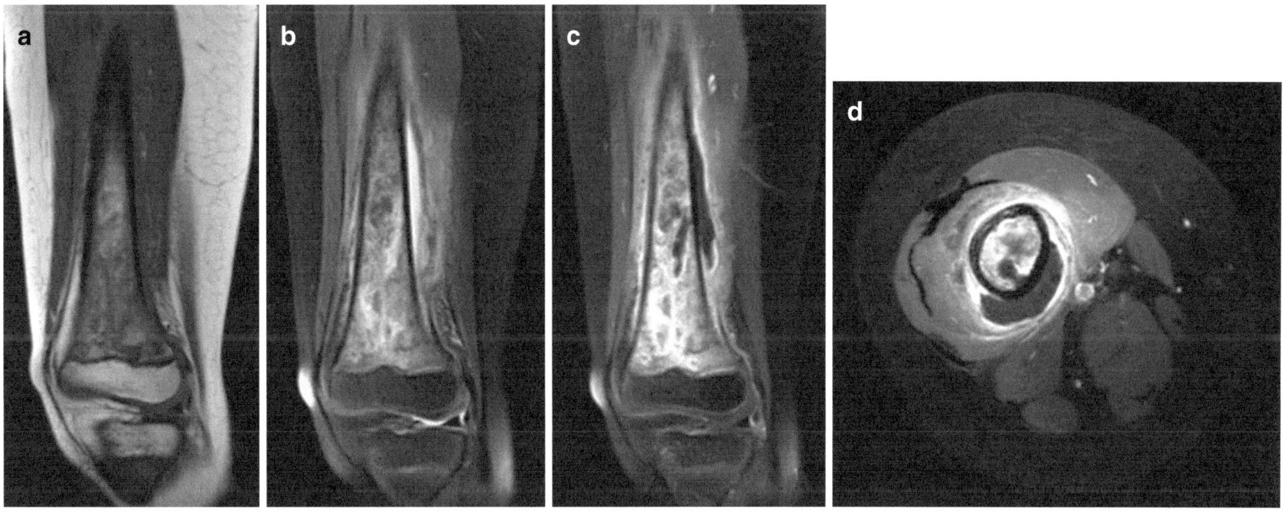

Fig. 6.18 Suppurative osteomyelitis at the distal end of right femur. Extensive bone destruction in the distal metaphysis of the right femur. (**a**) On MRI, T_1WI showed heterogeneous hypointense; (**b**) T_2WI and STIR sequences showed heterogeneous hyperintense, with strip-like hyperintense near the bone and peripheral soft tissue edema; (**c**, **d**) After potentiation, the bone destruction area was significantly enhanced in a heterogeneous way; irregular non-enhanced area was found in the marrow cavity; no enhanced abscess cavity was found in the side of the bone, the wall of the vomica was significantly enhanced, and the formation of an internal sinus was observed, with the surrounding soft tissue around ribbon-like enhancement

Fig. 6.19 Suppurative osteomyelitis of proximal right tibia. Radioactive concentration of the proximal right tibia

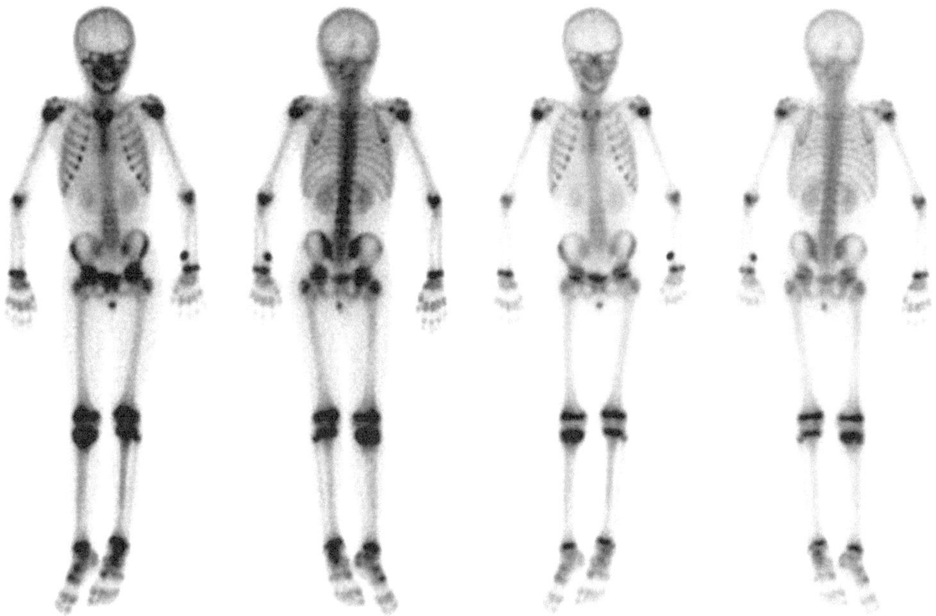

however, there are "cold zones" in the disease area, which are caused by significant ischemic damage to the bones resulted from increased tissue pressure due to the inflammatory response.

Key Points of Diagnosis

The imaging findings mainly depend on the development stage of the disease. The early diagnosis of acute suppurative osteomyelitis is very important. It is difficult for X-ray and CT examinations to meet the diagnostic requirements, and MRI examination is sensitive to the inflammatory changes of bone marrow and soft tissue, which has great clinical application value.

1. A definite history of purulent bacterial infection or a history of trauma is helpful in determining the diagnosis.
2. X-ray plain film shows extensive soft tissue swelling with a thick reticular shadow, which generally does not cross

the joint. Bone change is manifested as localized osteoporosis followed by scattered bone destruction, and subperiosteal abscess can be seen, or even the Codman triangle is formed. In severe cases, osteonecrosis and sequestrum can be seen.

3. Non-enhanced CT scan revealed diffuse soft tissue swelling and intermuscular lipodieresis. Small lesions were found in the bone, intraosseous and subperiosteal abscesses are formed, the Codman triangle is formed after extensive periosteal proliferation and destruction. In severe cases, the elongated and high-density sequestrum can be seen. The heterogeneous annular increased density shadow was formed by hyperostosis around the bone destruction area.
4. MR scan showed diffuse and irregular bone destruction area with the heterogeneous hypointense on T_1WI, the heterogeneous hyperintense on T_2WI and STIR sequences and the hyperintense on T_2WI for intraosseous vomica and subperiosteal abscess. The sequestrum presented the hypointense on both T_1WI and T_2WI and the proliferative periosteum showed stratified hypointense. After enhancement, the wall of the vomica was significantly enhanced, but no enhancement occurred to the vomica.
5. Acute onset; systemic symptoms of poisoning; persistent pain and obvious tenderness.
6. Blood biochemical examination: leukocytes are significantly increased, and the pathogens can be detected in the blood and the culture of diseased materials from puncture.

Differential Diagnosis

1. **Chronic suppurative osteomyelitis**. The lesions of acute osteomyelitis were mainly bone destruction, while chronic osteomyelitis had a long history, the lesions of which were mainly proliferation and sclerosis to the bone, and the destruction scope was limited, with the bone marrow cavity narrowed, and the local destruction could disappear, with the fusion of periosteal proliferation and bone cortex; the chronic osteomyelitis mostly had dead spaces and sequestra.
2. **Ewing's sarcoma**. It is common in adolescents, the age of onset is larger than that of acute suppurative osteomyelitis, and it usually occurs in the long bone diaphysis and is mostly seen in the middle part of diaphysis, which is mainly manifested as patchy infiltrating bone destruction centered on the marrow cavity, with the blurring margin of destruction area, and the marrow cavity can be slightly expanded, without the formation of sequestrum, often accompanied by localized onion-skin-like periosteal proliferation, which is manifested as Codman triangle formation after tumor puncture and rupture. For typical cases, thin and short vertical needle shadows appear, lacking the bone repair characteristics of proliferation and sclerosis for purulent osteomyelitis. The course of disease is slower and longer than that of acute suppurative osteomyelitis. In the early stage, there may be the formation of a large soft tissue mass, with smaller bone destruction area and obvious local pain, which can be multiple and metastasize to other internal organs such as bone or lung. The range of lesions can be narrowed after radiotherapy.
3. **Eosinophilic granuloma.** The age of onset was similar, but there were no systemic symptoms. Blood routine examination showed significantly increased eosinophilic granulocyte. The diaphysis showed cystic osteolytic destruction, with limited bone destruction area and clear boundary, rarely involving epiphysis, and the cortex was expanded and thinned, which could be accompanied by lamellar periosteal proliferation; the scope of periosteal proliferation was mostly larger than the bone destruction area, but the periosteum of proliferation was more complete and limited, without damage or fracture, and the surrounding soft tissue swelling was localized.
4. **Congenital syphilis of bone**. It is common in the long bone, more common in the bilateral long bone symmetry. The main manifestations were multiple moth-eaten and strip-like destruction areas in the bone cortex, and no sequestrum in the bone destruction areas and clear boundaries with normal bone, and most of them were accompanied by periosteal proliferation, which was linear or onion-skin, and the range of proliferation was larger, but the destruction area was relatively limited. There was no soft tissue mass around the bone lesion area, no osteoporosis, and also no epiphysis being involved.

Status Quo and Progress of Research

1. **DWI.** It can provide information for diagnosis and differential diagnosis of acute osteomyelitis, especially in the case of abscess formation. The pus of a bacterial abscess was composed of a variety of inflammatory cells, bacteria, necrotic tissue, and viscous fluid of proteins. The cells were more viscous and had a strong adsorption effect on water molecules. The diffusion of water molecules was significantly limited, and the ADC value was reduced, therefore, the abscesses tended to show hyperintense; With the reduction of the absorption of the abscess, the central necrotic area shrunken and disappeared, the bound water decreased, and the diffusion of water molecules was no longer limited. At this time, the abscess showed a slightly hyperintense and isointense. The presence and location of abscesses in acute suppurative osteomyelitis can be detected by DWI sequence. Imaging

diagnosis plays an important role when clinical manifestations and laboratory tests are atypical. DWI sequence can provide valuable information for the diagnosis of acute suppurative osteomyelitis and the differentiation of benign and malignant lesions [27].

2. **Enhanced MRI.** It is a useful supplementary means to the diagnosis of osteomyelitis, which can improve the diagnostic ability of bone infection and its complications [28]. When osteomyelitis involved in the epiphyseal plate, it could only be seen on the gadolinium-enhanced T_1WI sequence, but not on the non-contrast T_1WI liquid sensitive sequence, which was manifested as weakened epiphysis cartilage enhancement, or even no local enhancement, otherwise it should be uniformly enhanced. Since infection of the epiphyseal plate in infancy can cause growth disorders, the gadolinium-enhanced MRI is recommended for infants with suspected bone infections [29, 30].
3. **1H-magnetic resonance spectroscopy (^{1}H-MRS).** It can be used as an important supplementary imaging method for conventional MRI. The features of vomica without treatment were the absence of NAA, Cho and Cr, the increased levels of amino acids (AA, 0.9 ppm) and lactic acid (Lac, 1.3 ppm), with or without increased levels of acetic acid (1.9 ppm) and succinic acid (2.4 ppm). Amino acids are the result of proteolysis of polymorphonuclear leukocytes in pus and are considered as characteristic markers of purulent abscesses. Lac, acetic acid, and succinic acid are the products of glycolypurulentsis and fermentation of pathogens and are also important metabolites of purulent abscesses. ^{1}H-MRS can be used to identify the components in acute purulent lesions.

6.3.2 Chronic Suppurative Osteomyelitis

Overview

Acute suppurative osteomyelitis without timely treatment, or with incomplete treatment or unobstructed drainage, will remain infection focus, sequestrum or abscess in the bone, which will turn into chronic suppurative osteomyelitis [31, 32]. Chronic suppurative osteomyelitis in children is more complicated due to the fact that children cannot express the disease well, are not easy to find, and do not seek treatment in time. In particular, child patients with open bone trauma or after surgery not only have a longer course of disease, but also have a higher rate of treatment failure and recurrence, which has a great impact on such child patients' and their families' lives. The incidence of chronic suppurative osteomyelitis in developed countries is significantly lower than that in developing countries, and the incidence of chronic suppurative osteomyelitis in children under 3 years old is higher than that in children over 3 years old.

Chronic suppurative osteomyelitis is often a variety of bacteria mixed infection, but Staphylococcus aureus is still the main pathogens of chronic suppurative osteomyelitis in children, followed by pseudomonas aeruginosa, and other pathogens have enterobacter, staphylococcus haemolyticus, pyogenic streptococcus, pneumococcus, etc., and may also have Haemophilus influenzae. In recent years, increasing reports showed that the prevalence of methicillin-resistant Staphylococcus aureus (MRSA) varies geographically [32].

Chronic suppurative osteomyelitis can be resulted from that during the treatment period of acute suppurative osteomyelitis, the selected drugs are not sensitive to pathogens, or drug dose is not large enough, the course of medication is insufficient, or in the early stage of the disease or each relapse, the treatment is not in time or thorough [33]. Clinical manifestations are not typical, which are mainly manifested as the pain of local bone and joint, red and swollen skin, as well as exudation and abscess in sinus. Such manifestations can be mild or severe, which can be prolonged for several years, even decades, with repeated onset and lasting for a long time. If the residual focus in the bone is in a relatively stable state, most of the child patients have no obvious fever, and the systemic symptoms are mild, which are only manifested by local swelling and mild pain. Once the immunity of human body is reduced, the inflammation may develop again, causing acute osteomyelitis. The circulating disease can form a non-healing sinus, long-term intermittent flow of pus or fluid. Due to its long course and easy recurrence, it is prone to occurring to severe bone defects, bone nonunion, even malunion and other complications. Moreover, pyogenic infection can also invade the epiphyseal plate cartilage, and the epiphyseal plate invasion in the chronic phase can lead to osteogenic disorder. Epiphysis and epiphyseal plate damage will seriously affect bone development, resulting in severe deformity, which thus causes the disability of child patient [32].

The clinical diagnosis of chronic suppurative osteomyelitis in children mainly includes clinical manifestations of child patients, laboratory test, microbiological examination, and imaging examination. Diagnostic methods have their own value. As far as possible, specimens can be obtained for pathogen culture, including sinus secretions, pus and involved soft tissues, even scraping materials from bone lesion area, especially the culture of secretions around bone lesion area and in the marrow cavity is the most valuable [34]. Imaging examination of chronic osteomyelitis is the only method that is possible to find all residual active lesions, and it is non-invasive. Therefore, imaging diagnostic doctors should focus on the following signs of children's images, especially for child patients with prolonged disease: (1) whether there is soft tissue swelling in the lesion area or not; (2) whether there is periosteal reaction in the soft tissue swelling site or not; (3) whether there is bone texture in the proliferation and sclerosis area or not; (4) whether there is destruction area in the osteosclerosis area or not; (5) whether there is sequestrum imaging in the destruction area or not [1].

The clinical treatment of pediatric chronic suppurative osteomyelitis has great difficulty, with easy relapse. When the infected tissue and sequestrum are wrapped by the newly formed bone shell and fibrous tissue, clinical symptoms can be alleviated, but the disease will eventually relapse (as long as several years), and in severe cases, it will lead to complications such as fracture nonunion or bone defect, and even the shortening, deformity, or functional loss of the affected limb. Therefore, it is particularly important to timely and thoroughly treat the pediatric chronic osteomyelitis. The principles of treatment for chronic osteomyelitis are to thoroughly remove lesions, the sequestrum and as much hypertrophic scar and granulation tissue as possible, eliminate the dead space, improve local blood circulation, and create conditions for healing; therefore, surgical treatment should be performed on patients who, through imaging examination, are confirmed as manifestations of sequestrum, dead space, abscess in sinus, or have sufficient new bone to form an involucrum. The disappearance of the sequestrum or dead space is the sign of cure of chronic osteomyelitis; however, due to the cover of the high-density osteosclerosis and periosteal proliferation, it is not easy to find small residual dead spaces and sequestra, which need to be carefully found from the following aspects: the destruction area in the osteosclerosis area, bone destruction area near the periosteal proliferation, the area without bone texture in the bone near obvious soft tissue swelling or ruptured fistula, and when necessary, the intraoperative C-arm or CT scan shall be used to search.

Pathophysiology

Under the long-term presence and repeated stimulation of chronic inflammation, the hyperostosis and osteosclerosis, new bone formation and fibrosis, osseous tissue ischemia or hypoxia, and even the formation of dead space, marrow cavity occlusion, seriously hinder the blood circulation of the bone, thereby aggravating the lower bone resistance, leading to further osteonecrosis and bone absorption to form sequestra and local abscesses. During the onset of acute phase, osteolytic destruction was dominant, with the blurring margin of bone destruction area, and the periosteal reaction was also observed. After the acute inflammation subsided, the treatment focused on the restoration, and after the hyperostosis and osteosclerosis, the heterogeneous thickening and deformation was observed. Uniform osteosclerosis without bone trabecula structure has wider range and narrow marrow cavity, and in severe cases, may cause the occlusion of marrow cavity, which can be combined with extensive periosteal proliferation; In contrast, osteosclerosis with bone trabecular structure reflects new bone in remodeling. At the same time, due to the failure of some sequestra to discharge, the surrounding hyperostosis formed a dead space, and the sequestra were wrapped to form a bone involucrum. The involucrum was eroded by pus, forming a fistula. The abscess flowed out through the fistula, eroding the surrounding soft tissue of the bone, and forming fibrous scar under repeated stimulation. This persistent infection leads to chronic disease and a vicious circle in which the sequestrum makes the infection difficult to be removed.

Imaging Findings

1. **X-ray.** It has high value in the diagnosis of chronic suppurative osteomyelitis. Common signs of X-ray: soft tissue swelling, localized osteolytic bone destruction, local or diffuse hyperostosis and osteosclerosis, periosteal proliferation, bone involucrum, and sequestrum formation.
   (a) Changes in soft tissue: at the time of acute onset of chronic suppurative osteomyelitis, the soft tissue was mainly exudative with localized swelling, and subcutaneous fat may appear reticulated image. In the chronic stage, the soft tissue was mainly repaired by hyperplasia. In the severe site of periosteal proliferation with rupture, subperiosteal abscess was absorbed to form the localized soft tissue mass with clearer edges. With the control of the disease, the soft tissue mass was gradually reduced, and some cases may have defects or form fistulas. Due to repeated infection, the lesion site leads to ischemia, degeneration, necrosis, fibrosis, and increased density of soft tissue such as muscle (Fig. 6.20).

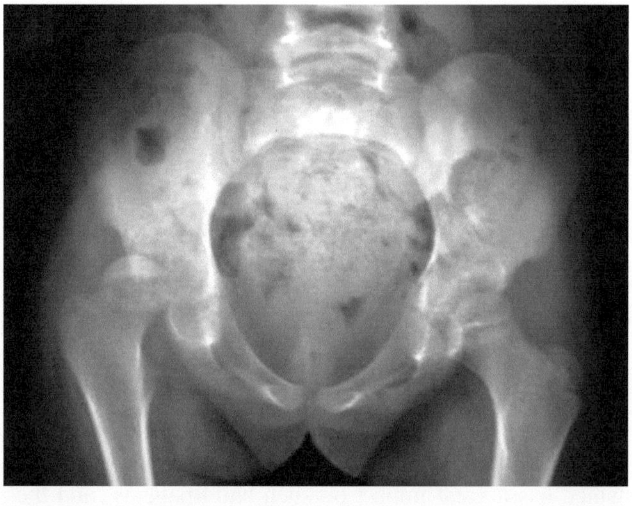

Fig. 6.20 Chronic osteomyelitis in the right femur. DR showed that the soft tissue of the right hip joint had local swelling and increased density, the epiphysis of femoral head was small and highly dense, the distal femoral metaphysis was deformed; multiple utricular bone destruction were observed, and the edge of the destruction area was slightly sclerotic

(b) Bone change: during the onset of acute phase, the osteolytic bone destruction was dominant, with decreased bone mineral density and blurring edges of bone destruction area, and the periosteal reaction may be also observed; in the chronic phase, due to reactive osteogenesis of the inner and outer membrane under the action of inflammatory stimulators. There were coarse and new bone trabecula in the destruction area, with increased density in the bone marrow cavity and osteosclerosis (Fig. 6.20), which was characterized by homogeneous or heterogeneous density increased, with the heterogeneous thickening and obvious deformation of bone form. This is an inevitable response in the repair process of chronic suppurative osteomyelitis. X rays showed homogeneous high-density shadows without bone texture, and active focuses were often present in the center of the new bone. After the lesion is cured, the proliferative osseous tissue can be completely absorbed and the marrow cavity can be recommunicated.

(i) Dead space and sequestrum: in the chronic suppurative osteomyelitis, there were osteolytic destruction areas with different sizes occurred in the bone, which is called as the dead space. It is manifested as the low-density area with clear edge and abscess formation, which is the remaining active lesion in the bone of chronic suppurative osteomyelitis. As chronic osteomyelitis has extensive bone proliferation and sclerosis, the dead space is not clear and is not easily found. High-density bone shadows of varying sizes can be seen in some of the dead space, known as the sequestrum (Fig. 6.21). The dead space of chronic osteomyelitis often contains the sequestrum, which was a specific sign of chronic osteomyelitis. The cause of the sequestrum is the ischemic or necrosis of bone arising from the fact that the periosteum is lifted by pus or thrombotic arteritis impedes the blood supply to the bone. The sequestrum tends to be surrounded by pus or fibrous granulation tissue, and may enter the surrounding soft tissue with exudate and pus, so the sequestrum may be distributed in the soft tissue inside or outside the bone or the soft tissue swelling outside the bone. The size of the sequestrum varies, and the small one is only the size of a grain of rice, which can be discharged out of the body through the sinus, or absorbed by granulation tissue. If the affected bone is accompanied by extensive periosteum destruction, the necrotic diaphysis will become a large naked sequestrum. The X-ray showed the dotted, quasi-circular, or strip-like high-density shadows in the central region. Around the sequestrum, there was often inflammatory exudation or granulation tissue hyperplasia, presenting a circular low-density shadow.

(ii) Periosteal reaction and bony shell: both periosteal reaction and bone involucrum are periosteal new bone caused by bone destruction and osteonecrosis. The periosteal reaction is formed outside the surviving bone cortex and is often extensive, multilayered, discontinuous, or even shell-like. The proliferative periosteum often fuses with the diaphytic cortex, making the density of affected bone increasing, and makes the bone thickening and deformation (Fig. 6.22). In the course of treatment, the periosteal reaction can be absorbed gradually and then be disappeared. And the bone involucrum is formed by the periosteum stripped around the large dead diaphysis. As long as the sequestrum exists, the bony shell is proliferated. After removal or absorption of the sequestrum, the bone involucrum is reconstructed and molded to replace the necrotic diaphysis and form a nearly normal bone cortex.

(iii) Sinus: After the formation of an abscess in the bone, the abscess spreads to the subperiosteal system along the Haversian system and forms a subperiosteal abscess, leading to periosteal reactive hyperplasia. The subperiosteal abscess spreads to the diaphysis and penetrates the periosteum into the soft tissue surrounding the bone,

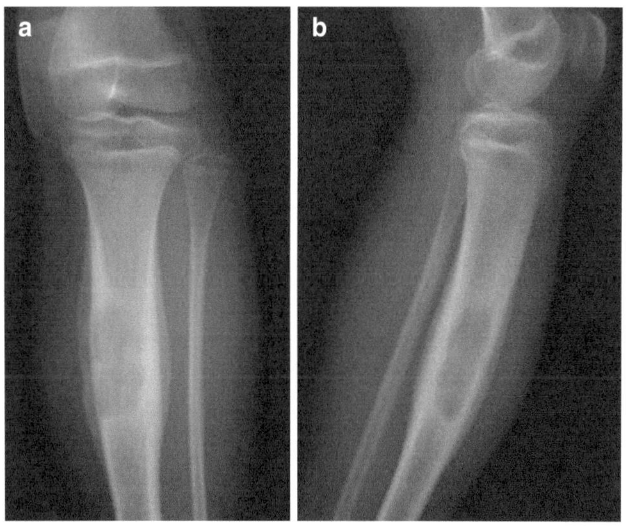

Fig. 6.21 Chronic osteomyelitis at the middle part of left tibia. DR showed oblong osteolytic destruction in the middle part of the left tibia, with clear edges, extensive osteosclerosis around, periosteal lamellar hyperplasia; the small bone blocks in the dead space can be seen and the surrounding soft tissue is swollen and highly dense

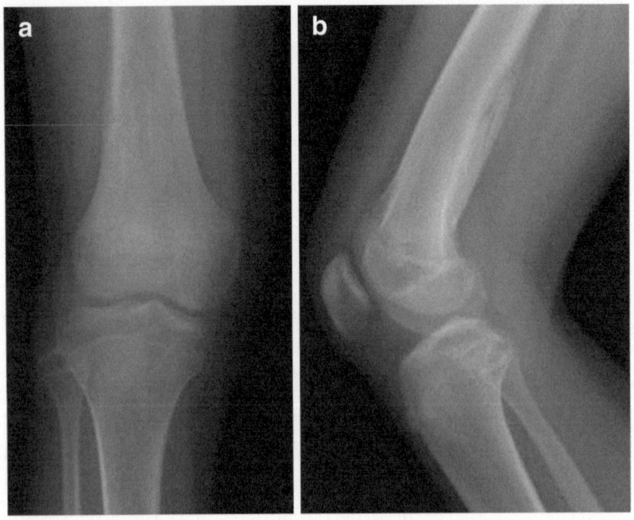

Fig. 6.22 Chronic osteomyelitis at the distal end of right femur. DR showed that the posterior lateral cortex of the distal part of the right femur was irregularly thinned with multilayer periosteal proliferation; both ends were fused with the diaphysis cortex, and the diaphysis was thickened and deformed

resulting in the formation of a soft tissue abscess. A soft tissue abscess may further penetrate the skin to form a sinus. After the formation of the sinus, the bone marrow cavity abscess and the subperiosteal space were connected with the periosseous soft tissue and the external body, and the intraosseous exudate or pus could flow to the external body along the channel.

Chronic suppurative osteomyelitis can be complicated by pyogenic arthritis. In case of no timely and thorough treatment, osseous ankylosis may occur.

2. **CT.** Similar with X-ray, CT is clearer in terms of osteosclerosis, narrowed marrow cavity, periosteal proliferation and cortical thickening, etc., and is more conducive to accurately determining the scope of lesion involvement. It is more accurate in showing bone destruction, sequestrum, pus and gas than X-ray plain film, and it is easier to find small sequestrum or dead space. Osteolytic bone destruction results in reduced bone mineral density with slightly blurred edges, accompanied by osteosclerosis and periosteal reaction (Fig. 6.23a). During the period of repair, the new coarse bone trabecula can be seen in the low-density bone destruction area. The density of marrow cavity is increased, which is manifested as homogenous or heterogeneous increase in density, heterogeneous thickening of bone morphology, and obvious deformation. High-density sequestrum mass shadows of varying sizes can be seen in some of the low-density lumen of the bone (Fig. 6.23b, e), which were distributed within or outside the bone or in the soft tissue swelling outside the bone (Fig. 6.23c). Extensive, multilayered, high-density

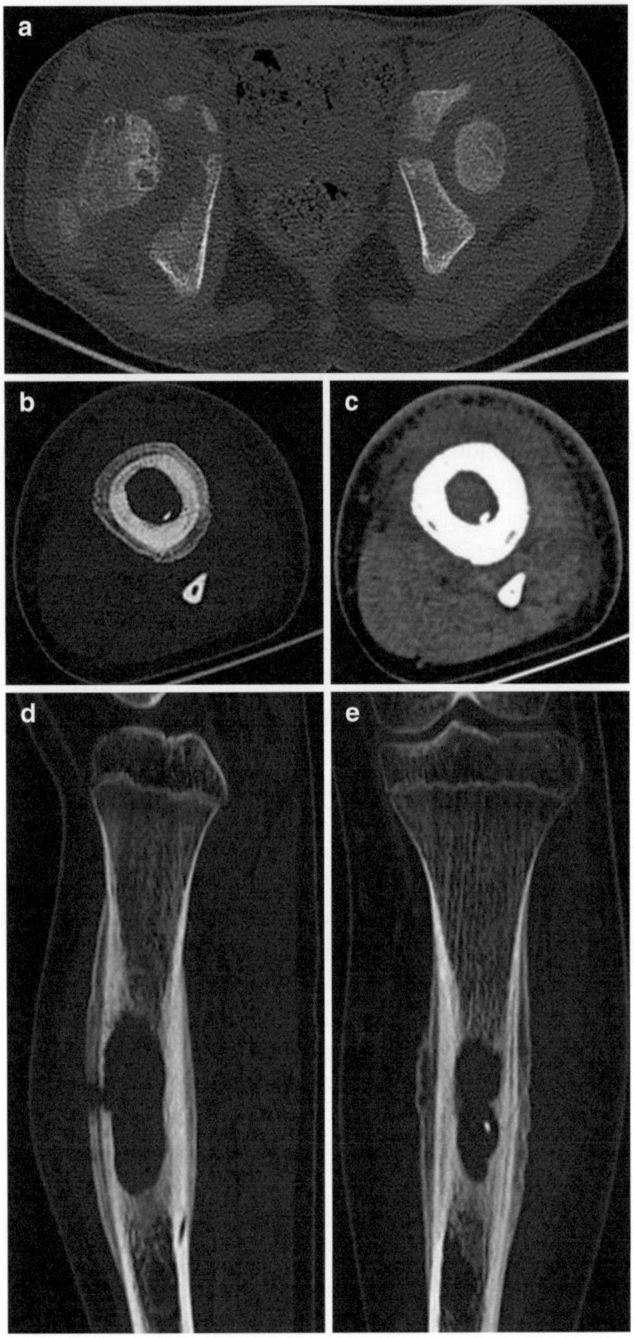

Fig. 6.23 Chronic osteomyelitis. (**a**) The bone window of CT transverse plane showed multiple hollow bone destruction in the metaphysis of the right femur, involving the bone surface. Some bone destruction foci were associated with the sclerotic edge. Acetabular bone was involved, and the hip joint space was widened; (**b**) The bone window showed the osteolytic bone destruction of the left tibia, with lamellar involucrum-like periosteal proliferation. No bone trabecula image but dotted small bone mass can be seen in the destruction area of marrow cavity; (**c**) The soft tissue window showed surrounding soft tissue swelling with homogeneous low density in the bone destruction area, and the grid-like shadow in subcutaneous fat. (**d**, **e**) The bone window reconstruction showed that the destruction area of the marrow cavity of the left tibia had clear boundary, accompanied by osteosclerosis; the periosteal proliferation and thickened and deformed diaphysis were observed; small sequestrum was found in the cavity, and the destruction area of the marrow cavity formed sinus towards the soft tissue near the bone through the bone cortex and periosteum fracture

shadows were formed outside part of the bone cortex and intermittent, even the periosteum of involucrum-like hyperplasia tends to fuse with the bone cortex, resulting in the affected bone was increased in density, thickened, and deformed (Fig. 6.23b, e). The low-density area in the bone is communicated with the soft tissue surrounding the bone through periosteum fracture to form sinus (Fig. 6.23d). Some can be communicated with the skin surface, presenting a strip-like low-density shadow with similar density. The moderate or marked enhancement can be seen in the low-density areas of the bone and surrounding soft tissue through the enhanced scan, and the boundary is not clear around the diseased bone. Multislice spiral CT can be used for multi-angle reconstruction with ultra-thin images and various post-reconstruction techniques, to determine whether there is bone texture structure in the sclerosis area, and the relationship between bone destruction, sclerosis, and periosteal reaction (Figs. 6.23d, e and 6.24).

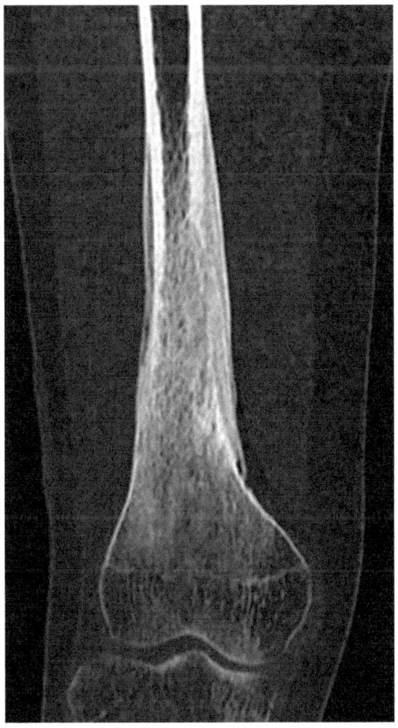

Fig. 6.24 Chronic osteomyelitis in the right femur. CT coronal plane reconstruction of the bone window showed irregular thinning and defect of the bone cortex at the distal end of the right femur, accompanied by lamellar periosteal proliferation; both ends were fused with normal bone cortex, with the diaphysis thickening and deforming, heterogeneous increase in the density of the marrow cavity, and the local and cortical boundaries were unclear

3. **MRI.** It has high resolution in soft tissue and wide application. It can distinguish periostitis, soft tissue inflammatory response, and epiphyseal lesions, but it is difficult for X-ray examination to distinguish.
   (a) Soft tissue swelling: In acute onset of chronic suppurative osteomyelitis, tissue edema, inflammatory response area, granulation tissue, and pus all displayed the hypointense on T_1WI, and the hyperintense on T_2WI, while the focus displayed hyperintense on T_2WI STIR sequences.
   (b) Bone destruction and proliferation and sclerosis: Most of the bone destruction was quasi-circular, showing hypointense on T_1WI and mixed signal intensity dominated by hypointense on T_2WI; there were sclerosis margins around the bone destruction area with clear boundary (Fig. 6.25). Heterogeneous thickened bone cortex showed hypointense on both T_1WI and T_2WI. The bone involucrum displayed a thin and strip-like hypointense on T_1WI and hypointense on T_2WI.
   (c) Sequestrum and dead space: The signal change of the sequestrum depends on the amount of bone marrow.

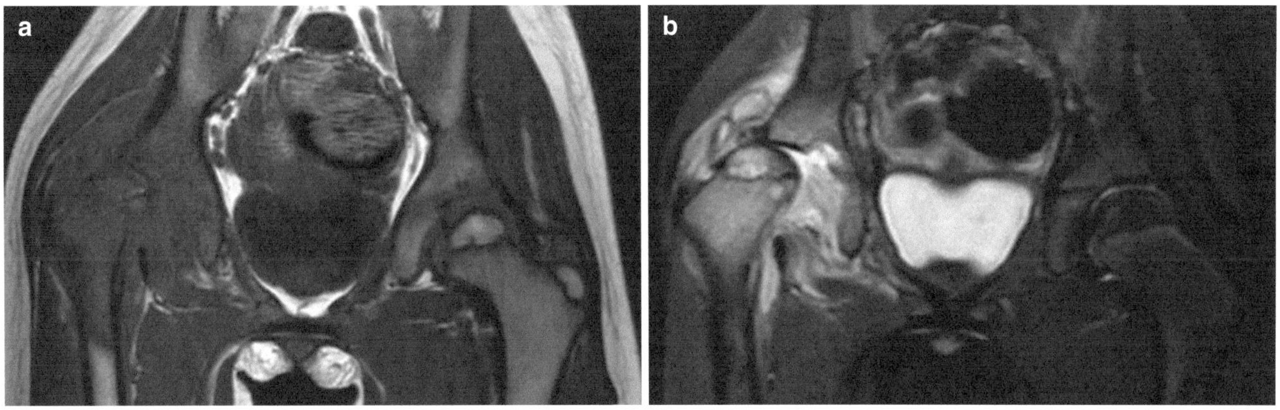

Fig. 6.25 Chronic osteomyelitis in the right femur and pyogenic arthritis in the right hip. (**a**) On T_1WI, the bone of the right hip joint displayed heterogeneous hypointense on T_1WI with the joint swelling; (**b**) On T_2WI fat-suppressed sequence, the multiple round hyperintense destruction foci in the bone of the right hip, and femoral metaphysis lesions displayed hypointense sclerosis margin; patchy hyperintense edema zone was observed around the bone destruction area, and the epiphysis became flat, the right hip joint space was widened, with synovial hyperplasia; extensive edema occurred to the surrounding soft tissues, accompanied by hyperintense microabscesses

Exudative changes or granulation tissue proliferation often occur around the sequestrum. Therefore, the signal of the sequestrum can be varied, showing hypointense, isointense, or hyperintense on T_1WI and hyperintense or hypointense on T_2WI. Dead space showed hypointense on T_1WI and hyperintense on T_2WI.

(d) Sinus: Manifested as local defect of bone cortex and soft tissue, internal and external communication of the marrow cavity, and generally displayed isointense on T_1WI and hyperintense on T_2WI (Fig. 6.26).

(e) After enhancement, granulation tissue was significantly enhanced, abscess wall was ring-enhanced, necrotic and pus were not enhanced, presenting hypointense. However, MRI could not accurately distinguish reactive bone marrow edema from bone marrow edema caused by osteomyelitis (Fig. 6.27), and the intensities of both edema were the same. MRI and enhanced examination showed the best results for active focuses or residual inflammatory lesions in chronic suppurative osteomyelitis, as well as clearly showing bone cloaca and soft tissue sinus. At the same time, the scope of involvement of osteomyelitis was shown, which provides an important reference for the scope of focus removal during surgery [30, 35].

4. **Radionuclide imaging.** During ^{99m}Tc-MDP bone imaging, for the chronic suppurative osteomyelitis, some radioactive tracers tends to accumulate in the diseased bone after being injected into human blood circulation, forming a concentrated "hot zone" (Fig. 6.28) due to abundant blood supply at the inflammatory response site and enhanced osteogenic activity after bone destruction (Fig. 6.28). Although radionuclide imaging has high sensitivity, its specificity was low.

Key Points of Diagnosis

To find residual focuses in chronic suppurative osteomyelitis is the main objective of imaging diagnosis. CT examination is sensitive to show the sequestrum. MRI examination is most valuable in showing residual focuses. Both X-ray and CT examination are difficult to fully meet the clinical needs, while MRI examination is very sensitive to the inflammatory changes in bone marrow and soft tissue, which has great clinical application value in the general diagnosis of chronic osteomyelitis.

1. A history of acute purulent bacterial infection, trauma, or surgery is helpful in determining the diagnosis.
2. X-ray plain film showed localized swelling of soft tissue, and bone changes were manifested as shadow of localized decrease in bone mineral density and increase in arc-shaped density beside the bone cortex, and in severe cases, the osteonecrosis and sequestrum can be seen.
3. Non-enhanced CT scan showed soft tissue swelling, or the shadow of narrow low-density sinus, increased bone mineral density, extensive periosteal proliferation and sclerosis, obvious bone deformation, and the formation of small damage focus and abscess in the bone, and in severe cases, the sequestrum and dead space can be seen.
4. MRI scan showed the hypointense on T_1WI in the bone destruction area, the heterogeneous hyperintense on T_2WI

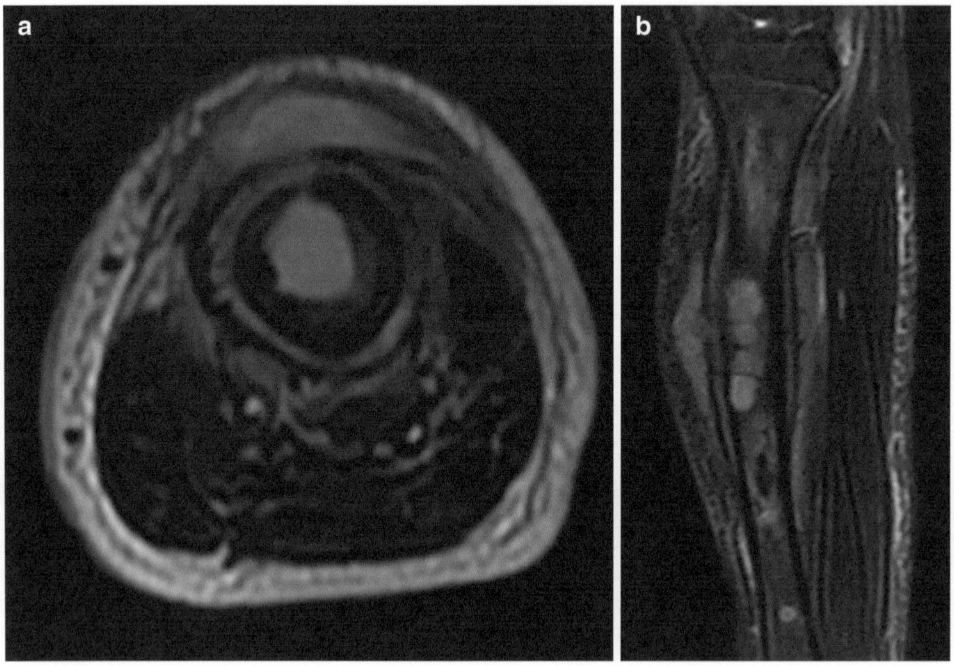

Fig. 6.26 Sinus formation of chronic osteomyelitis in the left tibia. (**a**) On MRI, T_2WI showed round homogeneous hyperintense shadow in the left tibia, the slightly hyperintense was seen in the cortex, and the vomica inside and outside the bone cortex was connected due to local fissure-like sinus in the ventral cortex; (**b**) The T_2WI fat-suppressed sequence showed multiple hyperintense in the middle and upper part of tibia, with hypointense septa; the tubular hyperintense sinus connected to external bone, subperiosteal abscess and intramedullary abscess can be seen in the ventral side, with extensive swelling and exudation of surrounding soft tissues

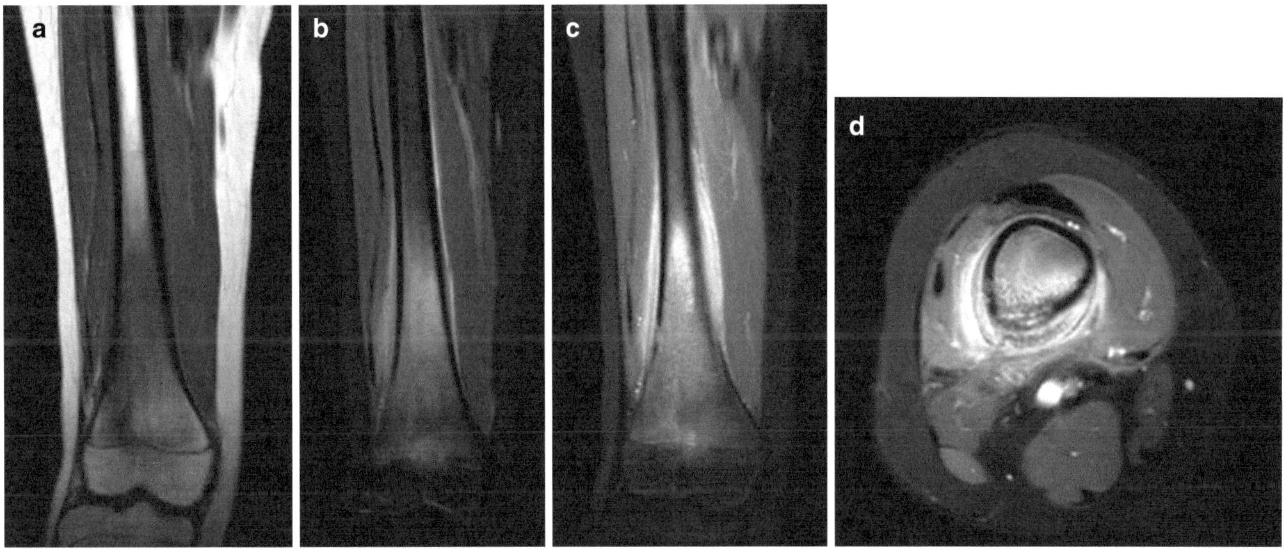

Fig. 6.27 Osteomyelitis at the distal end of right femur. (**a**) On MRI, the coronal plane T_1WI showed patchy heterogeneous hypointense area on T_1WI at the distal end of the right femur, with unclear boundaries; (**b**) The coronal plane T_2WI fat-suppressed sequence showed patchy heterogeneous hyperintense area at the distal end of the right femur, with unclear boundaries and swelling of the extraosseous soft tissue; (**c**) The enhanced scan of coronal plane T_1WI fat-suppressed sequence showed patchy enhancement zone at the distal end of the right femur, and strip-shaped enhancement was observed in the para-bone soft tissue; (**d**) The enhanced scan of transverse plane T_1WI fat-suppressed sequence showed patchy enhancement zone at the distal end of the right femur, accompanied by localized destruction of the dorsal bone cortex. The periosteal reaction can be seen, and the enhancement zone of soft tissue was surrounded outside the periosteum

Fig. 6.28 Chronic osteomyelitis at the upper part of left tibia. There was heterogeneous concentration of radioactivity in the upper part of the left tibia, with the lightness of the center part

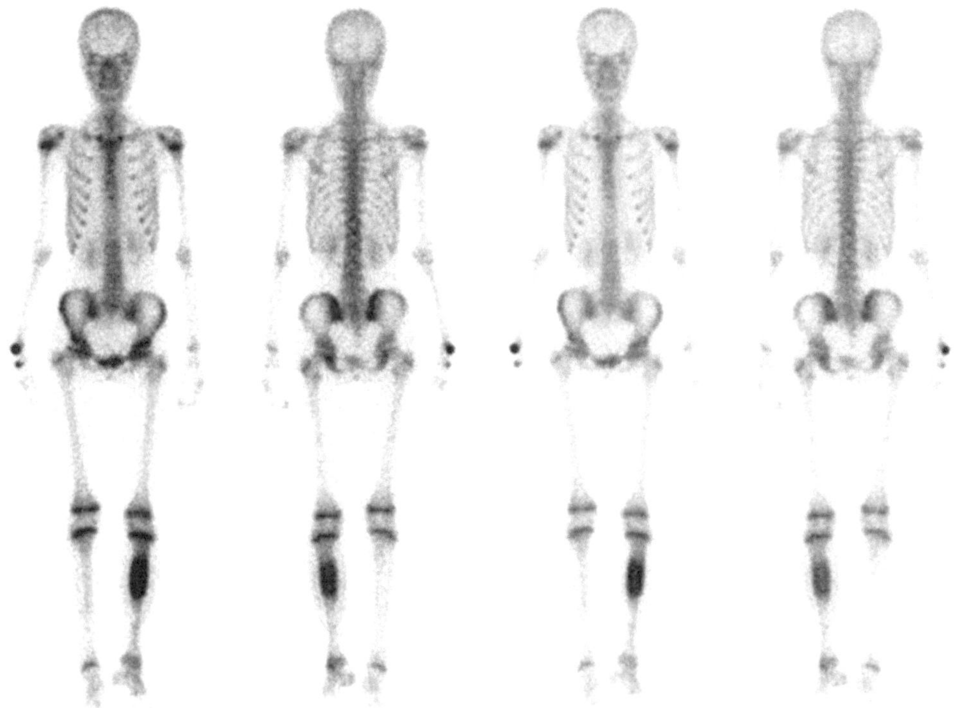

and STIR sequence, the hyperintense on T_2WI in the vomica of bone, and the narrow-strip hyperintense on T_2WI in the sinus. The sequestrum presented the hypointense on both T_1WI and T_2WI and the proliferative periosteum showed hypointense. The surrounding soft tissue showed irregular patchy hyperintense on T_2WI, and after enhancement, the enhanced vomica wall and sinus wall can be seen.

5. The onset is insidious, and the diseased site is in constant pain with obvious tenderness.
6. Laboratory test: The pathogens can be detected from the culture of fistula and lesion puncture.

Differential Diagnosis

1. **Chronic sclerosing osteomyelitis**. Without history of acute osteomyelitis, it is mostly considered as low-toxic bone infection, with no systemic symptoms, which may have a history of trauma, and the bone proliferation and sclerosis is limited relatively to the chronic suppurative osteomyelitis, with more regular bone shape, without dead space and sequestrum, and the hyperplasia periosteum is smooth and neat, without fracture, which generally does not involve the surrounding soft tissue, without formation of sinus.
2. **Ewing's sarcoma**. It usually occurs in the middle part of long bone diaphysis, which is mainly manifested as patchy infiltrating bone destruction centered on the marrow cavity, with the blurring margin of destruction area, and the marrow cavity can be slightly expanded, without the formation of sequestrum, often accompanied by localized onion-skin-like periosteal proliferation, which is manifested as Codman triangle formation after tumor puncture and rupture. For typical cases, thin and short vertical needle shadows appear, lacking the bone repair characteristics of proliferation and sclerosis for suppurative osteomyelitis. The course of disease is slower and longer than that of acute suppurative osteomyelitis. In the early stage, there may be the formation of a large soft tissue mass, with smaller bone destruction area and obvious local pain, which can be multiple and metastasize to other internal organs such as bone or lung. The range of lesions can be narrowed after radiotherapy.
3. **Osteosarcoma**. The age of onset is older, without the sequestrum and dead space, and the radiating or vertical tumor bone can be seen beside the bone; there are many hemispherical and ovoid soft tissue masses with clear boundaries, which can be accompanied by tumor bone or tumor cartilage.
4. **Acquired syphilis of bone**. It is common in long bones and can occur in multiple bones, long bones, or bilateral long bones symmetrically. It is mainly manifested as extensive lamellar and lacery periosteal proliferation in the diaphysis cortex, thick and hypertrophied bone cortex, proliferation and sclerosis in the spongy bone and marrow cavity, with no acute inflammation symptoms and no obvious bone destruction area in the bone, no dead space or sequestrum, no abnormal soft tissue change around the bone lesion area, no fistula and no epiphysis involvement.

Status Quo and Progress of Research

1. It may be used as a supplementary imaging method for conventional MRI. Amino acids are the results of proteolysis of polymorphonuclear leukocytes in pus, and Lac, acetic acid and succinic acid are the products of glycolysis and fermentation of pathogens and are important metabolites of purulent abscesses.
2. **Leukocyte bone imaging**. The leukocyte is an important part of the immune system. This imaging method is more sensitive to the inflammatory response mediated by neutrophil as the neutrophil accounts for 60% ~ 70% of leukocyte. To search for in vivo labeling way of leukocyte is the focus of current research. The blood flow phase reflects the blood flow velocity and perfusion concentration, the blood pool phase reflects the vascular permeability, and the delayed phase reflects the metabolism of osseous tissue. However, the leukocyte bone imaging has some defects, such as complex labeling process, easy occurrence of cross infection, and high cost, which limits its promotion and application.
3. **PET/CT.** The effective combination of functional and anatomical imaging is one of the most advanced imaging techniques for the diagnosis of bone infection, reflecting the pathological nature from the level of molecular metabolism and functional state. ^{18}F-FDG reflects metabolic changes through glucose uptake in inflammatory response tissues, reflecting the energy requirement level of inflammatory response cells. FDG is a small molecule that can quickly enter the perfusion area, so the inspection can be completed within 1 ~ 2 h. PET/CT has a high accuracy in the diagnosis of chronic suppurative osteomyelitis. Termaat et al. reported that the sensitivity and specificity of PET/CT in the diagnosis of chronic suppurative osteomyelitis were up to 96% and 91%, respectively. Wang et al. analyzed 23 studies on suspected osteomyelitis from 1980 to 2010, and the results showed that FDG/PET had the highest sensitivity and specificity, but it would also affect the results due to the interference of bone repair [36, 37].

6.3.3 Chronic Abscess of Bone

Overview

The localized purulent lesion in the bone is called a chronic abscess of bone, which in fact is a special type of chronic osteomyelitis. It was first described by British doctor Brodie in 1832 as a rare subacute or chronic localized intraosseous purulent inflammation, thus also known as Brodie abscess [38, 39]. Brodie abscess is more common in children and youth and in male. It is mostly localized to the local part of spongy bone of long tubular bone, and more common in the metaphyseal area of the tibia, femur and humerus [40].

The pathogens were mostly Staphylococcus aureus and Streptococcus aureus. The infection occurred when the low-toxic septic bacteria entered the bone through the blood stream. Due to the low virulence of the pathogens and the strong resistance of the child patient, the focus could not spread and became limited. Alternatively, the antibiotics were used during acute infection to temporarily control the disease, preventing the lesions from spreading to the subperiosteum or diaphysis marrow cavity, and in the lesion area, the localized bone destruction and bone abscess will be formed [41]. If the organism resistance is strong, the inflammatory focus can be confined to a small range for a long time and will be repeated with the fluctuation of the body resistance of the child patient.

Generally, the focus of Brodie abscess is small, 1 ~ 3 cm in diameter, with rounded or lobulated bone destruction. The lesions are mostly confined to the local part of the spongy bone of long tubular bone of the extremities or the metaphysis. As the epiphyseal small terminal arteries and capillaries curved into vascular loops, this slows blood flow and makes it easier for bacteria to linger in the area and form lesions. It is quite rare that Brodie abscesses involve the epiphyseal plate. As the epiphyseal plate has a barrier function, it mostly occurs at both ends of the tibia, the distal end of femur or the distal end of radius, and it is relatively rare for abscesses occurred at the diaphysis of long bone [42, 43]. The Brodie abscess was surrounded by a complete capsule with pus, which is manifestation for acute stage. Or there were different degrees of new bone around the lesions, with granulation tissue and pus inside, which is manifestation for chronic stage [39].

The onset of the disease was slow, which may be caused by local trauma or systemic blood spread, with low toxicity septic bacteria flowing into the bone through blood circulation and staying in the local part to multiply into infection foci. The course of disease was long with lack of specific clinical symptoms; there are no systemic symptoms of suppurative osteomyelitis, and the symptoms are generally mild, only local pain and tenderness existed at the affected bone, which can be accompanied by adjacent joint swelling and pain [44]. The pain tended to be paroxysmal, with short duration, and can be aggravated at night. With the treatment of antibiotics, the disease can be alleviated and the surgical injury can be avoided. After the lesion improves, the abscess will be absorbed by granulation tissue and the bone destruction area will shrink until it disappears.

Pathophysiology

In the early stage of the disease, the bone destruction area was purulent fluid, which was gradually replaced by granulation tissue. And then the fibrous capsule wall is formed due to the collagenization around granulation tissue, in which fibrous tissue gradually appears. The fibrous tissue may be replaced by osseous tissue and healed, and the bone substance around the bone destruction area was gradually proliferated and hardened, circumvoluting the vomica.

The pathological features include osteocyte necrosis, bone trabecula defect, inflammatory cell infiltration, multinucleated cell reaction, fibrous and purulent exudate and hyperplasia of granulation tissue. In addition to inflammatory exudate and granulation tissue, some detrital sequestra can be seen inside the abscess. As a result of repeated inflammatory stimulation, surrounding normal bone appears reactive proliferation and sclerosis, and the periosteal reaction also can be seen in some part of the bone.

Imaging Findings

1. **X-ray**. Generally, the focus is small, with a diameter of 1 ~ 3 cm, presenting round, ovoid, or lobulated bright area, and it was common in single-cystic lesions and occasionally multiple lesions were seen. It mostly located in the central or slightly off-center area in the metaphysis of long tubular bone, showing localized osteolytic bone destruction. The edge of destruction area in the early stage is fuzzy, with the progress of the disease, the surrounding area gradually formed a clear and more smooth sclerosis ring; there can be reactive osteosclerosis, and gradually transition into the normal bone and occasionally the granular sequestrum can be seen in the vomica. If the abscess is at the margin of bone, the localized cortical thickening and periosteal reaction can be seen. The adjacent soft tissue was generally normal, or there was only slight localized swelling. If the lesion involves the epiphyseal plate, it may cross the epiphyseal plate and is rarely confined to the epiphyseal plate (Fig. 6.29).
2. CT shows more clearly the small destruction area and the small sequestrum inside, showing the round or elliptic area of osteolytic bone destruction, with clear margin, which is surrounded by bone sclerosis strap with clear boundaries. More homogeneous fluid density was found inside the bone destruction area (Fig. 6.30). In a few cases, fine granular sequestrum and mild periosteal reaction were observed. In atypical cases, the area of bone destruction may be formed by fusion of two or more bright areas in lobulated form, with mild and localized swelling of the soft tissue surrounding the focus (Fig. 6.31).
3. **MRI.** It has important diagnostic value for Brodie abscess, which was characterized by "halo sign" in the

metaphyseal marrow cavity of long tubular bone, with 4 layers of concentric circles: (1) the central area, mainly the necrotic pus, showing hypointense on T_1WI, hyperintense on T_2WI, and significant hyperintense on fat-suppressed sequence; (2) the abscess wall, surrounded by a lamella ring of slight hyperintense on T_1WI and hyperintense on T_2WI near the vomica, which represents the granulation tissue with rich blood vessels and is called the inner halo ring; (3) the sclerosis strap, with thicker area of hypointense on T_1WI and hypointense on T_2WI outside the inner halo ring, which represents fibrous connective tissue and endometrial reactive hyperplasia and is called outer halo ring; (4) the bone marrow edema zone, appearing the diffuse area of hypointense on T_1WI and hyperintense on T_2WI with varying degrees in the bone around the lesions (Figs. 6.32 and 6.33). The soft tissue around the lesions may have different degrees of inflammatory edema changes, showing slightly hypointense on T_1WI and hyperintense on T_2WI [45].

4. **SPECT.** It is highly sensitive to the inflammatory lesions of bone, and the increased blood flow and abnormal bone metabolism at the inflammatory lesion area can lead to the concentration of imaging agents (Fig. 6.34). Fusion imaging showed that the bone destruction area displayed an abnormal concentration of clear "halo-like" radionuclides, and the concentrated shadows in the osteosclerosis area around the lesion were stronger while the concentrated shadows in the central destruction area were lighter.

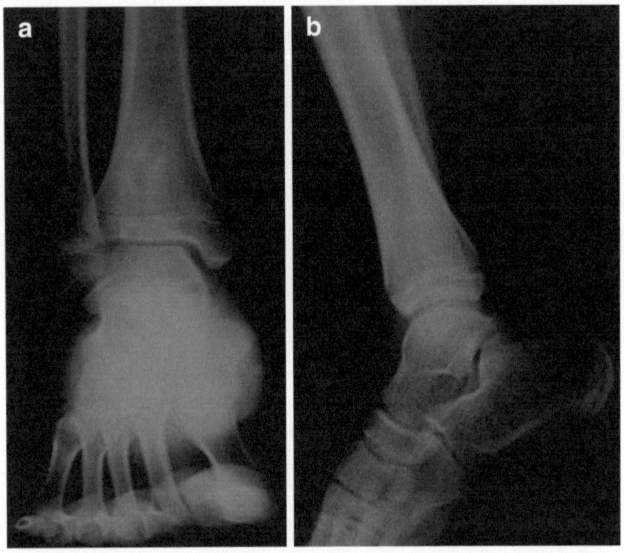

Fig. 6.29 Bone abscess in distal metaphysis of right tibia. The anterior and lateral images of the right ankle showed localized osteolytic bone destruction in the distal metaphysis of the right tibia, with smooth sclerotic edges, and there is reactive osteosclerosis around, with lesions across the epiphyseal plate involving the metaphysis

Key Points of Diagnosis

1 Characterized by insidious onset, slow progress, atypical symptoms, and mild pain.
2 The epiphysis of long tubular bone is the predilection site, located in the center or slightly to the side.
3 X-ray plain film shows that the focus is quasi-circular and low-density, edged with sclerosis margin, and the boundary is clear.
4 Non-enhanced CT scan shows that vomica has a low density, abscess wall has an equal or slightly high density, and reactive proliferation and sclerosis can be seen on edges.

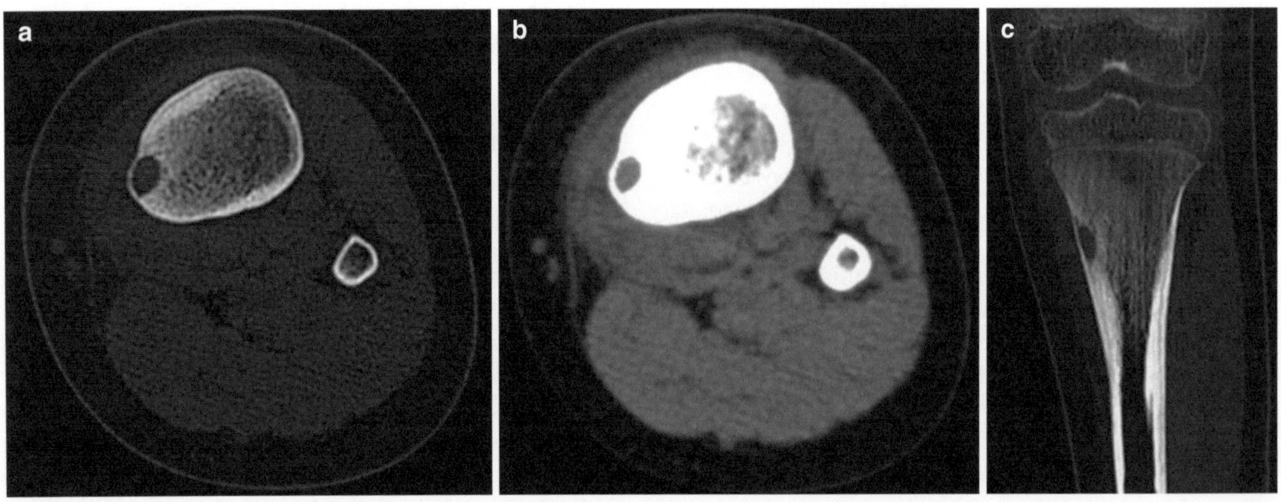

Fig. 6.30 Bone abscess at the proximal medial left tibia. (**a**) CT bone window showed the ovoid bone destruction of proximal medial left tibia, with clear margin; (**b**) Soft tissue window showed that in the bone destruction area, there was more homogeneous fluid density, and the surrounding soft tissue was accompanied by slight and localized swelling; (**c**) The coronal plane reconstruction of the bone window showed that the adjacent cortex of the bone destruction area was thin with clear boundary, and the surrounding bone was slightly hardened and moved into the normal bone marrow

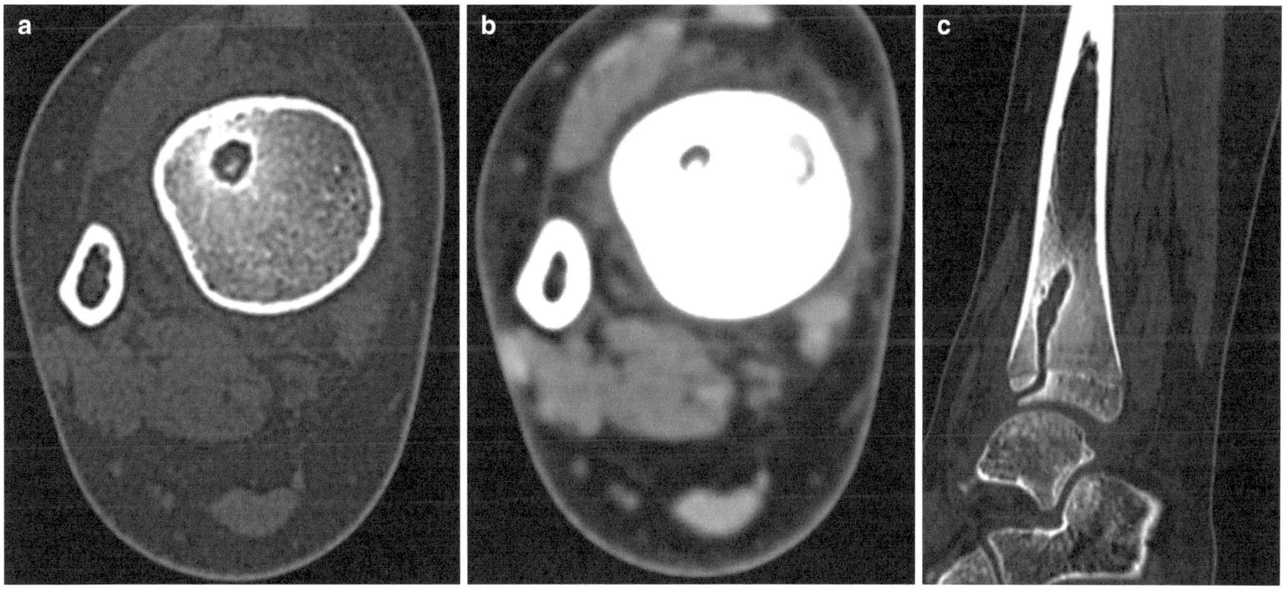

Fig. 6.31 Bone abscess in distal metaphysis of right tibia. (**a**) CT bone window showed round bone destruction at the distal end of right tibia, with clear margins, sclerosis edges, and small sequestrum inside. (**b**) Soft tissue window showed reduced density of bone destruction area and no swelling in surrounding soft tissue; (**c**) In the distal epiphysis of the right tibia, there was stripy osteolytic destruction with smooth sclerosis edges, and there was reactive osteosclerosis around. The lesions penetrated the epiphyseal plate and to involve in the epiphysis, and after penetrating the epiphysis, there was fine granular sequestrum

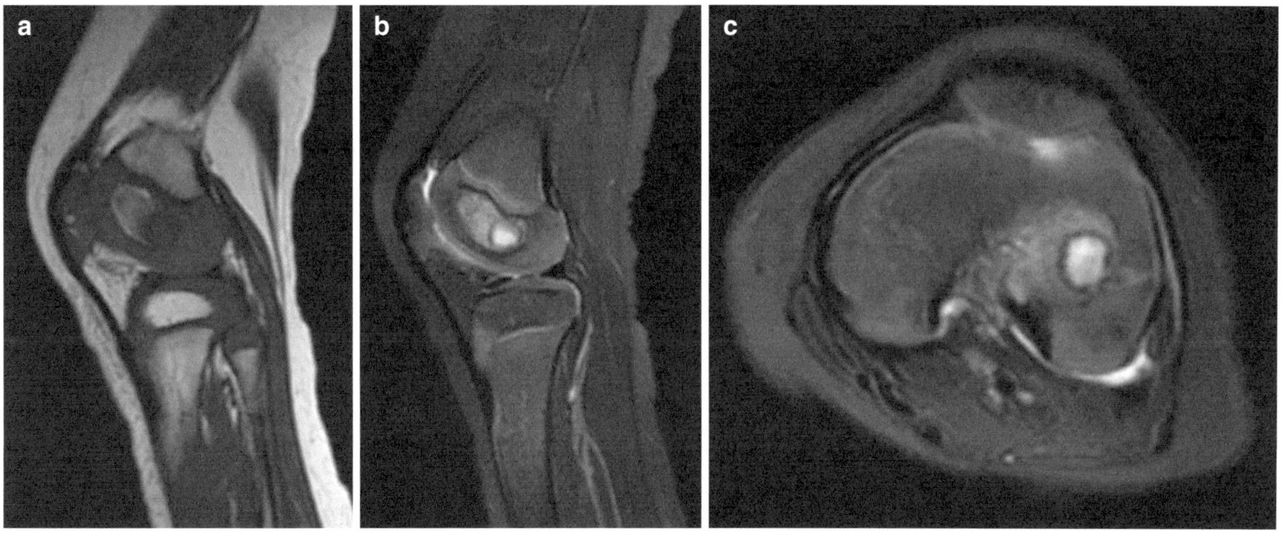

Fig. 6.32 Metaphyseal abscess at the distal end of the right femur. (**a**) On MRI, T_1WI showed a round focus of hypointense on T_1WI in the epiphysis at the distal end of the right femur, with a ring-like hypointense shadow around. (**b**) T_2WI fat-suppressed sequence showed obvious hyperintense in the center of the lesion, with a slightly hyperintense shadow surrounding it and a thinner signal halo ring of hypointense on T_2WI in the outer layer; (**c**) A slightly high intensity edema area was observed in the bone marrow around the halo ring of lesions

5 Non-enhanced MR scan shows that the pus presents hypointense on T_1WI and hyperintense on T_2WI, and the abscess wall presents isointensity or slightly hypointense on T_2WI, with the bone marrow edema accompanied around the lesion.

Differential Diagnosis

1. **Bone cyst.** Most of the cases were found in the irregular cyst-like bright area of metaphysis. Inside the bright area, there may be a few slender strip intervals. The local corti-

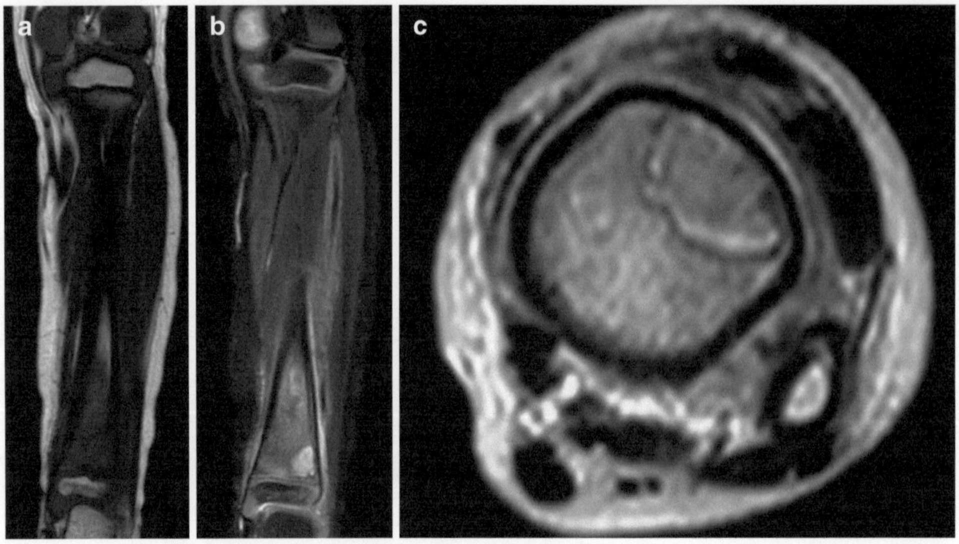

Fig. 6.33 Bone abscess at the distal metaphysis of left tibia (1). (**a**) On MRI, T_1WI showed a round lesion of hypointense on T_1WI at the distal metaphysis of the left tibia, with a slight ring-like hyperintense T_1WI around and a lamella hypointense shadow on T_1WI around; (**b**). T_2WI fat-suppressed sequence showed hyperintense in the center of the lesion, surrounded by a thin hypointense ring, with patchy slightly hyperintense edema area in the surrounding bone marrow; (**c**) The center of the lesion showed a slightly hyperintense on T_2WI, surrounded by a hyperintense area on T_2WI, and then a thinner hypointense ring on T_2WI in the outer layer

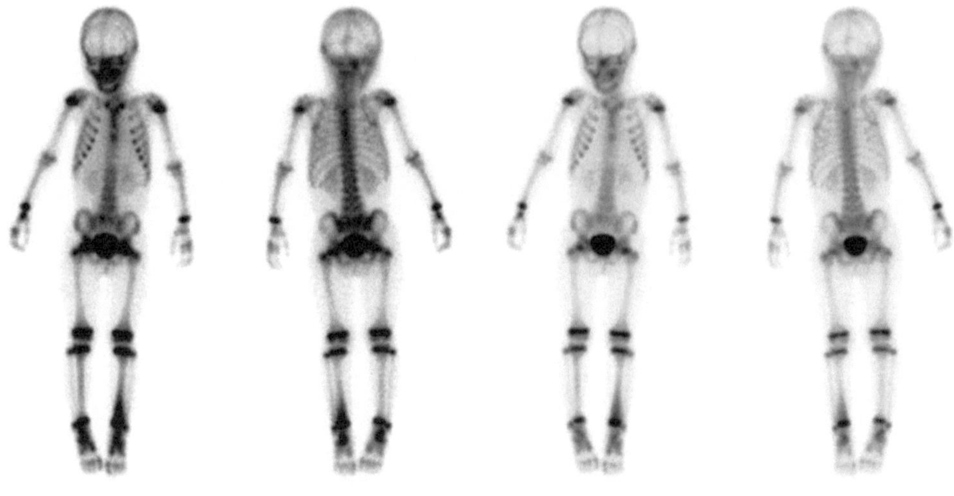

Fig. 6.34 Bone abscess at the distal metaphysis of left tibia (2). Radioactive concentration at the distal metaphysis of the left tibia

ces are thinned, and the surrounding sclerosis margins are thin. There is no periosteal proliferation or soft tissue swelling, and pathologic fracture is prone to occur. By contrast, Brodie abscess shows obvious osteosclerosis, with increasingly intensified sclerosis as history prolongs.

2. **Eosinophilic granuloma of bone.** It is most common in children under 10 years of age, single or multiple; for single cases, it is more common in the skull and femur and for multiple cases, it is more common in vertebral body. The lesions of long bone often involve the metaphysis and diaphysis, manifested as a single irregular bone destruction area, mostly located in the marrow cavity, showing expansive growth, with the border clear and well-defined; sometimes, the lamellar dense osteosclerosis can be seen in the destruction area, which is often accompanied by lamellar periosteal reaction and hyperostosis and osteosclerosis, and there may be soft tissue masses around, but the periosteal proliferation is less common than Brodie abscess, which can be diagnosed by laboratory test of eosinophilia.
3. **Osteoid osteoma**. It is common in teenagers under 30 years old with slow onset, manifested as pain at the site, which can be aggravated at night and relieved after taking salicylic acids and the like. It is a benign osteogenic tumor, composed of new osteoid tissues and arranged in a radial, reticular manner. The tumor is surrounded by proliferative and dense reactive bone. Imaging findings include small (typically less than 1.5 cm), circular or oval bright area in the focus, and irregular calcification or ossification shadows observed in tumor nidus,

surrounded by obvious proliferation and sclerosis rings, thickened bone cortex and periosteal reaction. According to MRI, the non-calcified part of the tumor shows hypointense to isointense on T_1WI and hyperintense on T_2WI, whereas the calcification part always shows hypointense. With the scan enhancement, the tumor is remarkably enhanced. Osteosclerosis surrounding the tumor nidus shows hypointense. Hyperemia is prone to occur in bone marrow and soft tissue surrounding the tumor, showing hypointense on T_1WI and hyperintense on T_2WI.

4. **Non-ossifying fibroma**. It is common in teenagers at the age of 8 ~ 20 years, typically located in the metaphysis of the limb long bone 3 ~ 4 cm away from the epiphyseal plate, especially the tibia, femur, and fibula. It is a benign tumor derived from bone connective tissues. If the focus is located in metaphysis or epiphysis of long bone, the single or multiple cystic radiolucent areas, which grow in a central, expansive manner in bones, can encroach on the bone along the most or entire transverse diameter, with homogeneous density and sclerosis margins, edged with thin shell of sclerotic osseous tissue that tends to grow outwardly. Proliferation and sclerosis are not as significant as Brodie abscess.

Status Quo and Progress of Research

1. CT boasts high resolution for soft tissue, without image overlap. Compared with X-ray plain film, it can better observe the lesions located at the site with complex structures. In particular, thin-slice 3D CT can clearly show the relationship between bone abscess lesions and peripheral tissues, and is the most sensitive to display of sequestrum in the vomica. For atypical cases or patients with extensive proliferation and sclerosis, CT examination can further reveal the internal conditions of the lesions.
2. MRI examination has important application value for the diagnosis of Brodie abscess due to multi-sequence and multi-azimuth imaging, which is more sensitive to early bone destruction than X-ray plain film and CT and can detect earlier periosteal reaction and soft tissue swelling. DWI imaging has high clinical application value in the detection of abscess within the lesions.

6.4 Fungal Infection

Junlin Li and Wei Li

Overview

The clinical manifestations of fungal infection are insidious, which may easily lead to misdiagnosis and delayed diagnosis, resulting in serious consequences. Fungal infections are extremely rare in the skeletal system of children, but strains such as aspergillus and blastomyces can also affect the skeletal system. There are many different kinds of fungi, and the main pathogens include coccidioides, candida, aspergillus, cryptococcus neoformans, and other rarer fungi, such as Fusarium mangiferae, etc. [46]. At present, the annual incidence of several major opportunistic fungal infections has reached (72 ~ 228)/million (candida), (30 ~ 66)/million (cryptococcus) and (12 ~ 34)/million (aspergillus), respectively. Candida and aspergillus are the two most common pathogens of fungal infection in children. Children and newborns with chronic granulomatous lesions are the most susceptible to infection. The incidence of candida in children was (10 ~ 47)/100,000 children, 37/100,000 children under 1 year of age, and 466/100,000 newborns. With the decrease of birth weight in newborns, the incidence of candidemia gradually increased, and the infection rate of ultra-low weight infants was as high as 12% ~ 15%. The overall case fatality rate of children is 40% ~ 71%. The rate of aspergillus infection in children is similar to that in adults, accounting for 5.9% ~ 12% of all fungal infections, and the mortality of aspergillus infection in children is similar to that in adults, which is more than 50%. Fungal infections are most common in child patient with low immune levels. In addition, the central venous catheterization, excessive or improper use of antibiotics, hormones, and trauma, joint surgery, and joint punctures can all increase the risk of fungal infections of the bones and joints. The most common cause of fungal infection in bone and joint system is the spread of primary infection foci to the bone and joint through hematogenous dissemination [47].

Invasive fungus can be divided into infectious pathogen and opportunistic pathogen. These infections can occur alone or as part of a systemic infection with multiple organs involved, usually as a result of hematogenous dissemination. Any bone or joint may be the site of infection, most often involving large weight-bearing joints and bones, and fungal infections of bones or joints may be resulted from direct spread of infection in adjacent tissues [48]. Most of fungal osteomyelitis and arthritis are a chronic, insidious process with no apparent symptoms in the early stages of the disease. Fungal arthritis usually occurs in single joints and is most common in the hip, knee, wrist, elbow, and other joints. The most common clinical symptoms are local pain, swelling and limitation of motion in respect of the affected limbs. In some severe cases, there may be erythema and joint swelling; the joint effusion may be accompanied by a sense of fluctuation, and local tenderness is obvious. The above inflammatory signs are the most common symptoms and signs [49]. In late stage, it leads to pathologic fracture. Chronic infections, such as coccidioidomycosis or blastomycosis, can cause cold abscess and sinus in soft tissues. At this time, it is easy to be associated with other bacterial infections, which is also accompanied by systemic symptoms with varying degrees, including fever, fatigue, appetite decrease, loss of weight, etc. Fungal septicemia may cause systemic spread and is often a cause of death.

The golden standard for the diagnosis of fungal infections of the bones and joints is the tissue culture of the pathogen, which may require tissue biopsy. Culture of synovial tissues, blood culture, bone marrow examination and culture, antibody tests (such as serum coccidioides antibody or histoplasmosis antibody), and inspection of fungal antigens in body fluids (such as serum cryptococcal antigen, urine tissue cytoplasmic antigen) can be used as auxiliary diagnosis methods [50]. GM [51] has been proven to be an alternative marker for invasive aspergillosis, and EIA detection of GM is a specific diagnosis of aspergillus infection.

Pathophysiology

The basic pathophysiology of fungal musculoskeletal infections is similar to that of common bacterial infections, but the fungi are generally less virulent, invading tissues when the body's resistance is reduced and multiplying to cause disease. When fungal pathogens arrive at the synovial membrane, they form granulomas (such as coccidioidomycosis) [52] or microabscesses (such as candidiasis and aspergillosis), which then proliferate in the synovial membrane, triggering inflammatory reactions that produce exudative joint effusion, and release collagenases and other proteolytic enzymes, to damage the joint surface. In case of chronic granulomatous synovitis, such as coccidioidomycosis, the joint swelling is mainly caused by synovial thickening, rather than joint effusion, wherein the vasculitis caused may erode articular cartilage, even subarticular bone [47].

The pathological changes of fungal infection lack specificity, and the pathogenic fungi do not produce any toxin, and mainly cause allergic reactions, which are different from those caused by different pathogens. Common basic pathological changes: (1) mild non-specific inflammation, with only a small number of lymphocytes and mononuclear cells in the lesions; (2) purulent inflammation, with a large number of neutrophils infiltrating to form abscesses, which mainly occurs when the number of infected fungi is large and the host reaction is strong. (3) necrotizing inflammation, with different size necrotic foci, accompanied by bleeding, less inflammatory cells; (4) granulomatous inflammation, often coexisting with purulent lesions. However, the tissue reactions of the same pathogen are also different at different stages. For example, coccidioidomycosis can cause necrotizing inflammation and purulent and granulomatous inflammations.

Imaging Findings

There is a lack of specificity in the imaging of fungal infections of the bones and joints, and all bones of the whole body can be affected. Different pathogens may involve different parts, for example, the sporotrichosis is often involved in the knee joint, hand, wrist joint, elbow joint, and shoulder joint, while the bone actinomycosis is usually secondary to peripheral soft tissue infection, with the mandible most often involved. At present, there is no summary of imaging findings of fungal infection in large samples.

1. **X-ray and CT**
   (a) Fungal osteomyelitis usually occurs in the metaphysis of tubular bone, with slow progress of the lesion, and the bone is mostly damaged by dotted erosion. The dotted destruction can be fused into large destruction foci, with clear margins.
   (b) In the early stage, there was no new bone formation, with mild periosteal reaction, and there was no sequestrum and proliferation and sclerosis. The adjacent bone edema was not obvious, and there could be abscess formation near the bone, and there was no soft tissue mass around.
   (c) In the early stage of joint disease, the joint space can be normal. With the development of the lesions, the joint space stenosis occurred [46], accompanied by joint effusion or synovial thickening, granulation tissue hyperplasia, and soft tissue swelling around the joint. The enhanced scan showed uneven enhancement.
   (d) Vertebral bodies and attachments can be involved in spinal diseases, with intramedullary and external abscesses and paraspinal abscesses, often damaging the anterior vertebral body and intervertebral disc. Aspergillus osteomyelitis is usually caused by direct invasion of pulmonary lesions into adjacent vertebral bodies, intervertebral discs, or adjacent ribs [47].
2. **MRI** can detect abnormal signals of bone and surrounding soft tissue lesions early, such as bone marrow edema and other inflammatory changes, and the T_2WI sequence and fat-suppressed sequence show slightly hyperintense; Joint effusion and thickened synovial tissues showed medium and hypointense on T_1WI image, similar to muscle intensity, and hyperintense on T_2WI and STIR sequence; Muscle tissue involvement showed blurred intermuscular space, slightly hypointense on T_1WI, diffuse increase on T_2WI, and mild to moderate muscle enhancement after enhancement, but not continuous. For early arthritis, the exudation, congestion, and edema are considered as specific changes. The soft tissue around the joint is swollen and the border is not clear.

Key Points of Diagnosis

1. Common in immunocompromised child patients.
2. Most of cases occur in the metaphysis of tubular bone, which is the localized punctate osteolytic bone destruction with well-defined margins and may accompany peripheral abscess formation.

3. In early stage, there is no new bone formation, little or no periosteal reaction, and generally no sequestrum.
4. In patients with joint disease, joint space narrowing, joint effusion, synovial thickening can be seen.
5. The diagnosis can take histological culture of fungal pathogen as a golden standard, supplemented by fungal antibody and antigen tests.

Differential Diagnosis

1. **Purulent inflammation of the bone marrow or joints caused by suppurative osteomyelitis and arthritis.** It mainly occurs in people with normal immune function, with acute clinical onset, local redness, swelling, heat and pain, and rapid development of lesions. The bone destruction can occur within 8 ~ 10 days, with irregular osteosclerosis surrounding, significant bearing surface, and joint space stenosis, and it is easy to be combined with joint dislocation. Fungal arthritis often occurs in immunodeficiency patients, child patients with long-term use of hormones and postoperative child patients, with slow and latent progress, clear boundary of imaging bone destruction, and less sclerosis.
2. **Fibrous dysplasia of bone.** Proximal femur is the most common for single-bone type and limb bone type. The typical manifestations are cystic expansible bone destruction in marrow cavity with clear sclerotic edges, ground glass like density and flocculent ossifying shadow.
3. **Tuberculosis of bone and joint**. Both images showed osteolytic bone destruction (with no sclerotic edge), the joint effusion, synovial thickening, and peripheral soft tissue swelling. Long bone epiphysis and metaphysis tuberculosis often involved in cartilage causing joint space narrowing. In tuberculosis bone destruction area, the sequestrum can be seen, and the fungal infection is relatively rare. Identification of difficult cases requires a combination of clinical symptoms, signs, and laboratory tests. Positive tuberculin test and T-SPOT tests are helpful in assisting the diagnosis of tuberculosis.
4. **Ewing's sarcoma**. It occurs often in long bone metaphysis, wherein invasive damage can be observed on the inner margin of the bone cortex, the bone cortex is intact, surrounded by obvious periosteal proliferation with onion-peel pattern and soft tissue mass. As the disease progresses, the edge of the bone destruction area becomes blurred. Fungal osteomyelitis bone destruction area usually has clear margins, with a periosteal reaction milder than that of Ewing's sarcoma.

Status Quo and Progress of Research

^{18}F-FDG PET/CT is a recognized imaging method that can reflect the function and metabolism of lesions, and in recent years, it has been used more and more in the diagnosis of inflammatory diseases. In the early stage, ^{18}F-FDG PET/CT can detect functional changes that occur prior to morphologic changes. In addition, since fungal infections of the bones and joints are usually a part of systemic infection, PET/CT can display the involved systems throughout the body. For example, it can identify whether there is occult involvement of the lungs, liver, spleen, or other organs. The research results of Leroy-Freschini et al. showed that ^{18}F-FDG PET/CT was highly sensitive (93%) and accurate (90%) in the diagnosis and treatment of opportunistic invasive fungal infections. The research results of Leroy-Freschini et al. further indicated that changes in ^{18}F-FDG intake intensity are associated with the clinical course of the infection, which can be used for treatment monitoring and efficacy assessment of fungal infection, thus helping clinicians provide therapeutic optimization during treatment [53].

6.5 Syphilis of Bone

The syphilis of bone is a special infection caused by Treponema pallidum, which is divided into 2 kinds by different ways of infection and onset time: (1) the Treponema pallidum in the maternal blood passes through the placenta and is introduced into the fetus, resulting in the corresponding bone infection, which is known as congenital syphilis of bone that occurs after 4 months of gestation. (2) the children were infected by contacting with Treponema pallidum through injecting the blood of syphilis patients or sexual abuse, kissing and other intimate contact or through chewing food for feeding and other ways, which is known as the acquired syphilis of bone.

Syphilis is a global public health problem, and its incidence is one of the important indicators to measure a country's public health level. All countries are actively carrying out epidemiological monitoring and studying management measures [54, 55]. The incidence of syphilis in China is on the rise year by year, becoming the third infectious disease after viral hepatitis and tuberculosis. In particular, the incidence in reproductive women increases the possibility of mother-to-child transmission.

6.5.1 Congenital Syphilis of Bone

Congenital syphilis of bone, also known as the congenital syphilis, can occur during the neonatal, infant, and pre-childhood years and can be divided into early-onset and late-onset according to the time of occurrence. The early-onset refers to the onset from birth to 4 years old and the late-onset refers to the onset after 4 years old. In mild cases, symptoms may appear 2–3 weeks after birth, such as swelling of skin mucosa, syphilis rash [56], irritable crying, interstitial pneumonia, hepatosplenomegaly, lymph node enlargement in all parts of the body; the pseudoparalysis may occur in limbs, and severe congenital syphilis of the fetus may cause abortion or death after birth [54].

Bone is one of the most frequently involved tissues of syphilis. Not all congenital syphilis have bone changes, and bone invasion accounts for about 90%. If the pregnant woman is a syphilis patient, the Treponema pallidum in the maternal blood can enter into the fetal bone and cartilage directly across the placenta. As the fetal cartilage has blood vessels, perichondrium, periosteum, cartilage, and bone can become infected. In particular, the fetal cartilaginous osteogenic sites, such as the metaphysis, ribs, flat bone and vertebral ossification center of the long and short tubular bone of the limbs, are more prone to suffer from syphilis bone destruction and the superficial bone is more easily affected [56].

6.5.1.1 Early-Onset Congenital Syphilis of Bone

Overview

It is an ossification process that Treponema pallidum forms granuloma of syphilis in bone and causes non-specific inflammation, which destroys the metaphysis and seriously damages cartilage. Clinical symptoms generally appear within 2–3 weeks after birth, such as extremity, palm and toe peeling, bullous dermatitis, skin rash, hepatosplenomegaly, involved joint swelling and limbs being unable to move autonomously, etc. When the baby is passively active, the baby cries, showing "pseudospasmodic paralysis." VDRL, USR, and RPR tests of serum syphilis were mostly positive. If the diagnosis is clear, systematic anti-syphilis treatment should be performed as soon as possible. In case of multiple organ complications or serious illness, corresponding treatment and timely symptomatic treatment should be provided to protect the liver, kidney, and other important organs. If congenital syphilis is not treated in the early stage, the mortality rate is as high as 25% ~ 30%.

Pathophysiology

The congenital syphilis of the fetal or the infant can invade any tissue of the whole body, for example, the fetus or the infant is infected before birth, the lesions are distributed more extensively, and the typical change is the fibrosis of visceral organ. Bone change is an ossification process that Treponema pallidum forms granuloma of syphilis in bone and causes non-specific inflammation, which destroys the metaphysis and seriously damages cartilage. Microscopically, the vascular wall in the lesion area was thickening, a large number of spirochetes were accumulated in the perivascular and/or endothelial cell areas, and the fibrous connective tissue hyperplasia, neutrophil and lymphocyte infiltration, and fewer plasma cells (PC), and single eosinophilic granulocyte were observed [57].

Imaging Findings

Bone abnormalities mainly include metaphyseal inflammation, periostitis, and osteomyelitis [56], among which the metaphyseal inflammation is the most important one. In fact, child patient with moderate and severe congenital syphilis of bone, the above three bone changes are often combined and difficult to distinguish. The ulna, distal radius, and proximal tibia and humerus are the most frequently affected parts, and the epiphysis is rarely affected. Skeletal changes of some child patients are not consistent with clinical symptoms. Although extensive bone changes occur within 6 months of birth, clinical symptoms may be insignificant or have only a mild rash.

1. **Metaphysitis**. It occurs in onset of symmetry. As the earliest invaded bone parts, it generally occurs in 3 ~ 6 months after birth and in the early stage, causes the early calcification band is widened and densified for about 3 mm due to the obstacle in the process of chondrogenesis, and there was an irregular layer of sparse bone across the metaphysis under the early calcification band, the components of which was granulation tissue, fibrous tissue and osteoid tissue, characterized by transverse bright belt (Fig. 6.35a, b). After the disease progresses, the metaphysis may have serrate protrusion deep in the metaphyseal cartilage, which is a limited irregular calcification. With the progression of the disease, severe destruction and fragmentation occurred in the metaphysis, with irregular margins, and the destruction area of proximal tibia was almost entirely in the medial side. If bilateral symmetry occurs, it is called Wimberger sign (Fig. 6.35c), which is characteristic. Some cases may be complicated by pathologic fracture, or epiphyseal plate, epiphyseal displacement.
2. **Osteomyelitis and periostitis.** They may occur alone, but they are mostly symmetrically found in long bones, mostly appeared with the development of metaphysitis.
   (a) Osteomyelitis: the manifestations are similar to suppurative lesions, mostly caused by metaphyseal inflammation spreading to the diaphysis. The early manifestations include spot-like and worm-eaten bone destruction in diaphysis and osteoporosis, and the edge of bone destruction area is relatively clear, which is the characteristic change of early-onset congenital syphilis of bone. With the progression of the disease, there is extensive destruction and sclerosis within the bone, but there is less sequestrum.
   (b) Periostitis: it is the commonest bone abnormality in early-onset congenital syphilis of bone, and the general range is more extensive, which can involve the 1/2 above of diaphysis length. In the first few months,

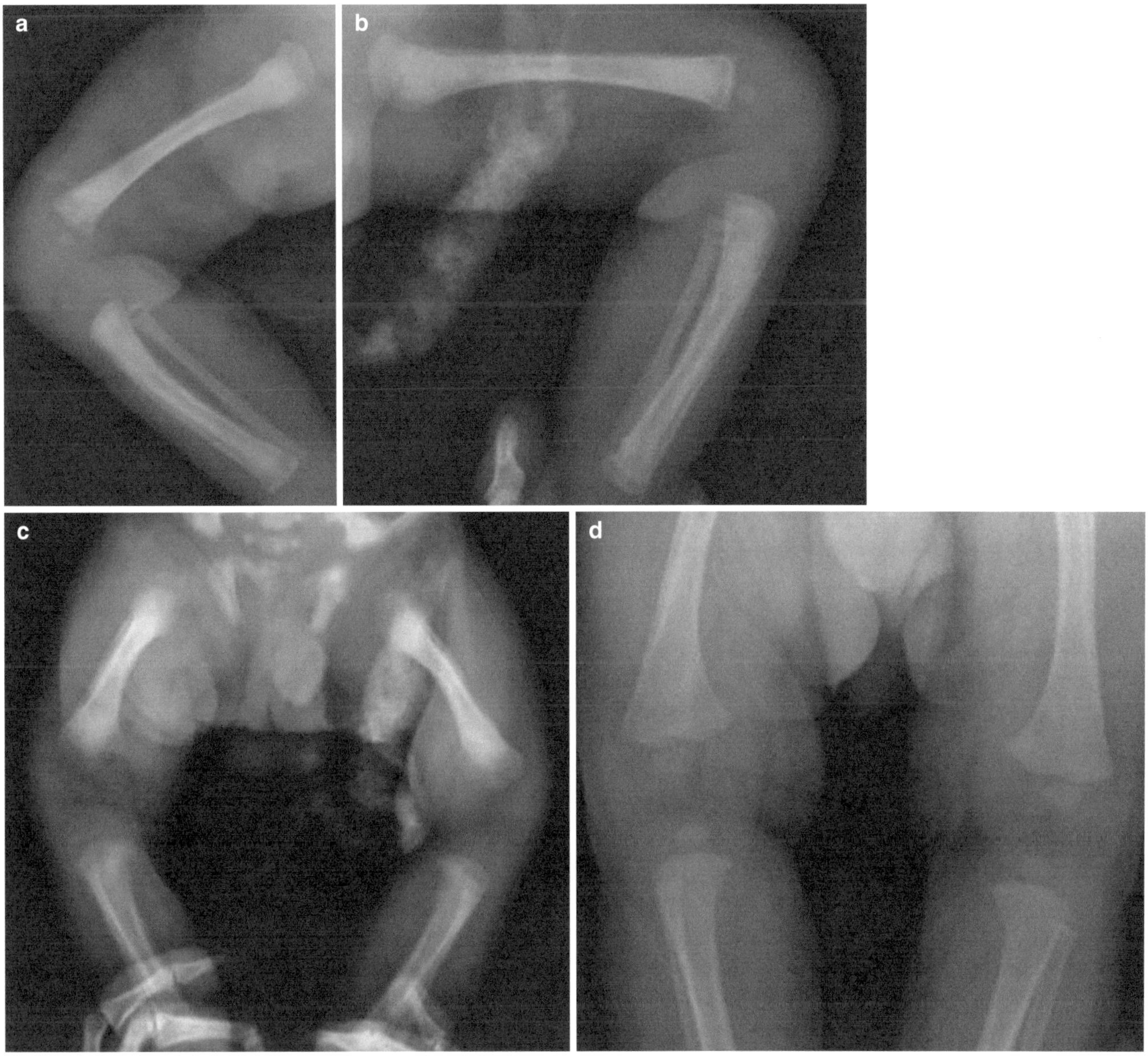

Fig. 6.35 Congenital syphilis of bone. (**a** ~ **c**) Symmetrical onset of long bones of both lower extremities occurred, with periosteum lamellar hyperplasia, uneven metaphyseal density, broadening and thickening of early calcification zone; a thin-layer radiolucent area under the metaphysis appeared, and serrate protrusions deep in metaphyseal cartilage may appear in the metaphysis; an irregular destruction area appeared in medial proximal tibia (Wimberger sign); (**d**) After treatment and review, the periosteal proliferation was significantly alleviated, the metaphyseal density was homogenous, and the destruction area was repaired

it is characterized by the "line" or "scallion" that is parallel to the diaphysis (Fig. 6.36). In late period, the diaphysis was thickened by partially laminated new periosteum fusing with the diaphysis (Figs. 6.35d and 6.37).

Key Points of Diagnosis

1. Symmetrical multiple bone disease foci occurred and the metaphysis is the first affected.
2. The early calcification zone of long tubular bone is widened and thickened, presenting Wimberger sign.
3. Often there have osteomyelitis and periostitis.
4. Severe cases may also be free from epiphysis involvement.

Differential Diagnosis

1. **Scurvy.** It is caused by the deficiency of Vitamin C, which mostly occurred in the artificial feeding infants less than

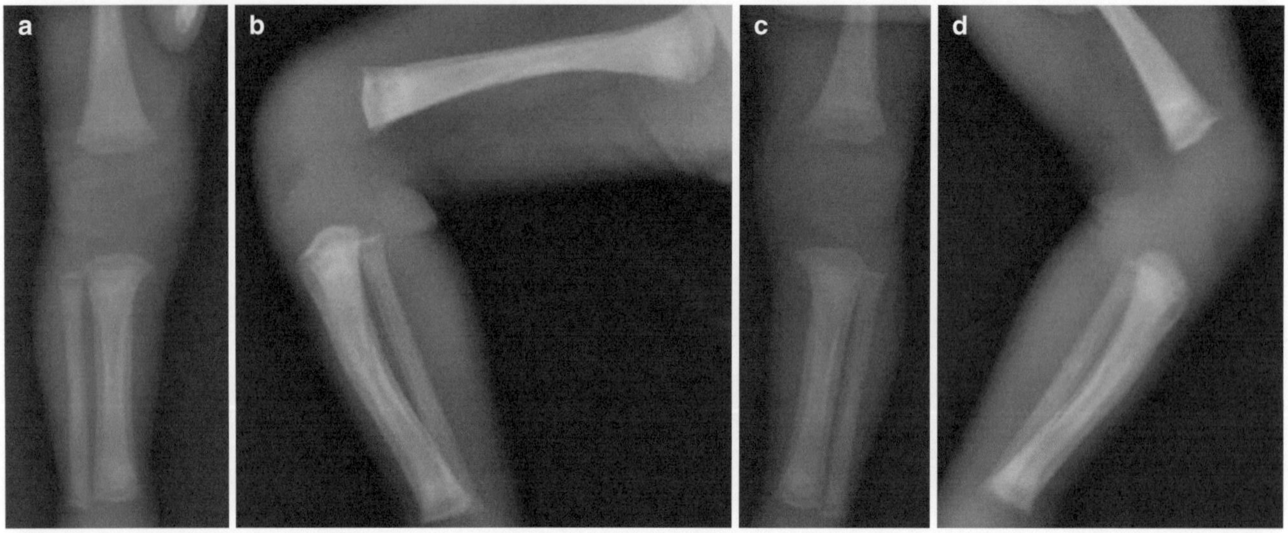

Fig. 6.36 Syphilis of bone (1). Symmetrical onset occurred in the long tubular bone of both lower limbs, with osteoporosis of diaphysis, mottled bone destruction and extensive linear periosteal proliferation, involving more than 1/2 of the length of diaphysis

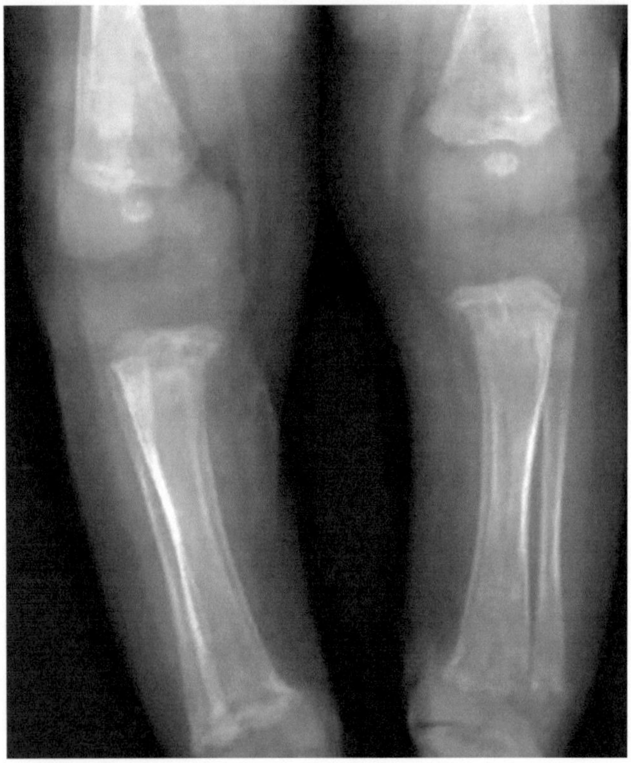

Fig. 6.37 Syphilis of bone (2). Partially laminated new periosteum fuses with the diaphysis to thicken the diaphysis

1 year old, with general osteoporosis and no bone destruction, and the epiphysis had "ring" sign with dense edges, while the syphilis epiphysis was normal, with no change in the bone mineral density.

2. **Suppurative osteomyelitis**. The systemic poisoning symptoms were obvious, characterized by rapid onset, main single-bone disease, rapid progression of bone destruction, involving a wide range, which was easy to cause large area of bone destruction and large sequestrum, with rare systemic multiple bone involvement and symmetrical onset.
3. **Infantile cortical hyperostosis**. Generally in 3 ~ 6 months, only the periosteum was thickened, there were no diaphysitis and osteomyelitis, and the epiphysis and metaphysis were not involved, with soft tissue swelling and tenderness. It can come on in succession of multiple bones and does not have symmetrical tendency to come on.
4. **Bone tuberculosis**. The bone was cystic destruction with slight swelling, accompanied by lamellar periosteal proliferation, and there was little hyperostosis. Sand-like sequestrum was found in the bone destruction area. The surrounding soft tissue was fusiform and swollen; although there were multiple cases, there was no symmetrical tendency.

6.5.1.2 Late-Onset Congenital Syphilis of Bone

Overview

Late-onset congenital syphilis of bone is rare in bone, mostly in the tibia, and may be caused due to fetal bone latent syphilis infection and reactivity. It is more common in infants, children or teenagers, and its clinical symptoms occur after 4 years of age and are more common in children aged 5 ~ 15 years. Child patients have physical development disorders, mental retardation, anemia, common keratitis, neurologic deafness, Holster teeth, saddle nose, saber leg, and intermittent osteodynia, and even joint swelling and difficulty walking. Diseases cannot heal themselves, often leaving bone and joint deformity [58].

Pathophysiology

The pathological changes were mainly periostitis and osteomyelitis, characterized by diffuse or localized subperiosteal cortical thickening with gumma.

Imaging Findings

1. **Periostitis**. It is more common in young patients with layered periosteum parallel to the diaphysis. In older children, only a few bones are invaded, especially the tibia, which is confined to the front of the tibia, resulting in thickening and anterior protrusion of the tibia diaphysis, reduced marrow cavity, causing the saber-like deformation of the tibia, which is called Saber leg.
2. **Osteomyelitis**. When long bones are involved, the tibia is the most common site. The lesions first affect the diaphysis, and the scope is relatively limited. Irregular bone destruction caused by gumma is accompanied by mild sclerosis; In diffuse cases, small speckle or flaky bone destruction can be seen in the osteosclerosis area, and the bone trabecula is dense and irregular, and the sequestrum is uncommon.

Key Points of Diagnosis

1. The pain of involved limb, and it is aggravated at rest.
2. Multi-bone symmetric lesions, and the tibia is the most common part.
3. X-rays showed periostitis, osteomyelitis, and osteosclerosis, with periosteal proliferation in front of tibia diaphysis forming a typical Saber leg.

Differential Diagnosis

Sclerosing osteomyelitis often has a history of inflammation, with more severe pain, mainly manifested as periosteal proliferation, bone cortex thickening, marrow cavity stenosis or occlusion, and osteosclerosis proliferation often surrounds the diaphysis. There is generally no or very slight irregular bone destruction in the bone destruction area, and there is no symmetrical tendency. A serum test for syphilis is helpful in differential diagnosis.

6.5.2 Acquired Syphilis of Bone

Overview

From the mid-nineteenth century to the mid-twentieth century, acquired syphilis in children was reported more abroad, and then decreased, but sporadic cases were reported in recent decades. China did not report acquired syphilis in children until 1995, but reports have been increasing gradually in recent years. According to preliminary statistics, a total of more than 40 cases were reported from 1995 to 2010. The detailed epidemiological data are not clear, and the ratio of boys to girls is about 3:1. As children syphilis basically comes from adults, as long as the incidence of adult syphilis continues to grow, the incidence of children syphilis, whether congenital or acquired, will increase accordingly. Especially the adult latent syphilis with often unclear history is potentially more infectious, more harmful and increases the risk of acquired syphilis in children. In recent years, with the acceleration of domestic sexual openness and aging, the incidence of syphilis is increasing not only among young people, but also among older age groups. Young couples are busy with work and mostly the elderly help to raise children. If the elderly have syphilis infection, the intimate contact between the two parties will undoubtedly increase the risk of acquired syphilis infection in children [59, 60].

Acquired syphilis of bone developed spirochetes septicemia 1 ~ 2 months after contact infection. The spirochetes entered periosteal vessels and caused perivascular inflammation. In the early stage, the most common inflammation is syphilitic periostitis, with the tibia and clavicle being the most common sites, other bones such as skull, ribs, sternum, femur, fibula and hands and feet all can be invaded. When the spirochete spreads to the cortical Haversian canal and bone marrow, it causes bone marrow infection, cortical destruction, and periosteal proliferation. Therefore, syphilitic osteomyelitis and periostitis are often mixed. Acquired syphilis can be divided into three clinical phases, with phase I for chancre and without bone and joint change; patients in phases II and III can appear long tubular bone involvement, the lesions are often multiple and easy to invade the long bone diaphysis. The Treponema pallidum forms a syphilitic granuloma under the periosteum, which lifts the periosteum and causes reactive new bone hyperplasia, presenting as periostitis, and the typical manifestation is saber-like tibia. The lesions may also cause osteomyelitis, and the gumma not only can erode bone to form a destruction area in which the sequestrum is rare, but also can form ulcer after breaking through the skin.

The incubation period for syphilis of bone may be several years to several decades. The clinical features are pain in affected limbs, aggravation during rest or sleep, and relief of symptoms after activity. Clinical symptoms often do not correspond to the degree of X-ray presentation.

Pathophysiology

Pathology was divided into gumma-like and non-gumma-like inflammation, with necrotic tissue inside. Microscopically, the syphilitic granulation tissue with a large number of neovascularization and connective tissue extending into the granulation tissue was observed, with caseous necrosis in the center, and lymphocyte and epithelioid cell infiltration and Langerhans giant cells around [11].

Imaging Findings

Lesions are often multiple, with more invasion of long bone diaphysis, less involvement of metaphysis and joint.

1. Periostitis is common in tibia and clavicle, presenting as lamellar periosteal proliferation.
2. Osteomyelitis is mostly common in phase II syphilis, with major features including: (1) extensive hyperostosis of long bone, osteosclerosis, bone cortex thickening and compact, diaphysis bulky deformation, and some cases accompanied by the disappearance of marrow cavity. In the marrow cavity, the transparent bone destruction area is occasionally visible, usually without sequestrum. (2) The localized bone destruction caused by gumma is mostly located in the thickened subperiosteum or dense cortex, and can also be seen in the marrow cavity, with osteosclerosis and periosteal proliferation around. The syphilitic gumma occurs in the diaphysis of the limbs, with common localized cortical destruction and defects, marrow cavity sclerosis, periosteal proliferation, cortical thickening, and diaphysis enlargement. Especially, the tibia changes are limited to the front, and the diaphysis is thickened and protruding, showing saber-like deformation, which is called Saber leg.

The lesions less invade the spine, skull, and joints. Skull invasion can occur in frontal bone, parietal bone, and occipital bone, mostly involving in the outer plate, but less involving in the inner plate, which manifested as multiple patchy or cribriform bone destruction with different sizes, accompanied by osteosclerosis. The sequestrum can be seen in some destruction areas, and bone destruction caused by gumma can also be found. Vertebral body was involved in many cases due to spinal invasion, which showed localized bone destruction in the vertebral body, accompanied by hyperostosis and osteosclerosis and ligament ossification, and subluxation of vertebral body can be seen in some cases. When the clavicle was invaded, symmetrical cortical destruction was observed at both sides of the extremitas sternalis claviculae, or osteolysis destruction of the bone marrow cavity at the sternal end was observed, with swelling of the surrounding soft tissue. Hyperplasia of the outer membrane of bone leads to thickening of the diaphysis, narrowing of the marrow cavity, and may invade the sternoclavicular joint and manubrium sternum. The invasion of the ribs is often manifested as bilateral multiple rib end punctate destruction and extensive periosteal proliferation. In the active stage of syphilitic osteomyelitis of metatarsal bone and metatarsal bone, the whole metatarsal bone, metatarsal bone, and tarsus joint can suffer from extensive osteolytic destruction and formation of sequestrum.

Key Points of Diagnosis

1. Bilateral symmetry of long bone periosteal proliferation, layered or lacy proliferation.
2. The cortex is thickened, the diaphysis is thickened, and the tibia in particular is arched forward, forming a typical saber sign.
3. Metaphysis and joint are rarely involved.
4. Localized bone destruction, defect, surrounding sclerosis, and soft tissue swelling.
5. A history of close contact with Treponema pallidum infections.

Differential Diagnosis

1. **Sclerosing osteomyelitis.** It often has a history of inflammation, with more severe pain, mainly manifested as periosteal proliferation, bone cortex thickening, marrow cavity stenosis or occlusion, and osteosclerosis proliferation often surrounds the diaphysis. There is generally no or very slight irregular bone destruction in the bone destruction area, and there is no symmetrical tendency. A serum test for syphilis is helpful in differential diagnosis.
2. **Bone tuberculosis.** It often occurs in the metaphysis of long bone, with osteoporosis. The bone was cystic destruction with slight swelling, accompanied by lamellar periosteal proliferation, and there was little hyperostosis. Sand-like sequestrum was found in the bone destruction area. The surrounding soft tissue was fusiform and swollen; although there were multiple cases, there was no symmetrical tendency. Acquired syphilis of bone occurs in long bone diaphysis, and osteosclerosis is more obvious than osteoporosis.

Status Quo and Progress of Research

The application of FDG PET/CT in brain, lung, gastrointestinal tract, adrenal gland, rectum, anus and other syphilitic lesions has been reported, and rare cases of syphilis of bone have been reported, and most cases are reported in adults, but few in children. Isolated osteolytic changes caused by syphilis are easily confused with other diseases such as tumors. PET/CT can also find reactive lymph nodes in hilum of lung and subcutaneous tissues, etc. Increased uptake of FDG has greater advantages in detecting lesions and determining biopsy sites. PET/CT is also helpful to the discovery of aortic inflammation and neural structure involvement, to determine the scope of disease involvement, to assess the degree of lymph node involvement, and is of great significance for the follow-up and evaluation of treatment options [61–64].

6.6 Pyogenic Arthritis

Wei Li, Xiaohong Lv, and Wei Zhou

Overview

The pyogenic arthritis refers to the suppurative inflammation of the joint that is caused by infection of the synovial membrane with suppurative bacteria, and the pathogens basically have Staphylococcus aureus, Bacillus influenzae, streptococcus, Pseudomonas aeruginosa, meningococcus etc., among which the Staphylococcus aureus is the most common one, while fungi or mycobacteria also can bring about the occurrence of pyogenic arthritis. The pyogenic arthritis is usually a single pathogen infection, but mixed infection with multiple pathogens is less common.

The pyogenic arthritis can occur at any age, most commonly in infants under 2 years old, which is highly likely to cause pyosepticemia. Susceptibility factors in children: joint open or penetrating injury, skin infection, respiratory tract infection, intestinal infection diseases, etc. The disease can occur at any joint, but the bearing large joint is more susceptible to disease, with hip joint and knee joint more common. The hip joint is one of the largest bearing joints and is the most frequent site of pyogenic arthritis. Its articular capsule is broad and has a high range of motion. A long section of the femoral head and neck is free in the articular capsule, and the blood vessels enter the joint, and by walking along the femoral neck synovial membrane are distributed in the femoral head. The pus produced after the pyogenic infection of the hip joint can easily destroy the articular capsule and lead to pathological dislocation. The incidence of pyogenic arthritis is more common in single joints, and sometimes multiple joints can be seen at the same time. The incidence of polyarticular pyogenic arthritis is most common in child patients with rheumatoid arthritis (RA) or other systemic connective tissue diseases and severe sepsis.

The route of infection was the same as that of acute osteomyelitis. Pyogenic bacteria directly invaded synovial membrane of joints, adjacent bone, and soft tissue infection foci through blood flow and directly infected the joints after open trauma. Suppurative osteomyelitis near the epiphysis of the diaphysis of the joints in children is primary. The pus can directly destroy the bone cortex to invade the joint or penetrate the epiphyseal plate to invade the subchondral bone of the joints, and then extend from the attachment point of articular capsule to the articular cavity. On the contrary, some scholars observed babies under one year old with the articular cavity effusion, if they found that there was enhanced display of decreased perfusion of femoral epiphysis on T_1WI fat-suppressed sequence, it was likely to develop into acute hematogenous osteomyelitis of the metaphysis, and in children after 1 year old, such signs were not observed, and acute hematogenous osteomyelitis was less likely to occur [35]. For children, the simultaneous incidence of acute osteomyelitis and pyogenic arthritis detected by MRI examination is more common than clinically suspected cases, because bacteria can spread from metaphysis to adjacent joints through blood vessels. Therefore, early diagnosis and treatment should be made for children with joint effusion to avoid sequelae [65]. The great importance shall be attached to the early diagnosis and early treatment of children's pyogenic arthritis, the joint debridement must be thoroughly cleared of bacterial colonization and reproduction of the residence-inflammatory synovial membrane, to protect the development and maintenance of joint functions. If the lesions are not removed early, both the entire bone and joint structure will be damaged to varying degrees, leading to joint dysfunction.

Clinical symptoms mainly depend on the site and scope of lesions as well as the type of pathogen. The disease usually occurs acutely. The joint with the disease swells. Surrounding soft tissues show acute inflammation manifestations such as redness, swelling, heat and pain, as well as systematic toxic symptoms such as chills, fever, and leukocytosis, with activity limitation and easy joint dislocation. Laboratory tests showed the elevation of leukocyte counts, neutrophils, and C-reactive protein and the acceleration of erythrocyte sedimentation rate. The auxiliary diagnosis of pyogenic arthritis includes hemoculture, bacterial culture of joint fluid and histological pathology; for joint and bone that is easy to obtain the specimens, the direct puncture aspiration is available; for ankle joint, hip joint, and other joints that are difficult to be operated, tissue specimens can be mediated by imaging and can be performed with stratified puncture in the articular capsule, periosteum, bone marrow cavity, and other suspected parts [24, 65, 66].

Pathophysiology

1. **Early stage**. It is also called as serous exudate stage, and the pathogens enter the joint to cause hyperemia and edema of synovial membrane, leukocyte infiltration, and serous exudate accumulation from the articular cavity first. There is no basement membrane as a barrier for synovial membrane tissue, and pathogens can quickly enter the synovial fluid, accelerating the process of pyogenic arthritis.
2. **Progressive stage**. It is the serous cellulose exudation period. The disease enters the progressive stage about 1 week after infection. The exudate from the articular cavity is pyogenic. Synovial cells are obviously prolif-

erated, and the inflammatory cell infiltration can be seen on the cartilage surface. A large number of proteases and cytokines released by leukocyte decomposition can degrade cartilage, dissolve and destroy subchondral bone, and inhibit the formation of cartilage, resulting in different degrees of articular cartilage damage or even destruction. Proteoglycan in cartilage matrix is lost during infection, mechanical strength of cartilage is reduced, and functional integrity is destroyed. The cartilage usually changes from the attachment point of articular capsule. As the disease progresses, the change scope expands gradually, chondrocytes degenerate and die, some cartilages fall off, chondrocytes at surface and middle layers gradually die but most of those at the deep layer are still alive.

In some cases, neutrophil infiltration can be seen in the subarticular bone, which may develop into an intraosseous abscess. Soft tissue with infection may form a large abscess in the tissue such as deep layer muscle.

3. **Late stage**. It is the purulent exudate period. The damage to articular cartilage will further lead to the infection and necrosis of subchondral bone. If there are exudated cartilage or bone fragments in the articular cavity, it can stimulate the aggravation of synovial membrane exudation, accelerate the process of articular capsule fibrosis and scar formation, and form granulation tissue in the articular cavity. After the lesion is improved or healed, the fibrosis and ossification occur, forming joint fibrotic or bony ankylosis [67].

The pathological characteristics of pyogenic arthritis for special ankle joint and wrist joint [1]: (1) the pyogenic arthritis of ankle joint can be divided into the osteomyelitis of the lower tibia invading the joint or calcaneus downward and talus osteomyelitis invading the joint upward, or synovial infection directly forming septic arthritis. There are many ligaments around the ankle joint, the anterior ankle has the extensor tendinous sheath passing through, and the posterior tibial medial malleolus has the posterior tibial tendon with the flexor digitorum longus and the flexor hallucis longus tendon passing through, and the lateral malleolus has the peroneal length and the peroneus brevis tendon passing through. There is only a thin fibrous membrane between the ankle joint and the posterior part of the subtalar joint, so the suppurative lesions of the ankle are likely to involve the above structures and destroy the corresponding tendons and tendinous sheath. In addition, ankle soft tissue is thin, and suppurative lesions are easy to puncture the articular capsule to form subcutaneous abscesses. (2) The wrist joint is composed of many bones, with many tendons and tendinous sheaths, and many surface of articular cartilage. The pus invades the tendon and spreads along the tendinous sheath, which will destroy the surrounding tendons and tendinous sheaths, causing irreversible joint adhesion or bone fusion. The pus damages the articular capsule, the dorsal metacarpal ligament, the ulnar and radial collateral ligaments, and the interosseous ligaments of the carpal bones, resulting in carpal bone separation and loosening. The blood vessels in the articular capsule are destroyed, and the carpal bones lose blood supply, leading to form osteonecrosis.

Imaging Findings

The soft tissue swelling of pyogenic arthritis indicates that the child patient has a very serious pathological change, not the common inflammatory response and edema, but the abscess in the joint, the spread of pus and the formation of soft tissue abscess, and the destruction of adjacent structures, such as ligaments, articular capsules, and blood vessels etc. by the spreading pus.

1. X-ray
   (a) Early stage: There were no obvious abnormal changes in most cases. Swelling and increased density of the articular capsule can be seen. Pus can be seen in the articular cavity within 2–3 days after infection. The soft tissue surrounding the affected joint has diffuse edema with unclear boundary and increased density (Fig. 6.38a). The subcutaneous fat layer may be accompanied by a thick strip-like and reticular septal shadows, and the fat in the intermuscular space may be displaced or blurred (Fig. 6.38b); A large amount of joint effusion showed obvious increase of articular capsule shadow and displacement of fat pad by pushing; The joint space is widened due to effusion, and subluxation may occur in children with severe disease (Fig. 6.38a).
   (b) Progressive stage: the articular cartilage was destroyed, the pus gradually invaded the subchondral bone, and the articular surface was blurred and eroded, which was gradually expanded from the initial small transparency area with the most obvious joint bearing surface (Fig. 6.39a). The disease progression showed massive bone destruction and sequestrum, and the joint space was narrowed after 1 ~ 2 weeks. In severe cases of infection, there may be epiphysitis, periostitis, and metaphysis osteomyelitis (Fig. 6.39b), which may also result in destruction of the epiphyseal plate, separation of the epiphysis, and secondary pathologic dislocation. At the same time of bone destruction, bone repair began to occur, which was manifested as irregular proliferation and sclerosis around the destruction area. The pus in the joints of some patients may run through the synovial membrane, articular capsule, subcutaneous tissue and skin to form sinus, resulting that it cannot

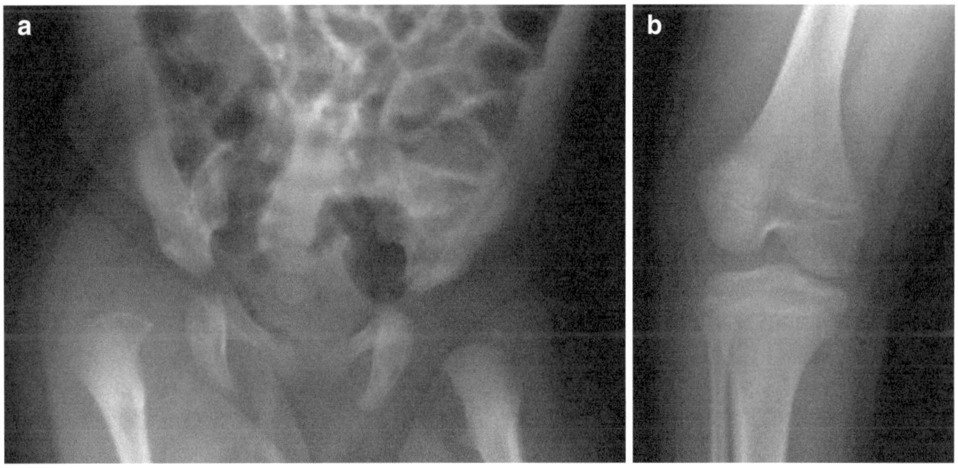

Fig. 6.38 Pyogenic arthritis (early stage). (**a**) Pelvis DR showed diffuse swelling of the right hip articular capsule, increased density, blurred intermuscular space, widened joint space, accompanied by joint subluxation. (**b**) The soft tissue around the joint was in diffuse edema with unclear boundary and increased density. The subcutaneous fat layer was accompanied by a thick reticular septal shadows, and the fat in the intermuscular space was displaced and blurred

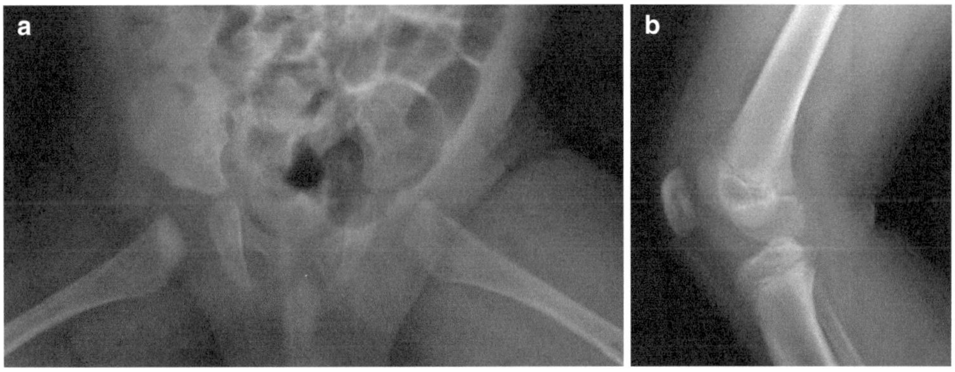

Fig. 6.39 Pyogenic arthritis (progressive stage). (**a**) DR showed swelling of the articular capsule of the left hip, increased density, decreased density of the left femur metaphysis, blurring, erosion, and destruction of articular surface and periosteal proliferation; (**b**) DR showed swelling of suprapatellar bursa, increased density, localized density reduction of femur metaphysis, and cortical destruction

heal for a long time. For example, the purulent lesions of the hip joint can perforate the bottom of acetabulum and enter the pelvic cavity, and the pus spreads along the obturator internus, resulting in the obturator internus sign; They spread along the obturator externus below the acetabulum, forming the obturator externus sign; After the pus destroys the articular capsule, it extravasates and forms a deep multiple abscess in the groin and pelvic cavity. If the epiphysis density is reduced, it indicates that the blood supply has not been damaged, and the prognosis is better.

(c) Restoration stage: the localized density of bone is reduced, and the edge of the bone destruction area is irregular, accompanied by osteosclerosis. In severe cases, various degrees of deformities are left, which are manifested as abnormal bone shape, loss of normal metaphysis, defect or expansion of bone structure, disordered structure, heterogeneous density (Fig. 6.40), and calcification of surrounding soft tissue. When the lesion is severe, the bony ankylosis may occur.

2. **CT.** CT is superior to ordinary X-ray examination, especially suitable for the examination of complex joint lesions, such as hip, shoulder, ankle, wrist joints, etc., and in the acute stage, it can show intra-articular and juxta-articular abscess, the soft tissue swelling, bone destruction and the range of abscess invasion is more accurate than plain film.

Soft tissue swelling is manifested as hypertrophy of the muscles around the diseased joints, but with reduced density; increased, blurred, or disappeared density of intermuscular fat space, and strip-shaped or grid high-density shadow in subcutaneous fat; Joint effusion is manifested as localized fluid density area in the articular cavity and surrounding soft tissue, with the density lower than that of normal muscles (Fig. 6.41a); The bone destruction is manifested as non-smooth and incomplete articular surface, thinning bone cortex, blurring edge. The lamellar low-density radiolucent area was observed in the bone under the articular surface, and the bone trabecula was interrupted and disappeared (Fig. 6.42), with hyperostosis and osteosclerosis, and small sequestrum shows the shadow of increased density in the vomica (Fig. 6.41b, c), with complete separation from the surrounding osseous tissue, and the big sequestrum density is higher, in which there is no bone trabecula, with the osteoporosis surrounding the joint; The proliferation of synovial membrane and granulation tissue is manifested that soft tissue density shadows in the articular cavity are mixed with the joint fluid. In severe cases, joint space stenosis and joint subluxation and dislocation can be seen.

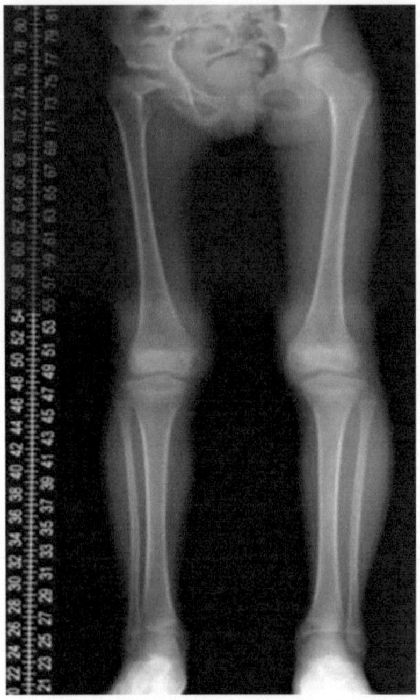

Fig. 6.40 Pyogenic arthritis (restoration stage). DR for the full length of both lower extremities showed that the right hip joint had pyogenic arthritis causing unequal length of both lower extremities, the right femur near the metaphysis was deformed, with irregular bone margin, obviously heterogeneous hyperostosis, osteosclerosis, and ossification. The underlying bone structure was disordered, the epiphysis structure was defective, and the osteosclerosis occurred to the acetabulum surface

3. **MRI.** MRI is obviously better than X-ray and CT in showing the pathologic anatomic details of pyogenic arthritis. In particular, MRI enhancement can be used for early detection of lesions, which is of high diagnostic value, can make the comprehensive evaluation of synovitis, cartilage or bone destruction, bone marrow edema, myositis, cellulitis, granulation tissue, abscess, fistula, fibrosis and other changes and especially is more sensitive in making early evaluation of abnormal changes in articular cartilage, epiphysis, metaphysis, bone marrow and synovial membrane, and other structures. It also can estimate the scope of affected soft tissue to provide the clinical doctors with reference for the operation, which has been recommended as a test for this disease [68, 69].

In the early stage of the disease, the joints were swollen, with a wide range and an unclear muscular hierarchy, presenting hypointense on T_1WI and hyperintense on T_2WI, and the fat-suppressed sequence was displayed more clearly; The detection rate of articular cavity effusion was up to 100%, which was manifested as hyperintense shadow on T_2WI in the articular cavity; Hyperemia, edema, and thickening of the synovial membrane, articular cavity effusion, and swelling of the articular capsule were shown as mixed intensity shadows in the articular cavity on the T_2WI fat-suppressed sequence (Fig. 6.43); The intensities in the epiphysis and metaphysis were heterogeneous, and the epiphysis morphology is abnormal. In the bone destruction area, spotted, patchy or linear and patchy T_1WI hypointense and T_2WI hyperintense crossing the bone cortex appear in the bone cortex with extremely hypointense (Fig. 6.44); Those involving the epiphyseal plate showed strip-like

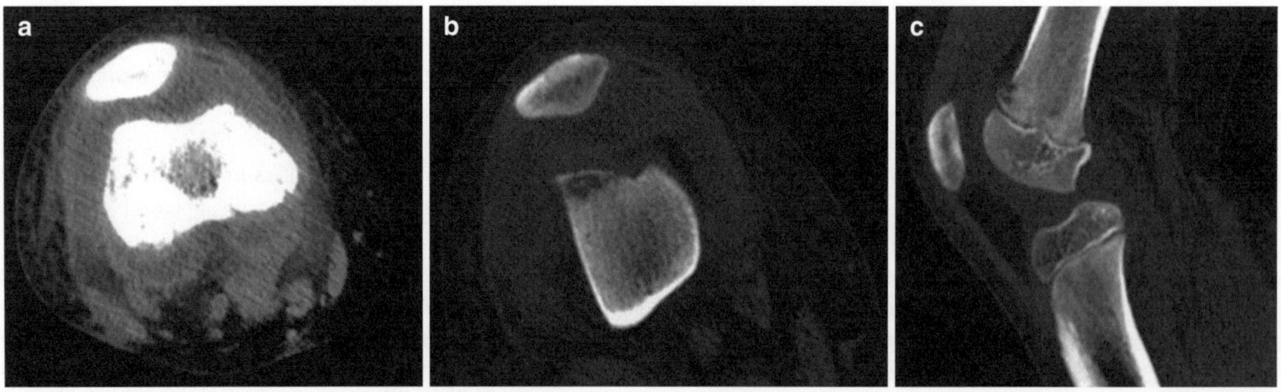

Fig. 6.41 Pyogenic arthritis of right knee joint. (**a**) The soft tissue window on CT showed increased density of peripheral intermuscular fat around knee joint, strip-shaped high-density shadow in subcutaneous fat, limited liquid density area in articular cavity and peripheral tissues; (**b, c**) The bone window on CT showed localized bone destruction in the metaphysis of the right femur, disappearance of bone trabecula, thinning of bone zortex, blurred edges, and hidden small sequestrum

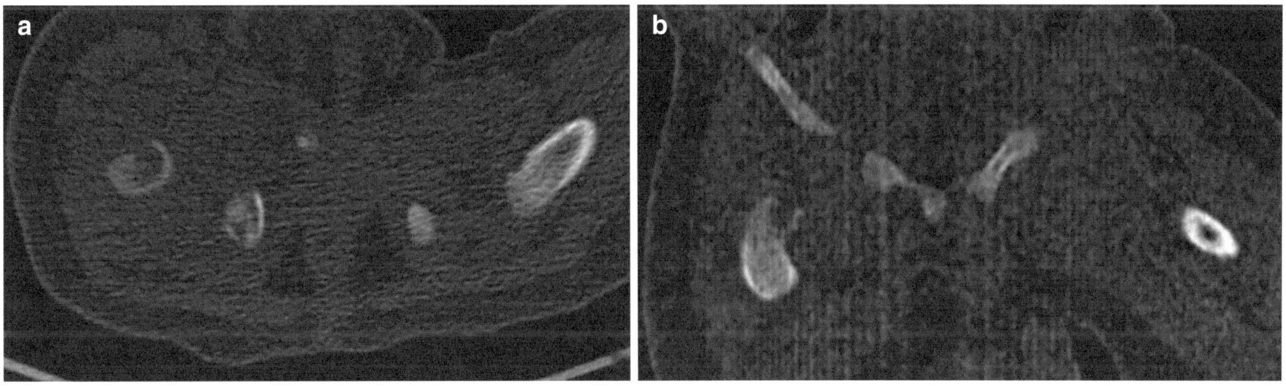

Fig. 6.42 Pyogenic arthritis of right hip joint. (**a**) The transverse section on CT showed the ovoid bone destruction in the metaphysis of the right femur, the disappearance of bone trabecula, and slight decrease in the surrounding bone density; (**b**) The coronal plane reconstruction on CT showed the bone destruction area was involving in articular surface, with thinning bone cortex and blurring edges

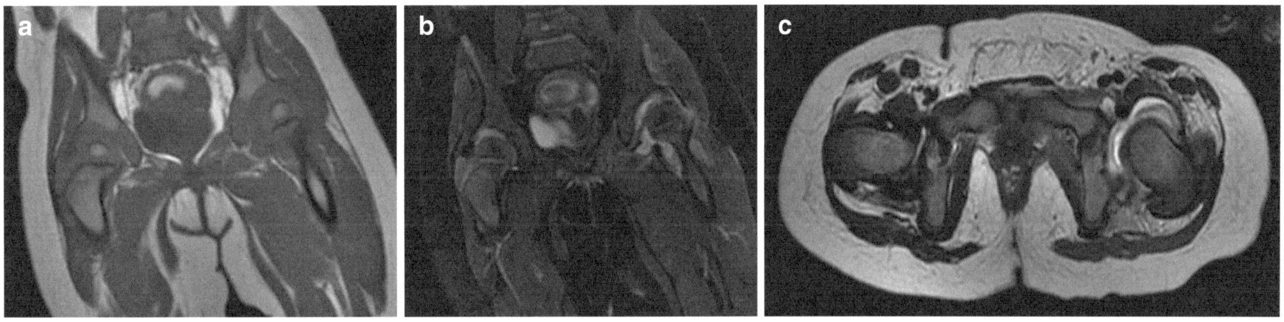

Fig. 6.43 Pyogenic arthritis of left hip joint. (**a**, **b**) MRI showed swelling of joint soft tissue, loss of intramuscular fat space, unclear muscle layers, hyperintense on T_2WI fat-suppressed sequence, with articular cavity effusion and heterogeneous intensity in metaphysis; (**c**) Transverse plane on T_2WI showed slight broadening of the joint space, space effusion, and synovial hyperplasia

T_2WI hyperintense shadow across the epiphyseal plate, while those involving the epiphyseal cartilage showed heterogeneous thickness of epiphyseal cartilage and abnormal intensity; the boundary between articular cartilage and epiphysis was unclear, with abnormal intensity, irregular cartilage surface and defect, and necrosis of articular cartilage. In the late stage, the bony articular surface was blurred, interrupted, destroyed, and disappeared, and the subchondral cystic destruction occurred. In a small number of patients, the intra-articular pus punctured synovial membrane, articular capsule, and skin, forming hyperintense sinus on T_2WI (Fig. 6.45), which could not heal for a long time. MRI can also show inflammatory reactions in bone marrow, manifested as hypointense shadow on T_1WI and hyperintense shadow on T_2WI. Follow-up review is required for bone marrow edema and osteomyelitis.

Enhanced examination with GD-DTPA showed that due to articular capsule hypertrophy and synovial hyperplasia, there were a large number of new blood vessels, with marked enhancement. If the epiphysis enhancement is weak during enhanced examination, it indicates reduced blood perfusion in the affected area [35], which is a characteristic manifestation of pyogenic arthritis and has diagnosis and differential diagnosis significance.

4. **Joint puncture and drainage angiography** is the most accurate method to diagnose the pyogenic arthritis in the early stage. The articular puncture will be performed within 3 ~ 5 days after onset. If the pus is extracted, the definite diagnosis is made immediately. Most of the pus is extracted as much as possible, and then an equivalent amount of iodine aqueous contrast agent is injected into the articular cavity for X-ray examination. The joint fluid extraction imaging also shows the site of the ruptured articular capsule and the extent of the spread of pus. If the purulent lesions invade the bone and the epiphysis, the contrast agent can also be developed in bone (epiphysis). X-ray film shows contrast agent surrounding the attachment point of articular capsule, joint structure, and space. If the articular capsule is punctured by pus, the contrast agent will synchronously spread to the soft tissue around the joint.

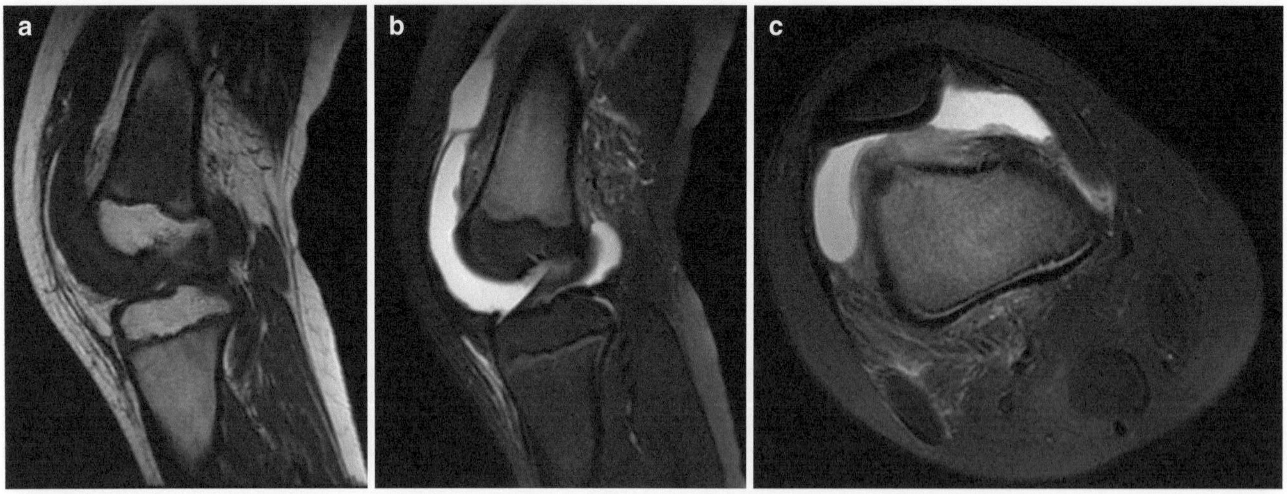

Fig. 6.44 Pyogenic arthritis of right knee joint. (**a**, **b**) Sagittal view on MRI showed articular cavity effusion, local synovial hyperplasia, large patellar hypointense on T_1WI in metaphysis of femur, and hyperintense on fat-suppressed sequence. (**c**) Local cortex was thinned in the articular surface of patellofemoral metaphysis of femur, with limited slightly hyperintense of the bone below

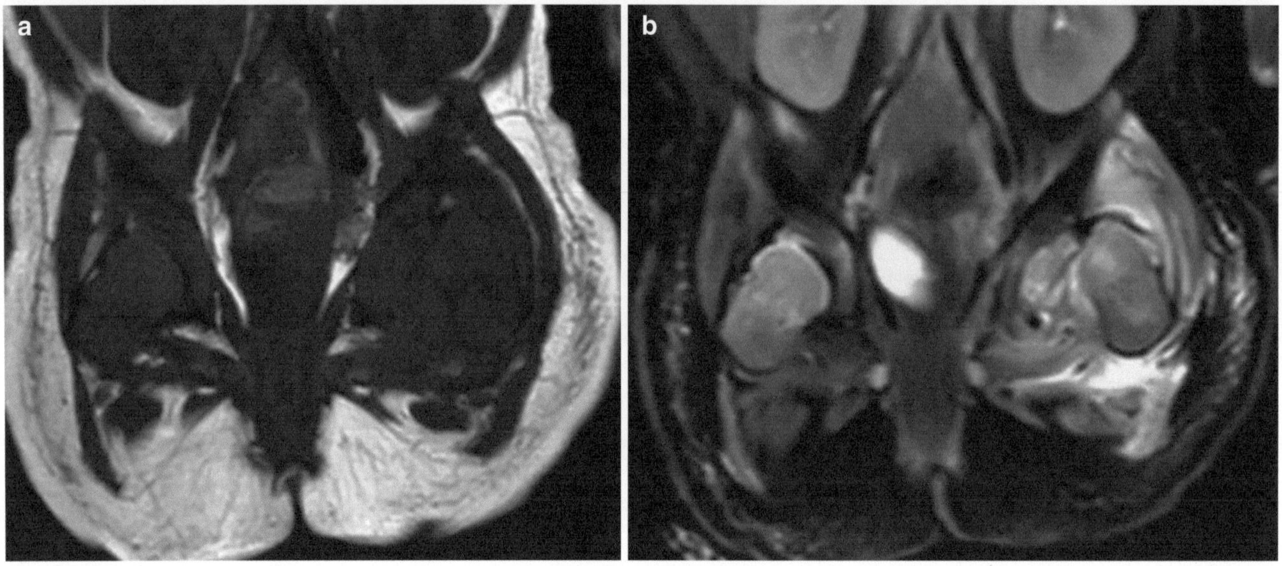

Fig. 6.45 Pyogenic arthritis of left hip joint. MRI showed extensive swelling of soft tissue of the left hip joint, loss of intramuscular fat space, unclear muscle layers, hypointense on T_1WI and hyperintense on T_2WI STIR sequence, with articular cavity effusion and synovial hyperplasia; The epiphysis cartilage was deformed, the epiphysis cartilage and metaphysis intensities were uneven, and the adjacent metaphysis and acetabulum bone marrow showed hyperintense on T_2WI STIR sequence; Left hip joint dislocation, and the round ligament of the femoral head became straight, with uneven intensity; The joint pus punctures the articular capsule to form the hyperintense sinus

Key Points of Diagnosis

1. Acute onset, systematic poisoning symptoms, local acute inflammation symptoms, large joints as predilection sites, onset of single joint and obvious swelling and pressing pain at affected parts.
2. X-ray showed extensive swelling of the joint and surrounding soft tissue, and in the middle stage, the joint space was widened, the articular surface was fuzzy and interrupted, and a radiolucent area was formed under the articular surface. Different degrees of proliferation and sclerosis occurred in surrounding areas, and symptoms such as abnormal joint morphology and bony ankylosis can be seen at the later stage.
3. Non-enhanced CT scan showed joint effusion, empyema, and swelling of surrounding soft tissue. In some cases, small sequestra in the bone destruction area and in the articular cavity can be seen, and in severe cases, joint subluxation occurred.

4. MRI showed synovial thickening, articular cavity effusion and empyema, and articular capsule, ligament, cartilage and other joint structures were damaged. T_2WI fat-suppressed sequence was shown more clearly.
5. Count of leukocyte, neutrophil and C-reactive protein increased, and the erythrocyte sedimentation rate was accelerated.
6. The purulent fluid was drawn from the joint for microscopic examination, gram staining and bacterial culture so as to establish the diagnosis.

Differential Diagnosis

1. **Synovial joint tuberculosis**. The joint tuberculosis starts slowly, with longer course of disease, which has the tuberculosis poisoning symptoms such as low fever and night sweat. The haemal lymphocyte is elevated and localized fusiform swelling of the soft tissue around the joint occurs with the atrophy of adjacent muscle; Osteoporosis appears later, the joint space is narrowed and the bone destruction of the articular surface on the non-weight-bearing side appears. However, the onset of pyogenic arthritis is rapid and progresses rapidly, with high fever and widespread swelling around the joints. The leukocyte and C-reactive protein were elevated, with early appearance of osteoporosis and no obvious muscle atrophy; the joint space can be narrowed in a short period of time, with the bone destruction of weight-bearing articular surface. The erosion and destruction of articular surface in case of tuberculous arthritis is more limited, cystic, less involved in the deep bone marrow, and the pyogenic arthritis is easy to be combined with osteomyelitis and bone marrow edema.
2. **Rheumatoid arthritis (RA).** RA is a systematic connective tissue disease. The disease starts slowly, most in years with multiple joint damage. It usually invades small joints such as hands and ankles symmetrically. The disease is usually found in more than one joint. Lesions begin in synovial membrane and the pannus is formed in the surface of articular cartilage to gradually undermine and absorb articular cartilage, with the bone erosion or cystic bone defect of joint edges, but the edges are sharp and clear, which are different from the fuzzy boundary of pyogenic arthritis, and the feather-like synovial hyperplasia occurs at the attachment point of tendons and ligaments or the laminar periosteal proliferation that is parallel to the diaphysis occurs. As the disease keeps developing, osteoporosis, cystic change under the articular cartilage and joint space stenosis may occur; the bone cortex margin of bony articular surface is less regular; and small cystic bone destruction area may occur below the bony articular surface. At the advanced stage, universal osteoporosis and joint subluxation may occur, and fingers may incline towards the ulnar. The pannus and granulation tissue show marked enhancement after enhancement. The amount of joint effusion is usually less than that of pyogenic arthritis.
3. **Hemophiliac joint hemarthrosis.** The symptoms occur, including joint swelling, space widening, often associated osteoporosis, osteoepiphysis hypertrophy and flat articular surface, which can be identified based on family history and laboratory tests.

Status Quo and Progress of Research

1. PET/CT with an optimal combination of functional and anatomical imaging has opened new frontiers in clinical molecular imaging. Its role in oncology imaging has been well demonstrated and its application in various infections of the musculoskeletal system is being investigated. FDG, ^{18}F-NAF, FDG labeled leukocyte, and ^{68}Ga citrate can be used for infection imaging. FDG PET/CT is not only used for imaging examination of various bone and joint infections, but also used for evaluation and diagnosis of various inflammatory diseases affecting muscles and nerves. In addition, PET/MR imaging, which provides finer details of cartilage, muscle, and nerves, is expected to be a leader in the imaging of musculoskeletal infection, but its use in pediatric patients has been largely limited.

2. MRI can not only show the changes of bone and soft tissue, but also the abnormal changes of synovial membrane, articular cartilage and bone marrow that cannot be shown by plain film or CT. Early assessment of articular cartilage changes by MRI examination is crucial for diagnosis and treatment of early pyogenic arthritis. It is of great value to make differential diagnosis of joint effusion and tendinous sheath effusion after static enhanced scan [70]. DCE-MRI uses the difference of tissue vascularization to identify the causes of synovial membrane involvement in joint lesions according to enhancement patterns and other quantitative derived biomarkers, which is helpful to understand the complex pathophysiological processes of different types of arthritis [71]. Some research results show that T_1-se-cor-water-fil, T_1-flash-3d-water-cor, T_2-me3d-cor, and T_2-me2d-cor are better than the conventional MRI sequence in terms of articular cartilage display, degree of defect and internal intensity [72].

6.7 Osteomyelitis in Infants

Junlin Li and Wei Li

Overview

Infantile osteomyelitis is a special type of osteomyelitis in children. It is a non-specific bone infection caused by pathogens. It is mostly blood-borne infection and occurs in the metaphysis of long bone of infants' limbs, especially in the metaphysis of tibia and humerus. It is secondary to respiratory tract, skin infection, especially the umbilical pyogenic infection, and there is a higher risk of bone infection. The risk of bone infection is higher in the premature and low birth weight infants and high-risk infants who are monitored. Especially, attention should be paid to the sterile operation of umbilical vein intubation and repeated intravenous infusion to prevent the occurrence of this disease. Staphylococcus aureus, group B streptococcus, and Escherichia coli were the most common isolates of bone infection in the neonatal and infant period.

Baby has a special blood supply in long bone metaphysis, the epiphysis, and the epiphyseal plate: the blood supply in the metaphysis originates from the nourishing arteries and perichondrium vessels, forming capillary loops in the metaphysis; the blood supply in the epiphysis originates from epiphyseal vessels (cartilaginous canals) and the metaphyseal vessels; the blood supply in the epiphyseal plate originates from epiphyseal vessels, metaphyseal vessels, and perichondrial vessels in Ranvier zone; therefore, the epiphysis in infancy is connected with the metaphyseal vessels [73, 74].

After 18 months of birth, when the epiphyseal plate is mature and the blood supply barrier is formed, the blood vessels in the epiphyseal plate become occluded and disappear, while the epiphyseal and metaphyseal vessels are not connected, and the epiphysis and the metaphysis have their own independent blood circulation. Therefore, the infection of infantile metaphysis of the long bone often affects the epiphysis and adjacent articular cavity, leading to the injury of epiphysis and epiphyseal plate and forming pyogenic arthritis [75]. At the same time, as part of metaphysis and epiphysis in the hip joint, shoulder joint and ankle joint is located within the joint, the pus, after penetrating cartilage or metaphysis area without periosteum, can directly spread to the articular cavity and be complicated by the pyogenic arthritis and then the articular capsule is damaged; the occurrence of pathological dislocation is the common complication of the disease, so the septic arthritis in infants is mostly caused by osteomyelitis.

In the early stage, the osteomyelitis in infants can form a large number of periosteal new bone and subperiosteal abscess, which is closely related to the infant's bone growth characteristics, because the infant bones are rich in spongy bone with the cortex thin and not dense and are very rich in blood supply and the periosteum is rich in cells and loosely attached to the bone cortex; thus, the bone marrow cavity is easy to communicate with subperiosteal space and the pathogens, in the early stage, are easy to perforate the bone cortex to form subperiosteal abscess, at the same time stimulate the proliferation of the outer membrane of the bone [76]. However, there are abundant osteoblasts and osteoclasts in infancy, which are in the stage of transformation from primitive bone to mature bone, and have strong repair and shaping ability. Generally, chronic osteomyelitis will not be developed, so the sequestrum is rare.

Unlike the clinical manifestations of osteomyelitis in children and adults, the clinical symptoms of osteomyelitis in infants are generally mild, characterized by low fever and local redness and swelling. In terms of physiology, the humoral and cellular immune functions of newborns and infants are not mature, and the body's resistance is low. The septicemia is easy to occur when bacteria enter the blood, and the local response ability to infection is also weaker than that of children. Pain in the affected limb and adjacent joints is a prominent symptom. Pain is caused by increased pressure in the bone marrow cavity due to inflammatory exudation of the lesions, which usually cannot be described by child patients; as a result, the osteomyelitis in newborns and infants is more likely to be missed diagnosis. As infants do not speak, the symptoms are only listlessness, restlessness, irritability, refusal of breasts, and refusal of activities. Careful physical examination can reveal soft tissue swelling, erythema, tenderness, and limitation of motion near joints. The child patients were crying during physical examination.

The erythrocyte sedimentation rate (ESR) and C-reactive protein (CRP) were not significantly accelerated and increased in child patients in the acute stage. However, in the child patient with chronic osteomyelitis, only 65% had changes in erythrocyte sedimentation rate and C-reactive protein, and the count of leukocyte was generally within the normal range. Therefore, pathogen culture results are still one of the golden standards for the diagnosis of epiphysis and osteomyelitis. Due to late visit of infants with acute epiphyseal osteomyelitis, some cases had been treated with antibiotics, so the positive rate of blood culture was very low. Improper collection of culture specimens or preoperative application of antibiotics could also affect the culture results. Culture of wound secretions alone is not enough for diagnosis. More specimens should be taken for culture during surgery, including sinus secretions, pus, soft tissue, and bone scraping objects, especially it is very necessary to culture the secretions around osseous tissue and in the marrow cavity.

Before the epiphyseal ossification of infants in the developmental stage, there are abundant cartilage canals in the epiphyseal cartilage, which are connected with the blood circulation of the whole body. The cartilage canals are the blood supply of supplying the epiphyseal cartilage, and also the base of providing chondroblasts and the birthplace of secondary ossification center. After entering the cartilage canal, bacteria form inflammation and destroy the primary base of chondroblasts, leading to disorder of secondary ossification center and even completely damaged [77, 78].

The formation of inflammatory thrombus in the cartilage canal leads to bad blood supply to the epiphysis, especially to the sites near the epiphyseal plate, and it often leads to the damage of the stationary cell layer and developmental disorder of the epiphyseal plate, resulting in a series of damage to the epiphysis and the epiphyseal plate, which can cause serious posterior deformities that are difficult to treat and often cause lifelong disabilities. For example, the acute osteomyelitis in the proximal femur results in partial destruction, even disappearance of femur epiphysis and femoral neck, causing the growth disorder of femoral head and femoral neck, the varying degrees of limb shortening and hip joint dysfunction, especially the pathological hip joint dislocation caused by the serious damage to the acetabulum is a severe sequela, and the prognosis is poor, which can cause disability in child patients. Therefore, the key to the treatment of osteomyelitis in neonates and infants is early detection and early intervention. Broad-spectrum antibiotics should be used in the early stage of inflammation until the bacterial culture results are obtained and medication should be adjusted. Once clinical diagnosis is made, surgical decompression should be considered to avoid further infection affecting epiphysis or even articular capsule [79].

Pathophysiology

The pathological changes are directly related to the invasion of bacteria. After the bacteria arrive at the local osseous tissue, they can cause the body to produce acute inflammatory reaction in the early stage. The capillaries in the marrow cavity were expanded due to stimulation of various inflammatory factors, resulting in congestion, exudation, and edema of the medullary tissue, and infiltration of a large number of neutrophils, which causes increased pressure in the marrow cavity. As the disease progresses, the local bone trabecula of metaphyseal spongy bone is absorbed and may be accompanied by accumulation of necrotic material, which forms abscesses. Metaphyseal exudate spreads to the subperiosteums along Haversian system and eventually forms subperiosteal abscess, which leads to periosteal reactive hyperplasia. The subperiosteal abscess may further spread to the diaphysis and enter the marrow cavity through the Haversian canal. Bacteria and necrotic materials in the spongy bone of metaphysis can also spread directly to the marrow cavity of diaphysis. Subperiosteal abscesses may also penetrate the periosteum and enter the surrounding soft tissue, leading to soft tissue inflammation and/or abscess formation. The latter can penetrate the skin to form sinus.

Imaging Findings

The long bone metaphysis of infants is rich in spongy bone, in which the blood supply is rich and the blood flow is slow. Therefore, the blood-infected bacteria often stay in the area of metaphyseal spongy bone after entering the nutrient vessels, causing metaphyseal infection. Different directions of expansion for infection focus in metaphysis can lead to inflammation in different sites. The abundant communication blood vessels between the epiphysis and the metaphysis of infants are important bridges for bacteria to invade the epiphysis and even joints. Osteomyelitis in infants less than 1 year old tends to develop to the epiphysis side, leading to joint inflammation. In older children, osteomyelitis is more likely to progress to the diaphysis [73].

1. **Epiphyseal osteomyelitis**. In the early stage, the metaphyseal inflammations were mainly caused by the congestion, edema, and exudation of marrow cavity, while the spread of inflammation through Haversian canal could lead to the cortical destruction, forming subperiosteal abscess, lamellar periosteal reaction, and soft tissue abscess, which may be related to abundant blood supply of infants and loose attachment of periosteum and cortex. MRI has good resolution for soft tissue and is easy to distinguish inflammatory infiltration in the marrow cavity, with slightly hypointense on T_1WI, slightly hyperintense on T_2WI and STIR, and fuzzy boundary (Fig. 6.46a); After the formation of abscess in the marrow cavity, the hypointense is displayed on T_1WI, and the hyperintense is displayed both on T_2WI and STIR (Fig. 6.46b); The involved bone cortex showed fuzzy and coarse hypointense, while subperiosteal abscess, periosteal reaction, and soft tissue abscess were common near bone cortex, with isointense or slightly hypointense on T_1WI and hyperintense on T_2WI [80].
2. **Epiphyseal osteomyelitis in the epiphysis.** The epiphyseal lesions in the long bone involve the epiphysis, the epiphyseal plate, and the joints. X-ray and CT showed low-density lesions in the bone with blurred margins (Fig. 6.47a). In severe cases, epiphysis separation and migration can be seen. The bone cortex of the long bone metaphysis is fuzzy and coarse. In severe cases, lamellar periosteal reaction and soft tissue swelling can be seen near the bone cortex. MRI mainly showed slightly hypointense on T_1WI and slightly hyperintense on T_2WI in the secondary ossification center within the epiphysis, and the

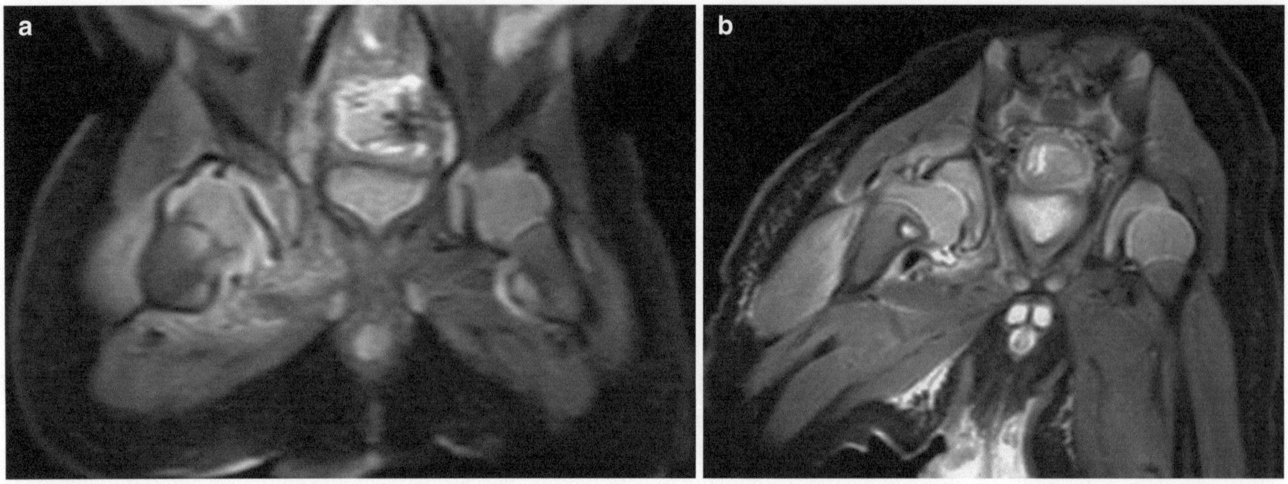

Fig. 6.46 Osteomyelitis near metaphysis in right femur. (**a**) MRI showed inflammatory infiltration in the metaphyseal marrow cavity of the right femur with slightly hyperintense on STIR and fuzzy boundary; (**b**) In the same child patient, small abscesses were formed from the lesions near the metaphysis of the right femur, with hyperintense in the center of STIR sequence and annular slightly hypointense around. Mild dislocation of the hip joint was observed, and edema of peripheral tissues was aggravated in the hip joint, presenting flaky hyperintense

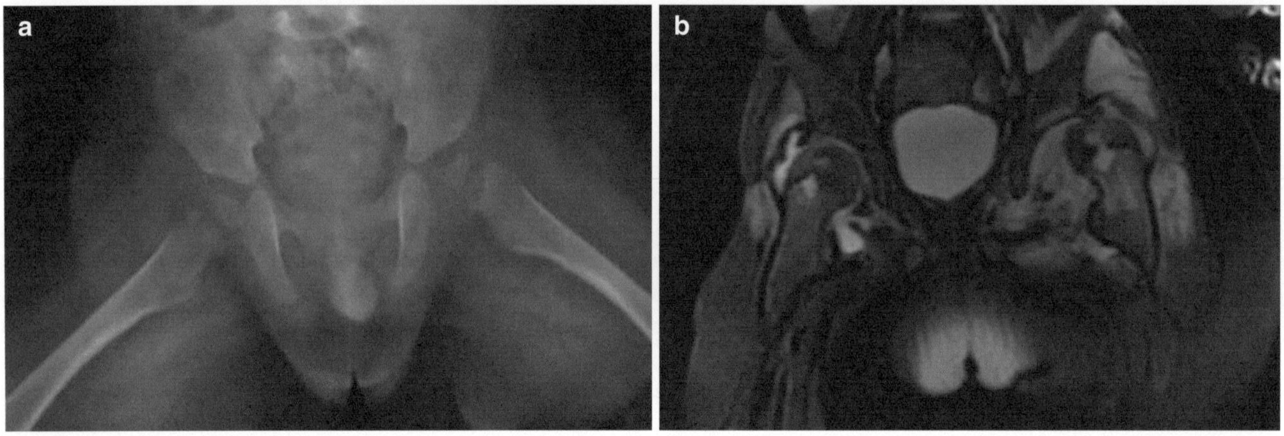

Fig. 6.47 Epiphyseal osteomyelitis in the proximal epiphysis of both femurs. (**a**) Frog DR showed that there were orbicular-ovate low-density shadows in the proximal epiphysis and metaphyseal bones of both femurs, with fuzzy margins, the metaphyseal bone density of femur was slightly decreased, and the soft tissue density around hip joint was increased; (**b**) T_2WI STIR sequence showed irregular hyperintense shadow on T_2WI in proximal epiphysis and metaphysis bones of both femurs, and the metaphysis plate was perforated and connected, with the peripheral bones presenting slightly hyperintense on T_2WI; synovial hyperplasia and effusion were observed in the hip joint; the edema of peripheral tissues in the hip joint was heavy, with patchy hyperintense, especially in the left hip joint, accompanied by joint subluxation

lesions in epiphyseal cartilage and epiphyseal plate present isointense or slightly hypointense on T_1WI and hyperintense on T_2WI and STIR sequence, with blurring or clear margins, and some lesions break through epiphyseal cartilage to communicate with the articular cavity. The focus of infection in the bone can lead to synovial hyperemia, edema, and leukocyte infiltration after spreading to the articular cavity, with the exudate accumulated in the articular cavity. The main manifestations were expansion of articular cavity, joint effusion, and synovial thickening. The thickened synovial membrane presented isointense on T_1WI and slightly hyperintense on T_2WI (Fig. 6.47b). Enhanced scan showed marked enhancement of the thickened synovial membrane, with the width < 2 mm and regular margins [79, 81–83].

3. **Osteomyelitis in the diaphysis.** It is mainly caused by the metaphyseal inflammation expanding to the marrow cavity or the subperiosteal inflammation re-entering the distal bone marrow cavity through the bone cortex. X-ray and CT showed extensive bone destruction and layered and lacerated periosteal reaction in the diaphysis (Figs. 6.48, 6.49, and 6.50a). MRI showed extensive and slightly hypointense on T_1WI and slightly hyperintense on T_2WI in the marrow cavity of the diaphysis, with fuzzy and rough bone cortex, and a large amount of layered periosteal reaction can be seen in the margins of diaphy-

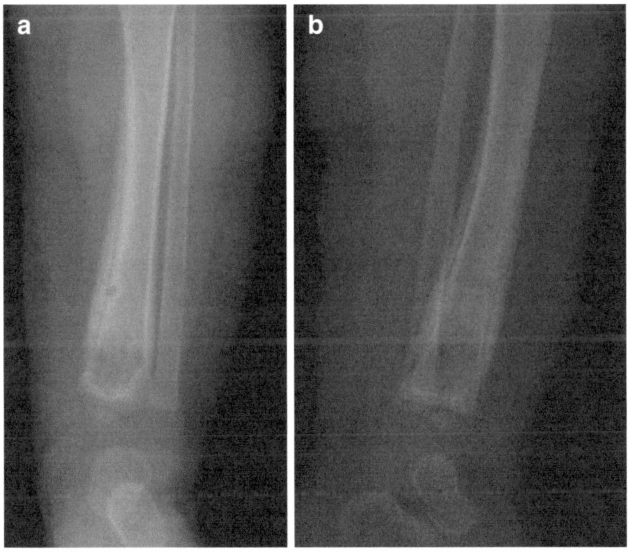

Fig. 6.48 Diaphyseal osteomyelitis in the left tibia (1). Worm-eaten bone destruction in the distal diaphysis of the left tibia can be seen, the metaphysis density was reduced, with extensive lamellar periosteal reaction in the diaphysis

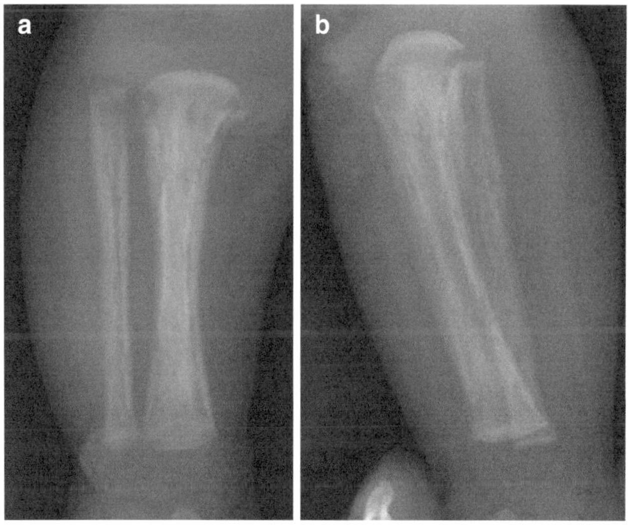

Fig. 6.49 Diaphyseal osteomyelitis in the right tibia (2). In the diaphysis of right tibia, there were multiple worm-eaten bone destruction, with obviously heterogeneous bone mineral density and extensive layered periosteal reaction in the diaphysis

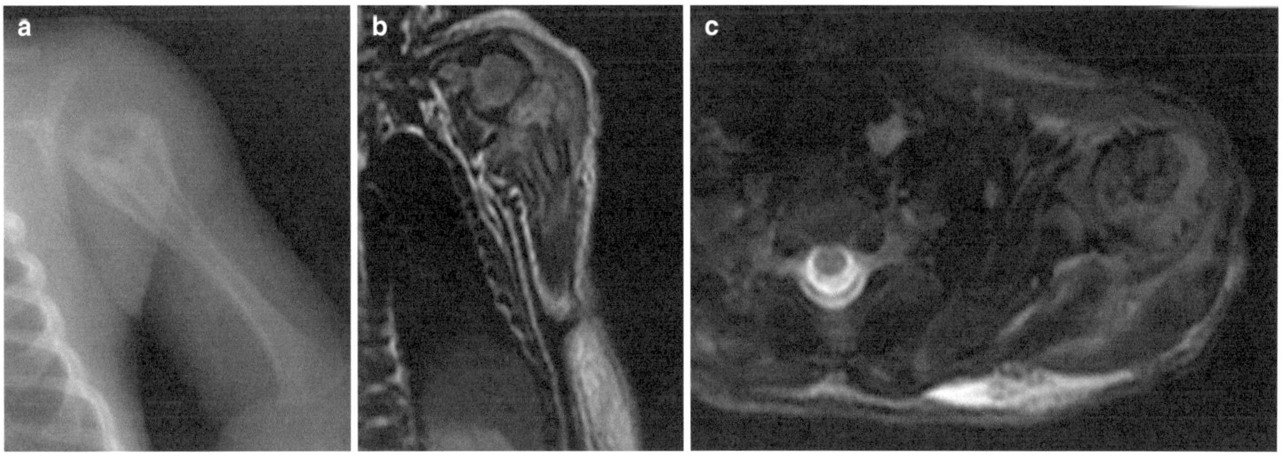

Fig. 6.50 Diaphyseal osteomyelitis in the left humerus (2). (**a**) DR showed that there was multiple irregular bone destruction in the metaphysis and diaphysis of the left humerus, with significantly heterogeneous bone mineral density, heterogeneous decrease of the density of the marrow cavity, extensive lamellar periosteal reaction, swelling and increased density of surrounding soft tissue; (**b**) MRI T_2WI showed that the morphology of diaphysis and proximal metaphysis of the left humerus were incomplete, presenting a heterogeneous slightly hyperintense on T_2WI, and the surrounding soft tissue presented a patchy hyperintense on T_2WI; (**c**) T_2WI showed an heterogeneous increase in intensity of left humerus, a rough bone cortex, and a patchy heterogeneous hyperintense on T_2WI in the surrounding soft tissue

sis; The surrounding soft tissue was swollen, with isointense or slightly hypointense on T_1WI and hyperintense on T_2WI [84] (Figs. 6.50b, c and 6.51).

Key Points of Diagnosis]

1. It usually occurs in the long bone of extremities, especially the tibia, femur, and humerus.
2. In the early stage, soft tissue swelling and massive periosteal new bone and subperiosteal abscess can be seen.
3. The sequestrum is rare.
4. It is easy to involve epiphysis and invade adjacent joints, forming pyogenic arthritis.
5. Sometimes pathologic fracture and joint dislocation can be seen, and the diseased bones can grow or shorten and also can produce obvious deformity.

Differential Diagnosis

1. **Metaphyseal tuberculosis in the epiphysis**. In the early stage, it has the local osteoporosis, followed by blotchy, round, or ovoid bone destruction with clear margins, and

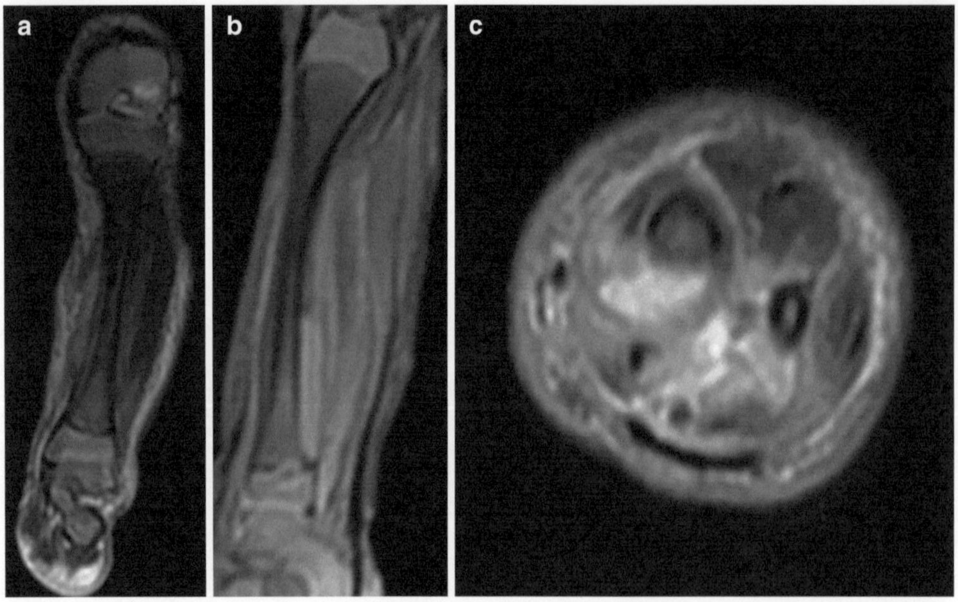

Fig. 6.51 Diaphyseal osteomyelitis in the left tibia (2). (**a**) MRI T_1WI showed a slightly hypointense on T_1WI in the diaphysis of left tibia and a heterogeneous hypointense on T_1WI in the surrounding soft tissue; (**b**) The sagittal plane of T_2WI showed the intensity of left tibia was heterogeneous and increased, and the strip-like hyperintense on T_2WI was observed beside the lower segment of bone, and the surrounding soft tissue presented patchy and inhomogeneous hyperintense on T_2WI. (**c**) The transverse plane of T_2WI fat-suppressed sequence showed the intensity of the left tibia was heterogeneous and increased, with heterogeneous cortical thickness, patchy hyperintense on T_2WI at the side of the bone, and patchy heterogeneous hyperintense in the surrounding soft tissue

clastic sequestrum can be seen in the area of bone destruction with rare periosteal reaction, mild soft tissue swelling, but significant osteoporosis; The periosteal reaction and soft tissue swelling of epiphyseal osteomyelitis in the epiphysis of infants are obvious, and less sequestrum is formed.

2. **Infantile cortical hyperostosis**. The lesions are self-limited. New bone is formed in the swollen soft tissue adjacent to the affected bone. The density increases progressively and the massive deposited bone is fused with osseous tissue, and the bone marrow cavity becomes narrowed.
3. **Ewing's sarcoma**. It usually occurs in the long bones of children and adolescents aged 10 ~ 15 years, and the characteristic manifestations are the infiltrative osteolytic changes with scallion skin, vertical radiating and cuff-like periosteal reaction. The onset age is older, and the middle part of diaphysis of long bones is more common, which is mostly manifested as patchy infiltrating bone destruction centered on the marrow cavity, without the formation of sequestrum, often accompanied by the formation of Codman triangle, and for typical cases, there are thin, short, and vertical shadows of bone spicule. The course of the disease is slower than acute osteomyelitis, and there are large soft tissue masses in the early stage, which are smaller than the range of bone destruction area. The range of lesions can be narrowed after radiotherapy.

Status Quo and Progress of Research

Enhanced MRI is a useful supplementary means to the diagnosis of osteomyelitis, which can improve the diagnostic ability of bone infection and its complications. When osteomyelitis involved in the epiphyseal plate, it could only be seen on the gadolinium-enhanced T_1WI sequence, but not on the non-contrast T_1WI and liquid sensitive sequence, which was manifested as weakened epiphysis cartilage enhancement, or even no local enhancement, otherwise it should be uniformly enhanced. Since infection of the epiphyseal plate in infancy can cause growth disorders, the gadolinium-enhanced MRI is recommended for infants with suspected bone infections [29, 85].

References

1. Zhenhua W, Lijun Z. Clinical imaging of pediatric bone and joint. Beijing: People's Medical Publishing House; 2012.
2. Zhenhua W, Xu D. Atlas of imaging diagnosis for osteoarticular disease. Hefei: Anhui Science & Technology Press; 2001.
3. Jingxue L, Dingyuan S. X-ray diagnostics of bone and joint. Beijing: People's Medical Publishing House; 1982.
4. Qiyong G. Practical radiology. 3rd ed. Beijing: People's Medical Publishing House; 2007.
5. Koo KH, Dussault R, Kaplan P, et al. Age-related marrow conversion in the proximal metaphysis of the femur: evaluation with T_1-weighted MR imaging. Radiology. 1998;206(3):745–8.
6. Wu Z, Yang B, Pan S, et al. MRI evaluation of bone marrow of normal lumbar vertebra in the Chinese: normal patterns and preliminary quantitative study. Chin Med J. 1999;112(9):646–8.

7. Zawin JK, Jaramillo D. Conversion of bone marrow in the humerus, sternum, and clavicle:changes with age on MR images. Radiology. 1993;188(1):159–64.
8. Hong S, Yuhua L, Wang Q, et al. Conversion of bone marrow signal of normal children's femur on MRI. Chin J Med Imag Technol. 2006;22(4):597–9.
9. Lattar SM, Tuchscherr LP, Centron D, et al. Molecular finger printing of Staphylococcus aureus isolated from patients with osteomyelitis in Argentina and clonal distribution of the cap5(8) genes and of other selected virulence genes. Eur J Clin Microbiol Infect Dis. 2012;31(10):2559–66.
10. Mc Carthy AJ, Lindsay JA. Genetic variation in Staphylococcus aureus surface and immune evasion genes is lineage associated: implications for vaccine design and hos-pathogen interactions. BMC Microbiol. 2010;10:173.
11. Lingxia Z, Xianzhi Z. Modern Epidemiology. 2nd ed. Beijing: People's Military Medical Press; 2010.
12. Adetunji SA, Ramirez G, Foster MJ, et al. A systematic review and meta-analysis of the prevalence of osteoarticular brucellosis. PLoS Negl Trop Dis. 2019;13(1):e0007112.
13. Zheng R, Xie S, Lu X, et al. A systematic review and meta-analysis of epidemiology and clinical manifestations of human brucellosis in China. Bio Med Res Int. 2018;1:1–10.
14. De Backer AI, Vanhoenacker FM, Sanghvi DA. Imaging features of extraaxial musculoskeletal tuberculosis. Indian J Radiol Imaging. 2009;19(3):176–86.
15. Nouroallahian M, Bakhshaee M, Afzalzadeh MR, et al. A hydatid cyst in an unusual location-the infratemporal fossa. The Laryngoscope. 2013;123(2):407–9.
16. Melissa DJ, John RP. Fungal infections of the bones and joints. Curr Infect Dis Rep. 2007;3(5):450–60.
17. Chen S, Chen Y, Zhou YQ, et al. Candida glabrata-induced refractory infectious arthritis: a case report and literature review. Mycopathologia. 2019;184(2):283–93.
18. Elias JA, Michael RM, Michael AP. Clinical mycology. 2nd ed. Amsterdam: Elsevier; 2009. p. 525–45.
19. Hung CY, Hsu AP, Holland SM, et al. A review of innate and adaptive immunity to coccidioidomycosis. Med Mycol. 2019;57(Suppl1):S85–92.
20. Fuquan L, Qianqiu W. Acquired syphilis in children. Chinese Journal of Dermatology. 2012;45(5):372–3.
21. Johnston JJ, Murray-Krezan C, Dehority W. Suppurative complications of acute hematogenous osteomyelitis in children. J Pediatric Orthop B. 2017;26(6):491–6.
22. Keren R, Shah SS, Srivastava R, et al. Comparative effectiveness of intravenous vs oral antibiotics for postdischarge treatment of acute osteomyelitis in children. JAMA Pediatr. 2015;169(2):120–8.
23. Santiago RC, Giménez CR, McCarthy K. Imaging of osteomyelitis and musculoskeletal soft tissue infections: current concepts. Rheum Dis Clin North Am. 2003;29(1):89–109.
24. Dodwell ER. Osteomyelitis and septic arthritis in children: current concepts. Curr Opin Pediatr. 2013;25(l):58–63.
25. Yagupsky P. Microbiological diagnosis of skeletal system infections in children. Curr Pediatr Rev. 2019;15(3):154–63.
26. Willegger M, Kolb A, Windhager R, et al. Acute haematogenous osteomyelitis in children: diagnostic algorithm and treatment strategies. Orthopade. 2017;46(6):541–56.
27. Douis H, Davies MA, Sian P. The role of diffusion-weighted MR (I DWI) in the differentiation of benign from malignant skeletal lesions of the pelvis. Eur J Radiol. 2016;85(12):2262–8.
28. Averill LW, Hernandez A, Gonzalez L, et al. Diagnosis of osteomyelitis in children: utility of fat-suppressed contrast-enhanced MRI. Am J Roentgenol. 2009;192(5):1232–8.
29. Pugmire BS, Shailam R, Gee MS. Role of MRI in the diagnosis and treatment of osteomyelitis in pediatric patients. World J Radiol. 2014;6(8):530–7.
30. Browne LP, Guillerman RP, Orth RC, et al. Community-acquired staphylococcal musculoskeletal infection in infants and young children: necessity of contrast-enhanced MRI for the diagnosis of growth cartilage involvement. Am J Roentgenol. 2012;198(1):194–9.
31. Leclair N, Thörmer G, Sorge I, et al. Whole-body diffusion-weighted imaging in chronic recurrent multifocal osteomyelitis in children. PLoS One. 2016;11(1):e0147523.
32. Dartnell J, Ramachandran M, Katchburian M. Haematogenous acute and subacute paediatric osteomyelitis:a systematic review of the literature. J Bone Joint Surg Br. 2012;94(5):584–95.
33. Gigante A, Coppa V, Marinelli M, et al. Acute osteomyelitis and septic arthritis in children: a systematic review of systematic reviews. Eur Rev Med Pharmacol Sci. 2019;23(2 Suppl):145–58.
34. Ceroni D, Cherkaoui A, Ferey S, et al. Kingella kingae osteoarticular infections in young children: clinical features and contribution of a new specific real-time PCR assay to the diagnosis. J Pediatr Orthop. 2010;30(3):301–4.
35. Merlini L, Anooshiravani M, Ceroni D. Concomitant septic arthritis and osteomyelitis of the hip in young children: a new pathophysiological hypothesis suggested by MRI enhancement pattern. BMC Med Imaging. 2015;15:17.
36. Warmann SW, Dittmann H, Seitz G, et al. Follow-up of acute osteomyelitis in children: the possible role of PET/CT in selected cases. Pediatr Surg. 2011;46(8):1550–6.
37. Horger M, Eschmann SM, Pfannenberg C, et al. The value of SPET/ CT in chronic osteomyelitis. Eur J Nucl Med Mol Imaging. 2003;30(12):1665–73.
38. Foster CE, Taylor M, Schallert EK, et al. Brodie abscess in children: a 10-year single institution retrospective review. Pediatr Infect Dis J. 2019;38(2):32–4.
39. van der Naald N, Smeeing DPJ, Houwert RM. Brodie's abscess: a systematic review of reported cases. J Bone Jt Infect. 2019;4(1):33–9.
40. Abdulhadi MA, White AM, Pollock AN. Brodie abscess. Pediatr Emerg Care. 2012;28(11):1249–51.
41. Qi R, Colmegna I. Brodie abscess. CMAJ. 2017;189(3):117.
42. Heng Z, Fei C, Yi L, et al. A case of brodie abscess involving epiphyseal plate. Chin Med J. 2018;98(17):1366–7.
43. Hourston GJ, Kankam HK, Mitchell PD, et al. Brodie abscess of the femoral capital epiphysis in a 2-year-old child caused by *Kingella kingae*. BMJ Case Rep. 2017;2017:bcr2016217663.
44. Ogbonna OH, Paul Y, Nabhani H, et al. Brodie's abscess in a patient presenting with sickle cell vasoocclusive crisis. Case Rep Med. 2015;2015:429876.
45. Dangman BC, Hoffer FA, Rand FF, et al. Osteomyelitis in children: gadolinium-enhanced MR imaging. Radiology. 1992;182(3):743–7.
46. Taj-Aldeen SJ, Rammaert B, Gamaletsou M, et al. Osteoarticular infections caused by non-aspergillus filamentous fungi in adult and pediatric patients: a systematic review. Medicine (Baltimore). 2015;94(50):e2078.
47. Dotis J, Roilides E. Osteomyelitis due to Aspergillus species in chronic granulomatous disease: an update of the literature. Mycoses. 2011;54(6):e686–96.
48. Henry MW, Miller AO, Walsh TJ, et al. Fungal musculoskeletal infections. Infect Dis Clin N Am. 2017;31(2):353–68.
49. Taj-Aldeen SJ, Gamaletsou MN, Rammaert B, et al. Bone and joint infections caused by mucormycetes: a challenging osteoarticular mycosis of the twenty-first century. Med Mycol. 2017;55(7):691–704.
50. Caro AK, Stanley CD. Fungal infection of bone and joint. Infect. 2018;3(2):525–45.
51. Davies G, Rolle AM, Maurer A, et al. Towards translational immune PET/MR imaging of invasive pulmonary aspergillosis: the humanised monoclonal antibody detects aspergillus lung infections in vivo. Theranostics. 2017;7(14):3398–414.

52. Belthur MV, Blair JE, Shrader MW, et al. Musculoskeletal coccidioidomycosis. Curr Orthop Pract. 2018;29(4):400–6.
53. Leroy-Freschini B, Treglia G, Argemi X, et al. 18F-FDG PET/CT for invasive fungal infection in immunocompromised patients. QJM. 2018;111(9):613–22.
54. Marinho de Souza J, Giuffrida R, et al. Mother-to-child transmission and gestational syphilis: spatial-temporal epidemiology and demographics in a Brazilian region. PLoS Negl Trop Dis. 2019;13(2):e0007122.
55. Simms I, Tookey PA, Goh BT, et al. The incidence of congenital syphilis in the United Kingdom: February 2010 to January 2015. BJOG. 2017;124(1):72–7.
56. Liang X, Liu T, Yuan C, et al. The disappearance of femoral head and neck resulting from extensive bone defect caused by secondary syphilis: a case report and literature review. BMC Musculoskelet Disord. 2018;19(1):251.
57. Fuquan L, Qianqiu W. Acquired syphilis in children. Chin J Dermatol. 2012;45(5):372–3.
58. Greenall J, Kumar N, Abdelmagid E. Early congenital syphilis in a premature baby. Eur J Pediatr. 2011;170(5):667–9.
59. Jun L, Shitai L, Donglai M, et al. A case of acquired syphilis in children. Chin J Dermatol. 2003;36(5):280.
60. Qing Z, Hejian S, Minhua S, et al. A case of infant acquired syphilis caused by chewing food feeding. Chin J Pediatr. 2010;48(9):679.
61. Wang LJ, Wu HB, Zhou WL, et al. Gummatous syphilis mimicking malignant bone tumor on FDG PET/CT. Clin Nucl Med. 2019;44(4):313–6.
62. Gameiro VS, Labronici PJ, Rosa IMA. Congenital syphilis with bone lesion: case report. Rev Bras Ortop. 2017;52(6):740–2.
63. Chen JH, Zheng X, Liu XQ. Usefulness of positron emission tomography in patients with syphilis: systematic review of observational studies. Chin Med J. 2017;130(9):1100–12.
64. Kim JM, Lee SM, Bae SB, et al. The role of PET/CT in diagnosing generalized lymphadenopathy in asymptomatic secondary syphilis. Hell J Nucl Med. 2016;19(1):60–2.
65. Manz N, Krieg AH, Heininger U, et al. Evaluation of the current use of imaging modalities and pathogen detection in children with acute osteomyelitis and septic arthritis. Eur J Pediatr. 2018;177(7):1071–80.
66. Ben-Zvi L, Sebag D, Izhaki G. Diagnosis and management of infectious arthritis in children. Curr Infect Dis Rep. 2019;21(7):23.
67. Qiyong G. Applied radiology. 3rd ed. Beijing: The People's Medical Publishing House; 2007.
68. Pineda C, Espinosa R, Pena A. Radiogra phicimagingin osteomyelitis: the role of plain radiography, computed tomography, ultrasonography, magnetic resonance imaging, and scintigraphy. Semin Plast Surg. 2009;23(2):80–9.
69. Goto H, Iwama Y, Fujii M, et al. A preliminary study of the T1 rho values of normal knee cartilage using 3T-MRI. Eur J Radiol. 2012;81(7):e796–803.
70. Yuming Y, Shinong P. Clinical application of MR arthrography. Chin J Radiol. 2012;46(3):197–202.
71. Martín Noguerol T, Luna A, Gómez Cabrera M, et al. Clinical applications of advanced magnetic resonance imaging techniques for arthritis evaluation. World J Orthop. 2017;8(9):660–73.
72. Crema MD, Roemer FW, Marra MD, et al. Articular cartilage in the knee: current MR imaging techniques and applications in clinical practice and research. Radiographics. 2011;31(1):37–61.
73. Ogden JA. Pediatric osteomyelitis and septic arthritis: the pathology of neonatal disease. Yale J Biol Med. 1979;52(5):423–48.
74. Kaye JJ, Winchester PH, Freiberger RH. Neonatal septic "dislocation" of the hip: true dislocation or pathological epiphyseal separation. Radiology. 1975;114:671–4.
75. Ogden JA, Light TR. Pediatric osteomyelitis: III. Anaerobic microorganisms. Clin Orthop Relat Res. 1979;145:230–6.
76. Allwright SJ, Miller JH, Gilsanz V. Subperiosteal abscess in children: scintigraphic appearance. Radiology. 1991;179(3):725–9.
77. Offiah AC. Acute osteomyelitis, septic arthritis and discitis: differences between neonates and older children. Eur J Radiol. 2006;60(2):221–32.
78. Sheikh HQ, Aqil A, Kirby A, et al. Panton-Valentine leukocidin osteomyelitis in children: a growing threat. Br J Hosp Med (Lond). 2015;76(1):18–24.
79. El Houmami N, Minodier P, Bouvier C, et al. Primary subacute epiphyseal osteomyelitis caused by Mycobacterium species in young children: a modern diagnostic approach. Eur J Clin Microbiol Infect Dis. 2017;36(5):771–7.
80. Agarwal A, Gupta N, Mishra M, et al. Primary epiphyseal and metaepiphyseal tubercular osteomyelitis in children a series of 8 case. Acta Orthop Belg. 2016;82(4):797–805.
81. Green NE, Beauchamp RD, Griffin PP, et al. Primary subacute epiphyseal osteomyelitis. J Bone Joint Surg Am. 1981;63(1):107–14.
82. Hara H, Akisue T, Kawamoto T, et al. Sequential MR images and radiographs of epiphyseal osteomyelitis in the distal femur of an infant. Case Rep Radiol. 2013;2013:672–81.
83. Sorensen TS, Hedeboe J, Christensen ER, et al. Primary epiphyseal osteomyelitis in children. Report of three cases and review of the literature. J Bone Joint Surg Br. 1988;70(5):818–20.
84. Kim BK, Dan J, Lee YS, et al. Salmonella osteomyelitis of the femoral diaphysis in a healthy individual. Am J Orthop (Belle Mead NJ). 2014;43(10):E237–9.
85. Browne LP, Guillerman RP, Orth RC, et al. Community-acquired staphylococcal musculoskeletal infection in infants and young children: necessity of contrast-enhanced MRI for the diagnosis of growth cartilage involvement. AJR Am J Roentgenol. 2012;198(1):194–9.

AIDS-Related Musculoskeletal Diseases

7

Li Li, Jing Zhao, Shi Qi, and Dechun Li

Patients with HIV infection/AIDS are more prone to a series of musculoskeletal complications, and their clinical manifestations are similar to those of non-AIDS patients. In contrast, patients with HIV infection/AIDS may present with atypical sites of involvement, incomplete arthritic manifestations, and/or infrequent organ involvement. As the effectiveness of reverse transcriptional therapy, the survival time of AIDS patients is prolonged and the incidence of musculoskeletal diseases in AIDS patients is rising; therefore, the prevalence of AIDS-related musculoskeletal diseases is increasingly associated with non-AIDS-identified comorbidities.

Complications of musculoskeletal system include infection, inflammation, tumor, etc. Among them, infection is the most common. A variety of factors may lead to the occurrence of musculoskeletal system complications, including the immunosuppression of the patient, the virus itself and other immune, environmental, and genetic factors. HIV infection impairs T lymphocytes responses and weakens the body's defense mechanisms, which causes the patients to opportunistic infections, immune-related tumors, and inflammatory lesions.

Soft tissue infections include superficial and deep cellulitis, necrotizing and non-necrotizing fasciitis, soft tissue abscesses, and pyomyositis. Osteoarthritis infection can cause osteomyelitis and pyogenic arthritis. The most common pathogen is staphylococcus aureus, but other pathogens have also been reported.

Imaging diagnosis of musculoskeletal disease in patients with HIV infection/AIDS is the same as routine imaging findings in patients with other infections, joint diseases, or tumors. The differential diagnosis of HIV infection/AIDS needs to be extended, especially in terms of infection, because it may threaten the lives of patients with HIV infection/AIDS.

X-ray plain film is the primary imaging examination for suspected musculoskeletal disease in patients with HIV infection/AIDS. In case of suspected infection, X-ray plain film may show soft tissue swelling, pneumatosis, and blurry and/or destruction of the bone cortex. As X-ray signs of acute osteomyelitis may be delayed by 2 weeks, CT examination is necessary. Although X-ray plain film has limited sensitivity to fasciitis and muscle infection, it may show the edema and the ambiguity of soft tissue layer and may also show soft tissue gas shadows in some cases. X-ray plain films of pyogenic arthritis often present soft tissue swelling and joint effusion, or without erosion and loss of cartilage. When fungi or Mycobacterium tuberculosis invades the joint, effusion and periarticular osteoporosis are not easily detected and diagnosed on X-ray plain film.

CT helps to show calcification, multiple osteolytic lesions, soft tissue gas, and abscesses and to differentiate sequestrum from active chronic osteomyelitis. Its advantages lie in its convenience, feasibility, and rapid examination in an emergency, as well as its assistance in planning and guiding puncture and drainage.

Although MRI may not be as feasible as CT in emergency situations, it can provide better contrast of soft tissue in images of muscles, joint structures, tumors, and bone marrow. When a tumor or infection is suspected, CT or MRI enhanced scans can show more clearly the lesions, including fistula, fluid accumulation, and the extent of soft tissue invasion. MRI enhanced scan also helps in the identification of blood vessel inactivation and/or necrotic tissue. The capsule and pseudomembrane were shown more clearly after the contrast agent is injected, which can better display the abscess, bursitis, and fasciitis.

L. Li (✉) · J. Zhao · S. Qi
Department of Radiology, Beijing Youan Hospital, Capital Medical University, Beijing, China
e-mail: 15001017169@139.com

D. Li
Department of Radiology, Xuzhou Central Hospital, Xuzhou, Jiangsu, China

H. Li et al. (eds.), *Radiology of Infectious and Inflammatory Diseases - Volume 5*,
https://doi.org/10.1007/978-981-16-5003-1_7

7.1 Osteomyelitis

Shi Qi and Jing Zhao

Overview

Osteomyelitis in AIDS patients is generally caused by bleeding, injury, and adjacent soft tissue infection. Although immune system of AIDS patients is damaged, opportunistic pathogens are not the main pathogens causing AIDS osteomyelitis. Staphylococcus aureus is the most common pathogens, and some patients are infected with a variety of microorganisms [1], which, for example, Staphylococcus aureus can be combined with Cryptococcus neoformans and Nocardia asteroides to cause disease. Wang Qing et al. [2] reported a case of infection with two kinds of opportunistic pathogens, including Haemophilus aphrophilus and anaerobe. Some scholars also believe that patients with HIV infection are often complicated by Mycobacterium tuberculosis infection, so Mycobacterium tuberculosis is the most common pathogen of AIDS complicated with osteomyelitis [3]. The wrist, tibia, femur, thoracic cage, and thoracolumbar segment of the spine are the most frequently affected sites.

Sudden onset occurs in patients, and in the acute phase, they may have high fever, chills, and other systemic symptoms. The local pain of the affected limb was severe. Examination showed that the skin was red, swollen, hot, and painful, with significant tenderness and limitation of motion.

Pathophysiology

1. **Prophase of subperiosteal abscess**. On the 2nd ~ third day after onset, extensive inflammatory infiltration occurs in the bone marrow, the venous sinuses are destroyed, and there is a small amount of pus and blood.
2. **Stage of subperiosteal abscess**. On the 3rd ~ fourth day after onset, more pus was formed in the bone marrow cavity, which reached the periosteum to form the subperiosteal abscess through the Haversian canal of bone cortex. The periosteum is stripped and the branches into the bone where the periosteum vessels enter are completely interrupted.
3. **Periosteum destruction period.** On the 5th ~ sixth day after onset, the periosteum ruptures and the pus spreads. At this point, extensive bone and soft tissue necrosis may occur, and pyemia may easily occur.

Imaging Findings

1. **X-ray.** Within 2 weeks of the onset, there were no obvious abnormalities on X-ray examination of acute suppurative osteomyelitis. 10 ~ 14 days after onset, bone changes may occur when cytolytic enzymes cause obvious periosteal reaction [4]. In the early stage, there were tiny cracks in the cortex with villous changes, which were caused by bone marrow edema, venous stasis, and osteoclast activity. In the late stage, lesions were not significantly different from the common osteomyelitis, with bone destruction, sclerosis, sequestrum formation, periosteal proliferation, and other changes (Fig. 7.1).
2. **CT** shows the lesions very well, especially early lesions. CT findings include periosteal reaction, change of bone marrow density, local destruction of bone cortex, bone trabecula thickening, formation of sequestrum, and soft tissue swelling.
3. **MRI** is the best imaging method for soft tissue and bone marrow lesions. The general sequences include T_1WI, T_2WI, and STIR. MRI can clearly show the range of inflammatory infiltration and edema in bone, showing hypointense on T_1WI and hyperintense on T_2WI. MRI is superior to CT in the display of intra-osseous and subperiosteal abscesses and soft tissue abscesses. The abscess on the enhanced T_1WI sequence was hypointense, surrounded by enhancement rings; The edema and fibrous tissue present hypointense, and the granuloma and pannus present hyperintense (Fig. 7.2). The enhanced scan can improve the assessment of the extent of bone and soft tissue infection. In addition, the SESS and FSE sequences of MRI can form a significant contrast between normal and pathological tissues. IR sequences help to show slight changes in fat, water, or bone marrow caused by inflammation by inhibiting the adipose tissue in the bone marrow.

Key Points of Diagnosis

1. Its clinical manifestations include fever, chill, pain and swelling of the affected limb and obvious tenderness.
2. The images showed varying degrees of bone destruction, formation of periosteum new bone and sequestrum, and secondary ulcers, fistulas, cellulitis, and abscesses around the affected bone.
3. Laboratory tests showed an elevated total count of leukocyte.

Differential Diagnosis

Osteomyelitis should be distinguished from osteosarcoma. Osteosarcoma is mainly characterized by bone destruction, mass, and tumor bone. Due to its aggressive and destructive nature, osteosarcoma often penetrates periosteum and grows outward, forming a Codman triangle. Osteomyelitis often presents extensive periosteal proliferation, mainly lamellar periosteal reaction, even though the destruction of bone cortex is small. Although the bone destruction was also considered as the main manifestation, the repair and hyperostosis were almost simultaneous, and the increase of bone

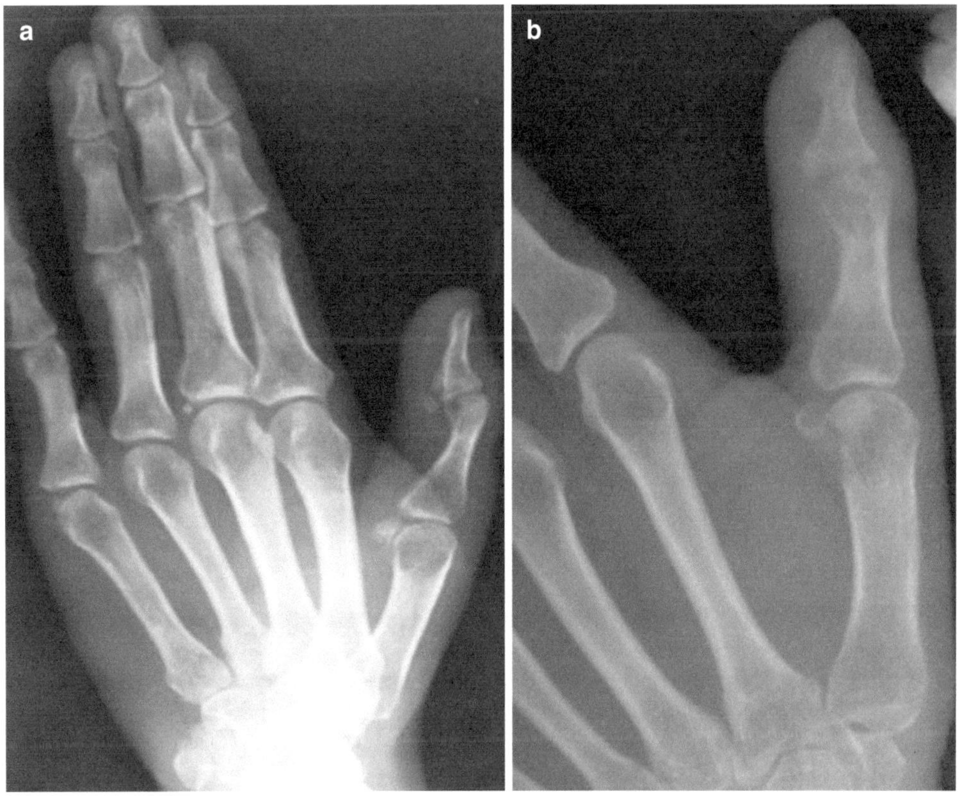

Fig. 7.1 AIDS-associated osteomyelitis (1). (**a** and **b**) X-ray plain film showed swelling of soft tissue around the interphalanx joint, osteoporosis around the joint, blurring of joint space, worm-eaten changes of articular surface, multiple small cystic low-density areas

mineral density around bone destruction was its important characteristic.

Status Quo and Progress of Research

MRI is an important technique for staging the infection and for monitoring the development of soft tissue and bone infections. The transverse plane, coronal plane, and sagittal plane images of liquid sensitive sequences such as T_1WI and T_2WI fat-suppressed sequence or STIR should be collected. Because all infection processes lead to increased blood flow, the gadolinium enhancement is rarely used as a diagnostic tool.

7.2 Bacillary Angiomatosis

Li Li and Jing Zhao

Overview

Bacillary angiomatosis (BA) is a special type of osteomyelitis caused by Bartonella infection, which mostly occurs in immunosuppressed people, especially AIDS patients. Cases of AIDS complicated with BA were first reported in the early 1980s. Compared with staphylococcal osteomyelitis, BA is relatively rare.

Bartonella is a group of gram-negative aerobic bacteria with strict nutritional requirements and facultative intracellular parasitics. It mainly takes mammals as its natural host and arthropods as the vector of transmission and can cause a variety of zoonosis [5]. At present, more than 40 species and subspecies of Bartonella have been identified, and more than 10 of them have been recognized as new zoonotic pathogens that cause life-threatening infections in animals and people. For example, B. henselae can cause cat-scratch disease, BA, bacitoid purpura, endocarditis, optic neuritis, and bacteremia; B. *quintana* can cause trench fever, BA, bacitrin-purpura, and endocarditis.

B. henselae and *B. quintana* are the main pathogens of BA, and when they parasitize the human red blood cells, they can cause long-term hematogenous infection and lead to a large number of endothelial cell proliferation, leading to hemangiomatoid changes [6, 7]. Koehler et al. [8] found through research that although both *B. henselae* and *B. quintana* may lead to BA in skin and deep tissues and cause angiogenic lesions in AIDS patients, *B. quintana* may mainly cause skin infection and bone lesions, while *B. henselae* may mainly lead to bacillary purpura and lymph node lesions. It reflects that although the two kinds of pathogens have highly consistent genetic material, there are differences in tissue specificity and etiology.

Focal angiogenesis is characteristic of BA and can invade the skin, trachea, mucous membrane, internal organs, bone, and brain. Clinical manifestations include fever, anemia, hepatosplenomegaly, multiple pale red papules, and vascular endothelial injury. Cutaneous and subcutaneous lesions are

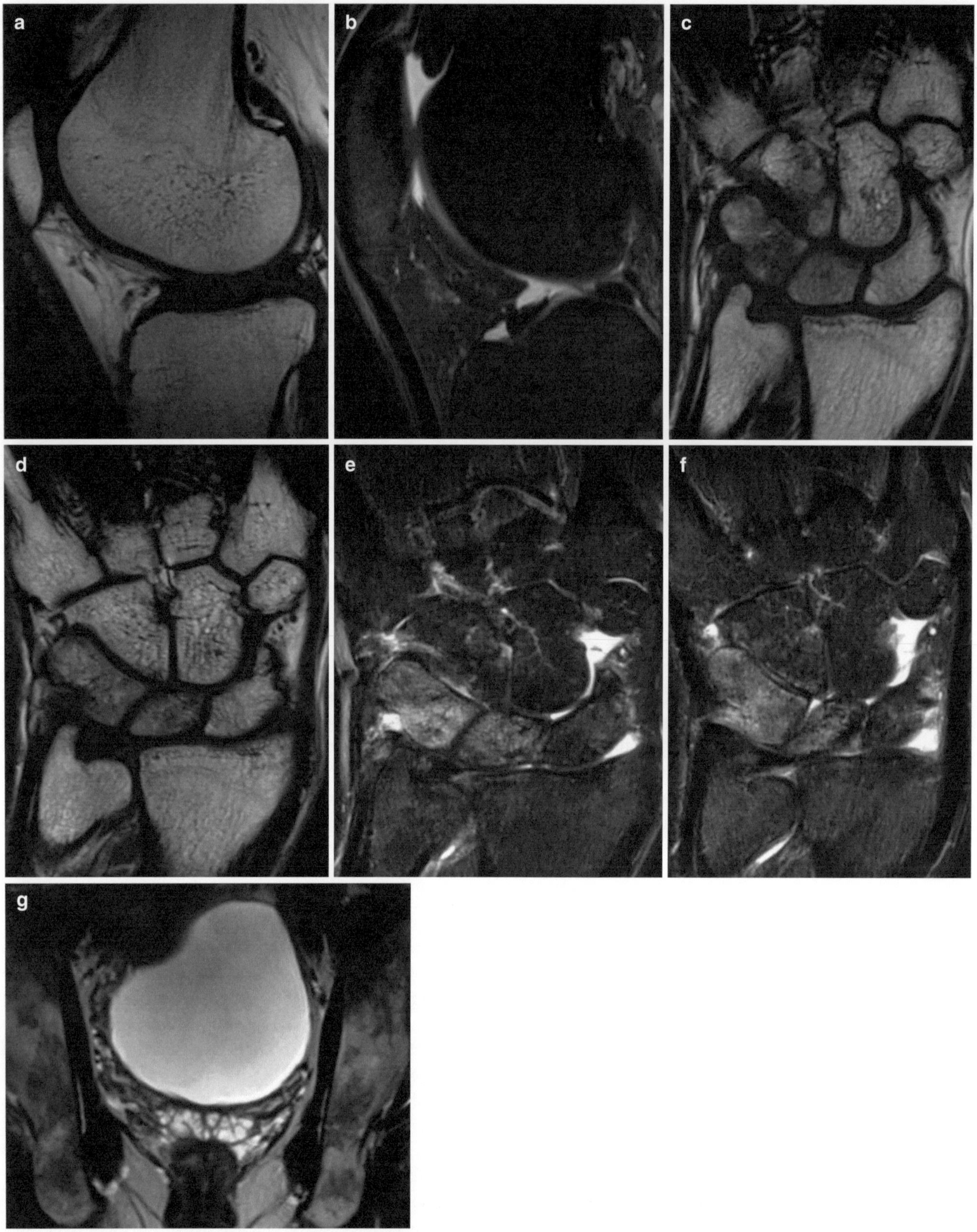

Fig. 7.2 AIDS-associated osteomyelitis (1). (**a** and **b**). MRI showed ribbon-like hypointense on T_1WI and hyperintense on T_2WI in the articular cavity of both knees; (**c**–**f**) The intensity of bone marrow of lunate bone and triangular in the right wrist was reduced on T_1WI, while there is hyperintense on T_2WI fat-suppressed sequence, with intact bone cortex. The ribbon-like hyperintense on T_1WI and hyperintense on T_2WI could be seen in the small polyhedral bone, cephalic bone, and scaphoid bone of the right wrist. The ribbon-like hypointense on T_1WI and hyperintense on T_2WI were observed in the joint space of radius. (**g**) There was extensive worm-eaten bone destruction on both sides of the pelvis

most common and resemble Kaposi's sarcoma (KS). The BA in the bone accounts for about 35% of BA secondary to AIDS. About 25% of BA presented as osteolytic lesions, most of which were not accompanied by sclerosis. The diagnosis can be confirmed by serologic examination of Bartonella, and a definitive diagnosis requires a biopsy. The positive Warthin-Starry stain is the golden standard for histological examination.

Pathophysiology
Skin and subcutaneous lesions are characterized by lobular vascular hyperplasia composed of abundant epithelioid endothelial cells. The lesions contain dense neutrophil granulocytes and eosinophilic particles containing bacilli clustered around the lesions, with positive Warthin-Starry stain [9].

Imaging Findings
Characteristic osteolytic changes are the most common imaging manifestations of BA, ranging from osteolytic lesions with clear boundaries to extensive cortical destruction, medullary infiltration, and periosteal reaction with blurred boundaries [10, 11]. Both CT and MRI could clearly show osteolytic lesions, and MRI showed hypointense on T_1WI and hyperintense on T_2WI. There is also a vascularized soft tissue mass. Radionuclide scans showed increased accumulation at the infected site.

If BA occurs in the skin, CT enhanced scan can clearly show obvious nodular enhancement lesions in the skin and subcutaneous tissues, as the lesions contain rich vascular structures. The lesions in soft tissue also present marked enhancement [11]. Angiography can show obvious neovascularization in the lesions, MRI can show infiltration of muscle septum, and T_2WI shows obvious hyperintense mass shadows and multiple cavitation vascular shadows in the mass [12].

Key Points of Diagnosis

1. It may be caused by suspected animal contact history, and there are fever, anemia, hepatosplenomegaly, multiple pale red papules, and other clinical manifestations.
2. Imaging examination showed osteolytic lesions without sclerosis.
3. A positive Warthin-Starry stain may confirm the diagnosis.

Differential Diagnosis

1. The osteolytic lesions on KS imaging play an important role in the differentiation of BA and KS.
2. **Osteomyelitis.** The osteomyelitis caused by Mycobacterium haemophilus infection is also one of the causes of osteolytic lesions in AIDS patients, but it is often accompanied by skin ulcers.

Status Quo and Progress of Research
Among over 40 species and subspecies of Bartonella that have been confirmed at present, 14 are recognized as new zoonotic pathogens [13], and 9 kinds of pathogenic Bartonella are distributed in China. In 2002, *B. Yunnannensish* was discovered in Yunnan, China, and in 2015, *B. heixiaziensis* and *B. fuyuanensis* were discovered in Heilongjiang. Such three new species were all found in the rat groups.

7.3 Septic Arthritis

Shi Qi

Overview
Pyogenic arthritis, also known as septic arthritis, is the most common musculoskeletal infection in HIV patients [14], which is common among intravenous drug users. Joint infections can be caused by hematogenous dissemination or direct spread of adjacent bone or soft tissue infections. Staphylococcus aureus is the most common pathogen, and Mycobacterium, Pneumococcus, Streptococcus, Salmonella can also cause disease. Pyogenic arthritis often occurs in weight-bearing joints of unilateral lower limb, such as the knee joint and hip joint, and the sacroiliac joint and acromioclavicular joint in intravenous drug users. Clinical manifestations include fever, pain, erythema, soft tissue swelling, and limitation of motion of joints [4, 14, 15]. Clinical treatment includes identification of the pathogens by culturing the joint effusion with needling aspiration and antibiotic therapy. If no treatment has been received, pyogenic arthritis can lead to rapid joint destruction and eventually ankylosis will occur.

Pathophysiology
In the early stage, the symptoms of pyogenic arthritis are synovial inflammation, synovial congestion, edema, inflammatory cell infiltration, and effusion in the articular cavity; as the exudate and pus increase, the articular capsule tears and forms a pericapsular abscess of articular capsule, and such pus destroys the articular cartilage and erodes the bone beneath the articular cartilage. In the late stage, the destruction of articular cartilage leads to joint space stenosis, erosion destruction in the bone beneath the articular cartilage, and fibrous granulation tissue proliferation and eventually leads to articular fibrotic ankylosis and bony ankylosis.

Imaging Findings

1. **X-ray** is not sensitive to early pyogenic arthritis, and no abnormalities can be found. As the lesion progresses, soft tissue swelling, joint effusion, periarticular osteoporosis, bone cortex erosion, and sclerosis may occur. Worm-eaten or patchy osteolytic bone destruction can also be seen.

Joint spaces can be normal, narrow, or widened depending on the degree of cartilage destruction and effusion.

2. **CT** can be used as the main examination method of pyogenic arthritis. There may be effusion in the articular cavity, worm-eaten or patchy bone destruction, nonunion of bone cortex, soft tissue swelling around the joint, fat space turbidity, and other changes that can be seen.
3. **MRI** is more sensitive to the early diagnosis of pyogenic arthritis and can show abnormal signal intensity of bone marrow and soft tissue, both of which have edema-like signal characteristics, namely hypointense on T_1WI and hyperintense on fat-suppressed sequence. Septic bursitis may also occur in the sites including olecranon, prepatellar bursae, and subdeltoid bursa. The spread of infection from the articular cavity to the surrounding lumen is easily recognized by MRI.

Key Points of Diagnosis

The diagnosis of pyogenic arthritis should be conducted based on the clinical symptoms and imaging manifestations. Joint effusion is its characteristic manifestation. Positive culture of joint puncture fluid is the golden standard for diagnosis.

Differential Diagnosis

Pyogenic arthritis is mainly distinguished from tuberculous arthritis. The onset of tuberculous arthritis is slow, the symptoms are mild and it often takes several months for a significant change; Osteoporosis is obvious, and the bone destruction develops slowly, often starting from the edge of the non-weight-bearing bone; There is no or very little reactive hyperostosis and periosteal proliferation. It can be seen that the enhanced abscesses have a thin and well-rounded walls as the abscess forms around the joints.

Status Quo and Progress of Research

It will be specified in Sect. 8 of Chap. IV.

7.4 Soft Tissue Infection

7.4.1 Cellulitis

Overview

Cellulitis is a diffuse, pyogenic infection occurred in the subcutaneous, subfascial, intermuscular space, or deep cellular tissue. It usually occurs in the lower extremities and is often indistinct from the normal skin. The main pathogens are Staphylococcus aureus, including methicillin-resistant Staphylococcus aureus (MRSA). Other pathogens include pseudomonas, pyogenic streptococcus, and mycobacterium. Helicobacter pylori can cause multifocal cellulitis and bacteremia, and about 40% of cases are infected with multiple microorganisms. The clinical manifestations were characterized by swelling, erythema, fever, and local pain. MRSA strains can cause acutely progressive and sharply painful pyogenic infection, with pain like spider bite as the patients commonly and mainly complain. Cellulitis may spread in progressive wildfire or through lymphatic vessels, producing red lines or marks in the area of inflammatory lymphatics. Reactive lymph nodes can be seen in the area of drainage.

Pathophysiology

As the hemolytic streptococcus, after infection, can release hemolysin, streptokinase, and hyaluronidase, the inflammation is not easy to be limited, and the boundary with normal tissue is unclear with rapid spread. In a short period of time, it can cause extensive subcutaneous tissue inflammation, exudation, edema, leading to systemic inflammatory reaction syndrome and endotoxemia, and the blood culture is often negative. If it is caused by Staphylococcus aureus, the lesions are relatively limited due to coagulase action produced by bacteria.

Imaging Findings

1. **CT**
   (a) Superficial cellulitis: superficial inflammation of soft tissues. CT showed fine reticular density shadows of soft tissue, which were contrasted with the low-density subcutaneous fat shadows. The skin thickens with edema, and the boundary between the fatty layer and the fascia space between muscle fascicles disappears. In addition, the subcutaneous fat septa and superficial fascia thickening can be seen.
   (b) Deep cellulitis: a sign of deep soft tissue infection in the early stage. CT features blurred soft tissue masses with displacement of surrounding structures. The boundary between the muscle fascicles and the subcutaneous fat disappears and is replaced by a shaggy hair-like density shadow of soft tissue. The lesions may contain bubblets.
2. **MRI.** Lesions showed hypointense on T_1WI, hyperintense on T_2WI, and hyperintense on STIR sequence. The thickened lymphatic vessels showed scattered hypointense on MRI T_1WI with fuzzy boundary and reticular hyperintense on T_2WI. The enhanced scan presented as diffuse medium enhancement.

Key Points of Diagnosis

The diagnosis of cellulitis mainly depends on the clinical features of the lesions, aspirate of diseased tissue or blood culture, and imaging findings.

Differential Diagnosis

Cellulitis needs to be distinguished from a soft tissue abscess.

7.4.2 Soft Tissue Abscess

Overview

Soft tissue abscess is also a common complication of HIV/AIDS patients, which mainly occurs in intravenous drug users and is mostly caused by the use of unclean needles. Other causes include hematogenous dissemination or direct spread (adjacent osteomyelitis or pyogenic arthritis). Most infections are caused by bacteria and are more limited. Common pathogens have Staphylococcus aureus, Streptococcus pyogenes, Salmonella, Mycobacterium tuberculosis, etc. The extent and progression of the abscess lies in the immune status of patients. The major clinical manifestations are fever and local pain. The abscesses can be treated by using needle aspiration, subcutaneous drainage, and antibiotic therapy.

Pathophysiology

Soft tissue abscesses often have well-defined fluid accumulation, thicker abscess walls, and an inflammatory response in the surrounding soft tissue.

Imaging Findings

The imaging examination plays an important guiding role in determining abscess location and scope, abscess aspiration biopsy, and drainage.

1. **CT** typically shows a low-density vomica in the center of lesions, and the density may increase when bleeding or containing protein. The abscess wall is composed of inflammatory granulation tissue and fibrous tissue, presenting a high-density annular shadow around the vomica. By enhanced scan, it can show that the abscess wall is thickened and presents ring enhancement, and the sinus wall may also be strengthened, thus it can clearly display the soft tissue sinus and its relationship with peripheral tissues. The gas density shadow in the soft tissue is an important manifestation of an abscess, showing several small scattered bubblets, or large bubblets that accumulate, which are located between low-density reticular shadows. CT examination can accurately locate the site of deep soft tissue abscess to facilitate puncture and drainage.
2. **MRI.** For abscess lesions with clear boundaries, hypointense or isointense on T_1WI and hyperintense on T_2WI, with slight changes in intensity strength due to different contents of proteins and necrotic debris in abscesses. The surrounding soft tissue edema shows a feather-like hyperintense with unclear boundaries. Hypointense pseudocystic changes and enhanced ring enhancement surrounding lesions were observed on all sequences. MRI has a good effect in determining the scope of abscesses, especially the relationships between bone and nerve, vascular structure. The display ability of T_2WI FATSAT or STIR is significantly better than that of other sequences, while the enhanced scan is the best choice in terms of the overall delineation and structural detail display of abscess walls and septa [16–18].

Key Points of Diagnosis

In terms of muscle tissue swelling, imaging examination of the center of the lesion showed low density or hypointense on T_1WI and hyperintense on T_2WI, with ring enhancement, and the diagnosis can be determined based on the clinical manifestations.

Differential Diagnosis

1. **Soft tissue hematoma.** The CT manifestations of soft tissue abscess and soft tissue hematoma are similar, but the latter has a history of trauma. With the evolution of the hematoma, the hematoma signals in different periods are different, and the hyperintense on T_1WI and hyperintense on T_2WI are the most common.
2. **Tuberculous abscess.** It is often accompanied by clear vertebral body destruction, and often multiple.

7.4.3 Pyomyositis

Overview

Pyomyositis, also known as bacterial myositis, is a primary bacterial infection involving the striated muscles. It is also known as tropical pyomyositis because of its prevalence in warm and humid environments. In recent years, more and more temperate regions have been reported, so there are non-tropical pyomyositis, infectious myositis, and other different names. This disease is all primary bacterial infection of skeletal muscle, excluding abscesses between muscles, abscesses caused by the spread of infection in adjacent tissues such as bone and subcutaneous tissues, and abscesses secondary to septicemia [19, 20].

Pyomyositis is one of the common musculoskeletal complications of AIDS. It mostly occurs in patients with CD4 T lymphocytes below 200 cells/μl and is associated with high incidence of intravenous drug abuse, rhabdomyolysis, and repeated trauma. Pyomyositis can also be seen in diabetes, malnutrition, or other systemic diseases. Staphylococcus aureus is the main pathogen of this disease, 90% of cases are caused by Staphylococcus aureus infection, and other pathogens include Streptococcus pneumoniae, Salmonella, Cryptococcus neoformans, Mycobacterium tuberculosis, etc.

The pathogenesis of this disease is still unclear. It has been reported in the literature that 20% ~ 50% of patients have a history of blunt injury or sports injury of diseased muscle tissues, so local trauma is considered as an important factor, and the large amount of iron in myoglobin after trauma is an essential substance for bacterial reproduction, leading to a large number of bacterial growth and causing disease [21, 22].

Pyomyositis is characterized by multiple pyogenic infections of the muscles. The infections are more likely to occur in the large muscle groups of thigh or buttocks, especially in the quadriceps and lower extremities, which tends to develop along the long axis of muscles. The symptoms are fixed cramp-like pain, local tenderness, and rigidity (wood-like sclerosis), accompanied by fever, leukocytosis, and systemic symptoms. The skin and subcutaneous tissue are relatively unaffected. It begins with inflammatory myositis, followed by muscle necrosis and abscess formation. In the late stage, lesions may affect adjacent joints and bones, and in a few cases septicemia may be developed, leading to shock and death, with a mortality rate of 1% ~ 20%. In the early stage, the use of antibiotics is effective. Blood culture was positive in 20% ~ 50% of patients. Treatment includes surgical drainage and appropriate long-term therapy of antibiotics.

Pathophysiology

In the early stage, the symptoms are muscle congestion and edema, followed by local necrosis and dissolution, which finally form a cavity filled with pus. When acrogenic bacterium infection occurs, there may be bubbles in the cavity, and the abscess wall is composed of granulation tissue and fibrous tissue. Peripheral muscle septum has edema or empyema, and when serious, spreads to adjacent muscle.

Some scholars [23] believe that pyomyositis is a process of acute pyogenic inflammation of skeletal muscle. If the body resistance is low or the treatment is not complete, it can turn into subacute or chronic pyomyositis or develop into a typical muscle abscess dominated by vomica. Therefore, there is no absolute limit between pyomyositis and muscle abscess. In addition, the formation of abscess is closely related to the type of pathogen, and it is more likely for Staphylococcus aureus infection to form abscess.

Imaging Findings

CT and MRI are helpful in defining the scope of infection and guiding the drainage of the infected area.

1. **CT**. Due to muscle edema and swelling, CT showed low density and blurred margins; The intramuscular effusion shows clearly. The enhanced scan can distinguish between necrosis and abscess of muscle tissues, where necrotic muscle tissue lacks enhancement and abscess presents a ring enhancement with clear boundaries.
2. **MRI.** It is the most effective imaging examination method for pyomyositis and it is sensitive from diffuse inflammatory response to abscess formation. In the early stage, T_1WI usually presented isointense or slightly hypointense or slightly hyperintense; The enlarged muscles with hyperemia and edema showed large area of fuzzy hyperintense and significant hyperintense on T_2WI and STIR, respectively, which often involved the whole muscle. Due to the uneven development of inflammation, the manifestations included hyperintense of different degrees and loose interfascicular tissues, which resulted in more hyperintense, and the adjacent intermuscular space also presented hyperintense. When inflammations developed and formed induration or mass, it presented hyperintense on T_2WI with relatively limited range and was surrounded by relatively low linear signal intensity around the periphery, with the interior septa also presenting linear signal intensity, and fuzzy edema signal intensity around the mass. T_1WI presented isointense or slightly hypointense or slightly hyperintense with unclear boundaries. In the stage of suppuration, the characteristic MRI features of this disease can be seen, that is, single or multiple vomicas of different sizes, with unclear boundaries. The pus on T_1WI showed hypointense, the abscess wall shows ring-like much hyperintense, and the interval showed relatively hypointense. The vomica showed higher hyperintense on T_2WI and STIR, and the abscess wall showed relatively low hypointense (Fig. 7.3). After T_1WI was enhanced, edema and inflammatory muscle showed obvi-

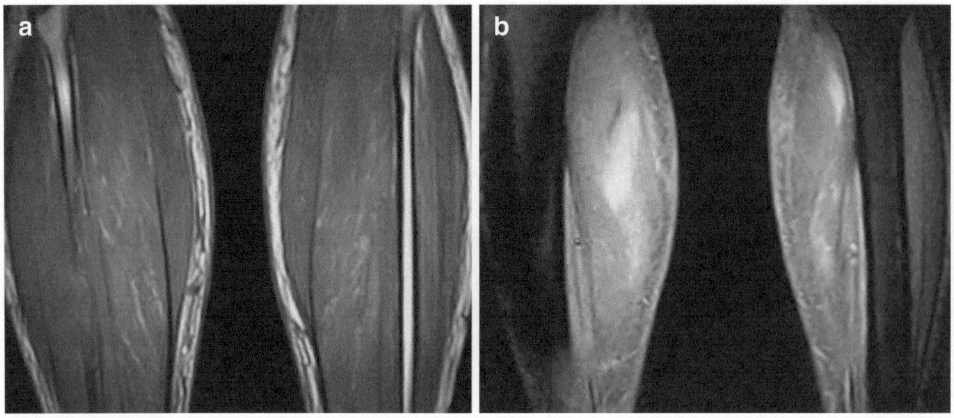

Fig. 7.3 AIDS-related pyomyositis. (**a** and **b**) MRI showed diffuse swelling of the diseased muscles in the posterior group of the shank, with ribbon-like hypointense on T_1WI and hyperintense on T_2WI

ous diffuse heterogeneous enhancement, no enhancement in the necrotic area and vomica was found, and abscess wall showed obvious ring enhancement. In patients with AIDS, gas may appear during myonecrosis, which was often caused by non-clostridium bacteria, especially in intravenous drug users. CT and MRI can easily identify abnormal gases in necrotic tissue.

Key Points of Diagnosis

1. For patients with AIDS, the symptoms include local muscular pain, tenderness, sclerosis, accompanied by fever.
2. Muscle edema can be seen on CT and MRI. Intramuscular effusion and/or abscess can be seen after enhanced scan. Microabscesses can be also seen on MRI.

Differential Diagnosis

1. **Soft tissue malignant tumor**. Local masses are the main lesion, and the lesion usually presents isointense on T_1WI and mixed hyperintense on T_2WI, which is relatively limited and does not develop along the long axis of muscle and does not take the intermuscular space as the boundary, and there is no capsule around tumor necrosis and liquefaction.
2. **Muscle hematoma**. There is a history of trauma, hematoma signal changes with time, sometimes the liquid–liquid plane can be seen, without capsule around. Local symptoms gradually improve with the extension of time, generally without systemic symptoms.
3. **Diabetic muscle infarction**. Severe pain is characteristic of diabetic muscle infarction. MRI showed isointense or hypointense on T_1WI and hyperintense on T_2WI, with marked enhancement by enhanced scan. There was no enhancement in the necrotic liquefaction area within the infarcted muscle, but there was surrounding ring enhancement, similar to the formation of myositis abscess. If MRI found multiple muscle edema or swelling in thigh or calf, the possibility of this disease should be considered. In addition, diabetic muscle infarction has post-infarction hemorrhagic point with hyperintense on T_1WI, and there was no such manifestation on pyomyositis.
4. **Muscle abscess**. The pathological tissue density of pyomyositis was heterogeneous, with the peripheral enhancement, but it did not form typical ring enhancement; The muscle abscess showed ring enhancement of the abscess wall, with more homogeneous low density inside.

Status Quo and Progress of Research

Unal et al. [24] believed that the sensitivity and specificity of soft tissue abscess diagnosed as hyperintense on DWI were 92% and 80%, respectively. DWI can be used as an important auxiliary sequence for MRI evaluation of the formation of vomica in soft tissue infection, especially for contraindications of MRI contrast agents. Other scholars believed that the dispersion state and distribution of water molecules in the vomica may be different due to the different period of soft tissue abscess, treatment process, initial fluid nature associated with infection, and uneven distribution of proteins or other macromolecules in the pus [25].

7.5 Necrotizing Fasciitis

Li Li and Jing Zhao

Overview

Necrotizing fasciitis (NF) is a soft tissue disease characterized by progressive infection and necrosis of deep fascia, superficial fascia, skin, and subcutaneous tissue caused by pathogens invading the organism. It is more likely to occur in patients with intravenous drug injection, alcoholism, diabetes, HIV carrier/AIDS, and leukemia.

NF is usually the result of a mixture of pathogens such as gram-positive, gram-negative, aerobic, or anaerobic bacteria. It is also known as carnivorous disease because it causes rapid tissue destruction. Bacterial infections are associated with susceptibility factors, such as Clostridium difficile and trauma, Staphylococcus aureus and diabetes, pseudomonas, Escherichia coli and immunosuppression, and malignant tumors. NF can involve soft tissues in all parts of the body, most of which are perineal genitalia, buttocks, and extremities, but rare in the chest, abdomen, and other torso parts.

The clinical manifestations of NF can progress rapidly within 24 ~ 48 hours. Fever and pain are the manifestations of NF in the early stage, and in addition, skin damage, ele vated skin temperature, soft tissue swelling, tenderness, and palpable soft tissue induration may occur. About 80% of patients initially present only with symptoms of cellulitis [26]. Most patients experience intense pain beyond clinical signs. In the progressive stage, it is characterized by diffuse swelling, erythema, blister formation, and skin gangrene. Systemic symptoms include septic shock, multi-organ failure, etc. and are often out of proportion to local changes. The dark skin area is smaller than the subcutaneous tissue and fascial infection area, and the skin can be intact. As tissue necrosis occurs, the pain progresses until loss of sensation. Cutaneous blisters and palpated crepitus are the manifestations of complete necrosis of subcutaneous tissue. Clinical manifestations of NF can range from slight skin changes to full-thickness skin necrosis. These symptoms and signs may rapidly progress to more typical clinical manifestations, such as ecchymosis, blisters or bullae, crepitus, and skin necrosis. In addition, reinfection may occur at the original site of NF. The mortality of this disease is as high as 30% ~ 70%, and the causes of death include sepsis, respiratory failure, renal failure, multi-organ failure, etc.

NF is a surgical emergency requiring immediate debridement. Thorough surgery and debridement are key to the treatment of the disease, and antibiotics are needed to control the infection. However, it is very difficult for patients with NF secondary to AIDS to use antibiotics for treatment, and the disease progresses rapidly, which can cause sepsis and systemic multi-organ failure. It's a very difficult clinical problem, even if the operation is difficult to recover.

Pathophysiology

NF is characterized by the spread of infection along the deep and superficial fascia, which may involve the skin and muscles as the disease progresses. The formation of subcutaneous fibrinoid thrombosis of arterioles and venules is a pathological marker of NF. Subcutaneous tissue and fascia inflammatory edema, necrosis, inflammatory cells, bacterial infiltration, fetid purulent secretion cover the necrotic fascia and muscle, accompanied by adjacent lacuna effusion and empyema.

Imaging Findings

The X-ray and CT imaging findings of NF are bubble shadows in soft tissue.

1. **X-ray**. The X-ray manifestation of NF is similar to cellulitis with swelling and blurring of the diseased soft tissue. Gas in the deep fascia is rarely shown until infection and necrosis are sufficiently advanced. The X-ray changes of NF are nonspecific; therefore, they are of limited value for diagnosis in the early stage.
2. **CT.** Deep fascial effusions and gaseous density shadows in soft tissues are characteristic manifestations of NF [27]. Extensive pneumatosis is considered as a marker of NF, but is related to the type of bacteria infected. Pneumatosis is distributed continuously along the fascia surface. No isolated gas accumulation is observed in soft tissues such as muscles. The thickening and strengthening of fascia are also the characteristic changes of NF. The superficial fascia may be affected, while the shallow, middle, and deep layers of the deep fascia may be affected to different degrees. In the early stage, the muscle is often not affected, followed by the adjacent muscle involvement with varying degrees, and appear thickening, destruction and other changes. In addition, the thickening of the diffuse edema in the skin and subcutaneous tissue and strip-like and reticular enhancement of subcutaneous fat and other changes can be seen.
3. **MRI.** Necrotic tissue liquefaction and inflammatory edema together result in increased fluid content in the fascia, leading to increased signal intensity on T_2WI and hyperintense along the thickened deep fascia layer on T_1WI. When the fascia is thickened and effusion occurs, T_2WI usually presents as a dome-shaped hyperintense area with clear margins. For example, deep fascia has large block-like hyperintense on T_2WI, which can be diagnosed as NF. T_2WI fat-suppressed sequence was superior to gadolinium-enhanced T_1WI in showing inflammatory lesions. Gas is manifested as loss of local foci signals on T_1WI and T_2WI [28]. When subcutaneous tissue was involved, T_2WI showed reticular hyperintense, with visible enforcement. T_2WI showed a mild diffuse increase in muscle signal intensity, and the enhanced scan showed discontinuous enforcement of muscle, which was less severe than fascia due to edema.

Compared with the surgical approach, the MRI scan often shows a larger scope of infections, i.e., the scope of soft tissues involved in the deep area is overestimated, some non-necrotizing deep fascia shows a mildly to moderately increased signal intensity on the T_2WI, which is caused by the non-infectious edema of the NF adjacent to the infected zone. Yet, the involvement of the deep fascia still indicates that the disease should be diagnosed with NF. In addition, MRI can be used to perform dynamic observations on non-NF to evaluate an NF that may occur.

Key Points of Diagnosis

1. For patients with AIDS, diabetes, and other relevant predisposing factors and risk factors, soft tissue pain, tenderness, skin erythema, fever, and obvious crepitus occur.
2. The image shows pneumatosis in the soft tissues, edema, effusion, and thickening in the fascia, strip-like, and reticular enhancement in subcutaneous fat.
3. Tissue biopsy and tissue culture help to make a diagnosis.

Differential Diagnosis

1. **Cellulitis** involves subcutaneous tissues only, and the fascia is normal. The image shows that the subcutaneous tissues thicken and the fat density increases, with strip-like and irregular enhancement, with or without effusion in the subcutaneous and superficial fascia, and the deep structure is normal. Most cases can be cured with the administration of antibiotics.
2. **Myositis** The myositis is featured by the involvement of muscles, which is clinically manifested as pain, hyperesthesia, and systemic poisoning. The imaging findings mainly include the thickening of muscles with or without heterogeneous enhancement. The pyomyositis or subcutaneous abscess shows a fusiform or round muscular or subcutaneous high intensity zone with clear borders.

3. **Fasciitis-panniculitis syndrome** Known as eosinophilic fasciitis, fasciitis-panniculitis syndrome (FPS) is common in muscular fascia adjacent to the elbows, knees, and other joints. It often occurs in a symmetrical manner and its clinical manifestation is similar to scleroderma. The MRI T_1WI shows symmetrical thickening and enhancement of the superficial fascia and less involvement of deep fascia. FPS is a specific connective tissue disease, and good efficacy may be realized through therapies of hormone and immunosuppressive agents.

Status Quo and Progress of Research

In the laboratory risk indicator for necrotizing fasciitis (LRINEC) scoring system, application of the laboratory risk indicators such as C-reactive protein, WBC, hemoglobin, serum Na concentration, creatinine, and blood glucose is of great value in the screening and diagnosis of NF. NF may occur when the total score is ≥6, and NF is highly likely to occur when the total score is ≥8. Serum lactic acid is considered as a novel diagnostic tool for NF. Studies of Murphy et al. [29] show that when the lactic acid level is ≥2, the sensitivity for the diagnosis of NF is 100% and the positive predictive value is 82%. Studies of Weng et al. [30] show that elevation in the red blood cell distribution width (RDW) can be used as an independent predictor of in-hospital mortality rate of patients with NF.

7.6 Osteoporosis

Li Li and Dechun Li

Overview

Osteoporosis is a systemic and metabolic bone disease characterized by osteopenia and poor bone quality, leading to increased bone fragility and susceptibility to fracture. About 50% of patients infected with HIV present osteoporosis as HIV infection may result in decrease in bone mineral density. The deficiency of 1,25-dihydroxyvitamin D_3 is the key mechanism of abnormal bone metabolism in AIDS patients.

Arnsten et al. [31] conducted a control study on 328 patients infected with HIV and 231 patients without HIV infection and found that the HIV-infected group had a decrease in bone mineral density and an increasing risk of fracture. The difference is statistically significant. Whether receiving highly active antiretroviral therapy (HAART) or not, HIV-infected patients generally have a decrease in bone mineral density. Hence, HIV infection itself may be a risk factor of abnormal bone metabolism. Possible mechanisms include persistent chronic inflammatory reactions caused by HIV infection, which are often accompanied by elevation in certain inflammatory factors such as tumor necrosis factor-α (TNF-α) and interleukin-6 (IL-6). These inflammatory factors can stimulate and increase osteoclast activity, raise the levels of osteoprotegerin, or reduce the level of 1,25-dihydroxyvitamin D_3 [32].

Tebas et al. [33] reported HIV-infected patients treated with antiviral drugs had low bone mass and an increased risk of osteoporosis. Some studies showed that an obvious loss of bone mass was observed in HIV-infected patients at 24 to 48 months after initial administration of antiviral drugs; and according to some studies, the loss of bone mass may reach 2%-6% [34], and the loss of bone mass in the treatment group was 2.5 times that of the control group.

Kinai et al. [35] conducted a study on 184 HIV-infected men through dual-energy X-ray absorptiometry (DXA) and found that bone mass decrease and osteoporosis were diagnosed in 46% and 10% of the patients at the lumbar vertebrae, and 54% and 12% at the femoral neck, respectively. Regression analysis and correlation analysis showed that bone mineral density (BMD) decrease mainly correlated with the application of protease inhibitor (PI), and HIV-infected patients who discontinued PI had a significantly lower BMD than those who continuously used PI at lumbar vertebrae but not at the femoral neck. The application duration of antiviral drugs significantly correlated with BMD decrease.

Patients with osteoporosis in the early stage do not present any clinical symptoms or signs, while those in the middle or advanced stages may successively present various symptoms. Pain, the most common and major symptom, includes muscular pain and osteodynia. Osteodynia may attack all over the body, and low back pain is most common. In addition, patients with osteoporosis are prone to fracture, which is sometimes even the reason for first visit. As the disease progresses, patients present height loss, with a hunchback and activity limitation.

Pathophysiology

The histological changes of osteoporosis include thinning of bone cortex, enlargement of Haversian canals and perforating canals, reduction, thinning, and even disappearance of bone trabeculae.

Imaging Findings

1. **X-ray.** The sign of osteoporosis can be observed on the plain film X-ray only when the bone loss exceeds 30%, which is, however, the manifestation of osteoporosis in the advanced stage. On the X-ray film, the main manifestation is BMD decrease. Other manifestations include thinning, a decrease in the number of, dilation of the gap of long bone trabeculae along with the thinning and stratification of the bone cortex. In serious cases, the BMD is similar to the peripheral tissues, the bone tra-

beculae almost disappear, and the bone cortex is as thin as a string. In the spine, the cortex thins, the transverse bone trabeculae decrease or disappear; and these symptoms are relatively obvious in the longitudinal bone trabeculae, and most of which are arranged in irregular longitudinal order. In serious cases, the disappearance of vertebral structure, flattening of the vertebral body, and indentation of superior and inferior borders of the vertebral body may be observed; and the intervertebral space widens and is biconvex, the vertebral body is biconcave and often compressed and in wedge-shaped due to minor trauma.

2. **Dual-energy X-ray absorptiometry (DXA)** DXA has been used in clinical practice for a long time and has been established by WHO as a gold standard for the diagnosis of osteoporosis and the follow-up of the therapeutic effect of osteoporosis. The lumbar vertebrae, femoral neck, and wrist are generally the observation sites. Bone mass in the healthy population aged 30 years (*T* value) compared with patients of the same age (*Z* value): normal: > −1; osteopenia: −2.5 - -1; osteoporosis: < −2.5.

Key Points of Diagnosis

According to the WHO diagnostic criteria, the diagnosis basis for osteoporosis is mainly the BMD measured through DXA. Compared with the peak value of BMD in healthy adults of the same gender and ethnicity, patients are diagnosed with normal if the value of BMD does not reduce or decrease by less than 1 standard deviation (SD); patients are diagnosed with osteopenia if the value of BMD decreases by 1-2.5 SD; patients are diagnosed with osteoporosis if the value of BMD decreases by more than 2.5 SD; and patients whose degree of BMD decrease meets the diagnostic criteria of osteoporosis accompanied by one or more fractures are diagnosed with severe osteoporosis [36].

Differential Diagnosis

1. **Multiple myeloma.** Patients with multiple myeloma (MM) are generally at an older age. Typical cases present multiple round, permeative, and osteolytic bone destruction on X-ray film; Beading changes are observed when tumor cells invade the junctions of costal bones, clavicles, and sternums. Intraosseous scallop-like lacy changes are seen in diffuse MM.
2. **Metastatic tumor of bone.** It is more common in the elderly. The foci differ in size, progress rapidly, and present complete bone destruction; and soft tissue masses and primary foci can be observed. Most patients with osteoporosis present osteopenia without complete bone destruction, the foci progress slowly, and no obvious changes are observed from the re-examination in the short term.
3. **Bone hemangioma.** Solitary bone hemangioma is common. Vertebral hemangioma is characterized by vertical striae or multiple locular osteolytic lesions on X-ray film, with significant enhancement.

Status Quo and Progress of Research

1. **Quantitative computed tomography (QCT).** QCT is the only method that can measure the density of spongy bone and bone cortex, respectively, and provides a new approach for the early diagnosis of osteoporosis, the analysis of different causes of osteoporosis, and the monitoring of the therapeutic effect. According to the recommendations of the International Society for Clinical Densitometry (ISCD) in 2007, QCT is available for BMD measurements and can be used for diagnosis of osteoporosis. The diagnostic criteria are as follows: for low bone mass or osteopenia, the threshold value of BMD is 120 mg/cm^3 (equiv. DXA-measured BMD—1.0); and for osteoporosis, the threshold value of BMD is 80 mg/cm^3 (equiv. DXA-measured BMD—2.5) [37].
2. **^{1}H-MRS.** The MRS of the lumbar vertebra conducts quantitative analysis of specific atomic nuclei and compounds by utilizing chemical shift and magnetic resonance phenomenon. H-MRS is the only non-invasive method to determine metabolic and biochemical indexes of in vivo tissues. The parameters commonly used for evaluating the fat content of bone marrow for osteoporosis include lipid water ratio (LWR) and fat fraction (FF) [38].
3. **DWI.** In the diffusion-weighted imaging (DWI) examination for lumbar vertebra, for osteoporosis, the accumulation of bone marrow adipocytes may cause a corresponding decrease in extracellular space and limit the diffusion of water molecules. DWI can reflect the dynamic changes of bone marrow components from the perspective of the microscopic motion of water molecules, providing a new perspective for the study of osteoporosis.
4. **DCE-MRI.** Through DCE-MRI, the bone marrow microenvironment can be understood from another perspective by observing the bone marrow perfusion in osteoporosis. This approach is expected to play a role in the early evaluation of therapeutic targets or therapeutic effect of osteoporosis [39].
5. **PET/CT.** This method can be used to indirectly determine the changes of bone marrow blood flow and osteoblasts by monitoring the uptake of tracer in the bone marrow. The higher the peak value of the tracer within the same period, the faster the metabolism of the tracer, which indicates that the more the bone marrow blood flow, the more active the bone metabolism. Therefore, PET can be used to evaluate the dynamic changes in the therapeutic effect of osteoporosis from the perspective of metabolism [40].

7.7 Hemophilic Arthropathy

Shi Qi and Dechun Li

Overview

Hemophilia is a hereditary and hemorrhagic disease caused by a lack or dysfunction of blood coagulation factors. It is marked by joint injury. Hemophilic arthropathy (HA) refers to the degenerative changes of joints caused by repeated hemarthrosis. Bleeding easily occurs at knee joints, elbow joints, ankle joints, and other weight-bearing joints, and is most common in knee joints. The main cause of HA is synovial hemosiderin deposition (SHD) due to hemarthrosis.

Patients with hemophilia may be infected with HIV from transfusions of contaminated blood coagulation factors. It is reported that in some countries, those infected with hemophilia in combination with HIV account for 70% ~ 85%. The main clinical manifestation of HA is bleeding. Mucosal bleeding mainly manifests as nasal bleeding and gingival bleeding. Hemarthrosis is accompanied by joint swelling, arthralgia, dysfunction, and other symptoms. In the advanced stage, osteoarthritis or ankylosis and deformities may occur secondary to hemarthrosis.

Pathophysiology

The course of HA can be divided into three stages: acute stage, subacute stage, and chronic stage [41], which mainly differ from each other in the duration of hemarthrosis, degree of joint damage, and severity of inflammatory reactions.

1. **Acute stage** (early stage, stage of hemarthrosis). The synovial hemorrhage enters the articular cavity, resulting in hemarthrosis; the intra-articular pressure (IAP) rises, resulting in the swelling of the synovial membrane and the articular capsule; and the joint space widens and joint structure remains basically normal.
2. **Subacute stage** (middle stage, stage of panarthritis). Repeated long-term hemarthrosis without timely absorption leads to synovial hyperplasia, the formation of a large number of new granulation tissues, organization of hematoma, and hemosiderin deposition, which further results in erosion and absorption of articular cartilage, roughening and sclerosis of articular surfaces, subchondral cystic change, joint space stenosis, and hypertrophy of the articular capsules.
3. **Chronic stage** (advanced stage, recovery stage). Gradual absorption and organization of hemarthrosis can be observed with bone destruction and proliferation and sclerosis of the surrounding bone; the proliferation of a large number of intra-articular fibrous connective tissues can be seen with limitation of motion of joints. In mild cases, the joint function gradually recovers; and in severe cases, secondary osteoarthritis or ankylosis and deformities may occur.

Other pathologic changes: massive intra-osseous hemorrhage and liquefactive necrosis may lead to cystic or geographic bone destruction, forming hemophilic pseudotumor.

Imaging Findings

Plain film X-ray is the earliest and most basic method for the examination of HA. Yet, it can only reveal the bone destruction of joints in the advanced stage and is limited in displaying the lesions of HA in the early stage. CT is valuable in evaluating mild bone erosion. In addition, it can further determine the size and scope of pseudotumor, calcification, and gas in the lesion and muscle involvement. MRI is uniquely advantageous in the display of cartilage lesions. It can detect the early erosion of cartilage, and some special MRI sequences can even show the changes in cartilage composition before the morphological changes in articular cartilage.

1. **X-ray, CT** Acute stage: HA manifests as joint swelling, increased density, and widening of a small number of joint spaces. Subacute stage: HA is accompanied by damage to the joint structure in addition to repeated hemarthrosis, resulting in osteoporosis (Fig. 7.4); and it also manifests as subchondral bone destruction and cystic changes, enlargement and squaring of the extremities, widening and deepening of intercondylar fossa of the femur, and square patella; and these characteristic changes of HA can be displayed on X-ray and CT films. Chronic stage: HA manifests as proliferation and sclerosis of the bone articular surface (Fig. 7.5), formation of osteophyte, intra-articular corpus liberum, soft-tissue calcification; and joint deformity and dislocation and ankylosis for severe cases.
2. **MRI** Acute stage: HA manifests as hemarthrosis only, and the lesions appear hypointense or isointense on T_1WI and hyperintense on T_2WI due to the short duration of bleeding; and it also manifests as synovial membrane widening, and swelling of the articular capsule and surrounding soft tissues. Subacute stage: HA manifests as repeated hemarthrosis, enlargement of bleeding scope and aggregation of bleeding severity, accumulation of hematoma in the articular cavity, bones or surrounding muscles which are formed at different stages; and the lesions appear mildly hyperintense or heterogeneous on T_1WI and hyperintense or heterogeneous on T_2WI. It also manifests as joint space narrowing, widening and deepening of intercondylar fossa of the femur, etc. Chronic stage: The bleeding reduces, the hematoma is gradually

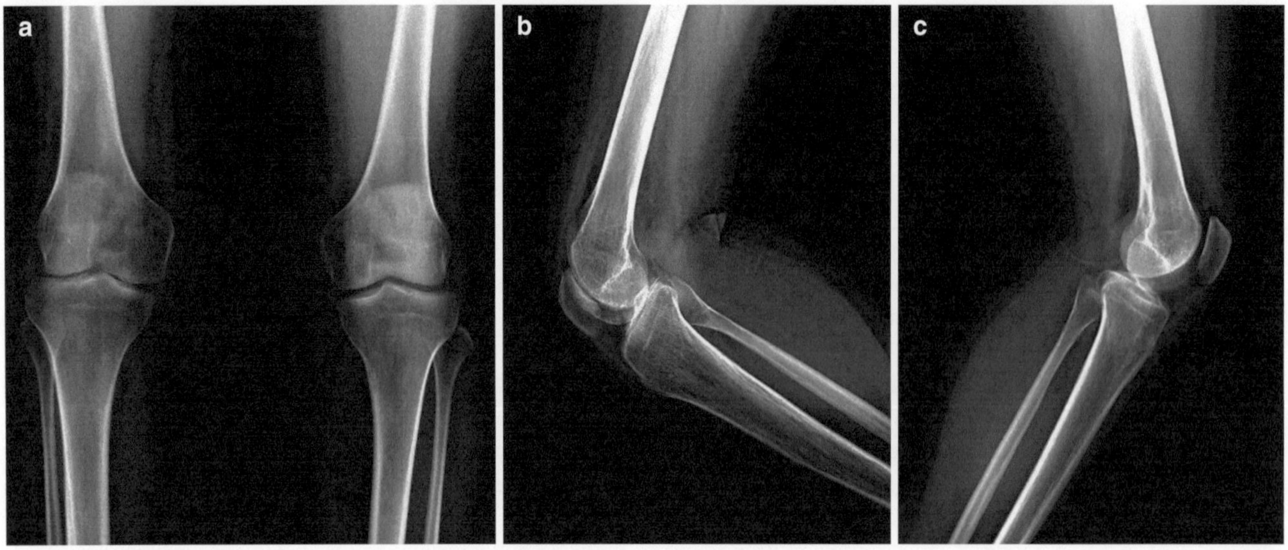

Fig. 7.4 AIDS-related HA (1). (**a–c**) X-ray film reveals that trabeculae are sparse in the bilateral knee joints, bone mineral density decreases, and the bone cortex becomes thinner

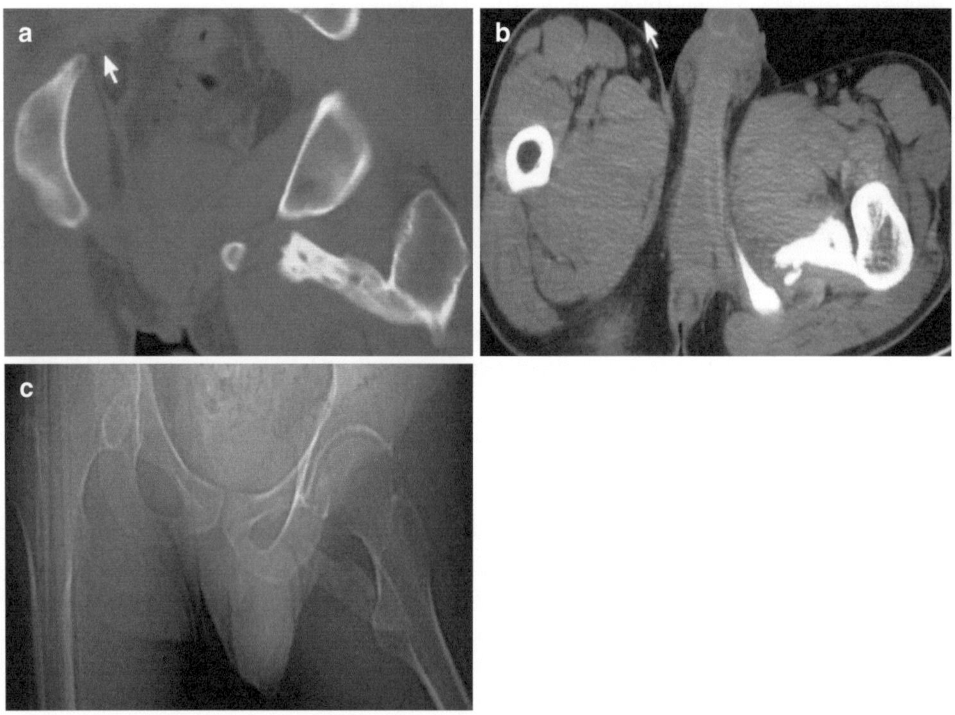

Fig. 7.5 AIDS-related HA (2). (**a**, **b**) CT film reveals that stripped ossified plaques are connected in the junctions between the left femoral intertrochanter and the pubic symphysis, forming a bone bridge; (**c**) X-ray film reveals that the trochanter of the left femoral intertrochanter is connected with the pubic symphysis to form a bone bridge

absorbed, and the lesions appear heterogeneous (hypointense dominated) or hypointense on both T_1WI and T_2WI due to hemosiderin in the synovial membrane of the articular capsule. The degree of swelling of articular capsules, muscles, and ligaments decreases, with atrophy and degeneration present; and there is secondary osteoarthritis or residual ankylosis and deformities [42].

Key Points of Diagnosis

1. The diagnosis of HA is based on clinical manifestation, genetic family history, and laboratory tests.
2. A definite diagnosis can be given when a lack of blood coagulation factors VIII and IX is found through the laboratory test.

3. Characteristic changes of HA can be observed with X-ray scan and MRI scan, such as osteoepiphysis hypertrophy and squaring, broadening and deepening of intercondylar fossa of the femur, and square patella.

Differential Diagnosis

1. **Purulent osteoarthritis.** It involves one or a few joints, with local persistent inflammatory reactions (redness, swelling, fever, and pain and systemic poisoning symptoms).
2. **Rheumatoid arthritis (RA)** It has long-term chronic medical history and involves small joints of the limbs, with symmetric onset in bilateral joints, but free of history of bleeding. In the laboratory tests, antistreptolysin O (ASO) and rheumatoid factor (RF) are tested positive, and accelerated erythrocyte sedimentation rate (ESR) is detected.
3. **Degenerative osteoarthropathy.** It is most frequent at an older age, with obvious hyperostosis.
4. **Joint tuberculosis.** It has long history, can be accompanied by history of tuberculosis, and most frequent in the knee and hip joints. Swelling of diseased joints, formation of cold abscesses, and ring enhancement of synovial edges of joints can be observed in the image. Mild bone erosion and destruction may be seen at the edge and non-bearing surface of the osseous articular surface, with significant osteoporosis in the adjacent bones.

Status Quo and Progress of Research

1. **MR scoring scheme.** Quantitative research is required to determine the severity of HA. At present, the most common scoring methods include Denver scoring Scheme [43], European scoring method [44], and a compatible MRI scoring scheme including a progressive scale and an additive scale [45]. In the Denver scoring scheme, the disease is evaluated based on the progressive changes of joint lesions. Each item is scored from 1 to 10 according to the severity of the disease, with the highest score of 10 being the most severe level of progression of the joint lesion. Denver scoring scheme is widely used as it can be used to conduct a semi-quantitative evaluation on the synovial and cartilage changes of joints at the early stage and show the severity of joint effusion and synovial hyperplasia at the early stage. In the Denver scoring scheme, "6" suggests severe synovial hyperplasia and "7" suggests bone change. Thus, the score of "6" is considered as the cut-off value to distinguish whether the lesion of hemophilic arthropathy is mild or severe. For joints with a Denver score below 6, the most severe signs include severe synovial hyperplasia/hemosiderin deposition; for joints with a Denver score above 7, the signs include subchondral bone and cartilage changes in addition to joint effusion/hemarthrosis, soft-tissue swelling, synovial hyperplasia/hemosiderin deposition. As a result, the Denver score is significantly correlated to the course of the disease and the total number of bleeding. The longer the course of the disease and the more frequent the bleeding, the higher the Denver score of the joint, and the more severe condition visualized in the MRI scan [46].
2. **T_2 mapping.** It can sensitively detect the injury of articular cartilage of HA in the early stage; the elevated level of cartilage defect causes prolonged T_2 relaxation time [47].
3. **DWI.** According to some studies, the apparent diffusion coefficient (ADC) value of cartilage in patients with HA is higher than that in the healthy volunteers and increases with the elevation of the grade of articular cartilage defect, which indicates that DWI is of value for the diagnosis of articular cartilage lesion in patients with HA and can be considered as a reliable new approach for diagnosis of the degeneration of articular cartilage in the early stage.
4. **SWI.** Susceptibility-weighted imaging (SWI) sequence is more sensitive to hemosiderin deposition than the conventional sequence, especially for small or even trace amounts of hemosiderin deposition that cannot be detected by conventional sequence. Therefore, it is of great significance for the accurate evaluation of hemosiderin deposition in HA, which is conducive to the accurate clinical evaluation of HA.
5. **Sodium MRI (^{23}Na-MRI) technique.** It mainly shows the area of proteoglycan depletion via sodium imaging. High sodium concentration is present in the normal cartilage, while the sodium concentration decreases in the cartilage of the lesion. Hence, sodium MRI technique is quite sensitive to the decrease of proteoglycan concentration in the cartilage in osteoarthritis at the early stage [48–50] and can be used as a new method to detect the pathological changes in HA at the early stage.
6. **Spectral CT.** Repeated hemarthrosis and progressive aggravation in patients with HA are mainly caused by synovial inflammation with a large amount of hemosiderin deposition. The iron-based (water) diagram of spectral CT examination can be used to quantitatively determine the iron concentration (FeC) in the region of interest (ROI) and pseudo-color image can be used to label the region with iron deposition. Therefore, it is possible to utilize the value of CT and FeC in spectral CT examination to evaluate the hemosiderin deposition more intuitively [51].

References

1. Zalavras CG, Gupta N, Patzakis MJ, et al. Microbiology of osteomyelitis in patients infected with the human immunodeficiency virus. Clin Orthop Relat Res. 2005;439:97–100.
2. Wang Q, Zhu W, Lu P, et al. A case of AIDS-complicated with osteomyelitis in the upper part of right tibia. Radiologic Practice. 2012;27(2):63.
3. Songfeng J, Jinxin L, Bihua C, et al. X-ray and CT findings of soft tissue and bone infections secondary to AIDS. Chinese J Radiol. 2011;45(12):1162–5.
4. Restrepo CS, Lemos DF, Gordillo H, et al. Imaging findings in musculoskeletal complications of AIDS. Radiographics. 2004;24(4):1029–49.
5. Billeter SA, Levy MG, Chomel BB, et al. Vector transmission of Bartonella species with emphasis on the potential for tick transmission. Med Vet Entomol. 2008;22(1):1–15.
6. Dehio C. Bartonella-host-cell interactions and vascular tumour formation. Nat Rev Microbiol. 2005;3(8):621–31.
7. Seubert A, Schulein R, Dehio C, et al. Bacterial persistence within erythrocytes: a unique pathogenic strategy of Bartonella spp. Int J Med Microbiol. 2001;291(6-7):555–60.
8. Koehler JE, Quinn FD, Berger TG, et al. Isolation of Rochalimaea species from cutaneous and osseous lesions of bacillary angiomatosis. N Engl J Med. 1992;327(10):1625–31.
9. Dawei Z, Hongjun L. Clinical and imaging findings of bacillary angiomatosis secondary to AIDS. Radiol Practice. 2009;24(10):1072–4.
10. Baron AL, Steinbach LS, Leboit PE, et al. Osteolytic lesions and bacillary angiomatosis in HIV infection: radiologic differentiation from AIDS-related Kaposi sarcoma. Radiology. 1990;177(1):77–81.
11. Herts BA, Rafii M, Spiegel G, et al. Soft-tissue and osseous lesions caused by bacillary angiomatosis: unusual manifestations of cat-scratch fever in patients with AIDS. AJR. 1991;157(6):1249–51.
12. Moore EH, Russell LA, Klein JS, et al. Bacillary angiomatosis in patients with AIDS: multiorgan imaging findings. Radiology. 1995;197(1):67–72.
13. Breitschwerdt EB. Bartonellosis, one health and all creatures great and small. Vet Dermatol. 2017;28(1):96–e21.
14. Tehranzadeh J, Ter-Oganesyan RR, Steinbaeh LS. Musculoskeletal disorders associated with HIV infection and AIDS. Part I: infectious musculoskeletal conditions. Skelet Radiol. 2004;33(5):249–59.
15. Plate AM, Boyle BA. Musculoskeletal manifestations of HIV infection. AIDS Read. 2003;13(2):62. 69-70, 72, 76
16. Turecki MB, Taljanovic MS, Stubbs AY, et al. Imaging of musculoskeletal soft tissue infection. Skelet Radiol. 2010;39(10):957–71.
17. Sepahdari AR, Aakalu VK, Kapur R, et al. MRI of orbital cellulitis and orbital abscess: the role of diffusion-weighted imaging. AJR Am J Roentgenol. 2009;193(3):W244–50.
18. Yu Z, Luo X, Dasheng L, et al. Diffusion weighted imaging in detecting abscess formation on soft tissue infection. Chin J Med Imag Technol. 2011;27(5):1030–4.
19. Chauhan S, Jain S, Varma S, et al. Tropical pyomyositis (myositis tropicans): current perspective. Postgrad Med J. 2004;80(943):267–70.
20. Ovadia D, Ezra E, Ben-sira L, et al. Primary pyomyositis in children: a retrospective analysis of 11 cases. J Pediatr Orthop B. 2007;16(2):153–9.
21. Amar T, Vilhekar K, Gupta S. Primary pyomyositis in a child. Int J Infect Dis. 2009;13(4):e149–51.
22. Huang HJ, Yc H, Lin CL, et al. Primary pyomyositis complicated by bilateral pyelonephritis in a healthy adolescent boy. J Emerg Crit Care Med. 2009;20(1):22–6.
23. Guo J, Lu Y, Guoyong S, et al. MRI diagnosis and clinical significance of gluteal pyogenic infection. J Bethune Med Sci. 2009;7(2):65–7.
24. Unal O, Koparan HI, Avcu S, et al. The diagnostic value of diffusion- weighted magnetic resonance imaging in soft tissue abscesses. Eur J Radiol. 2011;77(3):490–4.
25. Herneth AM, Ringl H, Memarsadeghi M, et al. Diffusion weighted imaging in osteoradiology. Top Magn Reson Imaging. 2007;18(3):203–12.
26. Hussein QA, Anaya DA. Necrotizing soft tissue infections. Crit Care Clin. 2013;29(4):795–806.
27. Fugitt JB, Puckett ML, Quigley MM, et al. Necrotizing fasciitis. Radiographics. 2004;24(5):1472–6.
28. Struk D, Munk P, Lee M, et al. Imaging of soft tissue infections. Radiol Clin N Am. 2001;39(2):277–301.
29. Murphy G. Raised serum lactate: a marker of necrotizing fasciitis. J Plast Reconstr Aesthet Surg. 2013;66(12):1712–6.
30. Weng CL. Red cell distribution width is an independent predictor of mortality in necrotizing fasciitis. Am J Emerg Med. 2014;32(10):1259–62.
31. Arnsten JH, Freeman R, Howard AA, et al. Decreased bone mineral density and increased fracture risk in aging men with or at risk for HIV infection. AIDS. 2007;21(5):617–23.
32. Kwan TS, Padrines M, Theoleyre S, et al. IL-6, RANKL, TNF-alpha/IL-1: interrelations in bone resorption pathophysiology. Cytokine Growth FR. 2004;15(1):49–60.
33. Tebas P, Powderly WG, Claxton S, et al. Accelerated bone mineral loss in HIV-infected patients receiving potent antiretroviral therapy. AIDS. 2000;14(4):63–7.
34. Brown TT, Qaqish RB. Antiretroviral therapy and the prevalence of osteopenia and osteoporosis: a meta-analytic review. AIDS. 2006;20(17):2165–74.
35. Kinai E, Nishijima T, Mizushima D, et al. Long-term use of protease inhibitors is associated with bone mineral density loss. AIDS Res Hum Retrovir. 2014;30(6):553–9.
36. Huang JS, Hughes MD, Riddler SA, et al. Bone mineral density effects of randomized regimen and nucleoside reverse transcriptase inhibitor selection from ACTG A5142. HIV Clin Trials. 2013;14(5):224–34.
37. Engelke K, Adams JE, Armbrecht G, et al. Clinical use of quantitative computed tomography and peripheral quantitative computed tomography in the management of osteoporosis in adults: the 2007 ISCD official positions. J Clin Derisitom. 2008;11(1):123–62.
38. Qiu Y, Yao J, Wu X, et al. Longitudinal assessment of oxytocin efficacy on bone and bone marrow fat masses in a rabbit osteoporosis model through 3. 0-T magnetic resonance spectroscopy and micro-CT. Osteoporos Int. 2015;26(3):1081–92.
39. Zhu J, Guangyu T. Research progress of quantitative dynamic contrast-enhanced MRI in osteoporosis. Int J Med Radiol. 2014;37(4):347–50.
40. Dyke JP, Aaron RK. Noninvasive methods of measuring bone blood perfusion. Ann N Y Acad Sci. 2010;1192(1):95–102.
41. Jingxue L, Dingyuan S. X-ray diagnostics in bones and joints. Beijing: People's Medical Publishing House; 1993.
42. Pingyou C, Xueqiang C, Xuanmin Z, et al. MRI features of hemophilic arthropathy. Radiologic Practice. 2017;22(7):731–3.
43. Nuss R, Kilcoyne RF, Geraghty S, et al. MRI findings in haemophilic joints treated with radiosynoviorthesis with development of an MRI scale of joint damage. Haemophilia. 2000;6(3):162–9.
44. Lundin B, Pettersson H, Ljung R. A new magnetic resonance imaging scoring method for assessment of haemophilic arthropathy. Haemophilia. 2004;10(4):383–9.
45. Lundin B, Babyn P, Doria AS, et al. Compatible scales for progressive and additive MRI assessments of haemophilic arthropathy. Haemophilia. 2005;11(2):109–15.

46. Meixia L, Yinghui G, Yuxia Z, et al. MRI appearance of hemophilic arthropathy and correlation with haemorrhage as well as course of disease. Chinese J Med Imaging. 2012;20(11):817–8. 822
47. Melchiorre D, Milia AF, Linari S, et al. RANK-RANKL-OPG in hemophilic arthropathy: from clinical and imaging diagnosis to histopathology. J Rheumatol. 2012;39(8):167–8.
48. Madelin G, Poidevin F, Makrymallis A, et al. Classification of sodium MRI data of cartilage using machine learning. Magn Reson Med. 2015;74(5):1435–48.
49. Zbyn S, Brix MO, Juras V, et al. Sodium magnetic resonance imaging of ankle joint in cadaver specimens, volunteers, and patients after different cartilage repair techniques at 7T: initial results. Investig Radiol. 2015;50(4):246–54.
50. Zbyn S, Mlynarik V, Juras V, et al. Evaluation of cartilage repair and osteoarthritis with sodium MRI. NMR Biomed. 2016;29(2):206–15.
51. Shufang W, Minghua S, Gao F, et al. CT spectral imaging assessment of synovial hemosiderin deposition in knee joint in patients with hemophilic arthropathy. Chin J Med Imag Technol. 2018;34(6):924–8.

Soft Tissue Infection

8

Junyan Yang, Jiye Song, Peng Zhang, and Na Su

8.1 Bacterial Infection

Jiye Song and Na Su

8.1.1 Congenital Malformation with Infection: Fistula and Sinus

Fistula may be caused by various reasons, it is a pathological duct between the in vitro organ and hollow organ or between two hollow organs. The former is called external fistula, with external and internal openings. The external fistula usually has at least two openings, such as intestinal fistula and anal fistula. The latter is called an internal fistula, with only internal openings, such as rectovesical fistula and gastrocolic fistula. Fistula does not heal over time and its condition is not stable. It varies in types. The fistula drainage may vary depending on the organ to which it is connected, such as digestive fluid, bile, urine, pus, or other secretions [1].

Sinus is a tract from deep body tissue to the body surface or a pathological blind tract that is only connected with the external opening but not the internal opening. In ancient times, it is called "Lou" (in Chinese, it literally means leakage). Sinus is a blind tract formed after infection and necrosis of deep tissue, with an opening in the mucous membrane or skin. It can occur in soft tissues, fat, muscles, and even bones, etc. The sinus can be short or long, thinned or interrupted. Yet, it has only one opening and is not connected with the in vivo hollow organ, such as the one formed due to chronic osteomyelitis. The sinus formed in the lumbosacral skin connects the skin to nervous tissue, accesses to the cranial cavity or vertebral canal, and often causes recurrent spinal pachymeningitis, which requires attention. Self-healing is possible for sinus infection to some extent, but it is not applicable to all. Severe sinus infections may lead to long-term coma and even death [2].

In most cases, fistula and sinus infections occur because the soft tissues are infected with bacteria. Therefore, fistula and sinus infections are similar to bacterial infections involving soft tissues. At the initial stage of sinus infection, the skin around the opening of the sinus may appear swelling and redness, with obvious pain occasionally. With further progression, the epidermis appears round or cone bulge. Evident necrosis may be seen a few days after infection, i.e., the duration that fistula or sinus takes to form. As the condition progresses, necrosis is further aggravated, and the bulge formed on the surface of the skin gradually evolves into a small pustule, which is manifested as redness and swelling of the external openings of the sinus. Purulent drainage is often seen to flow out, with an obvious foul odor. It is accompanied by fever and other systemic symptoms, which are especially prone to occur in sites with rich blood flow [3]. Most cases get improvement after receiving antibiotic therapy. While the disease is characterized by recurrent attacks and may evolve to chronic inflammation. In the laboratory test, most peripheral blood leukocyte count is usually increased, with an elevation of neutrophil count. The bacteriological examination includes taking wound drainage for a smear test and bacterial culture. Drug sensitive test is also practicable. The therapeutic regimen shall be developed and adjusted based on the related results.

Imaging examination can be used to further analyze the location, shape, content, scope, and the blood supply of fistula and sinus, along with their anatomical relationship with peripheral tissues, providing an important basis for clinical diagnosis and treatment. It can also be used to distinguish sinus and fistula from other similar cystic lesions, and be conducive to the selection of surgery pathway. X-ray radiography in fistula and sinus can be used to make a definite diagnosis and understand the course of the tracts, yet, it is poor in revealing the changes in peripheral tissues and their anatomi-

J. Yang (✉)
Department of Radiology, The Sixth People's Hospital of Shenyang, Shenyang, Liaoning, China
e-mail: yang.jyan@163.com

J. Song
Department of Radiology, The Sixth People's Hospital of Shenyang, Shenyang, Liaoning, China

P. Zhang · N. Su
Department of Radiology, The Sixth People's Hospital of Shenyang, Shenyang, Liaoning, China

H. Li et al. (eds.), *Radiology of Infectious and Inflammatory Diseases - Volume 5*,
https://doi.org/10.1007/978-981-16-5003-1_8

cal relationship herein. Ultrasonography is a technique frequently used, characterized by convenience and strong repeatability. It is of great value in observing the course of sinus and fistula and their relationship with the adjacent tissues as well as the follow-up before and after the treatment. However, the shortcoming is that it is related to the skill level of the operator. CT with multiplanar reconstruction can show the morphology and course of sinus and fistula and co-infection of sinus, fistula, and adjacent tissues more intuitively. MRI can produce a higher resolution for the soft tissues and clearly shows the co-infection of sinus and fistula and peripheral tissues. Multi-sequence and multi-dimensional imaging can identify the components of contents in the lesions. MRI is superior to ultrasonography and CT examination in the diagnosis for co-infection of sinus, fistula, and abscess. In addition, it can determine the relationship of fistula and sinus with the adjacent tissues without injection of the contrast agents, showing unique strength in diagnosis.

In the acute stage of infection, the diseased tissues appear lytic necrosis, mainly represented by the formation of pus, and the shape is regular. The cyst cavity is filled with pus and the cyst wall is intact. It is mainly composed of necrotic inflammatory tissue and fibrous granulation tissue, accompanied by a large number of capillaries and proliferative connective tissue. The inflammation, if not controlled, may further progress and lead to the formation of sinus and fistula. The tracts vary in shapes, mostly thin and long and narrow. Fistula and sinus are filled with unhealthy granulation tissue and the surrounding fibrous connective tissue is gradually proliferated and hypertrophic under the stimulation of chronic inflammation, abscess, or foreign body. The proliferation of fibrous tissue, inflammatory cell infiltration, and foreign body giant cell reaction may be observed under the microscope. The external openings of sinus and fistula appear obvious dark red granuloma, with a small amount of drainage overflowing. Sometimes the external openings of fistula and sinus may be temporarily closed. Yet, after a period of time, if the fistula and sinus are not completely cleared, it will result in the accumulation of residual foreign bodies or necrotic tissue, which will lead to recurrent attacks or make the sinus and fistula not heal over time. Sinus or fistula may experience cystic enlargement in the local area and form a cyst, which can be divided into an epidermoid cyst or a dermoid cyst according to the content in the cavity.

Sinus and fistula may be congenital or secondary. A congenital fistula develops at birth, while secondary sinus and fistula are formed mainly because cysts that are repeatedly infected and the wound infections caused by various reasons are not treated in time, which may be related to specific and iatrogenic infection. A congenital malformation is an anomaly in the size, shape, or structure of tissues and organs resulting from abnormalities in fetal development. This section mainly describes the fistula and sinus caused by a congenital malformation in combination with infection and mainly introduces the following several common malformations and infections.

8.1.2 Thyroglossal Cyst

Overview

The thyroglossal cyst is one of the most common types of congenital malformations in the neck region. It occurs due to the inability of thyroglossal duct to degenerate or to completely degenerate and disappear during the development of the thyroid gland. The thyroglossal cyst accounts for 70% of congenital neck masses. Thyroglossal cysts can occur anywhere from the foramen cecum of the tongue to the suprasternal notch, most commonly located adjacent to the hyoid bone. Thyroglossal cyst classically elevates with tongue protrusion. It is generally located on the midline, thus also called midline neck mass [4]. This disease is mostly seen in males and common in early childhood or adolescence. It is generally located superior or inferior to the hyoid bone. Clinically, about 1/3 of the thyroglossal cysts are accompanied by infection, which is mostly caused by infection of adjacent pharynx. Epithelial secretions generally accumulated in the cyst may rupture or be infected and form a fistula connected to the area below the skin of the neck and the base of the tongue after incision and drainage, namely thyroglossal fistula. Under the laryngoscope, the blue liquid may be seen spilling from the base of the tongue after an injection of methylene blue into the external openings of the fistula. The fistula may present as redness, swelling, tenderness in local areas, and overflow of (purulent) secretions at the openings of the fistula. Pus entering the respiratory tract may induce pulmonary abscess [5].

Imaging Findings

1. **X-ray** In the neck X-ray examination, the positive contrast agent is injected into the fistula. The development of high-density contrast agents in the tract is conducive to the diagnosis of the disease.
2. **Ultrasonography** It can clearly show the position of the internal opening of the fistula and achieves over 94% accuracy in the diagnosis of thyroglossal cyst. An ultrasound-guided needle biopsy may be performed before the operation. The cysts appear as a cystic and sonolucent area filled with anechoic fluid below the plane of the hyoid bone in the anterior neck, most of which are single cysts, few of which are separated by thin walls, and enhancement of echo can be observed in the rear of the cysts. When the cyst is accompanied by infection, it appears as an unclear border, and echo with heterogeneous patterns (cystic, solid, or solid-cystic) in the lesion. Bright floating hyperechoic spots with heterogeneous

patterns can be visualized in the cyst. When the cyst is formed to a fistula, it presents as a stripe-like structure with a tortuous and irregular tubular course. Along the course of the tract, it may be detected that the fistula is connected with the hyoid bone. On sonography, the fistula appears as a sonolucent area with hypoecho or without echo, fine echogenic dots are seen in the tract, and thickening of local soft tissues and enhancement of echo can be observed; a reticular hypoechoic line representing inflammatory exudation can also be seen; fistula containing gas appears as a repetition artifact with hyperecho.

3. **CT** The cyst can occur anywhere and appears as a cystic space-occupying lesion from the foramen cecum of the tongue to the jugular notch of the sternum in the midline of the anterior neck. The cyst has a thin wall and smooth edge, with low-density contents. When the cyst is accompanied by infection, the cyst wall is thickened and roughened, and the density of the contents is uneven; thyroid tissue mass may be seen in some lesions. When a fistula develops, it appears as a stripe-like and tubular soft tissue density lesion, necrotic tissues in the tract may show lower-density area, edema of tissues around the lesion is seen; the subcutaneous fat layer is thickened, presenting as patchy and vague high-density shadow, or a thick and stripe-like reticular structure. The enhanced scan shows significant enhancement of the tract wall and peripheral tissues, high-density shadows can be observed with the CT examination after the injection of the contrast agent into the external opening of the fistula, which helps to make a definite diagnosis.
4. **MRI** A routine non-enhanced MRI may show T_1 hypointense signal and T_2 hyperintense signal in the cyst; when the cyst is accompanied by infection, the cyst wall is thickened and roughened, with an irregular shape. An abscess is formed in the local area, the vomica shows a hypointense signal on T_1WI and a hyperintense signal on T_2WI; the cyst wall shows an isointense or slightly hypointense signal on T_2WI; the enhanced scan shows significant enhancement of the cyst wall, and the vomica shows a significant hyperintense signal in DWI. The fistula appears as a stripe-like and tubular lesion with a soft-tissue signal; MRI can clearly reveal the internal and external openings of the fistula as well as the direction and range of the discharge of pus. Thickening and edema of soft tissues around the opening of the fistula are observed, the subcutaneous fat space is blurred and disappears, showing abnormal signal shadows interwoven into a reticular or patchy pattern, the scan shows slightly hypointense on T_1WI and slightly hyperintense on T_2WI (Fig. 8.1), the enhanced

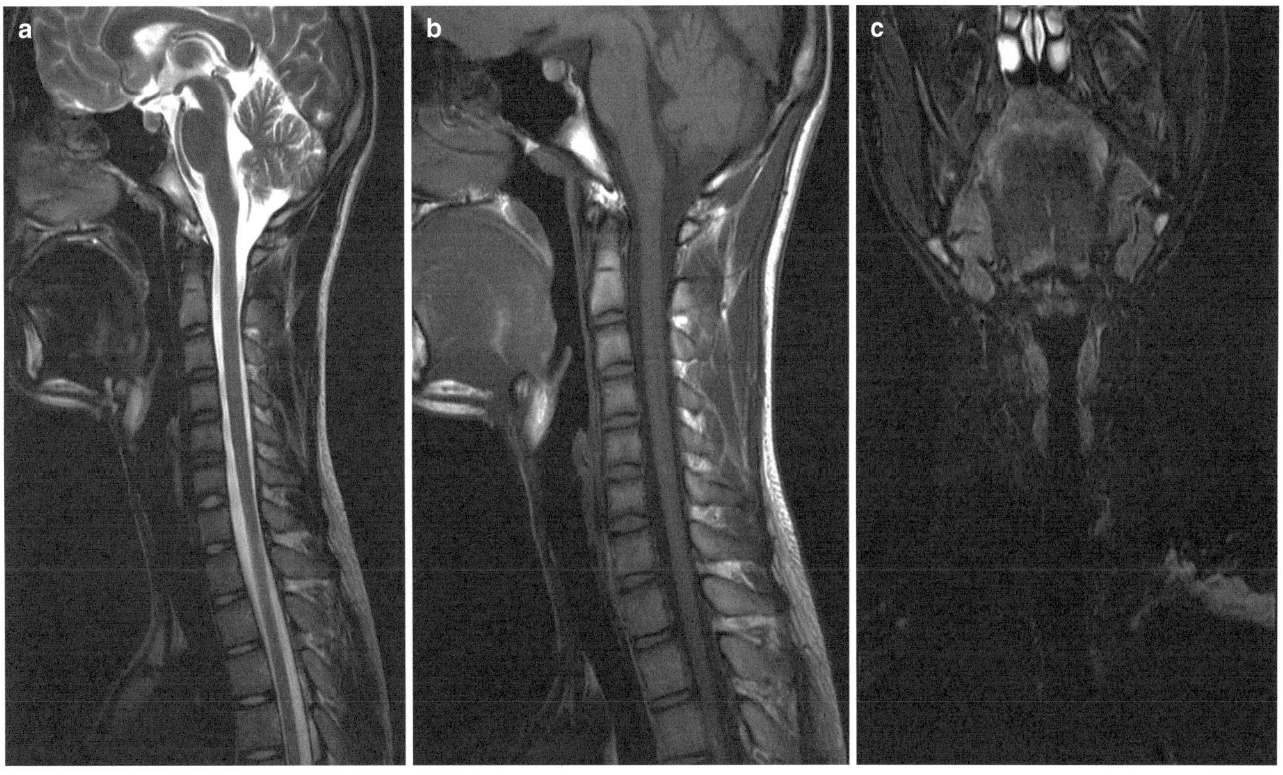

Fig. 8.1 Thyroglossal fistula accompanied by infection. The sagittal plane and coronal plane from MRI show tubular shadow from the anterior hyoid bone to the area under the skin, with local skin discontinuity, the peripheral subcutaneous tissues show hypointense on T_1WI (**b**) and hyperintense on T_2WI (**a**) with an irregular patch pattern, the fistula shows the hyperintense signal on T_2WI fat-suppressed sequence (**c**)

scan shows significant enhancement of co-infected cyst wall and tract wall.

Key Points of Diagnosis

1. Cystic mass near the midline area before the neck, the cyst spontaneously ruptures or is infected and forms a fistula after incision and drainage, a strip-like lesion is palpable below the skin of the neck and the base of the tongue, such lesion is common in early childhood or adolescence.
2. Under the laryngoscope, the blue liquid may be seen spilling from the base of the tongue after an injection of methylene blue into the external openings of the fistula.
3. On ultrasonography, the fistula appears as a sonolucent area with hypoecho or without echo, the course is tortuous, fine echogenic dots are seen in the tract, and thickening of local soft tissues and enhancement of echo can be observed; a reticular hypoechoic line with inflammatory exudation can be seen; fistula containing gas appears as a repetition artifact with hyperecho.
4. The neck CT and MRI scan show cystic cyst in the midline of the neck; when the cyst is accompanied by infection, the cyst wall is thickened and roughened, with an irregular shape. When a fistula develops, it appears as a stripe-like and tubular soft tissue density (signal) lesion, tissues with concurrent necrosis and pus in the tract cause heterogeneous density (signal); enhanced scan shows significant enhancement of the cyst wall and tract wall, edema of tissues around the lesion is seen; the subcutaneous fat layer is thickened, presenting as inflammatory exudation, which forms the abscess, the vomica shows a significant hyperintense signal in DWI.
5. The shape and course of the fistula can be clearly revealed after the injection of the contrast agent into the external opening of the fistula, which helps to make a definite diagnosis.

Differential Diagnosis

1. **Tuberculous fistula of the neck** It is mostly caused by the tuberculosis spread and rupture of mediastinal lymph nodes, and the openings of the fistula are mostly located in the suprasternal fossae; the patients may have a history of rupture of cervical and thoracic masses, with the discharge being caseous material rather than purulent fluid. Lesions with tuberculous infiltration can be observed with chest imaging, which can be distinguished from the thyroglossal cyst according to the clinical medical history and laboratory test.
2. **Midline cervical cleft** Congenital midline cervical cleft can also present as a fistula in the midline of the anterior neck. It is a rare clinically and exists at birth, with a length of 3 ~ 5 cm and a width of 2 ~ 5 cm. Congenital midline cervical cleft is often overlooked due to its vague appearance. The main clinical manifestations present as skin deformities along the longitudinal direction of the cervical anterior neck, most of which are located in the inferior end; occasional cyst combined with fistula in the superior end may be seen, which is not related to the hyoid bone; subcutaneous soft tissue shows a fibrotic change without skin appendages [6, 7]; the congenital midline cervical cleft can be distinguished from the thyroglossal cyst according to these features.

8.1.3 Branchial Cyst and Fistula

Overview

The branchial cyst and fistula is a cystic mass in the lateral area of the neck resulting from the congenital anomalies of embryonic development. Most scholars believe that it is caused by the failure of normal fusion or incomplete obliteration of branchial arch and branchial cleft during embryogenesis, and it can occur in anywhere of the neck, with a wide range, deep location, and complex structure. The unilateral neck can be divided into the upper, middle, and lower parts based on the origin of the branchial clefts. Among the branchial anomalies, second cleft lesions are the most common type, accounting for 95% [8]. The third branchial fistula is formed from the remnants of the third pharyngeal pouch not completely degenerated in the early embryonic period, accounting for 2 ~ 8%. Anatomically, it may originate in the internal opening at the base of the pyriform fossa (rostral end), would be likely to pass thyrohyoid membrane to superior laryngeal nerve before ending in the thyroid gland or its peripheral tissues. The third branchial fistula mainly presents as a sinus or fistula, with its external openings located below the anterior margin of the sternocleidomastoid. The mass is considered as a cyst when there is no internal or external opening; the mass is considered as an incomplete fistula when one side of the external or external opening disappears; the mass is considered as a complete fistula when the internal opening is connected to the external one. Clinically, the branchial cyst and fistula mostly appear as painless cervical mass, which grows slowly and develops in one side. It can occur at any age and is most common in children, showing no significant gender differences. When the body's immunity is low, the mass complicated with bacterial infection may rapidly enlarge accompanied by pain, and the inflammation will spread along the fistula, causing repeated infection or abscess formation in the local peripheral tissues, or even rupture and discharge of pus [9].

Imaging Findings

1. **X-ray.** Neck X-ray examination and barium swallow (or esophagram) are easy to perform and effective, which are

helpful for diagnosis. The X-ray visualizes air-fluid levels in the soft tissues of the unilateral neck, which is a specific manifestation of the disease.

2. **Ultrasonography.** The congenital branchial cysts are located under the skin of anterior skin, most of which are round or quasi-circular cystic anechoic lesions with regular shape; the lesion has a clear border and a thin cyst wall, with diversified internal echo; the manifestations of the lesions vary depending on the medical history and type of lined epithelium in the cyst wall; the cyst of the line squamous epithelium causes an increased exfoliation of the epithelium due to the persistence and repeated infection, resulting in dense acoustic shadows in the cyst, with uneven thickness and brightness; the lesion may appear as a solid echo when cheesy-looking or caseous discharge is observed in the central area [9]; the lesion may appear as a solid-cystic echo when yellow caseous discharge is seen inside. When the lesion is accompanied by infection, floating echogenic dots can be seen in the lesion, the mass is generally soft and will be deformed when being pressed; the echogenic dots move as the mass is deformed; heterogeneous nodules with strong echo can be seen in the local area; it is hard to distinguish this lesion from other inflammatory lesions. That the strong echo caused by gas is present in the mass is highly suggestive of the disease. The branchial fistula usually appears as a hypoecho with a strip-like, tubular, large patchy or irregular pattern or a strong echo with a combined dotted and gas-like pattern, similar to the sign of a tadpole [10].
3. **CT** The branchial cyst presents as a cystic space-occupying lesion in the lateral neck, with clear border; the peripheral tissues move when being pressed; when the cyst is accompanied with infection, the cyst wall is thickened; the border is not smooth; increased and heterogeneous density of contents in the cyst is seen; the peripheral adipose tissues are vague; enhanced scan shows significant enhancement of the cyst wall. The fistula appears as tubular or strip-like shadow, the soft tissues around the external openings show inflammatory changes, presenting as thickened skin and a reticular high-density lesion in the subcutaneous fat. When the thyroid gland is involved, its border is not vague, and a lesion containing gas is seen in the soft tissue, which are the characteristic presentations [11]. The enhanced scan shows mild or moderate enhancement of the tract wall of the fistula and its peripheral soft tissues; the abscess lesion presents as a round or quasi-circular lobular shadow in the soft tissues with clear border; a hypodense necrotic zone is seen in the center of the lesion; the CT value is 10-20HU; the enhanced scan shows significant enhancement of the abscess wall, no enhancement of necrotic foci is observed in the center, and air-fluid levels can be visualized. The course, pathway, and scope of the fistula are revealed more clearly with the fistula CT angiogram subjected to after-treatment and reconstruction, which is conducive to the pre-operative evaluation.
4. **MRI** The branchial cyst appears as a round, oval, or irregular cystic mass, the signal in the cyst varies depending on the component of the contents. When the liquid in the cyst is clear and thin, the cyst shows hypointense on T_1WI and hyperintense on T_2WI, with a thin wall and a few septated lesions; When the cyst contains a mucous or jelly-like substance, it shows a slightly hyperintense or hyperintense signal on T_1WI and isointense, slightly hyperintense, or hyperintense signal on T_2WI; When the cyst is accompanied by infection, it may evolve to a secondary fistula, with the cyst wall thickened and roughened; the enhanced scan shows an irregular and significant enhancement of the cyst wall and the peripheral inflammatory lesions. On MRI scan, the branchial fistula appears as a T_1 hypointense or T_2 hyperintense signal with a strip-like, large patchy or irregular pattern, a heterogeneous signal in the tract is visualized; the lesion is more pronounced in a fat-suppressed T_2WI sequence (Fig. 8.2), the enhanced scan shows significant enhancement of the tract wall.

Key Points of Diagnosis

1. Typical predilection sites: most of the branchial cysts are located in the anterior triangle of the neck, the front or deep area of the sternocleidomastoid, the front of the carotid sheath, traveling into the angle of the mandible before ending in the thyroid cartilage [12].
2. Clinical presentation: painless cervical mass, slow growth, common in children. When accompanied by infection, the mass enlarges rapidly with pain, the peripheral tissues in the local area may be repeatedly infected and rupture.
3. Imaging findings: branchial cyst usually appears as an oval cystic or solid-cystic mass in the longitudinal orientation, with clear demarcation. When the cyst is accompanied by infection, the cyst wall is thickened and roughened; the enhanced scan shows an irregular and significant enhancement of the cyst wall and the peripheral inflammatory lesions.
4. When accompanied by infection, the cyst evolves to a secondary fistula, which appears as a tubular or strip-like soft-tissue shadow; on ultrasonography, the fistula presents as a sonolucent area filled with anechoic fluid, on CT scan, the fistula presents as a low-density focus, on MRI scan, the fistula presents as a T_1 hypointense lesion and T_2 hyperintense lesion; the echo, density, and signal in the tract are increased and heterogeneous; the lesions and its surrounding tissue structures are not well-demarcated,

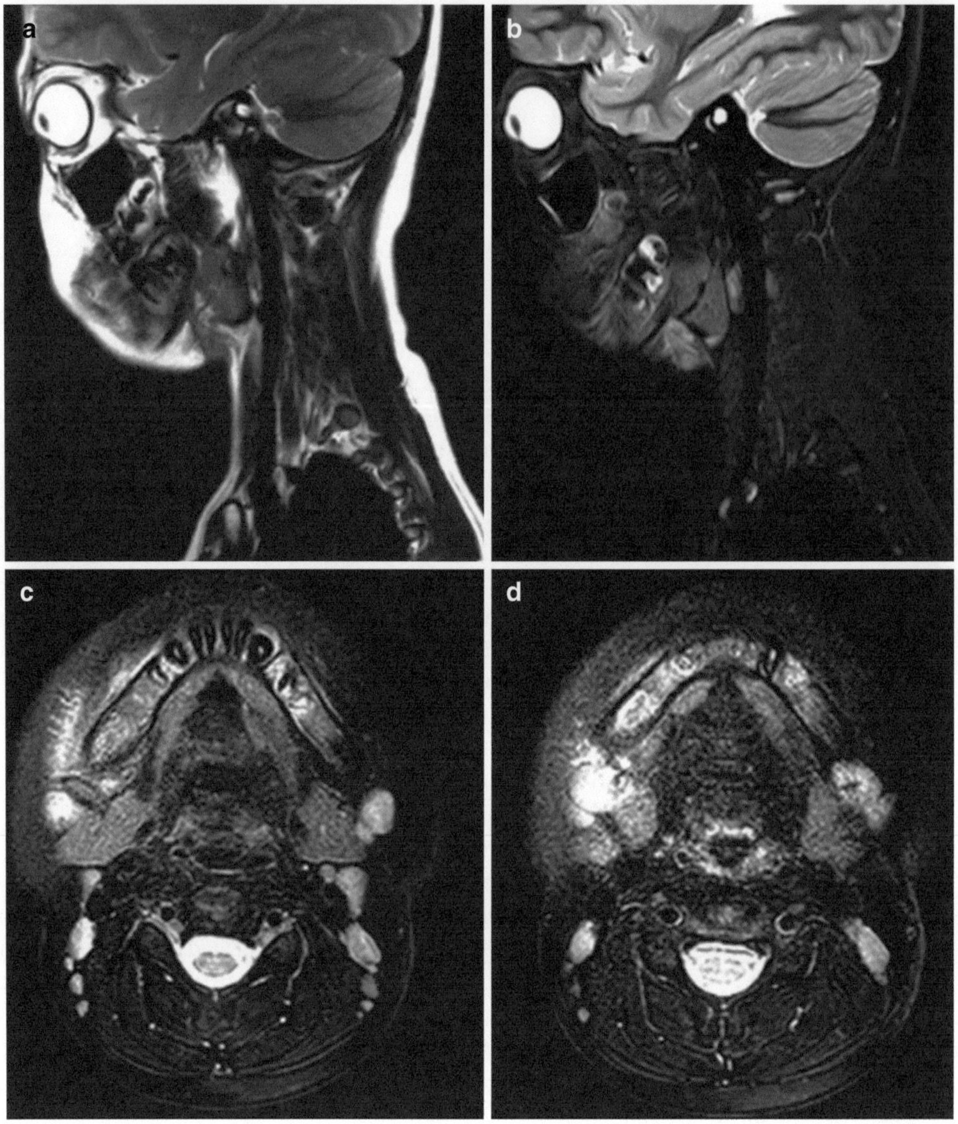

Fig. 8.2 (Right) Branchial cyst with infected fistula. According to the MRI obtained from the sagittal plane and transverse plane, a well-circumscribed cystic mass is observed below the right jaw, which shows a slightly hypointense signal on T_1WI (**a**) and a hyperintense signal on a fat-suppressed T_2WI (**b**) sequence; a tubular shadow is connected to the subcutaneous tissues, and subcutaneous tissues in the local area are locally thickened; the tubular shadows shows a reticular hyperintense signal on the fat-suppressed T_2WI (**c**, **d**) sequence; Inflammatory granulation tissue and necrosis below the skin are considered from the perspective of pathology

the enhanced scan shows a significant enhancement of the tract wall.

Differential Diagnosis

1. **Cystic lymphangioma.** It is common in children aged below 2 years; the cystic lymphangioma of the neck is usually located in the posterior border of the sternocleidomastoid, lateral neck, or supraclavicular fossa; on imaging examination, it appears as a multilocular or unilocular cystic lesion, showing infiltrating growth, without clear margins or significant enhancement.
2. **Cellulitis and abscess of the neck.** The cellulitis of the neck is an acute and diffuse pyogenic infection involving the skin and subcutaneous tissues; it is limited to the hypodermis, subcutaneous tissue, and superficial fascia, and mainly caused by the infection resulting from the ulceration and residual foreign body after skin or soft tissue injury. *Hemolytic streptococcus* and *Staphylococcus aureus* are the most common pathogens, non-spore-forming anaerobic bacteria can also cause the disease; the lesions spread directly or develop by spreading via the blood and lymph circulation. When the inflammation is limited and forms an abscess, it may appear as a lobed mass shadow on imaging examination; a gas shadow may be seen in the internal area of some lesions, the lesion may form a sinus due to persistence; it can be distinguished from the branchial cyst and fistula according to the clinical and imaging findings.
3. **Acute purulent thyroiditis** Infection is less likely to occur as the thyroid gland is well supplied with blood and lymph, and has a thick and complete capsule. Children, the elderly, and people with low immunity are susceptible to acute purulent thyroiditis; clinically, progressive enlargement of inflammatory mass in the neck is com-

monly seen in the neonatal period, which may be accompanied by an abscess and fistula. When the acute purulent thyroiditis occurs on one side of the neck and relapses frequently, it is hard to distinguish it from the co-infected branchial cyst and fistula; in such case, clinical presentations and imaging examination are used as the main approaches for distinction; the thyroid tissues of the branchial cyst and fistula are often pressed and invaded, while the thyroid gland itself is not diseased.

4. **Schwannoma.** Schwannoma of the neck is a benign nerve sheath tumor composed of Schwann cells, which normally produce the myelin sheath. It is located near the cervical vertebra, common in people aged 20–30 years. On imaging examination, it appears as a cystic tissue with a few solid parts; the enhanced scan shows marked enhancement of some solid parts in the lesion, which is characterized by a hypoechoic nerve trunk attached to one or both ends of the tumor. In terms of the branchial cyst and fistula, the fistula presents as a soft tissue shadow as well as necrosis, pus, and other components in the tract, which can be used to differentiate it from the schwannoma of the neck.
5. **Tuberculous fistula of the neck.** When the lymph node tuberculosis occurs with necrosis and liquidation, the fistula has a thick cyst wall, with an irregular inner wall and indistinct margins; the enhanced scan shows significant enhancement of the cyst wall and circular enhancement the thick wall. The patients may have a history of rupture of cervical and thoracic masses, with the discharge being caseous material. Lesions with tuberculous infiltration can be observed with chest imaging, which can be distinguished from the bronchial cyst and the fistula according to the clinical medical history and laboratory test.
6. **Dermoid cyst and epidermoid cyst.** A dermoid cyst is usually located in a specific site, mostly in the middle of the floor of the mouth; it often contains fat inside and shows characteristic changes in density or signal with a CT or MRI scan. An epidermoid cyst, common in adolescence, is a lesion close to the skin layer; the focus is usually small, with heterogeneous density (signal) in the cyst; the enhanced scan shows mild enhancement of the cyst wall.

8.1.4 Dermal Sinus

A dermal sinus is an epithelium-lined tract arising from the midline cutaneous region. It results from the failure of disjunction between the neural tube and the skin embedded on the surface in the early embryonic stage. A dermal sinus is common in children, usually accompanied by spina bifida and split cord malformation. Split cord malformation (SCM) refers to all double spinal cords that appear to have common embryogenesis, i.e., the spinal cord or filum terminale is characterized by a sagittal cleft. According to the recent theory, the formation of adhesions between ecto- and endoderm in the early embryonic stage leads to an accessory neurenteric canal around which condenses an endomesenchymal tract that bisects the developing notochord and causes the formation of two hemineural plates. The septum separating the spinal cord is osseous, cartilaginous, or fibrous, and runs backward through the spinal cord and may reach the vertebral lamina. There are two types of SCM. A Type I SCM consists of two hemicords, each contained within its own dural tube and separated by an osseocartilaginous (bony) median septum. A Type II SCM consists of two hemicords housed in a single dural tube separated by a nonrigid, fibrous media septum. This type of SCM is accompanied by typical thick dorsal hair, involving the dermal sinus in the vertebral canal and spinal cord.

A dermal sinus in children refers to sinus in the occiput and lumbar myeloid of the midline of the lower back; a dermal sinus usually consists of openings, a sinus, and a cyst. The external opening of the sinus is common in the dorsal, lumbar, sacral, parietal, and occipital midline. The internal and external openings of the sinus may be located at different horizontal planes, sometimes with 2–5 vertebral levels apart. When pressed, the inner opening of the sinus may dilate into one or more dermoid or epithelioid cysts and then form a blind end. The blind end is mostly located in the epidural space and outside the cerebrospinal meninges, with a few located in the sheath or outside the epidural space. About 50% sinus terminal is accompanied by dermoid cysts, which are rich in sebaceous glands and hair follicles and susceptible to bacterial infection. After being infected, the cysts may be accompanied by abscesses around the opening of the sinus, which may spread through the sinus for further infec tion, resulting in intraspinal infection and even purulent meningitis. The prognosis of the dermal sinus is associated with whether the central nervous system (CNS) is infected or not. Relevant studies show that the prognosis of patients with co-infected dermal sinus and nervous system is worse than that of patients with recurrent skin infection only [13]. Whether patients with dermal sinus present co-infected nervous system requires a comprehensive judgment. Once diagnosed, surgery should be performed as soon as possible.

Imaging Findings

1. **X-ray.** Plain film of the spine may suggest spina bifida occulta, and spinal angiogram may reveal an intraspinal space-occupying lesion.
2. **Ultrasonography.** The sinus may be hypoechoic, with different thickness and length; the sinus outside the vertebral canal shows a vertical course and changes to a longitudinal course after entering the vertebral canal. The

shape and course of the sinus are discernible as the soft tissue outside the vertebral canal, epidural fat, and dura mater show hyperecho. Epithelioid or dermoid cysts are mostly elliptic, the cyst wall may be isoechogenic or slightly hyperechogenic; homogeneous or heterogeneous hypoecho is seen in the cyst. When accompanied by intraspinal infection, it is hard to distinguish the relationship between the lesion and the spinal cord due to the vague anatomic relationship resulting from infection and adhesion.

3. **CT.** Compared to MRI examination, a CT scan can be used to determine the localization and nature of the intraspinal dermoid cyst, which manifests as a round or oval hypodense mass with clear demarcation. The CT value is usually −80 to −20 HU due to the fat contained in the cyst. The dermoid cyst may be accompanied by calcification, and the enhanced scan shows no pronounced enhancement. On a non-enhanced CT scan, the sinus appears as a tubular shadow, some of which are usually not clearly revealed. After the injection of the contrast agent, the overall profile of the sinus can be shown, and with the 3D post-processing technique, the shape of the spina bifida and the condition of SCM can be clearly revealed.
4. **MRI.** MRI is the main means to check the dermal sinus. The intraspinal cyst shows a hyperintense signal on T_1WI and a heterogeneous hyperintense signal on T_2WI; the fat in the cyst shows no signal on a fat-suppressed sequence. The sinus shows a tubular or strip-like hypointense signal shadow on T_1WI, an isointense or hypointense signal shadow on T_2WI (Fig. 8.3). When the sinus contains pus, it shows a hyperintense signal on T_2WI; the enhanced scan shows a bright enhancement of the abscess wall and inflammatory tissues; the vomica shows a significant hyperintense signal on DWI, Characteristic changes can be observed. A scan from the sagittal plane can reveal the overall profile of the sinus. The SCM shows an abnormal signal shadow with a longitudinal course in the spinal cord, a hypointense signal on T_1WI, a hyperintense signal on T_2WI; on the transverse plane, the spinal cord is bisected into two hemicords, the fibrous median septum shows a hypointense signal on T_1WI and T_2WI; the signals may be reintegrated when reaching the distal end. When the dermal sinus is accompanied by the infection of the CNS such as concomitant cerebral abscess, cerebral infarction, and hydrocephalus, MRI examination may also help to make a definite diagnosis.

Key Points of Diagnosis

1. It refers to a tract in the occiput and lumbar myeloid of the midline of the back and usually consists of openings, a sinus, and a cyst. About 50% sinus terminal is accompanied by dermoid cysts, usually with concomitant spina bifida and SCM.
2. The diagnosis of this disease mainly depends on imaging examinations. Spina bifida occulta may be revealed with an X-ray plain film and CT scan subjected to reconstruction. As the dermoid cyst contains fat, characteristic changes can be observed with a CT and MRI examination.
3. The most effective examination method for this disease is spine MRI. MRI scan from multiplanes can clearly show the morphology of the spinal cord, the position of the cone, and the relationship between dermal, sinus, and cyst; when accompanied by an abscess, the vomica shows a significant hyperintense signal on DWI.
4. Concurrent infection, formation of an abscess around the opening of the sinus; easy to be accompanied by intraspinal infection and even cause purulent meningitis. A lumbar puncture may lead to infection and spread of the abscess, which should be performed after imaging localization.

Differential Diagnosis

1. **Purulent meningitis.** Clinically, typical purulent meningitis is characterized by acute onset, with symptoms of systemic poisoning and without inflammatory changes of the skin in the back; it is also not accompanied by spine malformation and other lesions.
2. **Tuberculous meningitis.** Patients have a history of tuberculosis in other areas, mostly presenting acute or subacute onset; the cerebrospinal fluid (CSF) is colorless, transparent, or yellowish. Meningitis caused by this disease is usually characterized by latent onset, persistent and repeated course, with no systemic symptoms; the CSF is turbid. Dermal sinus should be considered when clinical physical examination reveals that a latent external opening of the sinus is present in the back. The presence of a dermal sinus can be confirmed with the imaging examination.
3. **Sebaceous cyst.** A sebaceous cyst should be distinguished from the end of the sinus of dermal sinus accompanied by a dermoid cyst. The sebaceous cyst is a disease caused by retention and deposition of secretion of sebum and is common in adolescence. It mainly manifests as comedones and infection of cyst in the lesion. Face, chest, and back are common sites of sebaceous cysts. The surface of the cyst is closely adherent to sebaceous glands, but not to the deep tissue. The cyst has fragments of sebaceous glands inside, without infection of the CNS.
4. **Meningocele.** Severe congenital spinal cord malformation in newborns can be located anywhere from the cervical spine to the lumbosacral spine. It appears as a cystic mass in the midline of the back, with different size; the

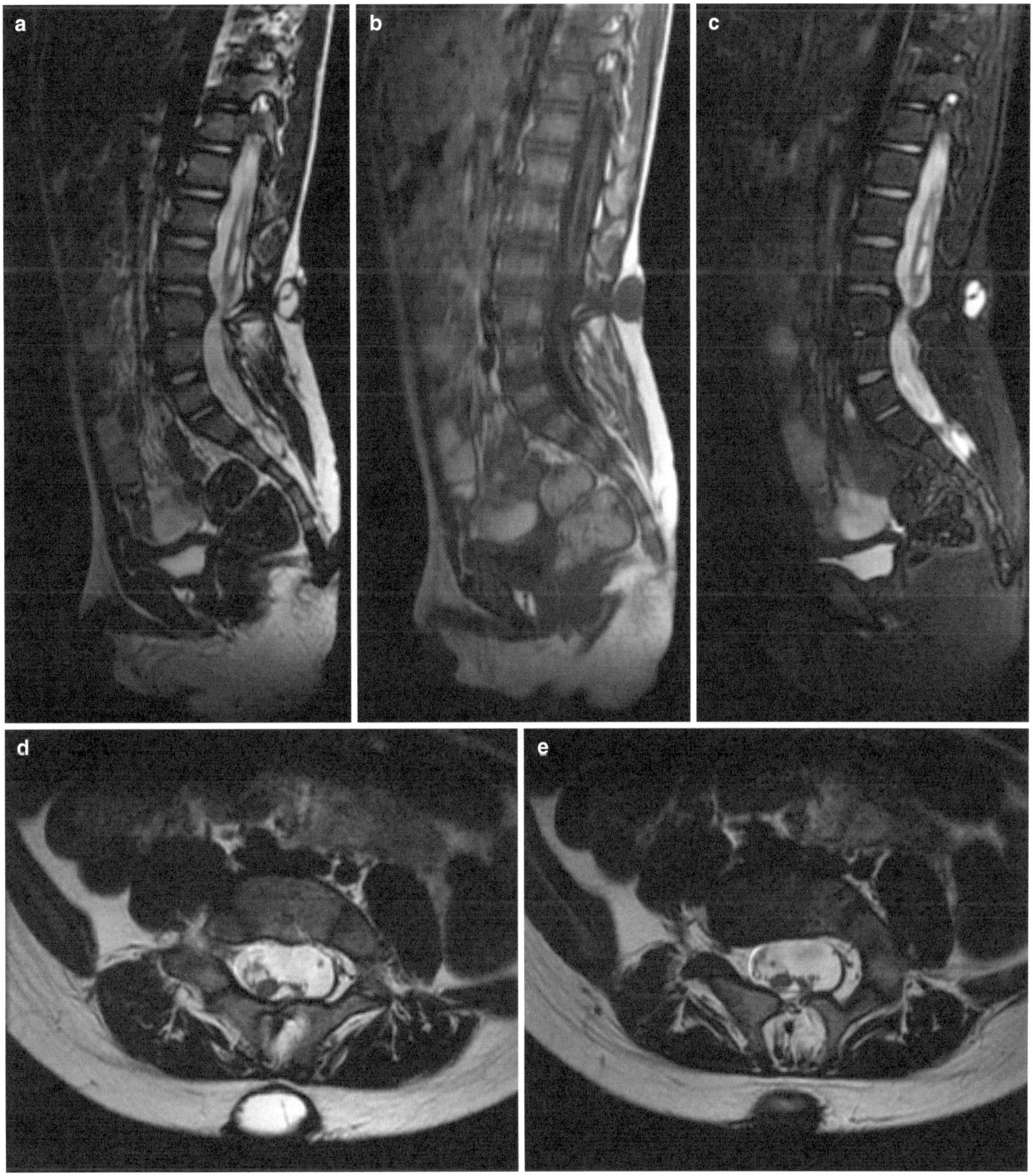

Fig. 8.3 SCM with dermal sinus in the lower back. The MRI (**a**–**e**) from the sagittal plane and transverse plane shows that the vertebral canals at the levels L_3 - L_5 are broadened, the posterior vertebral laminas are separated, and a shadow of the fibrous septum is visualized in the center of the spinal cord. A cystic lesion is observed on the midline cutaneous region of the back, showing a slightly hypointense on T_1WI (**b**) and hyperintense on T_2WI (**d**, **e**). On one end, the opening of the lesion starts from the skin, on the other end, a tubular sinus is connected to the epidural space (**a**–**c**)

base varies in width and is connected to the capsule of the meninges; the skin on the surface is normal; the disease is not accompanied by local infection; meningocele can be distinguished from the dermal sinus according to the above characteristics.

8.1.5 Panniculitis

Overview
Panniculitis is a non-purulent inflammatory disease primarily occurring in subcutaneous adipose tissue. It is most common in women aged 30–50 years. The etiology of panniculitis is unclear, and its incidence may be associated with infection, trauma, ischemia, autoimmune response, etc. Panniculitis has a higher incidence in patients with vasculitis, rheumatism, granulomatous diseases, and malignant tumors [14]. The adipose tissues of the whole body may be involved, most common in the subcutaneous fat layer and abdominal fat. The disease is mainly characterized by subcutaneous nodules, fever, and visceral injury. The clinical symptoms include recurrent general malaise, cough, joint pain, abdominal pain. Multiple, symmetrical, and clustered subcutaneous nodules are usually observed. Pain and tenderness are present in the nodules. The disease is mostly featured by a chronic course. After the lesion is healed, the skin may remain pigmentation and different degrees of depressed atrophy. It is easy to make a clinical misdiagnosis due to its lack of specificity in clinical manifestations and laboratory tests.

The panniculitis consists of cutaneous panniculitis and systemic panniculitis according to the lesion location and the scope of fat involved. The lesion of the formed only involves the subcutaneous adipose tissue. The latter is accompanied by the involvement of the viscera, showing multi-organ injuries. The liver and kidney are the most common organs involved, the occurrence of which is chiefly due to abnormal metabolism of fatty tissue and immune injury. Other systems involved include lung and heart. Patients with panniculitis and involvement of viscera are generally poor in the prognosis. This chapter mainly describes cutaneous panniculitis, namely subcutaneous panniculitis [15].

Several specific types of panniculitis:

1. Idiopathic lobular panniculitis (Weber-Christian disease): inflammation primarily occurring in the fat lobules, characterized by heterogeneity.
2. Cold panniculitis: a type of physical panniculitis directly caused by the cold environment [16].
3. Subcutaneous fat necrosis (SCFN) in newborns: this disease is common in the full-term neonates, and appears as a red, purplish, or dark purple subcutaneous nodule in the local areas, with the hardness similar to rubber. It is commonly located over the face, buttock, outer thighs, shoulders, and back. This disease is self-limited [17], with no formation of a scar.
4. Poststeroid panniculitis: this disease is common in nephritis, leukemia, and rheumatic fever in children and other patients requiring corticosteroid therapy; it occurs after withdrawal or a sudden reduction in the amount of medication taken, most commonly located over the face, shoulders, back, and thighs. The symptom usually resolves spontaneously after increment or reapplication of the corticosteroid.
5. Traumatic panniculitis: patients with traumatic panniculitis usually have a definite history of trauma; adipocytes in the lesion area become necrotic after trauma, resulting in edema, inflammation, and erythema in local areas; subcutaneous nodules are palpable; diagnosis can be made in combination with the pathological examination; this disease is self-limited, surgical removal is practical if a fibrous mass or larger nodule is formed.

Pathophysiology
The subcutaneous fat layer consists of the lobules formed by adipocytes and the interlobular connective tissue septa. Subcutaneous panniculitis can be divided into nodular panniculitis, liquefying panniculitis, and calcifying panniculitis due to different pathological changes. The nodular panniculitis present as a subcutaneous nodule of different sizes; most nodules are less than 2 cm, some may be larger. Pathologically, the disease manifests as the degeneration and necrosis of adipocytes in the lobules. As the course continues, some nodules of the nodular panniculitis may spontaneously rupture and evolve to the liquefying panniculitis. In the later stage, the disease shows fibrotic changes and thickening of the vascular walls and intima, which leads to a relatively decreased blood supply to subcutaneous adipose tissue; then the malnutrition occurs, resulting in metastatic calcification.

The pathological staging of panniculitis is of significant value to the early diagnosis of the disease. The course of the disease is divided into three stages according to the pathological progress [18]. In the first stage, namely the acute inflammatory stage, the main symptoms include hyperemia and edema, and the disease manifests as fatty degeneration and inflammatory cell infiltration. In the second stage, namely the phagocytosis stage, degeneration and necrosis occur on the basis of edema, accompanied by obvious fibrosis, sclerosis, and adhesion. The histiocytes engulf a large number of necrotic tissues and form macrophages. Infiltration of a small number of lymphocytes and plasmocytes and proliferation of fibroblasts can be observed in the surrounding areas; lipid granuloma is formed. In the third stage, namely the fibrosis stage, atrophy of adipose tissue, fibrosis, and deposition of calcium salts are visualized. Performing tissue biopsy in the early stage and excision of enough specimen for a pathological biopsy is especially important for the definite diagnosis of this disease [19].

Imaging Findings

It is of a certain value to diagnose this disease based on the imaging examination combined with clinical data. Yet, a pathological examination is required for a final diagnosis. A normal X-ray examination is of certain diagnostic value for the calcifying panniculitis, but not for the nodular and liquefying ones. Ultrasonography is an inexpensive, convenient, and effective tool that can be used to perform bedside and multiple examinations. It does not expose the patients to radiation and can clearly reveal the scope and morphology of subcutaneous lesions as well as the status of echo in the lesions, thus being widely used in clinical practice. CT with multiplanar reconstruction can show the scope and morphology of the lesion. MRI has a high resolution in the soft tissues and can clearly show the fat, components of the soft tissues, and the involvement of the peripheral tissues.

1. Ultrasonography.
   (a) Nodular panniculitis: the normal skin tissues show homogeneous hypoecho, a few spaced echoes are seen in the skin; the boundary between epidermis and dermis is clear and flat. In terms of the nodular panniculitis, the subcutaneous adipose tissue is thickened, with enhanced and heterogeneous echo; large patchy hyperecho is seen, within which a grid-like and strip-like hypoechogenic band with indistinct margin is visualized; the nodule shows hyperecho or heterogeneous echo; the CDFI shows dotted blood flow signal in the lesion area or no obvious blood flow signal.
   (b) Liquefying panniculitis: the liquefying panniculitis appears as a single or multiple irregular hypoechogenic areas; nodular or patchy lesions are observed with clear demarcation; the peripheral adipose tissues are not clearly revealed; no blood flow signal is detected with CDFI.
   (c) Calcifying panniculitis: the calcifying panniculitis manifests as tubular or irregular echogenic foci, with an acoustic shadow behind.
2. CT.
   (a) Nodular panniculitis: The lesion is only located in subcutaneous adipose tissue, some of which are closely associated with the skin. Local subcutaneous tissue is swollen and thickened, showing nodular and patchy high-density shadow, which is clustered and symmetrically distributed, with clear boundary. The surrounding adipose tissue shows a thick striped reticular structure, and the lesion has not invaded the muscularis, and the enhanced scan shows no marked enhancement. CT multiplanar reconstruction can clearly show the extent of lesion involvement (Fig. 8.4).
   (b) Liquefying panniculitis: subcutaneous adipose tissue is thickened and densified, with nodular focus, slightly high-density striped & patched shadow and grid-like shadow. The lesion shows irregular shape, uneven density, and blurred edge, and the view of necrotic area in the lesion is not enhanced by enhanced scan.
   (c) Calcifying panniculitis: There are many nodular and reticular high-density shadows in subcutaneous fat layer, which are complicated with heterogeneous calcification. The boundary between them and adjacent adipose tissue is clear, but there is no marked enhancement by enhanced scan.
3. MRI.
   (a) Nodular panniculitis: There are many patchy and nodular abnormal signals in subcutaneous adipose tissue, and they can also appear as quasi-circular

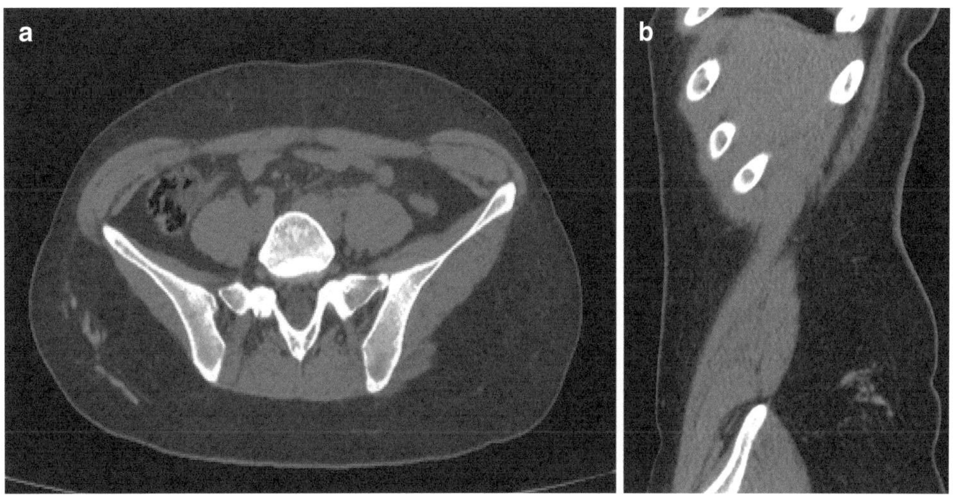

Fig. 8.4 Nodular panniculitis of right iliac region. The CT shows that the transverse plane (**a**) and sagittal plane (**b**) have nodular and patchy high-density shadow in subcutaneous fat layer of right iliac region, which is distributed in clusters and has clear boundary. The adipose tissue around the lesion shows a reticular structure, and the lesion does not invade the muscularis

masses, with obvious adhesion with epidermal tissue and some symmetrical changes. In acute inflammatory phase, T_1WI sequence shows hypointensity, T_2WI fat suppression sequence shows slight hyperintensity, unclear boundary, fuzzy subcutaneous fat and grid-like change; no obvious abnormal signal is found in adjacent muscle tissue, and enhanced scan shows mild or no obvious enhancement. When the lesion progressed to fibrosis stage, T_1WI and T_2WI shows slight hypointensity, or T_2WI shows slight flocculent hyperintensity, which has a clear boundary with normal adipose tissue.

(b) Liquefying panniculitis: shows heterogeneous abnormal signal in subcutaneous adipose tissue, indicating multiple nodular and patchy shadows, hypointensity on T_1WI, central hyperintensity in T_2WI fat-suppressed sequence, and hypointense shadow in the periphery, with blurred edge, unclear boundary with adjacent tissues, slightly grid-like hyperintense in subcutaneous adipose tissue, and no marked enhancement in necrotic area by enhanced scan.

(c) Calcifying panniculitis: MRI shows hypointense focus on T_1WI and T_2WI, which is easy to be missed by MRI examination, and can be confirmed by CT and X-ray examination.

Key Points of Diagnosis

1. This disease is a non-purulent inflammation involving subcutaneous adipose tissue, which is a rare disease, especially in women aged 30–50. The adipose tissues of the whole body may be involved, most common in the subcutaneous fat layer and abdominal fat [20].
2. Skin panniculitis only involves subcutaneous adipose tissue, but not deep fascia and muscle tissue. Its clinical manifestation is subcutaneous nodules, accompanied by general malaise and fever.
3. The main pathological changes are subcutaneous adipose tissue damage, degeneration, and necrosis caused by various reasons, and the pathological types consist of nodular panniculitis, liquefying panniculitis, and calcifying panniculitis.
4. The lesion is located in subcutaneous fat layer, which is closely related to the skin, showing nodular and patchy shadow, with multi-cluster, symmetrical distribution, clear boundary, and the surrounding fat tissue shows a thick striped reticular structure. CT shows a slight hyperintensity shadow, MRI shows a slightly lower value on T_1WI and a slightly higher value on T_2WI, but there is no obvious enhancement by enhanced scan. CT shows clearly calcifying panniculitis with high sensitivity.

Differential Diagnosis

1. **Panniculitis of other types**. Hard erythema is characterized by chronic subcutaneous nodules with ulcers and atrophic scar lesions, which cannot be cured for a long time, which can be diagnosed by conducting pathological biopsy on tissues with sufficient depth in the middle and late stage of skin lesions [21]; Erythema nodosa is characterized by repeated attacks and subcutaneous nodules appearing in masses. After the nodules subside, local skin is subject to concave and pigmentation with different degrees. Nodules recur every few weeks or months, which can be differentiated from this disease by clinical analysis.
2. **Subcutaneous panniculitis like T cell lymphoma (SPTCL).** SPTCL is a rare peripheral T cell lymphoma with subcutaneous tissue infiltration [22, 23], which is more common in people aged 20–50 years. The tumor often persists for several years, and skin damage often occurs in limbs, which often leads to extensive fat necrosis. It has no specific clinical features in the early stage of the disease, and is difficult to distinguish from nodular panniculitis. They are also characterized by high fever, pancytopenia, bleeding tendency, hepatosplenomegaly, multiple subcutaneous nodules, or masses without tenderness, but there are tumor cells infiltrating in SPTCL adipose tissue, which can be differentiated from panniculitis by histopathology.
3. **Subcutaneous cellulitis.** Cellulitis is marked with diffuse thickening and edema of the tissue in the lesion area. The subcutaneous fat layer is of a flaky fuzzy shadow or thick striped reticular structure; the boundary between subcutaneous fat and muscle is blurred, and the fat layer between muscle bundles is displaced, blurred, or disappeared. After injection of contrast agent, the lesion tissue can be obviously continuously strengthened, and even liquid density shadow between subcutaneous tissue and muscle can be seen when checked together with effusion. Nodular panniculitis lesions are limited to subcutaneous tissue, without invading muscle layer. The lesions are nodular or patchy, with clear boundary, and the affected skin can appear normal.
4. **Sebaceous cyst.** Differentiated from liquefying panniculitis, it is a sebum secretion retention and accumulation disease, which is common in young people, mostly of single occurrence, marked with round cystic density (signal) shadow, smooth surface, normal skin color, and no blood flow signal. Sebaceous cyst exists in the skin, and its surface adheres closely to sebaceous glands, but rarely invades the skin and adheres to deep layer tissues. The density (signal) of the cyst is heterogeneous due to mixed sebaceous gland fragments, which can be distinguished from this disease.

8.1.6 Cellulitis

Overview

Cellulitis is an acute diffuse pyogenic infection of skin and subcutaneous tissue, which is limited to dermis, subcutaneous tissue, and superficial fascia, and does not involve deep layer fascia and muscle. It is mostly caused by skin or soft tissue injury, ulcer, and foreign body residue, and the primary infection focus spreads directly or through blood and lymph circulation. Common risk factors include vascular insufficiency, diabetes, and immunosuppressive patients, which can also be secondary to venous or lymphatic damage caused by surgery, previous thrombophlebitis, previous trauma, or right heart failure. The disease can occur at any age and may recur in some patients. It often occurs in limbs and forehead of adults, while occurs in forehead and perianal area of children. It can be caused by various microorganisms. The main pathogens include hemolytic streptococcus and Staphylococcus aureus, and it can also be caused by non-spore forming anaerobic bacteria, among which purulent pyogenes and Staphylococcus aureus are the most common pathogens [24].

According to the infected area, cellulitis can be divided into two categories: (1) superficial cellulitis, which is characterized by obvious redness and swelling of local skin and rapid expansion to the surrounding area. The central area is of dark red and the edge is of slightly light red. There is no obvious boundary between the inflamed skin and the surrounding normal skin tissue, and the tenderness is obvious. (2) Deep acute cellulitis; although local skin redness is not obvious, there are swelling and deep tenderness in the affected area, and obvious systemic symptoms such as chills, high fever, and headache. If the disease is not controlled in time, blood vessel thrombosis and tissue necrosis may develop into necrotizing fasciitis. There are some soft tissue swelling caused by some low-toxicity pathogens, marked with atypical medical history, long course of disease, and lack of typical clinical signs, which are sometimes difficult to distinguish from tumors. Clinically, we should pay special attention to cellulitis occurring in the following two special areas. (1) Orbital cellulitis: It is a serious cellulitis, which can cause permanent vision loss, spread to the brain, cause septicemia and endanger life [25, 26]. (2) Cellulitis at submandibular area and mouth floor: Local infection causes diffuse swelling of subcutaneous tissue of neck, which easily leads to edema of vocal cords and larynx. The patient has hoarse voice and may have wheezing noise. In severe cases, it causes difficulty in breathing due to the compression of trachea and obstruction of inhalation, and the condition would be critical. When non-surgical treatment is ineffective, trachea should be cut for decompression as early as possible to prevent suffocation.

Laboratory test is helpful to the diagnosis of this disease. (1) Peripheral blood test: the total number of white blood cells increased, neutrophils increased, C-reactive protein increased, and erythrocyte sedimentation rate accelerated. (2) Etiological examination can identify pathogens, so as to carry out further targeted treatment. Rapid antigen detection test has higher specificity, which can generate results quickly, and is easy for clinical application, but its sensitivity is slightly lower than that of bacterial culture.

Pathophysiology

Simple acute cellulitis causes a wide range of lesions without boundary and spreads rapidly around, marked with obvious congestion and edema in local tissues, with unclear boundaries with normal tissues. Hyaluronic acid secreted by hemolytic streptococcus, the main pathogenic bacterium, can degrade hyaluronic acid in loose connective tissues, and streptokinase secreted can dissolve cellulose, allowing various bacteria to easily pass through interstitial spaces and lymphatic vessels and further spread; Local edema causes bacteria to retain here and becomes an excellent medium for their growth. Microscopically, a large number of neutrophils infiltrate diffusely, and the boundary between neutrophils and peripheral tissues is unclear. This type of cellulitis generally does not cause obvious tissue necrosis and dissolution, and generally leaves no trace after healing.

In advanced cases or for patients infected with strong toxicity, cellulitis can be characterized by pneumatosis and abscess formation: (1) Inflammation caused by anaerobic bacteria or aerobacter infection can produce gas in tissues, neutrophil infiltration can be identified under microscope, and the lesions may develop into tissue necrosis and dissolution. (2) High bacterial toxicity and improper use of antibiotics. Toxins produced by bacteria cause local tissue necrosis, which is mainly caused by Staphylococcus aureus. Thrombin in bacteria converts the fibrinogen into cellulose, and necrotic inflammatory tissue is dissolved by enzymes into pus. A large amount of cellulose oozes out from peripheral non-necrotic inflammatory tissue to form vomica wall, where there are a large number of capillaries and hyperplastic connective tissue. Once abscess is formed, pus should be drained immediately, otherwise it will easily spread and diffuse along the fascia space, forming multi-gap abscess, and it may also subject to lymphatic channel dissemination and hematogenous dissemination, which tend to cause sepsis [27].

Imaging Findings

X-ray plain film gives a very limited evaluation of soft tissue lesions, which should be used when the lesions are suspected to involve bone and joint tissues, or are complicated with calcification and pneumatosis, or when metal foreign bodies need to be excluded. Ultrasound is a convenient and mobile imaging technology, which can be examined at the bedside of patients, and is suitable for examination and follow-up for superficial or small focus. Because it involves no ionizing radiation, it can be used as the first choice for children and pregnant women. However, ultrasound has certain limitations due to its strong dependence on operators and nonspecific examination results. CT is highly sensitive to foreign bodies and gases in soft tissues, deep lesions, and calcified lesions. CT is isotropic, and its multiplanar soft tissue reconstruction can better display and evaluate various infectious lesions. Bone reconstruction can also be used to observe the changes in adjacent osseous substance and calcified focus in lesions. CT-guided percutaneous needle biopsy can be used to support a clear diagnosis. MRI can use different sequences to observe the changes of tissue signals. In particular, T_1WI enhanced examination can clearly show congestion and edema of cellulitis and can identify the infection scope and whether there are deep layer fascia and muscle involvement. It is more sensitive than X-ray plain film and CT, and its higher soft tissue resolution and absence of ionizing radiation make it the main choice for clinical examination.

Usually, different types of inflammation and different stages of pathological changes correspond to different imaging manifestations. In this section, the imaging manifestations of simple cellulitis and necrotizing cellulitis characterized by pneumatosis and abscess formation are described as follows.

1. X-ray.
   (a) Simple cellulitis: The lesion is localized or shows diffuse swelling, and the boundary between subcutaneous tissue and muscle is unclear. It occurs in limb lesions. It is manifested that the affected limb is obviously swollen and thickened, the fat gap is blurred and disappears, and the lesion area appears cord-like or subject to increased reticular density shadow, with unclear boundary and fuzzy tissue layers.
   (b) Complicated abscess formation: The boundary is relatively clear, the density is different, and the adjacent muscle bundle can be displaced under pressure.
   (c) Gas-producing subcutaneous cellulitis: Small beaded bubbles or striped translucent shadows between subcutaneous soft tissues or muscle bundles, which are inconsistent in size and can fuse with each other.
2. Ultrasonography.
   (a) Simple cellulitis: Ultrasonography shows that the soft tissue in the lesion area is swollen, and the diffuse echo of subcutaneous tissue is enhanced. In the meantime, it can be mixed with the reticular low echo vocal zone representing inflammatory exudation, with unclear lesion boundary. Follow-up examination shows that the lesion tissue and normal subcutaneous tissue gradually displace, and colored Doppler examination shows a few blood flow signals scattered around the lesion area.
   (b) Complicated abscess formation: The lesion area of abscess has a clear boundary with normal peripheral tissues, and it gives a sense of fluctuation by palpation. The ultrasonographic image shows round, oval, or irregular anechoic areas with rather clear boundary inside subcutaneous soft tissue. Ultrasonography offers good sensitivity in displaying liquefying lesions and can guide the direction of puncture needle to suck from the focus.
   (c) Gas-producing subcutaneous cellulitis: Local small bubbles can be found in diffuse swelling tissue, showing high echo reflection artifact.
3. CT.
   (a) Simple cellulitis: It can be seen that the tissue in the lesion area is thickened and edema is formed, and the subcutaneous fat layer is thickened. By plain CT scan, it appears as a flaky fuzzy slightly high-density shadow, or a thick striped reticular structure. The interface between subcutaneous fat and muscle is blurred, and the fat layer between muscle bundles is displaced, blurred or disappears. Enhanced scan shows obvious reticular and patchy continuous enhancement. Homogeneous liquid density shadow between subcutaneous tissue and muscle can be seen when effusion is merged (Fig. 8.5).
   (b) Complicated abscess formation: Abscess mostly occurs at the superficial part of the skin, and circular or quasi-circular mass shadows with different sizes, clear boundary and heterogeneous density can be seen in the swollen soft tissue. Low-density necrotic zone can be seen in the center of the focus, with CT value of 10 - 20HU. Enhanced scan shows heterogeneous enhancement of lesion tissue, homogeneous thickness of abscess wall, obvious annular enhancement by enhanced scan, and no abnormal enhancement of central necrotic focus. Some lesions can spread along the intermuscular septum, forming deep multiple abscess [28, 29]. CT can be used for puncture or incision and pus discharge under the locationing guidance.
   (c) Gas-producing subcutaneous cellulitis: CT plain scan can clearly indicate whether there is gas in the diseased tissue and the amount of pneumatosis. It is suggested to use the lung window to observe the gas, which gives high detection rate. It is mainly characterized by swelling and thickening of soft tissue, with circular, quasi-circular, or irregular gas-like density shadow in it, with CT value less than -150HU and clear boundary (Fig. 8.6). When gas enters between muscles, it is distributed along the long axis of muscle bundle, which widens the intermuscular space.

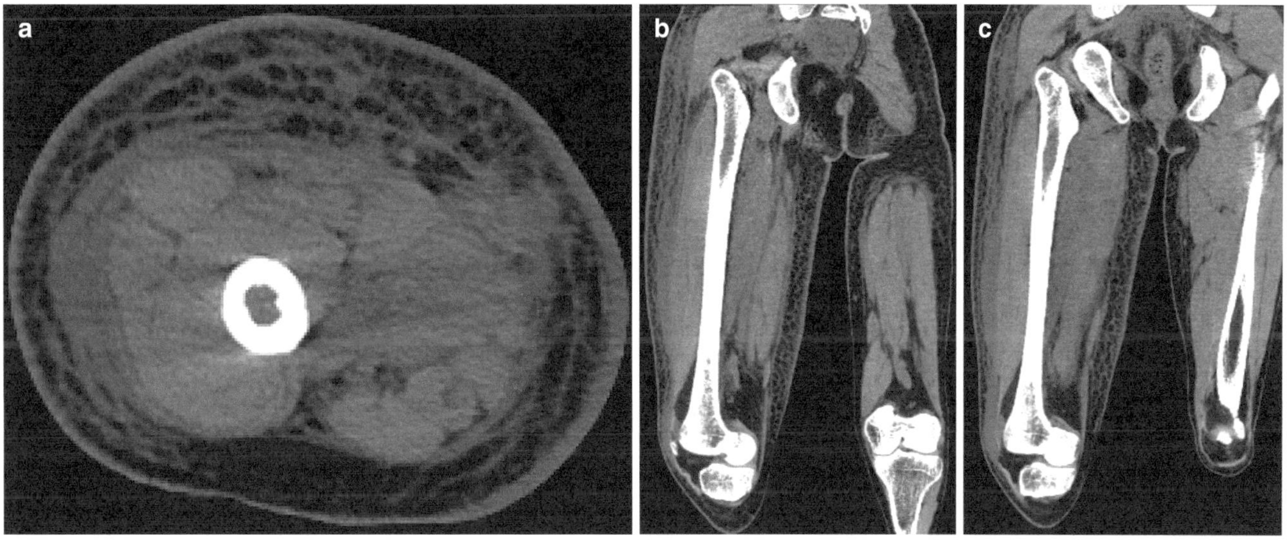

Fig. 8.5 Subcutaneous cellulitis of right thigh. (**a**) CT transverse plane shows that the affected limb is obviously thickened and swollen, subcutaneous fat is thickened, and thick striped and patchy shadows can be seen. The lesions involve the front and sides of the limb, and localized effusion is seen between the lateral subcutaneous and muscle tissues (**b**, **c**) Multiplanar reconstruction clearly shows the extent of lesion involvement

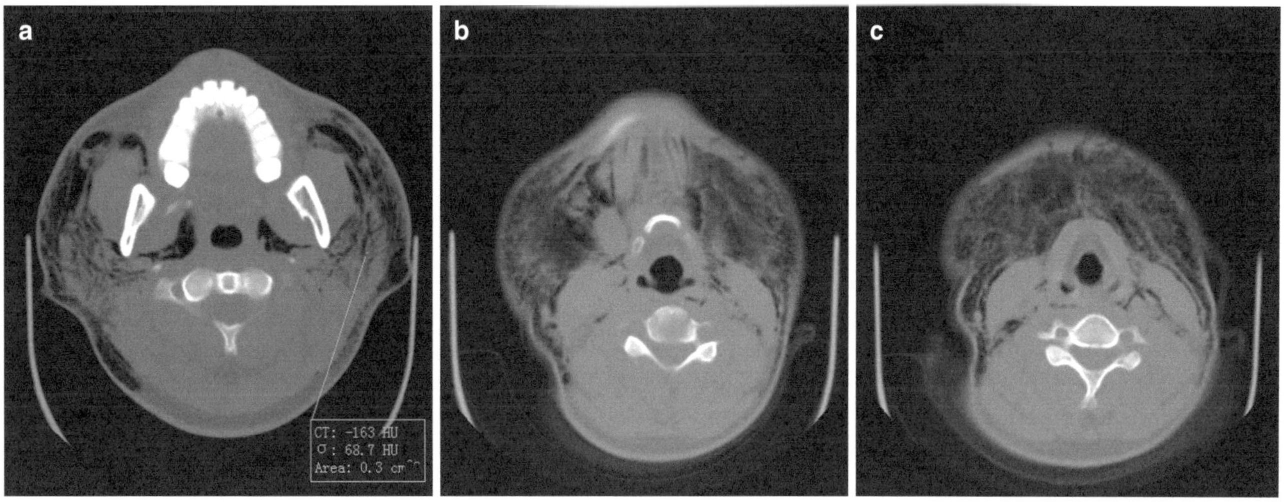

Fig. 8.6 Extensive cellulitis in submandibular area and neck. Male, 15 years old, cheek infection spreading to submandibular area and neck (**a**–**c**). CT indicates diffuse thickening and edema of subcutaneous tissue, increased density of fat layer, and shows thick reticular shadow complicated with multiple irregular gas shadows

4. **MRI** mainly uses T_1WI and T_2WI, fat-suppressed sequence and T_1WI enhanced scan. DWI sequence can be used for the diagnosis of abscess. In general, spin echo and fast spin echo sequences are most suitable for identifying and indicating soft tissue abnormalities. T_1WI shows the anatomical structure clearly, and the difference of T_2WI signals on diseased tissues is helpful for locating and qualitative diagnosis, and to find the spread of infection to deep tissues. Because inflammatory tissues are characterized by interstitial edema and increased mucus secretion, they contain a high amount of "water," which prolongs T_2 value, so T_2WI sequences are more conducive to the detection of lesions.
   (a) Simple cellulitis: diffuse thickening and edema of the lesion tissue, showing localized striped hypointensity focus in adipose tissue with hyperintensity on T_1WI; the corresponding lesion site on T_2WI sequence indicates hyperintensity, which can be patchy or feathery with unclear boundary; the T_2WI fat-suppressed sequence more clearly shows the lesion, indicating that the lesion and adipose tissue interweave into reticular abnormal signal (Fig. 8.7). The enhanced

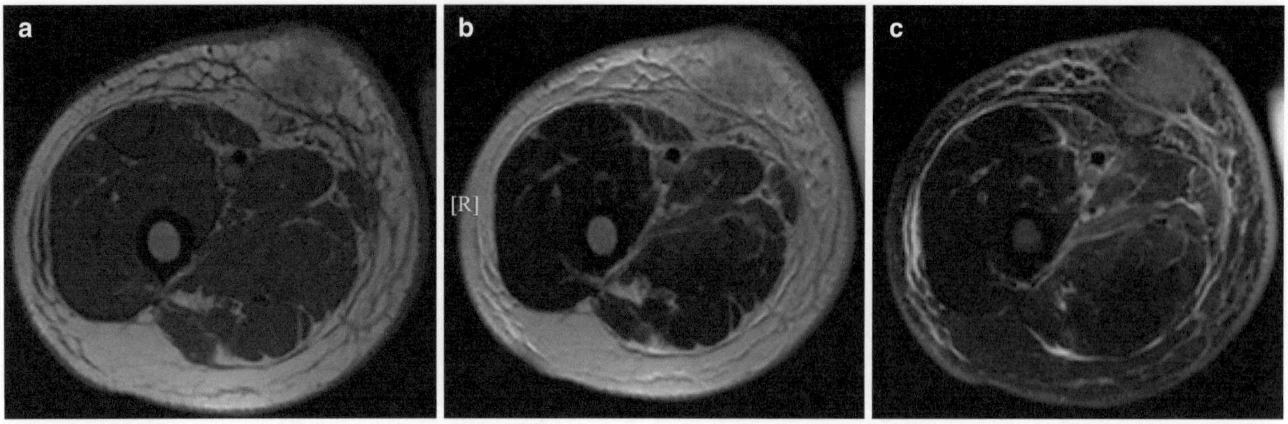

Fig. 8.7 Cellulitis. It is manifested with subcutaneous tissue at the right thigh diffusely thickened with edema, showing grid-like and linear shadow with unclear boundary. (**a**) The transverse plane T_1WI shows hypointensity; (**b**, **c**) T_2WI and T_2WI fat-suppressed sequence show hyperintensity

scan shows patchy or grid-like continuous enhancement The curved T_1 hypointense and T_2 hyperintense signal shadow between subcutaneous tissue and muscle can be seen when effusion is complicated, but the enhanced scan shows no obvious enhancement.

(b) Complicated abscess formation: The lesion continues to develop, and some inflammation is limited to develop into abscess. Abscess shows a round or lobulated mass shadow, with hypointense on pus T_1WI and hyperintense on T_2WI. The abscess wall is mainly composed of capsule of fibrous components, and its thickness is relatively uniform. On T_2WI, it shows equal or slightly hypointense, and its boundary is relatively smooth, which can be distinguished from tumor and venereal disease [30]. Edema zone can be seen in the periphery of abscess, with varying degrees, and hyperintense on T_2WI. On enhanced T_1WI, the abscess wall shows obvious ring enhancement, while the central necrotic area is not enhanced. If sinus was formed, the direction and scope of its deep multiple abscess can be clearly displayed. Because of the limited diffusion movement of water molecules in abscess, DWI shows obvious hyperintense in vomica with characteristic changes.

(c) Gas-producing subcutaneous cellulitis: both T_1WI and T_2WI show extremely hypointense [31], which is not as good as the examination methods mentioned above in terms of display.

Key Points of Diagnosis

1. Acute skin infection, limited to subcutaneous tissue, dermis, and superficial fascia, is characterized by erythema, diffuse swelling, obvious tenderness, blurred boundary, and lymph node enlargement.
2. In advanced cases or those infected with strong virus, cellulitis takes the form of the type characterized by pneumatosis and abscess formation.
3. The main pathogens include hemolytic streptococcus and Staphylococcus aureus.
4. Imaging shows swelling and thickening of subcutaneous tissue, diffuse echo enhancement by ultrasound, and mixed reticular low echo bands. CT shows fuzzy hyperdensity shadow in subcutaneous fat that is streaky and patchy, enhanced scan shows continuous enhancement, and extreme hypodensity bubbles or streaks can be seen together with pneumatosis. When abscess is formed, CT can be used for puncture or incision so as to discharge pus under the locationing guidance.
5. MRI has good soft tissue resolution, showing diffuse linear and grid shadows, hypointense on T_1WI and hyperintense on T_2WI, and continuous grid-like and plaque-like enhancement on enhanced scan. When taken together with abscess formation, the vomica shows ring enhancement, and DWI sequence shows that the vomica shows obvious hyperintense.

Differential Diagnosis

1. **Non-necrotizing fasciitis**: It is a set of diseases characterized by soft tissue inflammation and fascia thickening, usually characterized by skin thickening, soft tissue edema, fascia thickening, combined with abnormal signal in subcutaneous reticular, and no abnormal changes in adjacent muscles. The main distinguishing point between it and cellulitis is that the lesion is mainly centered on fascia, and the fascia of T_2WI fat-suppressed sequence is thickened, showing slightly hyperintense, and the fascia is obviously enhanced uniformly by enhanced scanning.

2. **Non-inflammatory soft tissue edema:** Congestive heart failure, diabetes-induced vasculopathy, and obstruction of lymphatic reflux can all be manifested as soft tissue swelling and pain, which is difficult to differentiate from cellulitis if complicated with infection. Clinical history and manifestation are very important. In terms of imaging changes, when edema occurs in tissues, the lesion area is larger. Both CT and MRI can show the existence of subcutaneous fat signal. Because it is not complicated with congestion, simple edema is not enhanced in contrast enhancement, while cellulitis can be remarkably enhanced. There may be gas in cellulitis area, and there may be gap or necrotic area adjacent to skin [32, 33].
3. **Deep vein thrombosis of lower limbs**: The systemic symptoms such as local skin and soft tissue changes and fever are similar to that of cellulitis. Intravascular thrombosis is found by ultrasound and CTV examination of lower limbs, and ischemia, sclerosis and necrosis may occur in muscle tissue complicated with vasculopathy, which can be distinguished from cellulitis.
4. **Changes in soft tissue after radiotherapy**: Radiotherapy causes skin thickening, erythema, and swelling in the corresponding sections, with subcutaneous edema similar to the case with cellulitis. Radiotherapy can also cause extensive edema of muscles in the corresponding areas, and enhanced scanning can also play a certain role in distinguishing the two. After radiotherapy, soft tissue has no marked enhancement, while cellulitis is obviously continuously enhanced.

Status Quo and Progress of Research

1. **DWI** is a kind of functional imaging, which mainly reflects the diffusion movement of water molecules in tissues. Diffusion is limited when the diffusion movement of water molecules is limited to a certain extent, which is related to the peripheral tissues environment. In recent years, DWI has been widely used in the differential diagnosis of muscle and soft tissue diseases. When cellulitis is complicated with abscess, the diffusion movement of water molecules is limited, and the pus shows hyperintense, which is beneficial to definite diagnosis and differential diagnosis.
2. **PET/CT:** In recent years, radionuclide technology has been widely used in the diagnosis of soft tissue infection, and infection-specific imaging agents have also become the research focus of nuclear medicine. Nuclear medicine for soft tissue infection imaging is based on local pathological changes of acute inflammatory tissues, which often appear before morphological changes. FDG is a glucose analogue transported to cells by glucose transporter, which is related to the increase of glucose transport quantity, and its uptake increases during inflammation and infection. ^{18}F-FDG can be used to effectively detect and reflect the characteristics of infection, which is of great significance in evaluating the therapeutic effect of infection.

8.1.7 Necrotizing Fasciitis

Overview

Necrotizing fasciitis (NF) is a widespread and rapid soft tissue infection characterized by subcutaneous tissue and fascia necrosis, which is often accompanied by systemic toxic shock. It is an important feature of this disease that it does not involve the muscle tissue at the infected section. If the development of the disease is not controlled in time, the infection will further spread to deep area and involve bones, which may lead to emphysematous osteomyelitis. If the diagnosis and treatment of this disease are not timely, the mortality rate can be as high as 52% [34]. The etiology of NF is not clear, usually bacteria directly infect deep layer soft tissues from skin surface, which is mostly caused by injection (drug injection), surgery, diverticulitis, furuncle, slight trauma, poisonous insect sting, and other factors. Most patients are elderly people, and the incidence of males is higher than that of females, where most of them are complicated with underlying disease. Diabetes is the main risk factor of this disease [35, 36], and other related factors include chronic consumptive diseases (chronic renal failure, immunosuppression, alcoholism, obesity), peripheral vascular diseases, etc. This disease most commonly occurs in limbs, accounting for about half of the cases, followed by perineum, trunk, and head and neck. When it involves male scrotum, it is named Fournier gangrene [37].

NF can be divided into 4 types according to different flora [38]infected. Type I is a mixed infection of many bacteria, including Gram-positive cocci, Gram-negative bacilli, and anaerobic bacteria, which accounts for the most cases, about 75%. NF is usually considered to be the result of the synergistic effect of aerobic bacteria and anaerobic bacteria [39]; Type II is β hemolytic streptococcus A infection [40], which can exist alone or mixed with Staphylococcus. This type of infection is invasive and often occurs in limbs; Type III is a single microbial infection involving Clostridium or gram-negative bacteria; Type IV is a fungal infection, mainly consisting of candida and associated bacteria. This type of infection usually occurs after trauma, and the disease progresses rapidly and widely. The clinical manifestations of NF include local skin changes and systemic symptoms: (1) Local skin manifestations may not be obvious. If there are skin manifestations like cellulitis pain, edema, and erythema, severe pain is usually not proportional to the degree of skin involvement. The lesion progresses rapidly, with a series of skin changes, which can affect the whole limb within

24 hours, including skin blackening, blisters, bullae, dotted & patchy ecchymosis or local ulcer necrosis, and the skin around the ulcer is subject to extensive stealth; When combined with subcutaneous gas, it gives crepitus, which may be accompanied by bloody exudation with intense stink. (2) The main feature of this disease is obvious systemic reaction with atypical local skin manifestations. Patients in the early stage of the disease may be accompanied by severe systemic poisoning symptoms such as chills, high fever, hypotension, anemia, and organ failure. If not treated in time, disseminated intravascular coagulation and toxic shock may occur. Laboratory test: the leukocyte count is increased, and bacteriological examination is of great significance to diagnosis. The best culture materials are collected from the edge of progressive lesions and blister fluid, smeared and cultured with aerobic and anaerobic bacteria, respectively; When the culture is negative, PCR technology is used to detect the B gene of pyrogenic exotoxin such as streptococcus, or serum antibody is used to detect whether there is antibody induced by streptococcus in blood, which is helpful for pathogen diagnosis. In the early stage of suspicious lesions, soft tissue biopsy by freezing microtome section can be used to provide clear and life-saving diagnosis.

Pathophysiology

NF is often accompanied with systemic and local tissue immune function damage and minor vasculopathy, which is an inflammatory disease involving deep fascia and having infectious characteristics. According to the different pathological manifestations and the development of local lesions, it can be divided into three stages: (1) Cellulitis, which is often the early stage of morbidity (1–3 days). Due to the rapid proliferation of bacteria and the release of toxins, local tissue damage is caused, which is manifested as edema and necrosis of subcutaneous tissue and shallow and deep fasciitis. Microscopically, a large number of neutrophil diffuse infiltrations are manifested, and the boundary with peripheral tissues is unclear. Complicated with aerogenic bacteria infection can lead to the generation of subcutaneous gas, forming effusion, and pneumatosis in soft tissue. Infection and soft tissue destruction progress rapidly, especially in limbs and trunk, because there is not much fibrous tissue between subcutaneous tissue and fascia in these sections to limit the spread of infection. (2) In the stage of fascia necrosis, that is, in the late stage of the disease, subcutaneous fat and superficial and deep fascia are destroyed progressively, and the epidermis can be intact, which is characterized by superficial fascia necrosis, inflammatory cell infiltration in deep fasciitis, and then extensive superficial and deep fascia necrosis. Toxins produced by bacteria can cause fibrin-like thrombosis in fascia venules and arterioles, leading to ischemia and necrosis of tissues. Microscopically, dead cells are completely digested and local tissues are rapidly dissolved. Thrombosis is considered as a pathological sign of NF, which can be seen in the obvious lesion area of imaging examination, and also in the unformed necrosis in periphery inflammatory tissues. With the further aggravation of infection, the necrotic fascia tissue is accompanied by effusion and empyema in the adjacent cavity, which can further involve muscles, where toxic organisms can cause toxic shock symptoms systematically. (3) During the repair stage, granulation tissue is formed in local wounds, and a large number of new blood vessels and neutrophils are observed under microscope. The occurrence and development of diseases is a continuous process, and the above changes cannot be completely staged, instead, there may be overlapping parts.

Imaging Findings

The course of the disease progresses rapidly and its clinical manifestations are unstable. Infection usually spreads rapidly and can lead to multiple organ failure, adult respiratory distress syndrome, and death [41]. If early diagnosis can be made, the survival rate of patients can be obviously improved. Although finger test, that is, making a small skin incision in the operating room for finger subcutaneous exploration, is considered as the best method for diagnosing NF [39], imaging examination still has great significance for early stage diagnosis of the disease. High-resolution ultrasound (HRUS), CT, and MRI can identify the structural disorder of subcutaneous soft tissue and determine whether there is gas formation, can determine the lesion scope, degree of effusion in soft tissue, and necrosis of fascia, so as to help clinicians understand the lesion progress. It is worth noting that enhanced examination should be used with caution or contraindicated in some patients with renal failure.

1. **X-ray:** The diagnostic value of NF is limited, and it mostly gives negative result in the early stage. Until the disease progresses to the late stage, it is characterized by swelling and thickening of soft tissue, thickening of affected limb, blurred boundary between subcutaneous tissue and muscle, streak-like or reticular increased density shadow in the lesion area; and some cases are manifested with small bubbles or banded gas density shadow in soft tissue.
2. **Ultrasound**: It is a simple and easy examination method, which can quickly observe the progress and changes of lesions at bedside repeatedly, and can also be used as an intraoperative guide to define the scope of debridement so as to avoid omission. Especially for special patients, such as children and patients with testicular diseases, it can be used as the first choice for examination. Its main manifestation is subcutaneous tissue inflammation, with soft tissue swelling subject to diffuse echo enhancement, disorder, and unclear boundary; When combined with

effusion and empyema, diffuse soft tissue swelling is manifested as a fluid sonolucent area (anechoic) with blurred or limited boundary. When combined with pneumatosis, it shows hyperechoic reflex artifact in diffuse swelling tissue. Ultrasonography shows no obvious characteristics of fascia thickening and necrosis.

3. **CT** can show fascia inflammation and necrosis in the early pathological stage, especially when combined with pneumatosis. Further multiplanar reconstruction can show necrosis more visually.
   (a) Cellulitis stage: diffuse swelling and thickening of subcutaneous tissue in the affected area, thick streaky & reticular shadow or fuzzy patchy shadow in subcutaneous fat, for which enhanced scan shows marked enhancement; The subcutaneous soft tissue is complicated with pneumatosis and effusion, which is characterized by small bubbles and liquid density shadow. The gas CT value is less than -150HU, the boundary is clear, and the gas can also be distributed in the deep and shallow fascia space, which is a characteristic change; Lesions may be limited, forming abscesses, manifested as circular or quasi-circular lobulated masses, with low-density necrotic areas visible in the center of the lesions. The abscess wall shows marked enhancement by enhanced scanning, but the central necrotic focus is not enhanced.
   (b) Fascia necrosis stage: The fascia in the lesion area is locally and asymmetrically thickened, and its boundary with the periphery soft tissue is unclear. The necrotic fascia tissue is not enhanced by enhanced scanning, while the unaffected fascia shows marked enhancement, which can be used as the main diagnostic basis. The lesion further expands and spreads along the course of fascia. When there is extensive gas shadow in the lesion area, it suggests gas gangrene [42], which should be noted clinically. The muscle tissue in the deep section of the lesion is often not affected, and there is no obvious swelling and enhancement.

   Secondary calcification can be formed after healing. CT can be used for diagnosis in recovery stage due to its high sensitivity to calcification.
4. **MRI**: Because of its high soft tissue resolution, it is considered as the first imaging examination method for NF, but it is not recommended in severe cases or emergencies. The T_2WI fat-suppressed sequence shows clearer lesions. Studies have shown that MRI tends to overestimate the degree of deep tissue involvement [43].
   a. In cellulitis stage, the subcutaneous tissue is thickened and edema is developed, which is manifested by localized banded hypointense focus in adipose tissue with hyperintense on T_1WI, and the T_2WI fat-suppressed sequence shows that the lesion and adipose tissue interweave into abnormal reticular signal, and the lesion area shows mild or moderate slow and continuous enhancement by enhanced scan. Shadow showing hypointense on T_1WI and hyperintense on T_2WI between subcutaneous tissue and shallow and deep fascia can be seen when combined with effusion. Pneumatosis is manifested as extremely hypointense shadows on T_1WI and T_2WI sequences; Partial inflammation forms limited abscess, showing circular or lobulated mass shadow. The pus shows hypointense on T_1WI and hyperintense on T_2WI. On enhanced T_1WI, the abscess wall shows obvious ring enhancement, and DWI shows marked hyperintense in vomica.
   b. Fascial necrosis stage: The disease further expands and spreads in a short period of time (several hours), showing that: (1) The involvement scope is extensive, and the periphery of the deep fascia and the deep intermuscular fascia can be involved, showing diffuse T_2WI hyperintense distributed along the deep fascia, especially the deep intermuscular fascia, with encapsulated or layered effusion; (2) Thickening of diseased fascia, usually $\geq$3 mm; thick; (3) More than 3 muscle compartments are involved in a single limb; (4) In enhanced scan, the deep fascia shows marked enhancement, which is mixed with or surrounded by unenhanced areas (necrosis). DWI sequence shows hyperintense or hypointense, and there is no characteristic change. (5) No marked involvement is found in deep muscle tissue, and no marked enhancement is found by enhanced scan. Some severe cases are complicated with edema and pneumatosis in fibrils.

Key Points of Diagnosis

1. Soft tissue infection characterized by extensive and rapid necrosis of subcutaneous tissue and fascia, where necrosis does not involve muscle tissue.
2. There are many pathogens involved, mainly due to the synergistic effect of Gram-positive cocci, Gram-negative bacilli, and anaerobic bacteria.
3. The early stage symptoms include severe pain and skin changes, and the disease progresses rapidly. The symptoms of systemic poisoning with change in consciousness occur and it may lead to multiple organ failure and death.
4. Imaging examination (CT, MRI) has important reference value for the diagnosis of lesions, showing thickening and edema in subcutaneous tissue. The most characteristic change by CT is multiple pneumatosis in subcutaneous soft tissue. T_2WI fat-suppressed sequence show diffuse hyperintense shadow distributed along deep fascia as the main sign by MRI.

5. In enhanced scan, the deep fascia is subject to abnormal marked enhancement, mixed with necrotic fascia tissue without enhancement.

Differential Diagnosis

1. **Cellulitis.** The difference between the two is mainly based on clinical manifestations. NF can have various manifestations of cellulitis and subcutaneous infection, and its development progresses more rapidly, with severe systemic poisoning symptoms and rapid deterioration; The main distinguishing point in imaging manifestation is that, in cellulitis, there is no diffuse T_2WI hyperintense focus distributed along deep fascia. Enhanced scanning is helpful to distinguish necrotizing fasciitis from simple infectious fasciitis. The former shows that there is no enhanced area (necrosis) in markedly enhanced fascial tissue.
2. **Gas gangrene**. It often invades deep or contaminated wounds, and muscle tissue is involved in the early stage, showing rapid necrosis, with marked local pain, accompanied with "bursting-like" severe pain, and there is "snow grip feel" around the wound, with severe systemic poisoning symptoms, often accompanied by changes in central nervous system. However, NF does not involve muscle tissue, and bacteriological examination is helpful in distinguishing them.
3. **Infectious myositis:** NF usually does not involve muscle tissue, which in some cases may cause inflammatory reaction of adjacent muscles, manifested as heterogeneous muscle edema. Infectious myositis not only complicated with fascia changes, but also showed general swelling and enlargement of muscle tissue. CT showed a density reduction area. MRI showed T_2WI hyperintense and formation of intramuscular abscess. Laboratory test showed that the increase of serum creatine phosphokinase could be distinguished from NF.
4. **Neonatal infectious gangrene of subcutaneous tissue.** It mostly occurs in lumbosacral region, buttocks, and other compression regions, usually occurs about one week after birth with superficia diseased regions, and can be found early and treated in time. NF usually occurs in the abdominal wall and limbs of newborns, with deep diseased regions and fascia necrosis as the characteristics. It progresses rapidly and occurs within 2 ~ 3 weeks. Most of them are already very serious at the time of onset, with a relatively high mortality rate.

Status Quo and Progress of Research

1. **CE-MRI.** Necrotic fascia tissue is not enhanced in gadolinium magnetic resonance enhanced scanning, which can clearly identify non-necrotizing infectious fasciitis. CE-MRI can better evaluate the range of non-enhanced necrotizing fascia, which is considered as a characteristic change with high sensitivity.
2. **PET/CT.** In recent years, radionuclide technology is widely applied in soft tissue infection, which often occurs before morphological changes. Early diagnosis of NF is of great significance for clinical treatment. Abnormally increased radionuclide uptake on radionuclide imaging indicates congestion and edema of local fascia tissue. Early clinical intervention can prevent further development of lesions.

8.1.8 Neonatal Infectious Gangrene of Subcutaneous Tissue

Junyan Yang and Jiye Song

Overview

Neonatal infectious gangrene of subcutaneous tissue is a unique acute pyogenic infection of subcutaneous tissue in neonatal period. It usually occurs in 6 ~ 10 days after birth, and occasionally within 24 hours after birth[45]. The disease has an acute onset and extensive necrosis of subcutaneous tissue after the onset, it progresses rapidly and spreads rapidly. If not treated in time, it can be complicated with toxemia, bronchitis, and lung abscess, and with a relatively high mortality rate. It is reported that the mortality rate can reach 5% ~ 8% [44]. Most of them occur in the back or lumbosacral part of the newborn, which is easily compressed, occasionally in the occipital region, shoulder, leg and perineal region, and are common in winter and spring. The main pathogens are Staphylococcus aureus, occasionally Pseudomonas aeruginosa, Streptococcus viridans, Proteus, etc. In recent years, with the improvement of medical conditions and the improvement of people's living standards, the incidence of this disease has a significant downward trend. If it can be diagnosed and timely treated at early stage, the complications and mortality rate can be reduced [45].

Etiopathogenesis: Poor skin barrier function of newborns, local nutritional disorders of their backs and buttocks caused by long-term lying position, friction of bedding and clothing, soaking of urine and feces or crying agitation, etc. can cause skin destruction, leading to bacteria invading the subcutaneous and infection, and a few of them are caused by the spread of infection in adjacent regions. For newborns with onset within 24 hours after birth, it is mostly closely related to intrauterine infection, hypoxia, local blood supply disorders, etc. [46] Clinical picture: (1) Local symptoms, at the initial stage of onset, the local skin temperature rises, showing red, slightly swollen and hard, with unclear boundary and whitening of the finger pressed region. The lesion expands rapidly within a few hours and can spread to most or all of the back within one day. The skin becomes soft, the color of the central region turns dark red, the subcutaneous tissue becomes necrotic and liquefied, the skin and subcutaneous tissue are separated, with a floating feeling in palpation, but rarely with fluctuation feeling. Some newborns have multiple blisters on their local skin and gradually fuse. The contents turn into bloody liquid, and the central skin turns black and gradually increases necrotic area. Necrotic tissue drops out to form a large ulcer and secretes a little pus. (2) Systemic symptoms include high fever, crying, breast refusal, or vomiting and diarrhea, can be complicated with toxemia and pneumonia, and severe toxic shock and death [47]. Laboratory test: increased leukocyte count in peripheral blood and increased neutrophils; Bacteriological test includes smear and bacterial culture. If it is complicated with toxemia, positive results can be obtained by blood culture [48].

Pathophysiology

According to the clinical pathological classification, neonatal infectious gangrene of subcutaneous tissue can be divided into gangrene, cellulitis, necrosis, and abscess [27, 49]. At the initial stage, the diseased skin and subcutaneous tissue show extensive congestion and swelling, with blurred boundary, unclear boundary with normal tissue, and cellulitis changes. Under the microscope, a large number of neutrophils can be seen to infiltrate diffusely, and further development of the lesion causes deterioration and necrosis. Bacterial infection leads to intravascular thrombosis and necrosis of subcutaneous tissue, mostly a mixture of coagulation necrosis and liquefied necrosis, with clear boundaries with peripheral tissues. The necrotic tissue is grayish yellow or grayish white, dry and solid due to the decrease of water content. The outline of tissue structure can be seen under microscope, but the fine structure of cells disappears. Congestion, hemorrhage, and inflammatory reaction zones are formed around the necrotic area [50]. Necrotic inflammatory tissue is dissolved by enzyme to form pus. Thrombin possessed by Staphylococcus aureus converts the exuded fibrinogen into cellulose. Cellulose formed vomica wall around necrotic tissue. The lesion is localized and abscessed, with a lot of capillaries and proliferative connective tissue in the vomica wall. Pus is easy to spread and diffuses along the fascia space, forming multi-space abscess or spreading along lymphatic and hematogenous dissemination, causing toxemia [51, 52]. Therefore, it is extremely necessary to drain pus immediately after abscess formation.

Imaging Findings

X-ray examination cannot provide valuable diagnostic information. Imaging mainly applies ultrasound, CT and MRI examination, the CT and MRI examination can help to determine the scope of lesion invasion and whether deeper muscle tissue is involved. It is characterized by cellulitis and abscess imaging changes. If the newborn's condition is serious and complicated with serious infection, active treatment should be carried out, and imaging examination should be taken as auxiliary diagnosis. The renal function of newborn is not perfect, so it is not suitable for CT and MRI enhancement examination.

1. **Ultrasonography.** The sonogram of cellulitis shows diffuse echo enhancement in subcutaneous tissue, during which reticular hypoecho cords can be mixed. The boundary between the lesion and normal subcutaneous tissue is unclear and gradually migrated. Color Doppler shows a little blood flow signal scattered around the lesion area. After the abscess is formed, there is a clear boundary with the surrounding normal tissues, which is manifested as a round, oval, or irregular anechoic area with a clear boundary. Ultrasonography has good sensitivity in displaying fluidity focus, but it is not suitable for ultrasonography when complicated with skin ulcer
2. **CT.** Cellulitis is characterized by thickening of subcutaneous fat layer, showing flaky fuzzy high-density shadow, or showing thick strip-like reticular structure, blurred boundary between fat and muscle, and relatively uniform liquid density shadow between subcutaneous tissue and muscle when combined with effusion. After the abscess is formed, there are many round or quasi-circular lobulated masses with different sizes, clear boundaries, and uneven density. Low-density necrotic zone can be seen in the center of the focus, with the CT value of 10 ~ 20HU, and the thickness of the abscess wall is relatively uniform.
3. **MRI.** Compared with the above two examination methods, MRI is more suitable for the diagnosis and differential diagnosis of soft tissue lesions.

Cellulitis is characterized by diffuse thickening and edema of pathological tissues. On T_1WI, hyperintense adipose tissue is localized with band-like hypointense foci, T_2WI sequence shows hyperintense at the corresponding diseased region, which can be flaky or feather-like, with unclear boundary. T_2WI fat-suppressed sequence shows clearer lesion, lesion and adipose tissue interwove into reticular abnormal signals, and hypointense T1 and hyperintense T2 signal shadows can be seen between subcutaneous tissue and muscle when combined with effusion. Part of the inflammation is localized abscess, showing round or lobulated mass shadow. The pus shows hypointense on T_1WI and hyperintense on T_2WI. The thickness of the abscess wall is relatively uniform. T_2WI shows isointensity or slightly hypointense, with relatively smooth boundary. The periphery is a hyperintense edema area on T_2WI, and the vomica shows obvious hyperintense on DWI, with characteristic changes.

Key Points of Diagnosis

1. About one week after the newborn is born, symptoms such as fever, crying, breast refusal, vomiting, diarrhea, or lethargy of unknown causes occur with severe systemic poisoning symptoms.

2. The main characteristics of the disease are acute, rapid, and severe onset. Skin changes can spread rapidly within a few hours. Subcutaneous tissues show extensive necrosis and with a feeling of floating during palpation. A few herpes turn into black eschar, deep ulcer occurs under the skin and fuses into large gangrene.
3. Lesions mostly occur in the back or lumbosacral parts and other frequently compressed regions.
4. The pathogen is mostly Staphylococcus aureus, and positive results can be obtained by blood culture.
5. The imaging showed diffuse thickening and edema of the lesion tissue with unclear boundary. MRI examination showed hypointense on T_1WI, hyperintense on T_2WI fat-suppressed sequence, and grid-like abnormal signal. If abscess was formed, the vomica on DWI sequence showed obvious hyperintense.

Differential Diagnosis

1. **Diaper rash.** It is mostly found in infants, especially in perineum, buttocks, and lateral thighs. The skin is red and may have red spotted rash. Exudate may appear and epidermis drops out to form ulcer if it continues to develop. Different from neonatal infectious gangrene of subcutaneous tissue, the disease usually occurs in hot and humid summer seasons, with red skin but no obvious swelling.
2. **Scleredema.** It is more common in winter and spring with the main cause of cold injury and is characterized by subcutaneous fat sclerosis and edema. Diffuse intravascular coagulation and pulmonary hemorrhage occur in serious cases. The skin is swollen and hard, but it is not red. Most of them are stiff in both lower limbs with no obvious systemic symptoms such as infection, and with low body temperature, which can be distinguished from neonatal infectious gangrene of subcutaneous tissue.
3. **Erysipelas.** The skin in the lesion area is obviously swollen and widely erythema, which is bright red, slightly higher than the surrounding skin surface, with no obvious boundary with normal tissues, and is mostly complicated with lymph node involvement. The lesion mainly occurs in lower limbs, common in children and the elderly, subcutaneous tissues have no floating feeling, and rarely occurs in newborns [53, 54].

8.2 Fungal Infection

Junyan Yang and Peng Zhang

Overview

Fungi widely exist in nature, with various types. They live in saprophytic or parasitic ways and reproduce in sexual or asexual ways. At present, there are more than 10,000 genera and 100,000 species of fungi that have been confirmed and described. Most of them are beneficial to human beings and a few are harmful to human beings [55]. The infection of skin and deep tissues caused by fungi is called fungus soft tissue infections. In recent years, due to the abuse of antibiotics, anti-tumor drugs, immunosuppressive agents, the development of diagnosis and treatment technologies such as organ transplantation, intervention and intubation, and the increase of AIDS, diabetes, malignant tumors, tuberculosis and other basic diseases has led to low immune function of the body, resulting in an obvious upward trend in the incidence of fungal infection [56]. Fungus soft tissue infections can be directly introduced (such as intravenous drug injection, trauma, surgery, or indwelling foreign bodies, etc.) or spread through blood sources. The disease infects more men than women, especially the elderly men. Fungal infection in children tends to increase year by year.

Fungi are an independent biological group, more than 400 species are related to medicine, with 50 ~ 100 of common species. Fungi are various in morphology and size. According to their morphology and structure, they can be divided into two types: unicellular fungi and multicellular fungi. (1) The number of unicellular fungi is small, with round or oval in shape, such as yeast-type and yeast-like fungi; (2) Multicellular fungi have a large number and are composed of mycelium and spores [57]. Fungi have strong resistance to dryness, sunlight, ultraviolet rays, and general disinfectants, but are not heat resistant. Studies have shown that many important fungi in medical fields, including candida, aspergillus, cryptococcus, and coccidiospores, form biofilms, reducing the efficacy of antifungal therapy, and may lead to refractory infections [58, 59].

Fungal infections are mostly caused by pathogenic fungi and opportunistic pathogenic fungi. According to the different regions of the human body invaded by fungi, they are divided into superficial mycosis and deep mycosis. (1) Superficial mycosis mainly invades keratinous tissues, such as skin, hair, and nails, and is mainly manifested as tinea capitis, tinea corporis and cruris, tinea manus and pedis, tinea unguium, and other tinea diseases. (2) Deep mycosis is also called invasive mycosis, mainly invades dermis, subcutaneous tissue, muscle, various internal organs, bone and joint systems and other regions, with great harm. The common pathogens of deep infection include candida, chromomycosis, sporotrichum, cryptococcus, aspergillus, fusarium, mucor, etc., of which candida is the main pathogen, accounting for more than 80%. Candida can form pseudohyphae and elongate into germ tube, which is not easy to be engulfed by phagocytes, with strong pathogenicity, and is easy to cause infection [60]. Deep soft tissue infection can be divided into specific and non-specific infections. The specific infection can be caused by direct spread of bone or vertebral fungal infection; and non-specific infection can be formed due to local soft tissue infection that cannot be controlled in time, and can also be caused by systemic diseases and low immune function of the body. Deep soft tissue infection is divided into subcutaneous cellulitis, fasciitis, pyomyositis, and soft tissue abscess according to the scope of involvement [61, 62]. If deep myositis and soft tissue abscess are not controlled in time, they can further spread to adjacent bones and joints, causing more serious body injury. Therefore, timely and clear diagnosis is particularly important.

Fungus soft tissue infections have various clinical manifestations and lack specific manifestations. The occurrence of deep mycosis is related to factors such as immune damage and low immune function. Fungal infection has a long course of disease and poor conventional treatment effect. The most serious symptom is AIDS complicated with fungal infection [63]. The main clinical manifestations are limited skin injury, with nodules, suppurations, ulcers, fistulas, or granuloma occurring locally, of which skin ulcers are the majority, accounting for 57.14% [64]. Fungal osteoarthritis and myositis can be the only manifestations of systemic infection. The disease changes at different speeds. Most patients have hidden onset, slow progress or only local pain and swelling. Late severe cases can cause systemic disseminated infection. Laboratory diagnosis of mycosis mainly depends on histopathology and mycological test. In recent years, serological test has become a laboratory test method for deep fungal infection, and histopathology is still the gold standard for diagnosis [65].

Pathophysiology

After entering the body, fungi are easy to be phagocytized by mononuclear-macrophages and neutrophils, but the phagocytized fungal spores cannot be completely killed. They can reproduce in cells, stimulate tissue proliferation, cause cell infiltration to form granuloma, and can also be carried by phagocytes to deep tissues and organs to proliferate and cause pathological changes.

A variety of tissue reactions can be seen in deep skin mycosis, including purulent reaction, eosinophilic reaction, necrotizing lesion, vasculitis, skin pseudoepithelioma-like hyperplasia, and granulomatous reaction. In the early stage, the lesion tissue can be normal without obvious reaction, and a few monocytes and lymphocytes infiltrate in the focus under microscope; Further development of the lesion may be accompanied by necrosis and abscess formation in different degrees. Necrosis foci in the focus are mostly accompanied by hemorrhage foci and hyperplastic blood vessels. Abscess is generally limited and can penetrate all around to form sinus tract with strong spreading force and can invade adjacent tissues. The most characteristic pathological manifestation of fungal infection is chronic granulomatous inflammatory reaction [66]. Microscopically, a small abscess with neutrophil formation is located in the center of the focus. Fungal spores are mostly located in small abscesses. The spore capsules have bud-like protrusions, the periphery is surrounded by radial epithelial cells and a few lymphocytes. The outermost layer is surrounded by plasma cells, lymphocytes, and fibroblasts, forming nodules with clear boundaries [67]. The above lesions can exist alone or simultaneously.

Imaging Findings

X-ray examination is simple and easy to carry out, but with poor soft tissue contrast and low sensitivity. CT examination has high spatial resolution. It can observe the lesions of different tissues and abnormal lesions in the same tissue by adjusting the window width, window level and measuring the difference of CT values, especially can clearly diagnose calcified lesions. MRI examination has high soft tissue resolution and can perform multi-parameter, multi-sequence, and multi-directional imaging, with the conventional scanning sequences of T_1WI sequence, T_2WI sequence, fat-suppressed sequence, DWI sequence, and enhanced scanning sequence, and can be used for diagnosis and differential diagnosis of soft tissue abscess. Ultrasonography is a routine examination method for soft tissue infection and can also be used to guide diagnostic puncture.

Superficial mycosis is mainly a variety of tinea diseases, fungal infection of the skin is superficial, generally, imaging examination is not required, and diagnosis can be made according to clinical manifestations and laboratory test. This section mainly describes the image changes of deep fungal infection.

1. Cellulitis and Fasciitis.
   (a) X-ray: The main manifestations are local soft tissue swelling, increased density, blurred fat space, cord-like or reticular increased density shadows in the progression of lesions, and small bubbles or band-like gas density shadows in soft tissues in some cases.
   (b) CT: In the early stage, inflammatory hyperemia and edema of soft tissues are mainly manifested as local soft tissue swelling, increased density of surrounding fat space, local cord-like shadows and grid-like shadows, showing honeycomb change; there can be pneumatosis and effusion change, manifested as irregular small bubbles and fluid density shadow distributed along the space, with CT gas value less than -150HU, with clear boundary; the fascia in the lesion area shows localized and asymmetric thickening, manifested as patchy high-density shadow which is poorly demarcated from the surrounding soft tissue; the necrotic fascial tissue shows no enhancement on enhanced scan, while the uninvolved fascia shows

marked enhancement. Inflammation further develops to form a soft tissue mass with heterogeneous density and blurred borders in the mass, which may present with liquefaction and calcification foci, and the lesion area shows heterogeneous enhancement or patchy enhancement on enhanced scan.

(c) MRI: Cellulitis is characterized by diffuse thickening and edema of diseased tissues, which are localized, banded, and hypointense in hyperintense adipose tissues on T_1WI. Lesions interwoven with adipose tissues show reticular abnormal intensity on T_2WI fat-suppressed sequences, and the lesion area shows enhancement on enhanced scan. When the lesion is combined with effusion, hypointense T1 and hyperintense T2 signal shadows are observed between the subcutaneous tissue and muscle; pneumatosis is manifested as extremely hypointense shadows on T_1WI and T_2WI sequences; The lesions further extend to involve fascia tissue, and both deep fascia and deep intermuscular fascia may be involved, showing fascia thickening, usually ≥3 mm in thickness. The diseased deep fascia is hyperintense in strip on T_2WI fat-suppressed sequences. Enhanced scan suggests local necrosis if there is no marked enhancement, and there is encapsulated or laminar effusion in the deep layer of the lesion, which is hyperintense or hypointense on DWI sequences without significant characteristic changes.

(d) Ultrasound: The main manifestations are diffuse swelling of soft tissues, increased echo, unclear boundary with peripheral tissues, local blood flow signals. Hyperplastic vessels are non-specific manifestations of local inflammation, with exudative inflammation in the focus. Follow-up exploration shows that the diseased tissue and the normal subcutaneous tissue gradually migrate, and the echo of infectious exudate is generally enhanced. When combined with effusion and empyema, diffuse soft tissue swelling is manifested as a fluid sonolucent area (anechoic) with blurred or limited boundary. When combined with pneumatosis, it is manifested as hyperechoic small bubble changes in the diffusely swollen tissue. However, ultrasound shows no obvious characteristics for fascial thickening and necrotic changes.

2. Soft Tissue Abscess.

   (a) X-ray reveals more significant local soft tissue swelling, blurred fat space, and increased density, and the surrounding muscles are squeezed and displaced when an abscess is formed, with irregular slightly hypodense shadows in the increased density area, clear margins, and a sense of fluctuation in the touched local area.

   (b) On CT, the necrotic tissue is localized, and when an abscess is formed, the boundary of the lesion is relatively clear. The central hypodense area reveals necrosis and liquefaction, surrounded by an isodense or slightly hyperdense abscess wall with a smooth inner wall (Figure 8.8a), and the abscess wall shows marked enhancement after enhanced scan, with no enhancement in the central necrotic area. The abscess may spread along the intermuscular space and progresses into deep multiple abscesses.

   (c) On MRI, the inflammation is localized or further develops into a soft tissue mass or abscess. The abscess, quasi-circular, or fusiform, with a localized extent and clear boundary with the peripheral tissues is heterogeneously hypointense on T_1WI, and the abscess wall is slightly more hyperintense than the pus (Figure 8.8b); On T_2WI sequences, the abscess wall is isointense or slightly hypointense, the pus is hyperintense, and the signal is homogeneous or heterogeneous, in which there may be septa (Figure 8.8c, d). On enhanced scan, the abscess wall or septa can be enhanced, the pus is not enhanced, and the pus is significantly hyperintense on DWI sequences. Abscesses can form deep multiple abscesses along the joint space, intermuscular space, or intervertebral space. Abscesses located beside the vertebrae can protrude into the vertebral canal to form intraspinal epidural abscesses. The dural sac may be compressed to varying degrees, and the adjacent spinal cord or nerve roots may also be compressed, presenting as intraspinal epidural fusiform or strip abnormal signals. The infection is protracted, the local soft tissue forms a sinus tract which can be of different thickness, and the sinus tract cavity is often accompanied by secretions, showing heterogeneous signals.

   (d) Ultrasound: When an abscess is formed, there is a sense of fluctuation during palpation, and the abscess is well-defined, manifested as a well-defined round, elliptic, or irregular sonolucent area filled with (anechoic) fluid in the subcutaneous soft tissue.

3. **Pyomyositis and periarthritis.** The infection further spreads to the deep layer and can invade the muscles, osteoarticular system, and peripheral soft tissues, causing periarthritis, with symptoms and signs such as fever, local soft tissue pain, and soft tissue swelling and masses, and in later stages, osteoarticular dysfunction and osteoarticular deformity [68, 69].

   (a) X-ray: Fungal osteoarticular soft tissue inflammation has no obvious specificity in early stage, and the osteoarticular space is normal or widened. Further development of the disease may result in swelling of periarticular soft tissues, increased soft tissue density, thickening of articular capsules, joint effusion,

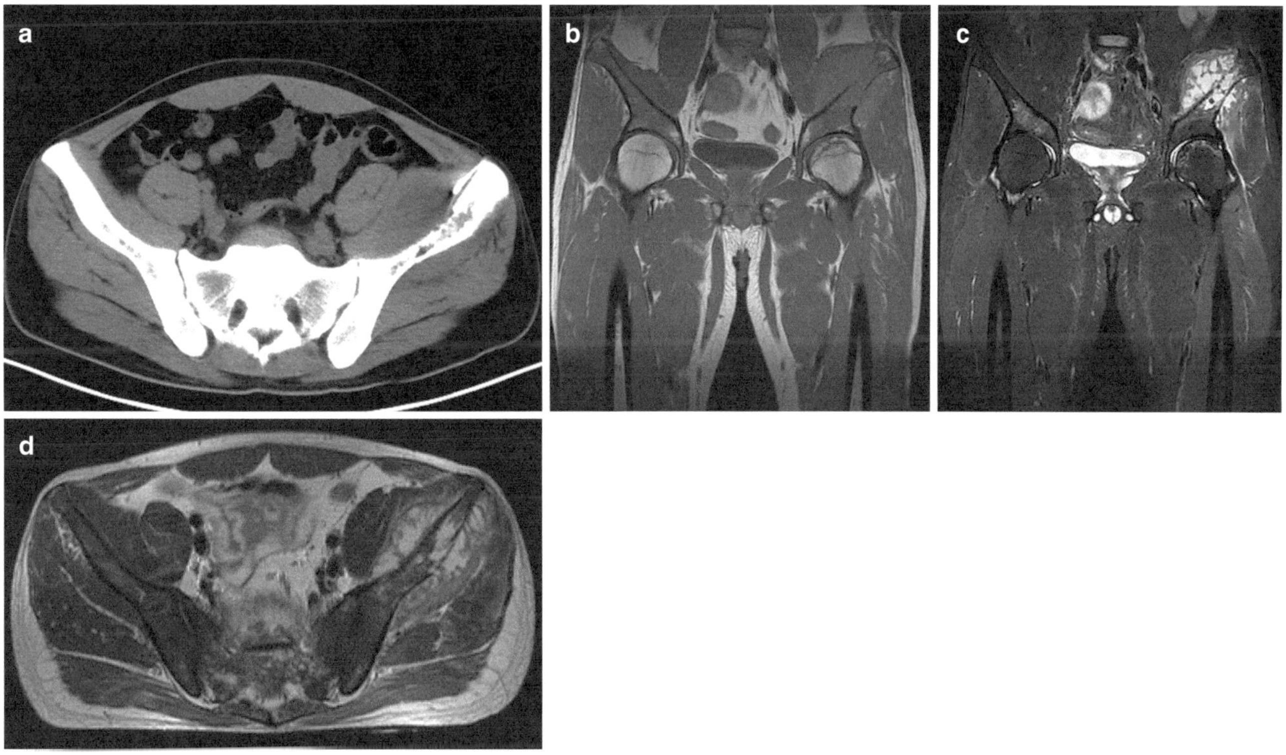

Fig. 8.8 Pelvic abscess (infection due to Talaromyces marneffei). An irregular soft tissue mass in the medial and lateral aspect of the left ilium. (**a**) Plain CT scan shows that the focus has reduced central density and slightly high density around them; (**b**) On coronal T_1WI sequences, the focus is hypointense, surrounding iliac and hip muscles are involved, with unclear boundaries; (**c**, **d**) T_2WI fat-suppressed sequences for coronal and transverse planes show multiple septa and hives in the lesion. Septa and abscess wall are hypointense, while pus is significantly hyperintense (the pictures are provided by Tang Yonghua, Ruijin Hospital, Shanghai Jiao Tong University School of Medicine, thank you)

articular cartilage destruction and joint space stenosis, bone destruction (mostly osteolytic), peripheral osteosclerosis and osteogenesis (rare), and periosteal reactions (rare).

(b) CT: Soft tissue reconstruction and bone reconstruction should be performed for peripheral inflammation involving the bone and joint, and the relationship between the bone and joint and soft tissue can be better visualized by CT image post-processing techniques such as multiplanar reformation. Diseased muscle tissues are diffusely enlarged due to edema, with unclear borders, uneven density, and low-density liquid accumulation in the center, which can have different degrees of enhancement on enhanced scan, combined with areas of liquefactive necrosis without enhancement. Edema can be associated with pneumatosis in muscular tissues and shows signs of very low-density small bubbles and strip gas. Inflammation may involve adjacent bones and joints, causing cystic destruction of bone, osteomyelitis and other changes, thickening of articular capsules, and joint effusion. The periarticular soft tissues are swollen with increased density and poorly defined borders, and show streak enhancement on enhanced scan. Vertebral body and intervertebral disc destruction and intraspinal epidural abscess may occur when the lesion involves the vertebral body.

(c) MRI: It can detect periarticular soft tissue lesions and abnormal signal changes in the spine and bone joints earlier. Muscle tissue involvement is characterized by edema of muscle fibers and blurred intermuscular space. Edema is slightly hypointense on T_1WI and shows diffusely increased signal intensity on T_2WI. Muscles show heterogeneous (mild to moderate) enhancement on enhanced T_1WI (Fig. 8.9). In some cases, edema is combined with signs of pneumatosis. In the early stage of osteoarticular soft tissue inflammation, exudation, hyperemia, and edema are the specific changes, manifested as periarticular soft tissue swelling with unclear boundary. Inflammation can spread around the tendon or muscle, bone and joint can be associated with bone edema, destruction, and other changes. There are bone marrow edema signals which are slightly hyperintense on T_2WI and fat-suppressed sequences, and lesion tissues show mild enhancement on enhanced scan.

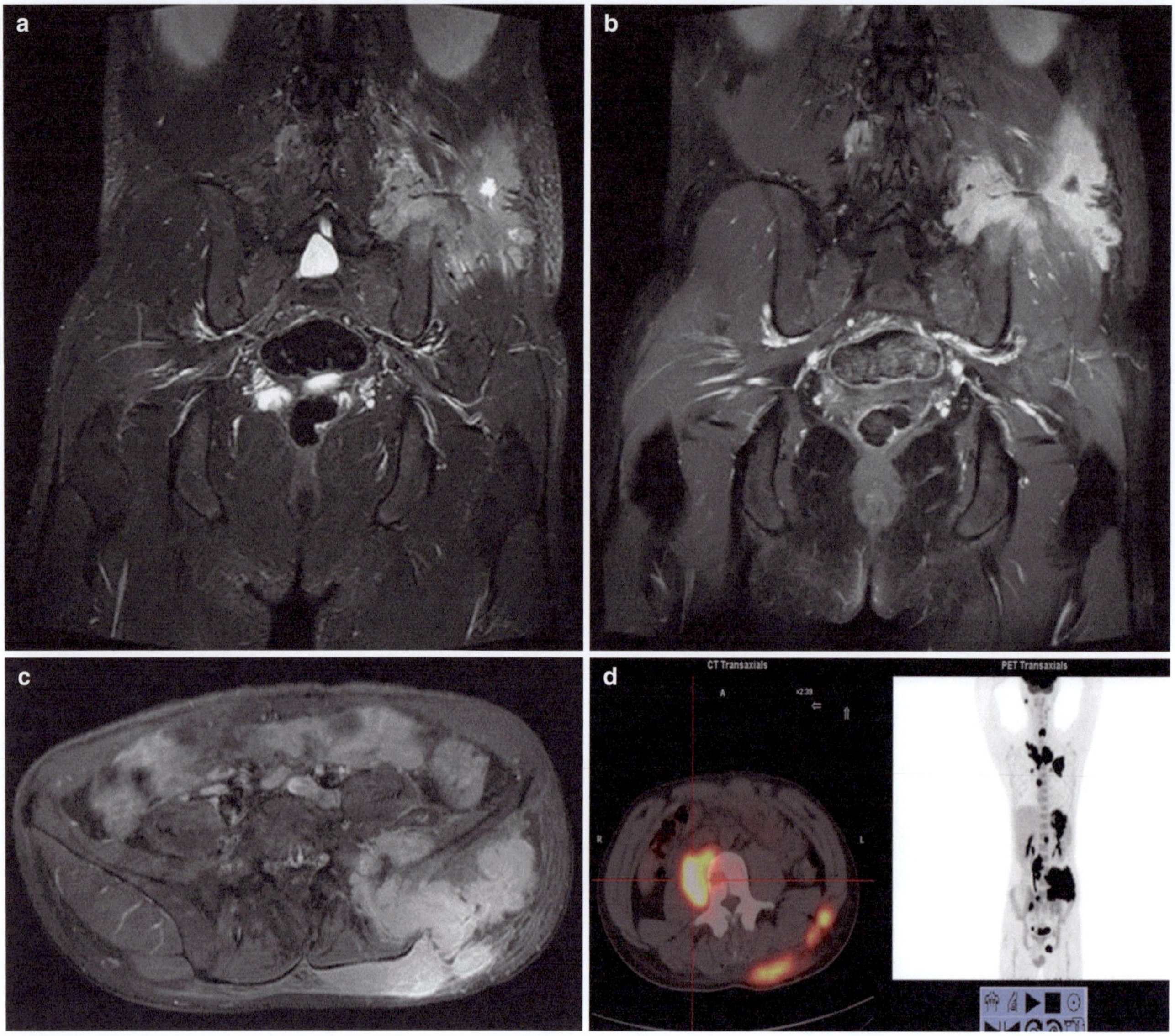

Fig. 8.9 Disseminated coccidioidomycosis (granuloma formation). There are multiple mass shadows in the subcutaneous, hip, and erector muscles of the left lower back. (**a**) Coronal T_2WI fat-suppressed sequences show swelling of diseased muscle tissues, blurred intermuscular space which is diffusely hyperintense; (**b**, **c**) Enhanced coronal and transverse T_1WI show significant heterogeneous enhancement of the affected muscle; (**d**) PET/CT shows concentration of multiple imaging agents throughout the body and increased uptake (the pictures were provided by Tang Yonghua, Ruijin Hospital, Shanghai Jiao Tong University School of Medicine, thank you)

(d) Ultrasound: It is less specific for inflammation of deep paravertebral soft tissues and invasion of the osteoarticular system, and the changes caused by inflammation of paraarticular soft tissues are the same as those above.

Key Points of Diagnosis

1. **Susceptible population.** Fungal soft tissue infection mostly occurs in immunodeficient or immunocompromised population, such as patients with autoimmune diseases, organ transplantation, severe burns, trauma, long-term use of antibiotics and glucocorticoids, AIDS, severe underlying diseases, the elderly and young children.
2. **Clinical manifestations.** Superficial mycosis is mostly manifested as a variety of tinea; deep mycosis tends to be insidious in onset, has a long course, and can cause multiple organ damage. Fungal soft tissue inflammation may present with changes such as subcutaneous soft tissue nodules, suppuration, ulcers, sinus tracts, or granulomas, in which skin ulcer is the most common manifestation.
3. **Laboratory tests.** Morphological examination (direct microscopic examination, fungal culture) and serological examination are mainly performed. Histopathological

examination is the gold standard for definite diagnosis, and molecular biology is used to detect nucleic acid when necessary.

4. **Imaging findings depending on the depth of involved soft tissue.** The main manifestations are cellulitis, fasciitis, muscle involvement, and periarthritis, which are subacute and chronic processes in clinical practice, and the lesion area shows heterogeneous mild to moderate enhancement on enhanced scan. Effusion and abscess formation may be associated in the focus, and sinus tracts may be formed locally when the infection is protracted. Periarthritis is associated with local bone changes. CT has a high sensitivity for combined pneumatosis and calcification changes; MRI can detect soft tissue involvement and abscess formation earlier, and identify the extent of inflammation and abscess. The pus is hyperintense on DWI sequences with a high specificity.

Differential Diagnosis

1. **Pyogenic soft tissue inflammation.** Pyogenic inflammation caused by fungal infection can be easily misdiagnosed as bacterial infection, and the use of a large number of antibiotics and hormone therapy makes the diagnosis difficult, which delays treatment and even leads to the death of the patient. The differential diagnosis of the two is therefore extremely important. Bacterial infections are mostly caused by Staphylococcus aureus and hemolytic streptococci, manifesting acute onset, wide range of lesions, rapid development, obvious local skin redness, and swelling which rapidly expand to the surrounding. The central area of the lesion is dark red, with slightly lighter edge. There is no obvious boundary between the red and swollen skin and the surrounding normal skin tissue. Tenderness is obvious, accompanied by chills, high fever, headache, and other systemic symptoms. The image findings show diffuse swelling of local soft tissues with blurred borders in early stage, which may be accompanied by lymphadenopathy. The infection may spread widely along the intermuscular bundle. The acute inflammation of the diseased tissue on enhanced scan shows marked enhancement, which may be associated with pneumatosis, effusion, and abscess formation. Fungal infection has a long course of disease, showing a subacute to chronic process. Redness, swelling, fever, pain, and other clinical manifestations are mild, mostly associated with skin ulcers, and local foci show heterogeneous, mild to moderate enhancement on enhanced scan.
2. **Granulomatous Inflammation**
   (a) Brucellosis: Susceptible populations are people who have a clear epidemiological contact history, residents living in animal husbandry areas or related occupational groups, people who have drunk dairy products that have not been disinfected and sterilized, or people with a history of eating raw beef and mutton, etc. Clinical manifestations are fever, fatigue, hyperhidrosis, muscle and joint pain, hepatosplenomegaly, lymph nodes, and testicular enlargement. Positive tube agglutination test (SAT), blood culture, or isolation of bacteria can confirm the diagnosis. Its soft tissue involvement occurs frequently around the thoracic and lumbar spine, hip joints, knee joints, and other major bearing joints. Adjacent vertebral bodies are mostly affected, and bone destruction and hyperostosis, sclerosis may exist at the same time. The periarticular area shows soft tissue swelling with a clear fat space around it. The lesion further develops to form a juxta-articular abscess, which is limited in extent, has a clear boundary with the peripheral tissues. The peripheral soft tissues and muscles are squeezed and displaced, and the abscess occurring in the paraspinal region usually does not exceed the length of the diseased vertebral body.
   (b) Tuberculous granuloma: Most of the patients have a relevant medical history such as pulmonary tuberculosis and intestinal tuberculosis, and present tuberculosis poisoning symptoms such as fatigue, night sweats, and afternoon low-grade fever. Tuberculin test is positive and erythrocyte sedimentation rate is accelerated. Bone destruction (mostly "skipping") and osteoporosis changes are predominant in the diseased osseous tissue in which sequestrum and calcifications are observed. In the late stage, joint space stenosis and fusion disappearance may occur, which may be accompanied by varying degrees of osteoarticular deformity. When the diseased bone tissue is combined with abscesses, they are mostly cold abscesses, with clear margin with peripheral tissues, occurring in the paraspinal region, mostly forming psoas abscess, with thin and smooth abscess wall, often accompanied by destruction of adjacent vertebral endplate and intervertebral disc. The extent of the abscess, in which sequestrum or calcification can be observed, often exceeds the length of the diseased vertebral body, and deep multiple abscesses can be developed. Soft tissue inflammation occurring in the paraarticular region, thickening of the articular capsule, swelling of the peripheral soft tissues, homogeneous enhancement of the joint capsule and abscess wall on enhanced scan, and extraction of purulent fluid from the joint can confirm the diagnosis by microscopic examination and bacterial culture [66, 70].

   The typical clinical history and imaging findings of the above two types of granulomatous inflammation can be differentiated from this disease.

3. **Soft tissue tumors.** They arise as inflammatory mass shadows in the deep soft tissues and soft tissue masses are differentiated from tumors of soft tissue origin. Inflammatory masses show diffuse and irregular changes, with clinical manifestation of infection such as fever and general malaise. Local masses are often palpable in soft tissue tumors, and malignant tumors can rapidly increase in size in a short period of time. Inflammatory masses occurring beside bone tissues are differentiated from synovial sarcomas and tumors of osseous tissue origin. Generally, the osseous substance adjacent to inflammatory masses shows sclerotic changes rather than bone destruction. Where there are inflammatory lesions, bone marrow cavity is extensively hyperintense in T_2WI fat-suppressed sequence, extensive edematous changes are around the bone and inflammatory masses, and tumor lesions are relatively localized.

Status Quo and Progress of Research

Fungal inflammation in soft tissues has different clinical manifestations and insidious symptoms can progress into rapid tissue destruction. It is difficult to diagnose insidious fungal infections, and because the host response to fungal infections is slow, there are no obvious clinical manifestations for physicians to refer to. For patients with fungal osteoarthritis and soft tissue inflammation, systemic inflammatory indicators are only slightly elevated, or completely normal. Therefore, the detailed history and physical examination of patients are very important for the diagnosis. Imaging cannot be used as the basis for the diagnosis of fungal pathogens, but the imaging findings of soft tissue inflammation and osteoarthritis can be used as the basis for indirect diagnosis.

1. **DWI.** It can detect the abnormal signal of soft tissue inflammation earlier by applying the multi-parametric, multi-sequential, and multi-directional imaging features of MRI and is of positive significance for the extent determination and diagnosis and treatment of soft tissue infection. DWI has been widely used in clinical practice, and according to different ADC (apparent diffusion coefficient) values, it is of great value in the diagnosis and differentiation of inflammatory masses, abscesses, and neoplastic lesions.
2. **MRS.** It can detect and analyze the metabolites of phospholipid metabolism, energy metabolism, and intracellular pH changes in skeletal muscles and is the only noninvasive method that can observe energy metabolism in muscle tissue in vivo. The substances that can be observed on P-MRS include PCr and Pi. When the inflammatory lesion involves the muscle tissue, the abnormal change of its metabolic rate can be reflected by the change of P-MRS. In most cases, the peak value of PCr decreases while the peak value of Pi increases, and the pH value of cytoplasm increases significantly, which can be used to judge the involvement of muscle tissues.
3. **Nuclear medicine and PET/CT.** In recent years, radionuclide technology has been widely used in soft tissue infections, and nuclear medical imaging of soft tissue infections is based on local pathological changes in inflamed tissues, which often occur before morphological changes. The rapid development of infection-specific imaging agents has become a research hotspot in nuclear medicine. Labeled leukocytes play an important role in the diagnosis and localization in the early stage of soft tissue infection, and may detect occult foci. Uptake of ^{18}F-FDG uptake is increased in the body under infection. PET/CT examination can provide information on early inflammatory foci such as osteoarthritis, soft tissue inflammation, epidural abscess, and other lesions. It is effective in detecting inflammatory foci and abscess formation. Differences in FDG uptake can be used to identify whether the lesion is infectious, but the diagnosis is less specific as to what pathogen is infecting the lesion. PET/CT is also of interest in the evaluation of treatment effects in infections.

8.3 Brucella Infection

Overview

Brucellosis, also known as Mediterranean fever or undulant fever, is a zoonotic allergic disease caused by Brucella and is specified as Category B infectious diseases in the *Law of the People's Republic of China on Prevention and Treatment of Infectious Diseases* [71]. Sick sheep, cattle, dogs, and other animals are the main source of brucellosis infection, and people are generally susceptible to the disease. People who have direct contact with sick animals or who eat undercooked beef or mutton are at high risk of contracting the disease. Brucella is divided into 6 species and 19 biotypes, and in recent years, scientists in the United Kingdom, Germany, and Czech have successively discovered new Brucella species.

Brucella is generally not easy to die in the external environment and is highly resistant to dry and low temperature environments. It can still survive in cold environments but is sensitive to hot and humid environments and has difficulty surviving in the environments with high temperature, ultraviolet irradiation, and disinfectants. It has weak resistance to antibiotics such as tetracycline and streptomycin [71, 72].

The clinical symptoms of brucellosis often vary in severity, show wavy changes, and are prone to recurrence and chronicity. The disease often invades tissues and organs such as the liver and spleen, as well as the nervous system and osteoarticular system [72]. The clinical stage is divided into acute, subacute, and chronic stages, and the chronic stage is divided into active and relatively stable stages. The osteoarticular damage is fixed in position and presents as joint enlargement and arthritis, mostly in large joints such as hip and knee joints, and persistent musculoskeletal soreness or dull pain. Symptoms in the chronic stable phase are stable, which can be aggravated by overwork or long-term depression. Patients may have low immunity, weakness, anemia, malnutrition, and other symptoms. In the laboratory test, the tube agglutination test is positive at 1:100 and above, and the isolation of bacteria from blood culture is the gold standard for the diagnosis of brucellosis [73].

Pathophysiology

Brucella enters the human body mainly through the skin, digestive tract, and respiratory mucosa, and conjunctival contact with germs can also lead to infection. After invading the host, Brucella mainly infects macrophages, placental trophoblastic cells, and dendritic cells. If it is not killed by macrophages, it can grow and multiply in host cells and form primary tumors in lymph nodes. Depending on the strength of the body's immunity, the amount of bacterial content in the body, and the use of antibiotics, it can cause acute and chronic allergic reactions, the formation of inflammatory exudation, granuloma, proliferation of fibrous tissues, and other acute and chronic diseases.

Brucellosis has extensive pathological changes which mostly occur in the liver, spleen, lymph nodes, heart, and kidney and can cause multiple organ injury. The main pathological changes are: (1) Exudation (mainly serous inflammatory exudation, mixed with a few necrotic cells), degeneration and necrosis changes. (2) Proliferative changes, mostly diffuse changes, which may be followed by fibrocyte proliferation in the focus. (3) Granuloma formation, granulomas composed of macrophages, lymphocytes, plasma cells and epithelioid cells may appear in the focus, and granulomas may further develop fibrosis, resulting in sclerosis of tissues and organs.

The soft tissue inflammation caused by Brucella can be divided into three stages by the occurrence and development of inflammation, that is, edema caused by inflammatory exudation of soft tissues, soft tissue mass, and abscess formation. The above lesions are mostly secondary to spondylitis, spondylodiscitis, and osteoarthritis. Its occurrence and development is a continuous process, and its pathological changes can be alternated from the acute phase to the chronic phase. The acute phase is characterized by inflammatory congestion, edema, and necrosis, accompanied by venular inflammatory embolism, which can cause soft tissue swelling; in the subacute and chronic phases, inflammation continues to spread to form mass-like lesions, and then the central necrotic area further develops into the vomica, and the surrounding abscess wall is composed of a large number of inflammatory cells and fibrous granulation tissues, with microscopic histiocytosis, proliferative nodules, and granuloma formation in the lesion area [72, 74].

Imaging Findings

X-ray examination is simple and feasible, and is mainly used to observe the changes of bones and joints in the late stage of brucellosis. However, its sensitivity of lesion detection is poor due to the superimposed images and the lack of good soft tissue contrast. CT is an important examination method for this disease. Large-range scanning and multi-directional reconstruction can clearly show the infectious lesions of soft tissues. When infectious lesions of soft tissue are combined with abscess formation, the extent and shape of abscess and its relationship with the peripheral tissues can be well displayed in combination with enhanced examination. It is not good for the display of intraspinal lesions and CT-guided biopsy can be used for lesions that are difficult to diagnose. MRI has high soft tissue resolution and is very sensitive to changes in water and protein content of tissues. It can show soft tissue involvement and abscess formation more clearly and detect abnormal signal changes in the spine and joints earlier. Compared with CT, MRI can detect lesions in soft tissues and the extent of lesions earlier and more clearly and is commonly used to diagnose and differentiate acute and chronic lesions. Conventional scanning sequences include: T_1WI sequence, T_2WI sequence, fat-suppressed sequence, and enhanced T_1WI sequence. Furthermore, DWI can be used for abscess diagnosis and differential diagnosis [75]. For special types of lesions such as intraspinal epidural abscess, MRI can better detect abscesses, as well as the involvement of the spinal cord, while MRI is recognized as the imaging examination of choice for the assessment of soft tissue infections due to its multi-directional, multifunctional, multi-sequence imaging, and absence of ionizing radiation [76, 77]. Radionuclide bone scan mainly reflects the blood circulation and local metabolic disorders of the lesions, with high sensitivity and low specificity.

1. **Paravertebral soft tissue inflammation.** It can occur in the soft tissues around the cervical, thoracic, and lumbar vertebral bodies, with lumbar paravertebral soft tissue inflammation being the most common.
   a. X-ray: There may be no obvious specificity in the acute phase. Calcification of the paraspinal ligaments can be observed in the chronic phase, which is more common in the lower lumbar vertebra and presents as cord-like calcification along the ligament, narrowing of each intervertebral space, formation of vertebral bone bridges, and blurred and widened shadows in the paraspinal soft tissues or psoas muscles.
   b. CT: Paravertebral soft tissue infection has different CT findings due to different disease severity and course of

disease, and imaging examination can identify the findings at each stage, which is very important for clinical treatment.

   i. Paravertebral soft tissue swelling or mass: Paravertebral soft tissues show different degrees of thickening and swelling, with a relatively limited range, clear peripheral fat space, uniform density, and no calcification. Granulation tissue mass is often serpiginous, spreading along the ligament, pushing against the peripheral tissues, and the lesion area shows marked enhancement on enhanced scan, with clear boundaries with the peripheral tissues.
   ii. Paravertebral abscess: After formation, it usually communicates with the corresponding vertebral destruction area. Abscesses are mostly in the shape of fusiform, quasi-circular, and strip, with different size and shape and irregular distribution. The boundary between abscess and peripheral tissues is clear, and there is significant difference in CT value. It is rarely combined with sequestrum and calcification. Multiple abscesses or large abscesses can push the adjacent psoas muscles, causing the distance between vertebral body and psoas muscle significantly widened. It is rarely combined with psoas abscess and there may be formation of deep multiple abscesses along the ligament. Abscesses are mostly small, multiple, and thick-walled, and the cyst wall shows ring enhancement on enhanced scans. When the lesion invades the vertebral canal, irregular soft tissue density shadows are observed in the vertebral canal, and the adjacent nerve roots and dural sacs are compressed to varying degrees.

c. MRI.
   i. Paravertebral soft tissue swelling or mass: It is an early manifestation of paravertebral soft tissue involvement, and mostly occurs in front of and on both sides of the vertebral body. Paravertebral soft tissues are characterized by inflammatory exudation. It manifests itself as thickened soft tissue shadow beside the vertebral body, surrounding the vertebral body in a stripe or fusiform shape. It is slightly hypointense on T_1WI and isointense or slightly hyperintense on T_2WI. The lesion can spread widely below the ligament, with clear boundary. The lesion invades posterior to the vertebral body, protrudes into the vertebral canal, and compresses the dural sac. The lesion tissue shows strip enhancement on enhanced scans; as the lesion further develops, it shows heterogeneous signal changes, and heterogeneous enhancement on enhanced scan [78–80] (Fig. 8.10).
   ii. Paravertebral abscess: Further development of paravertebral soft tissue inflammation causes degeneration and necrosis, and thus paravertebral abscess. The abscess has limited lesion extent that generally does not exceed the length of the adjacent diseased vertebral body. It is heterogeneously hypointense on T_1WI, probably less hypointense in the hypointense area, slightly hyperintense on T_2WI, hyperintense on fat-suppressed sequence. The abscess wall is isointense or slightly hypointense, and the vomica is significantly hyperintense on DWI sequence [81]. On enhanced scan, the abscess margin shows marked enhancement, and its wall is thick and irregular with a clear boundary with the peripheral tissues (Figs. 8.11 and 8.12). Special types of abscesses: (1) Intraspinal epidural abscess, which protrudes into the spinal canal in which abnormal intensity with unclear boundary can be observed. The abscess is slightly hypointense on T_1WI, hyperintense on T_2WI, heterogeneously hyperintense on fat-suppressed sequence, and the abscess wall shows marked enhancement on enhanced scan. Dural sacs and nerve roots are compressed to varying degrees. (Fig. 8.13). (2) Extensive paravertebral abscess. Long Brucella infection time and absence of systematic standardized treatment may worsen the condition and cause extensive paravertebral abscess, presenting as a large range of lesions, the formation of deep multiple abscesses along the vertebra, below the liga-

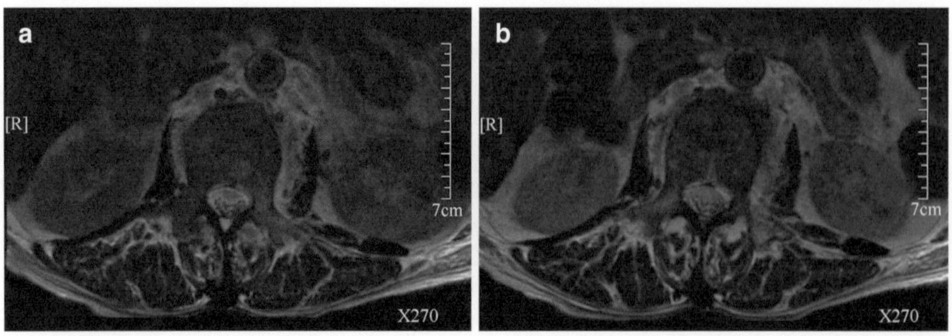

Fig. 8.10 Paralumbar soft tissue swelling. It is presented as a fusiform and slightly hyperintense shadow on the anterior margin and bilateral sides of the vertebral body on transverse T_2WI MRI, encasing the vertebral body with a clear boundary. The space between the vertebral body and the psoas muscle is widened

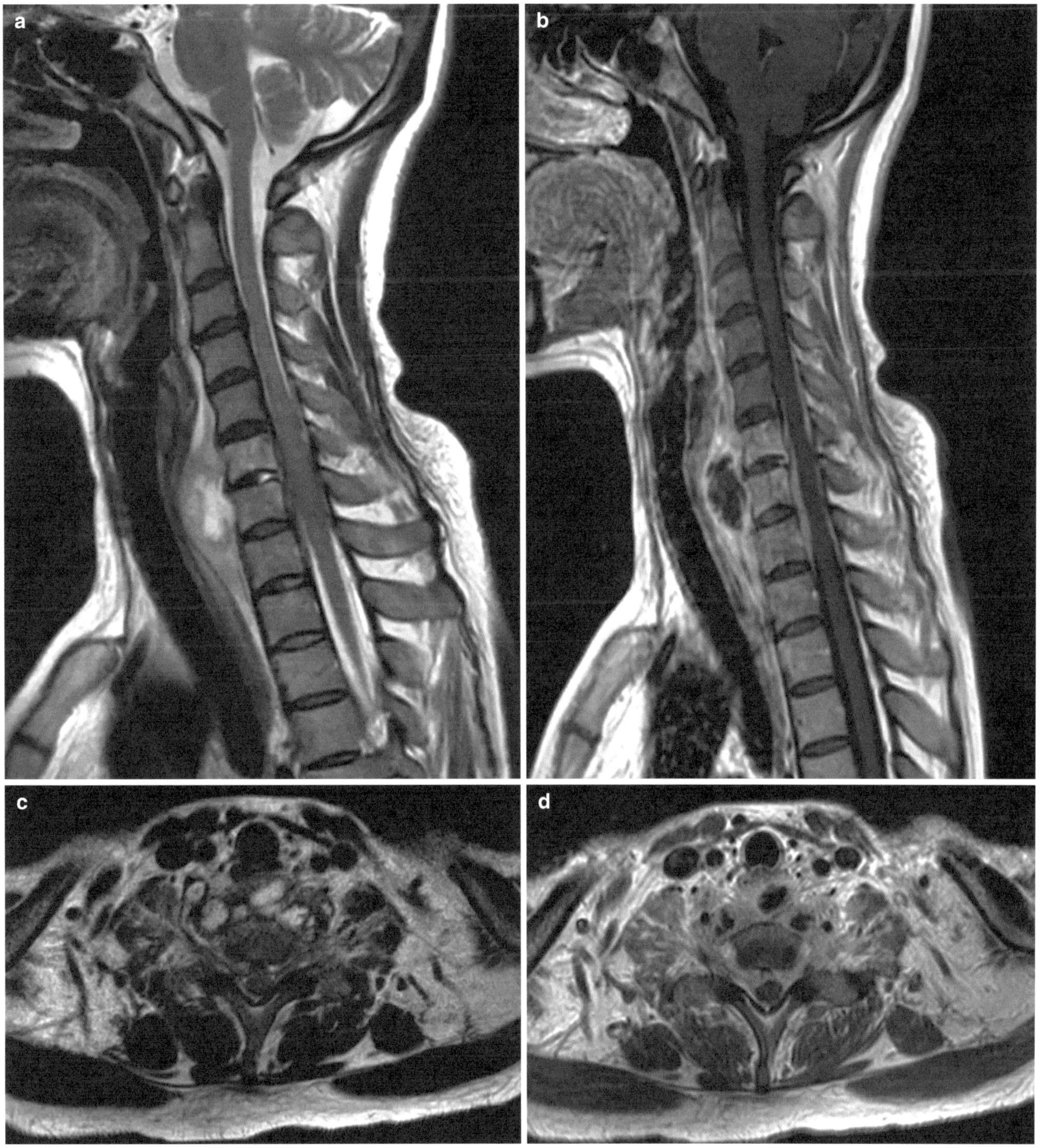

Fig. 8.11 Multiple small paracervical abscesses. There are multiple small, thick-walled abscesses below the anterior longitudinal ligament from C6 to C7 of the neck. (**a**, **c**) On T_2WI MRI, the pus is hyperintense and the abscess wall is hypointense; (**b**, **d**) The abscess wall shows ring enhancement on enhanced T_1WI sequence, with smooth inner wall, and the peripheral tissues are compressed

ments and between the interstitial spaces. It is more than 3 vertebral bodies in length and resembles a cold abscess of vertebral tuberculosis [82], so some scholars also call this disease "pseudotuberculosis." Such abscesses often require surgical resection (Fig. 8.14).

2. **Periarthritis.** It mostly occurs in the soft tissues around large joints such as the hip joint, knee joint, sacroiliac joint. The pain in the acute phase is migratory with unfixed location, while the joint damage is more fixed in location in the chronic phase in which bony ankylosis may even occur.

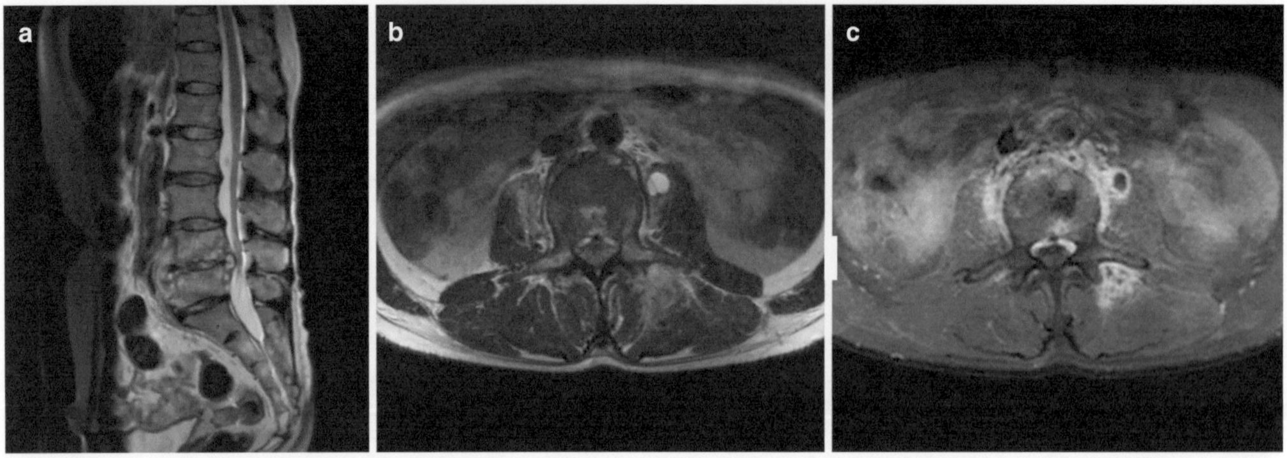

Fig. 8.12 Paralumbar mass and abscess. Soft tissue shadows and abscesses on both sides and in front of vertebral bodies L_4 - L_5. (**a**, **b**) On T_2WI MRI, the soft tissue mass is slightly hyperintense and the left vomica is significantly hyperintense; (**c**) On enhanced T_1WI sequence, the abscess wall and paravertebral soft tissues show marked enhancement, and enhanced soft tissue shadows are also observed around the facet joints after the left transverse process

Fig. 8.13 Cervical intraductal epidural abscess. (**a**) It is fusiform and slightly hyperintense in the anterior and posterior borders of the diseased vertebral body on sagittal T_2WI fat-suppressed sequence, spreading below the ligament; (**b**) Transverse T_2WI shows that the abscess protrudes into the spinal canal, forming an intraspinal epidural abscess, and the dural sac and bilateral nerve roots are compressed

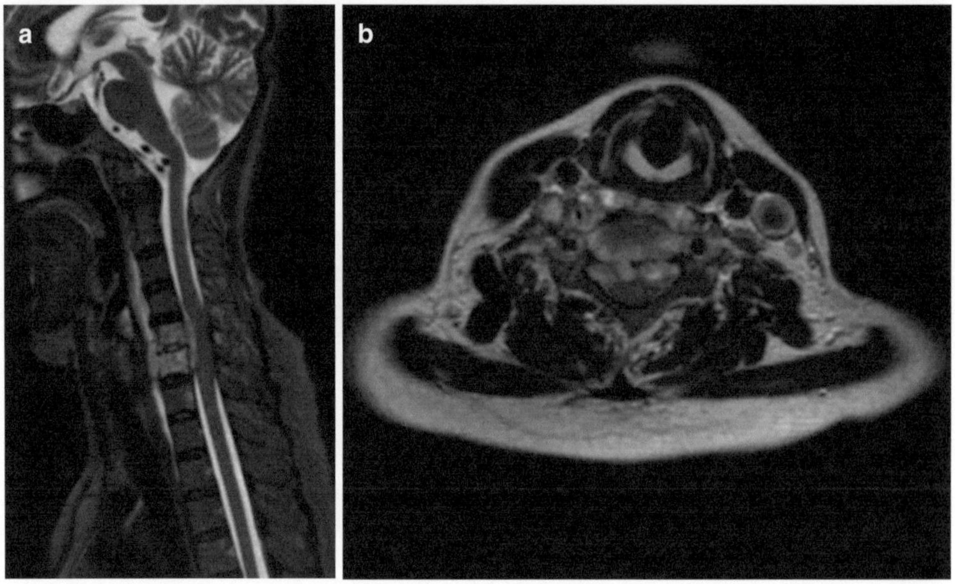

a. X-ray: Only the approximate location of the lesion and skeletal changes can be known due to the lack of good soft tissue contrast, which is difficult to meet the needs of clinical diagnosis. In the acute phase, X-ray only shows periarticular soft tissue swelling, increased density, and slightly widened joint space; in the chronic phase, it mostly invades large joints such as the hip and knee joints, with insignificant soft tissue swelling, joint space stenosis and disappearance, and even bony ankylosis.
b. CT: When it occurs around the Kashin-off segment such as the hip and knee joints, the articular capsule is significantly thickened, a slightly lower soft tissue density shadow is observed around the joint, which spreads along the periarticular space in a fusiform and irregular shape, and there is little to moderate amount of effusion in the articular cavity; further development of the disease can cause intra-articular abscesses which are multiple and small abscesses with thick cyst wall, hypodense vomica, and isodense or slightly hyperdense abscess wall. The abscess edge shows marked enhancement on enhanced scan, and there is no enhancement in the necrotic area (Fig. 8.15).
c. MRI: In the acute phase, inflammatory exudation and edema are specific changes, manifested as articular capsule thickening, joint effusion, periarticular soft tissue swelling, blurred interstitial space. Inflammatory exudation and edema are slightly hyperintense on

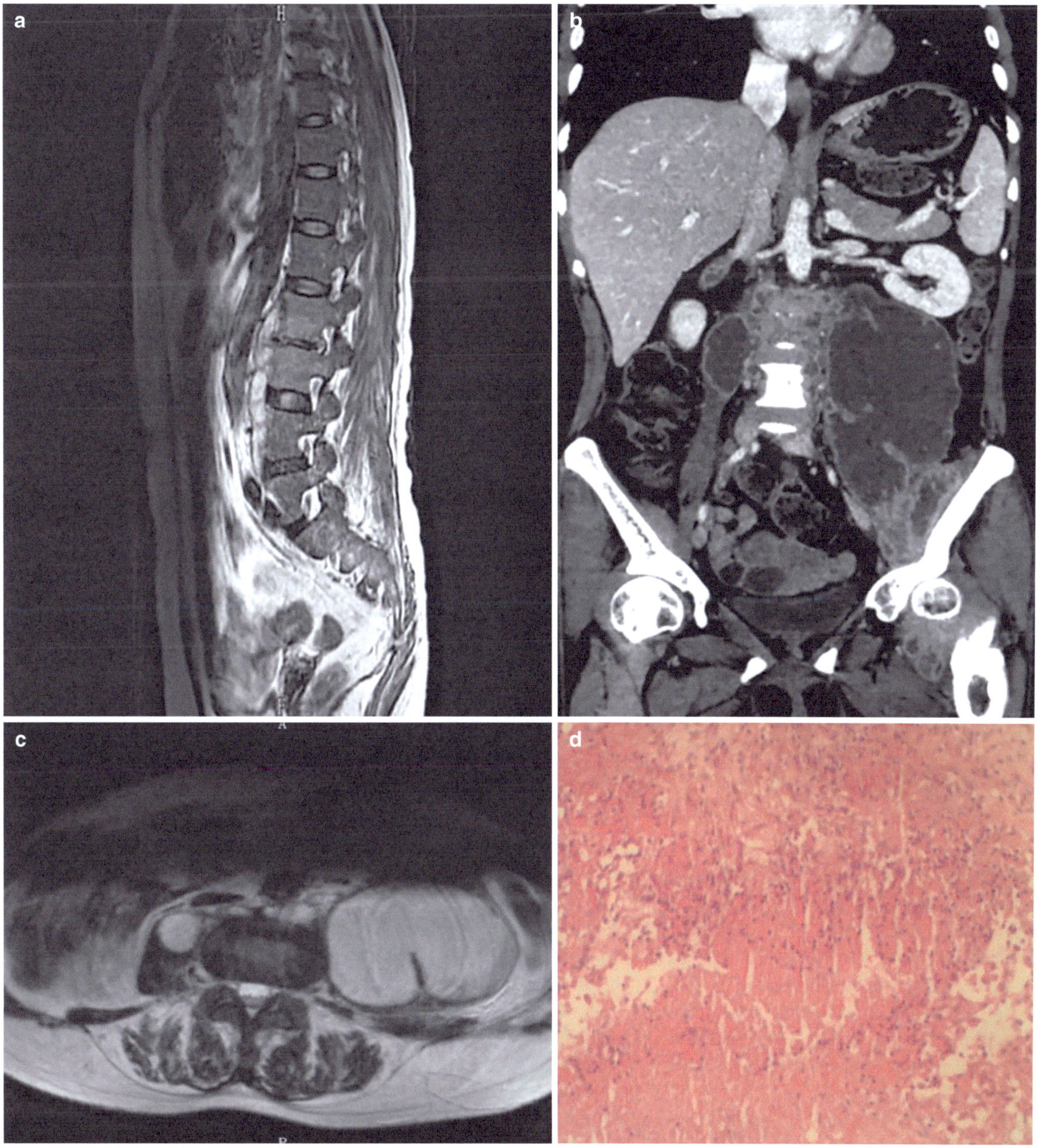

Fig. 8.14 Extensive paravertebral abscess. Extensive paravertebral abscess (Brucella agglutination test 1:200, positive), which is more than three vertebral bodies in length and has wide range of lesions, can progress into deep multiple abscesses. (**a**, **c**) On sagittal and transverse T_2WI sequences, the vomica is significantly hyperintense; (**b**) CT enhancement shows marked enhancement of the abscess wall, uneven thickness of the cyst wall, and multiple septa in the larger vomica on the left side; D. Pathological examination shows histiocytosis in the lesion area, and a large number of inflammatory cells and fibrous granulation tissues

T_2WI, fat-suppressed, and DWI sequences. Diseased tissues show patchy and strip enhancement on enhanced scan (Figs. 8.16, and 8.17); further development of periarticular soft tissue inflammation can cause abscess, and there may be a sense of fluctuation when the abscess is palpated. The abscess has relatively limited extent, with clear boundaries with peripheral tissues and bone joints and deep multiple

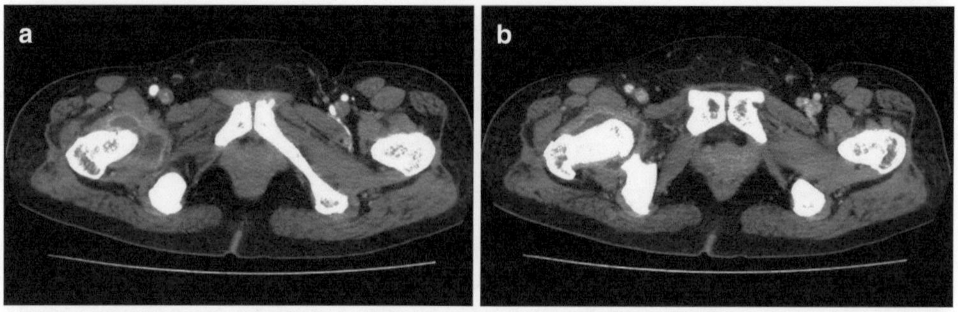

Fig. 8.15 Abscess formation in right hip joint cavity. Enhanced CT shows swelling of the right hip joint, multiple small abscesses in the space around the femoral head, and a thick cyst wall with marked enhancement (**a**, **b**)

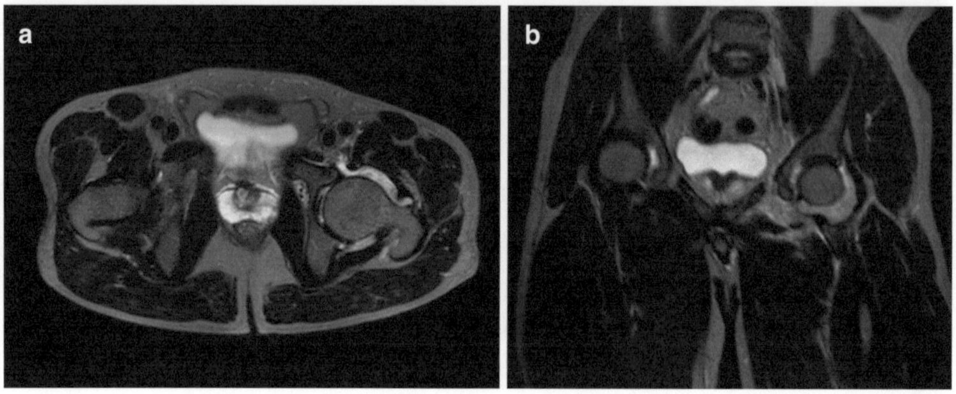

Fig. 8.16 Foci of inflammatory exudation in left hip joint cavity. MRI shows soft tissue shadow in the left hip joint space encasing the femoral head and showing slightly hyperintense on T_2WI, without significant destruction of adjacent bone

abscesses can be formed along the joint space. The abscess wall shows marked enhancement on enhanced scan, with heterogeneous thickness, and there was no enhancement in the central necrotic area. The peripheral bones and joints may be associated with changes such as edema and destruction, or there may be no significant change [83] (Fig. 8.18).

Key Points of Diagnosis

1. Patients are those who have a clear epidemiological contact history, close contact with livestock, livestock products or Brucella cultures before the onset of the disease, residents living in epidemic areas, and people who have drunk dairy products that have not been disinfected and sterilized to the standard or who have eaten immature beef and mutton.
2. The main clinical manifestations include fever, fatigue, hyperhidrosis, muscle and joint pain, enlargement of the liver, spleen, lymph nodes, and testis, which last for days or even weeks.
3. In the laboratory test, the tube agglutination test is positive at 1:100 and above, and the isolation of bacteria from blood culture is the gold standard for the diagnosis of brucellosis.
4. Brucellosis soft tissue infection is often secondary to inflammation of vertebral body and large joints, and the lesions are more common in the paraspinal and periarticular regions. Imaging findings show a fusiform or irregularly shaped soft tissue mass shadow, and paravertebral lesions can spread widely below the ligaments. Brucellosis soft tissue infection is manifested as isointense and slightly hyperintense shadows on non-enhanced CT scan, slightly hypointense on non-enhanced T1WI MRI, slightly hyperintense on non-enhanced T2WI and fat-suppressed sequences, and the lesion area shows marked enhancement on enhanced scan.
5. The abscess formed has a clear boundary with the peripheral tissues, and thick and irregular cyst wall that is hypointense on T_1WI and T_2WI sequences. The cyst cavity is hyperintense on T_1WI and hypointense on T_2WI, the abscess wall shows ring enhancement on enhanced scan, and the pus is significantly hyperintense on DWI sequence.

Differential Diagnosis

1. **Tuberculosis of vertebral body and joint that invades the surrounding soft tissues.** Most of the patients have a relevant history of pulmonary tuberculosis, intestinal tuberculosis, etc. with tuberculosis poisoning symptoms such as afternoon low-grade fever, fatigue, night sweats, positive tuberculin test, and accelerated erythrocyte sedimentation rate. Skip bone destruction and osteoporosis are predominant, and hyperostosis and osteosclerosis are not significant in the lesion area. Tuberculosis of vertebral body and joint is combined with cold abscess with thin and smooth wall. In the cold abscess, sequestrum and

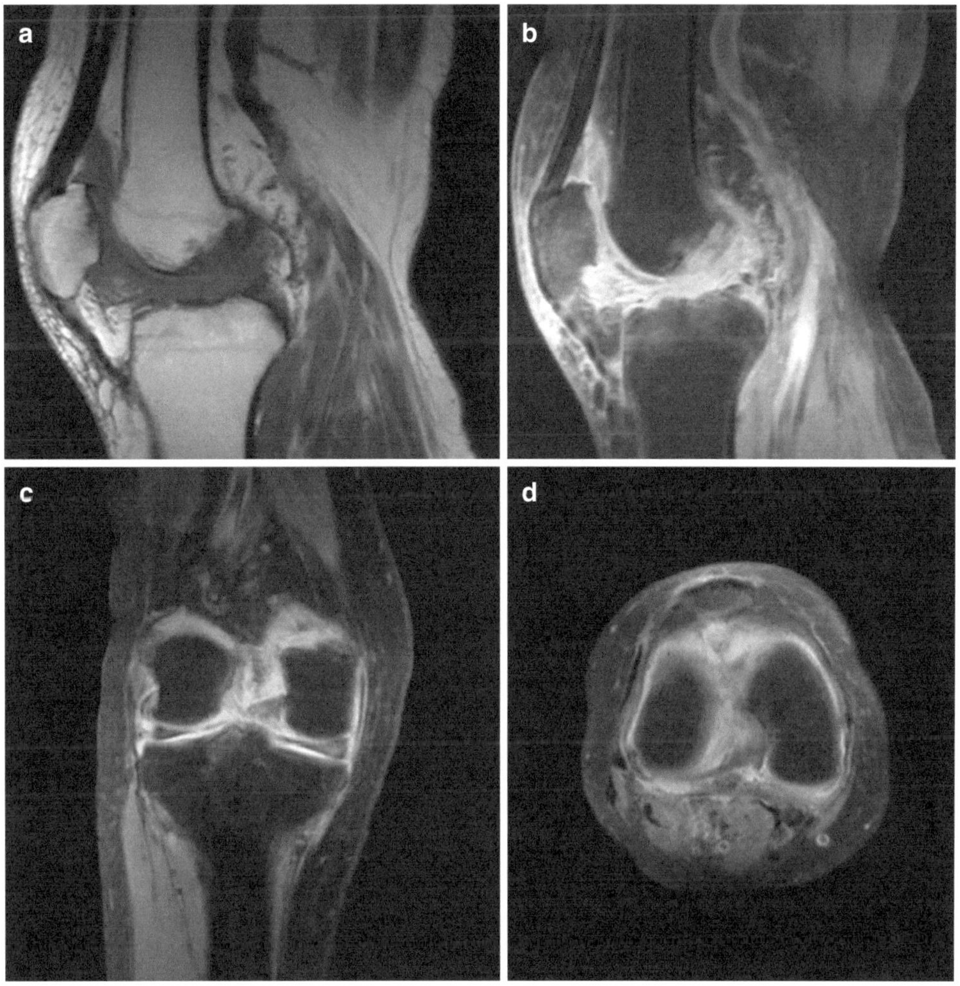

Fig. 8.17 Extensive inflammatory effusion in knee joint. The knee articular capsule is significantly swollen, the synovial membrane is thickened, and extensive effusion and soft tissue shadows are observed in the articular cavity. (**a**) Joint capsule and synovial membrane are slightly hypointense on sagittal T_1WI MRI; (**b**, **d**) Joint capsule and synovial membrane are slightly hyperintense on sagittal and transverse T_2WI fat-suppressed sequences; C. Joint capsule and synovial membrane are slightly hyperintense on coronal T_2WI fat-suppressed sequences

calcification shadow can be observed, which is different from the abscesses in Brucellosis. The tuberculosis abscess located beside the spine often has an extent exceeding the length of the diseased vertebral body. It is easy to be associated with psoas abscess, accompanied by destruction of the adjacent vertebral endplate and intervertebral disc, narrowing of the intervertebral space, and disappearance of fusion. Deep multiple abscesses can also be formed along the paraspinal space. Intraspinal epidural abscess mostly compresses the spinal cord or nerves to produce related symptoms, and its components are necrotic intervertebral disc tissues and sequestrum. Tuberculosis occurring around the joint causes cold abscesses and can be diagnosed by microscopic examination and bacterial culture of the aspirated fluid from the joint, which is differentiated from Brucellosis [84].

2. **Pyogenic osteoarthritis with surrounding soft tissue inflammation.** Most cases are caused by hematogenous infection, a few by trauma, surgery, and other infections. Pathogens are mostly Staphylococcus aureus. It has an acute onset, accompanied by systemic toxic symptoms such as high fever and chills. The lesions are extensive, develop rapidly, and expand circumferentially. There is no obvious boundary between the red and swollen skin and the surrounding normal skin tissues, and the total white blood cell count is significantly increased. Paravertebral soft tissue inflammation caused by purulent osteoarthritis and brucellosis can be characterized by paravertebral soft tissue involvement which is limited and does not exceed the extent of the diseased vertebral body. The difference is that the paravertebral soft tissues of purulent lesions show diffuse swelling with blurred borders, and bubble shadows can be observed in the lesions. The paravertebral soft tissues show hypointense changes on T_1WI and T_2WI sequences, and paravertebral soft tissue inflammation is rarely combined with paravertebral abscesses. Paraarticular soft tissue inflammation can be caused by purulent osteoarthritis and brucellosis. The difference is that purulent lesions have significant soft tissue swelling around, which may be accompanied by lymphadenopathy, and show gas shadows in a few cases. Purulent lesions cause irregular infection when they are outside the joint and cause joint effusion (empyema) when in the joint. The thickness of the abscess wall is

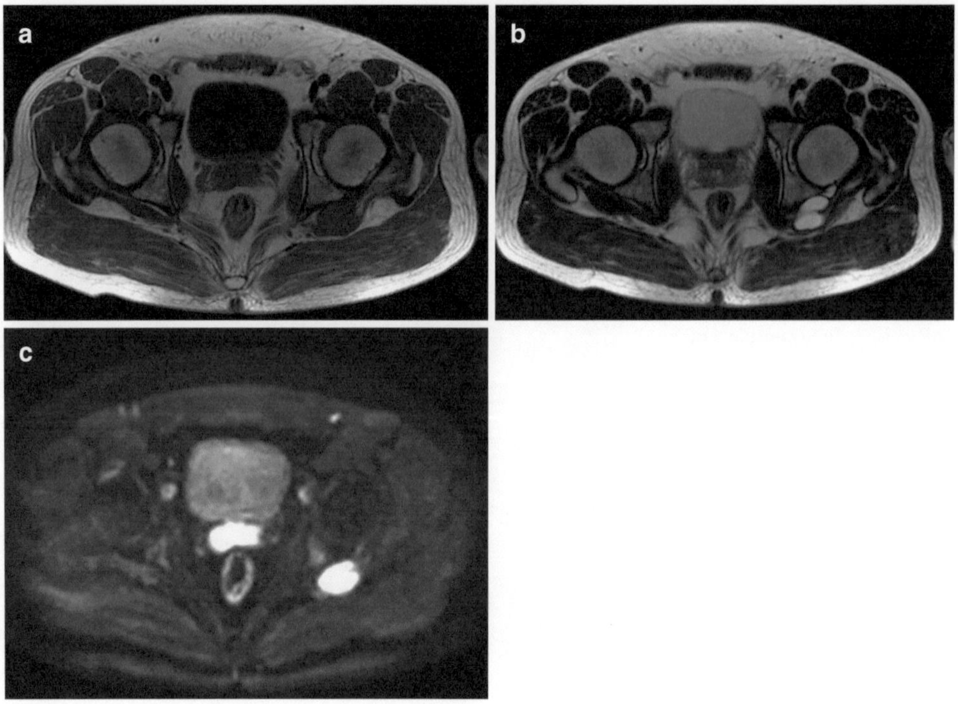

Fig. 8.18 Abscess in left hip joint cavity. Multiple small abscesses formed in the articular cavity. (**a**) The abscess is hypointense on T_1WI MRI; (**b**) The abscess wall is hypointense and the vomica is significantly hyperintense on T_2WI; (**c**) The abscess is significant hyperintense on DWI

uniform, the cysts are quasi-circular and lobulated, and the multilocular cysts are connected to each other. Bacterial culture of pus can be used for further differential diagnosis.

3. **Metastatic tumors in bone and surrounding soft tissues.** They are more common in the elderly who have primary lesions, irregular soft tissue masses around the bone and joint, and multiple bone destruction changes in adjacent bone and joint, but rarely have abscesses. The masses, in which soft tissue shadows can be observed, are with clear boundaries. The soft tissue mass caused by Brucella is fusiform or patchy, irregular in shape, spreads along the joint space, and is often associated with small abscesses which make the density (signal intensity) of the lesion heterogeneous.
4. **Periarthritis caused by other pathogen infections.** The X-ray and CT findings lack specificity, and MRI can detect local soft tissue swelling and abscess formation. It can be differentiated by asking about epidemiological contact history, clinical manifestations, pathogen isolation and blood culture, and diagnostic puncture.

Status Quo and Progress of Research

1. **DWI.** DWI, widely used in clinical and scientific research, can detect the abnormal signal of soft tissue inflammation earlier, which has positive significance for the extent determination and diagnosis and treatment of soft tissue infection. Diffusion changes can also be quantitatively evaluated with the ADC value. In the inflammatory exudation period, the diffusion of water molecules is not significantly limited, and the inflammatory exudation is isointense on DWI; in the abscess formation period, because the pus is composed of viscous fluid of a variety of inflammatory cells, bacteria, necrotic tissue, and proteins, the cell viscosity is increased and the diffusion of water molecules is significantly limited. The abscess is hyperintense on DWI, and the ADC value is decreased. The ADC value range of inflammatory masses is different from that of neoplastic lesions, so it is of great value in the diagnosis and differentiation. DWI plays an important role when clinical manifestations and laboratory tests are atypical [85].
2. **Dynamic contrast-enhanced magnetic resonance imaging (DCE-MRI).** It is a research hotspot in recent years. DCE-MRI reflects the morphological and physiological characteristics of the lesion at the microcirculation level by the degree of microvascular changes in the lesion, makes a quantitative analysis of the lesion tissue, and provides the basis for differential diagnosis. DCE-MRI can reflect the enhancement characteristics of the lesion more objectively than conventional enhanced MRI, thus providing important information for the staging of brucellosis [86].
3. **Magnetic resonance spectroscopy (MRS).** As an important supplementary imaging method for conventional MRI and DWI, it can detect the chemical composition and content of metabolites in living organ tissues. With the development of magnetic resonance technology, in vivo MRS has been further extended from H-NMR to P-MRS, C-MRS, F-MRS, K-MRS, and

Na-MRS, which can detect and analyze the metabolites of phospholipid metabolism and energy metabolism in skeletal muscle, as well as intracellular pH changes. The nature of the lesion adjacent to the affected soft tissue can be roughly evaluated by analyzing the composition of the diseased osseous tissue, thus providing a basis for the diagnosis of this disease.

4. **PET/CT and nuclear medicine.** They can provide lesion information such as paravertebral soft tissue involvement, arthritis, organomegaly, and epidural mass in early foci of brucellosis due to increased FDG uptake in inflammatory lesions, which are effective for early detection of lesions, very helpful for combined abscess localization, but have poor diagnostic specificity [87, 88]. Radionuclide bone imaging can reflect the degree of skeletal muscle damage caused by brucellosis at the molecular level, which is helpful for earlier detection of foci.

8.4 Hydatid Infection

Overview

Echinococcosis, also known as hydatid disease, is a zoonotic parasitic disease caused by the parasitic larvae of Echinococcus in the human body, which belongs to natural epidemic diseases and is specified as a Category C infectious disease in the *Law of the People's Republic of China on Prevention and Treatment of Infectious Diseases*. Domestic dogs, cattle, wolves, foxes, etc. are the main source of infection and definitive hosts. Their excreta contain eggs, and humans can be infected by close contact with infected animals or sharing the same water source, and can also be infected through the respiratory tract in arid and windy areas. Echinococcosis has a global distribution and is mainly endemic in countries and regions with developed animal husbandry. There are four types of pathogenic Echinococcus: Echinococcus granulosus, Echinococcus multilocularis, Echinococcus oligarthrus, and Echinococcus vogeli [89]. There are two types of echinococcosis in China, namely cystic echinococcosis caused by Echinococcus granulosus and alveolar echinococcosis caused by Echinococcus multilocularis, of which Echinococcus granulosus is the most common in clinical practice, accounting for about 98% [90], mainly distributed in agricultural and pastoral areas in the northwest, with the hepatic echinococcosis being the most common (70%), followed by the pulmonary echinococcosis (20% to 30%), and bone and soft tissue echinococcosis accounting for 0.5% to 1% [91], which can occur alone and is often accompanied by hepatic and pulmonary echinococcosis. Alveolar echinococcosis is slightly limited in distribution, mostly sporadic, and highly lethal.

The incidence of infection in various organ tissues is related to their blood flow and also directly related to the order in which the oncosphere passes through the tissues with the blood circulation. The organs with a cystic echinococcosis incidence from high to low are the liver, lungs, abdominal cavity, pelvic cavity, spleen, kidneys, brain, bones, muscles, subcutaneous tissues, etc. [92] Echinococcus multilocularis is similar to Echinococcus granulosus, but smaller. Its larvae mainly parasitize in the liver, also in lungs, brain, and other parts, and almost all the parasitized organs in 1 to 2 years are occupied by large and small vesicles, similar to malignant tumors, so echinococcosis is known as "worm cancer."

The disease has a long incubation period and develops extremely slowly. Infections often occur in childhood, but symptoms do not occur until adulthood. Soft tissue echinococcosis is divided into primary echinococcosis and secondary echinococcosis according to the site of involvement [93]. Primary soft tissue echinococcosis is rare and can be seen in muscle tissue, but also in tendons, fascia, periosteum, and even subcutaneous adipose tissue. Secondary soft tissue echinococcosis has no subjective symptoms in the early stage. Most patients present with soft tissue mass, often without obvious systemic symptoms. As the disease progresses further, it may present with soft tissue swelling, mass, pain, numbness, weakness, limited motion, local muscle atrophy, and dysfunction. In recent years, muscular hydatid infection has increased, and parasitic cyst growth in striated muscle is inhibited due to muscle contraction and the presence of lactic acid (5). Spinal and neurological involvement may present with corresponding clinical symptoms and even pathologic fractures. The pathogenesis of echinococcosis is mainly mechanical compression, followed by hydatid cyst destruction causing alloprotein allergic reactions, and cyst rupture can cause peripheral tissue infection and related complications. Biopsy or puncture for diagnostic purposes may lead to leakage of cystic fluid, spread of the scolex, and may cause severe allergic reactions, so this procedure should be used with caution in clinical practice. At present, the treatment of echinococcosis is mainly based on surgical resection, but the postoperative recurrence rate is still 2% to 10% [94].

Pathophysiology

Echinococcosis can be divided into cystic type, polycystic type, and calcified type according to its special pathological basis, occurrence, evolution, and outcome process. Necrotic tissue and cavities can be observed in the section of the diseased tissue. Vesicles of different sizes and irregular shapes are observed, around which inflammatory granulation tissues are formed, with infiltration of various inflammatory cells such as eosinophils, lymphocytes, and plasma cells. Foreign body giant cell reaction is observed locally in the necrotic fibrous cyst wall tissue, residual parasites, and egg tissue are observed between the giant cells, and calcium salt deposition may be observed in the cyst wall, showing granular amorphous calcification.

Secondary soft tissue echinococcosis is mostly caused by hydatid infection of the spine and bones, and the lesion perforates the bone cortex to form echinococcus cysts in the surrounding soft tissues and muscles. The disease is more common in the pelvis and lumbar vertebra, mainly caused by infection through blood circulation. The lesions usually occur in the spongy bone with abundant blood supply and vigorous growth, and in the metaphysis or marrow cavity of long diaphysis and grow along the spongy bone or the boundary of marrow cavity to form unilocular or multilocular cysts. The diseased bone shows cystic and expansive osteolytic bone destruction without surrounding fibrous capsule. With the gradual growth of the cyst, the pathological changes are mainly caused by compression on adjacent organs by space-occupying growth, and atrophy, degeneration, or necrosis of the surrounding soft tissues.

Imaging Findings

X-ray examination is simple and feasible and is mostly used for the detection of pulmonary and skeletal lesions, with poor soft tissue contrast and sensitivity. CT is an important method for the diagnosis of echinococcosis and related complications, which can be used for the examination of various organs throughout the body. CT examination has high spatial resolution. By adjusting the window width, window position and measuring the difference of CT value, it can clearly show the lesion site and lesion characteristics, as well as the cyst wall and intracystic structure of echinococcus, especially for calcified lesions. MRI has good soft tissue resolution, can detect lesions earlier, and show the size and extent of lesions and their spatial relationship with adjacent tissues better, as well as the pathological changes of diseased tissues to a certain extent, which plays an important role in the diagnosis of echinococcosis. Especially for soft tissue echinococcosis, it can clearly show the location, number, extent of echinococcus cysts, and the involvement of surrounding organs. Conventional scanning sequences include T_1WI, T_2WI, fat-suppressed sequence, and Gd-DTPA enhanced scanning sequence. Fat suppression can also distinguish fat and bleeding signals. Diffusion weighted imaging (DWI) plays an important role in differential diagnosis. Ultrasonography is a routine examination method for soft tissue infection, which can display the space-occupying lesions of hydatid without injury, safely and visually. It has the advantages of repeatable dynamic observation and simplicity.

1. X-ray.
   (a) Muscle echinococcosis: It has no obvious specificity in the early stage. As the disease progresses further, the local mass effect is produced after the echinococcus cyst becomes larger, and the peripheral tissues are compressed, presenting with soft tissue swelling, blurred and widened intermuscular space, and irregular or dot-like calcification around; when the lesion is located in the paravertebral soft tissue, it is manifested as symmetrical or asymmetric spherical shadow in the psoas muscle, and irregular or arc-like calcified shadow may also occur beside the vertebra.
   (b) Parosteal soft tissue echinococcosis: It is mostly caused by adjacent vertebral echinococcosis, presenting with irregular worm-eaten bone destruction in the vertebral body, compression and deformation, and even thinning and disappearance of most of the vertebral body. If echinococcus protrudes from the vertebral body and grows continuously, it will form a shadow similar to a paracervical abscess. Utricular radiolucent areas can be seen in the diseased spongy bone, followed by multiple connected round or irregular cystic radiolucent areas. There is no periosteal reaction, no erosive bone destruction and new bone, and the bone cortex is compressed and thinned. In the late stage, cystic cavity enlargement may involve the whole bone block, and pathologic fracture may occur.
2. CT.
   (a) Muscle echinococcosis: Echinococcosis is characterized by soft tissue swelling and blurring at the lesion and divided into cystic and polycystic types. CT is the most valuable method for its diagnosis. (1) Cystic type is characterized by single or multiple round or oval low-density mass lesions with clear boundary. The multiple foci vary in size, with sharp edge. The cyst, whose wall is 2–5 mm, has uniform density which is similar to that of water and clear boundary with the peripheral tissues, but has no daughter cyst structure. The adjacent tissue is compressed and pushed by the cyst. Calcification may occur in the cyst wall and interval, and there is no significant enhancement of the cyst wall on enhanced scan. (2) Polycystic type is characterized by multiple daughter cysts in clusters, botryoidal changes, and cyst septa formation which is a feature of echinococcus granulosus cysts. The daughter cyst has uniform density which is similar to that of water, but lower than that of the mother cyst. Daughter cysts appear as quasi-circular hypodense shadows of varying numbers and sizes in the mother sac, arranged in the periphery of the mother sac or filling the entire mother sac (Fig. 8.19). On enhanced scan, the cystic fluid shows no enhancement, and some parts of the cyst wall may have enhancement. The outer wall of echinococcus cysts with long disease duration is thick and may show various forms of calcification, arcs and ring shadows of varying lengths and thicknesses

(Figure 8.19b, d). The cyst wall is blurred when echinococcus cysts are combined with infection, and the density in the cyst is mixed and heterogeneous [95].

(b) Parosteal soft tissue echinococcosis: Bone hydatid disease is often associated with surrounding soft tissue echinococcosis and when skeletal lesions have no characteristic changes, image changes in adjacent soft tissues are the key to imaging diagnosis of bone echinococcosis [96]. Typical bone hydatid disease shows cystic bone destruction areas with honeycomb or botryoidal internal septa, in which the cystic fluid is clear and mostly without fibrous capsule. Advanced bone echinococcosis invades the surrounding soft tissues and forms a mixed large mass with echinococcosis in both the bone and soft tissues, which may present with pathological fractures and can cause pathologic fracture when invading the joints. Spinal echinococcosis is characterized by unilocular or multilocular quasi-circular, cystic masses with homogeneous density in the vertebral body, mostly in the anterior part of the vertebral body. The lesion may be cartwheel shaped, and dot-like calcified shadows may be observed in its cyst wall and septa. The cyst can invade the spinal canal along the intervertebral space or foramen, enlarge the vertebral canal, compress the surrounding spinal cord and nerve roots, while the intervertebral disc is generally not affected. In the late stage, narrowing of the intervertebral space may occur, and compression fractures may occur in the affected vertebral body. The lesion shows no enhancement on enhanced scan. Single or multiple quasi-circular and elliptic cystic shadows with low density and different sizes are observed in the paravertebral soft tissues, which are more common in the

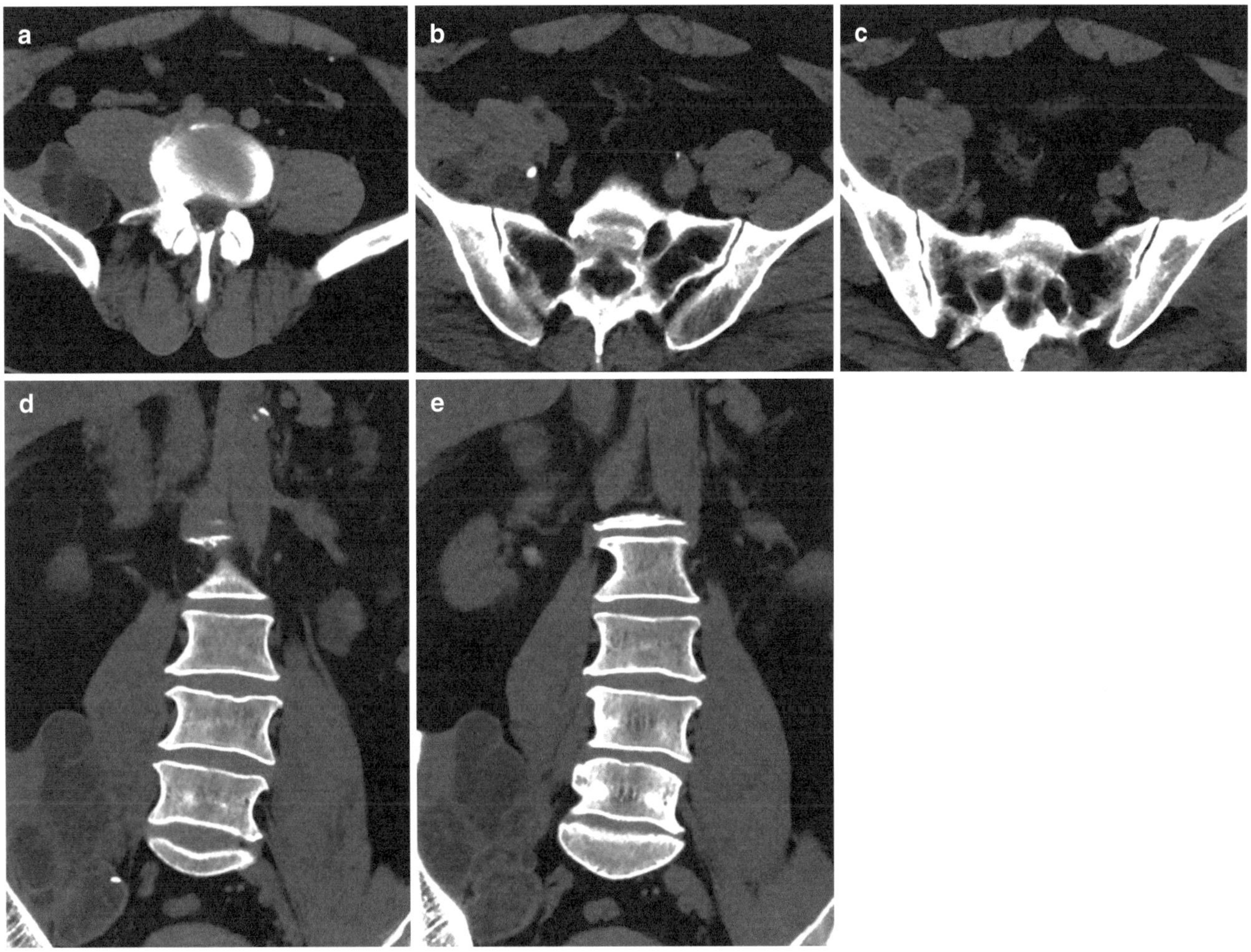

Fig. 8.19 Muscle echinococcosis (polycystic type). (**a**–**e**) Transverse and coronal CT scans show multiple elliptic cystic density foci in the right iliac muscle. In the foci, multiple quasi-circular daughter cysts with lower density which is similar to that of water are observed, with smooth and sharp edge, clear boundary. There is septa with different thickness in the cyst. The posterior cyst is less uniform in density, with the cyst wall thickened by about 4 mm, and spotty calcification at the edge (the picture was provided by Hui Guo from the First Affiliated Hospital of Xinjiang Medical University, thanks)

psoas muscle, with regular margin, clear boundary with the peripheral tissues. The lesion shows no enhancement on enhanced scan, and calcification can be observed in the cyst wall and septa of echinococcus cyst.

3. MRI.
   (a) Muscular echinococcosis: MRI findings also vary depending on the stage of lesion development. (1) Simple echinococcus cyst: It is characterized by round and quasi-circular lesions with smooth edges in the musculature. Multiple lesions are of different sizes, with the cyst fluid being hypointense on T_1WI and hyperintense on T_2WI, and the cyst wall being hypointense on both T_1WI and T_2WI. The adjacent tissues are compressed and displaced, and the surrounding soft tissues show diffuse edema. (2) Polycystic type: It is characterized by cystic and multilocular lesions. Daughter cysts are arranged in the mother cyst in a rose petaloid or mulberry pattern. The cyst wall and septa are clearly displayed, with clear boundary. The mother cyst is hypointense on T_1WI sequence, while the daughter cyst is less hypointense, which is similar to water; The mother cyst shows hyperintense on T_2WI, which is clearer on fat-suppressed sequence. Compared with the mother cyst, the daughter cyst has significantly higher and more uniform signal intensity, and the interval shows hypointense. The sac wall and septa show mild enhancement on enhanced scan (Fig. 8.20), and the adjacent muscles could show enhancement to varying degrees; cyst calcification manifests itself as dotted and arc-shaped shadows in the sac wall and shows isointense on T_1WI and hypointense on T_2WI. (3) Echinococcus cyst with infection: The cyst is irregular, with blurred boundary, and thickened cyst wall. It is hypointense on T_1WI and slightly hyperintense on T_2WI. Signal intensity on T_1WI is generally increased due to increased protein content in the cyst. (4) When complicated with cyst rupture: it is manifested as internal capsule dissection and floating in the cyst fluid, like "ribbon sign." Larger hydatid will compress the muscle and cause local tissue ischemia, and muscle necrosis, which shows localized signal intensity reduction or no signal intensity on T_1WI sequences, increased signal intensity on T_2WI sequences, and a wide edema signal around the necrotic tissue.
   (b) Parosteal soft tissue echinococcosis: Intraspinal echinococcosis can occur in any part of the vertebral canal, and the lesions have clear boundaries. The cyst can compress the spinal cord and cauda equina and cause corresponding clinical symptoms. The intervertebral disc is generally not affected, showing normal signal intensity, and intervertebral space stenosis may occur in the late stage. Echinococcus cysts can be located on one side of the spine after growing up, forming a pseudoabscess which presents as a round or elliptic cystic mass in the paravertebral soft tissue, is slightly hypointense on T_1WI and slightly hyperintense on T_2WI. Psoas major involvement is common. Bone hydatid disease is mostly characterized by the formation of cysts of different sizes and with sharp and clear margins in the spongy bone, and thinning or dilatation of the bone cortex. In the late stage, bone echinococcus cysts can break through the osseous tissue and enter the surrounding soft tissues, forming soft tissue echinococcus cysts which show hypointense on T_1WI and hyperintense on T_2WI. There may be septa and fluid-air levels of different sizes in the cysts, and the lesions rupture extracutaneously to form unhealed fistula, sometimes with the outflow of daughter cysts [97].

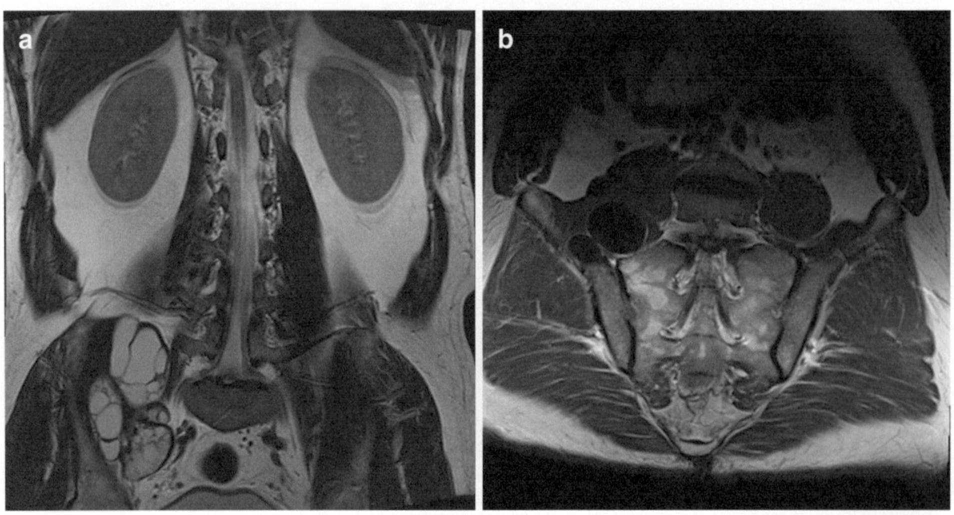

Fig. 8.20 Muscular echinococcosis (polycystic type). (**a**) T_2WI MRI shows multiple daughter cysts of different sizes in the mother sac, with visible septa, hypointense in the cyst wall and septa, higher signal intensity in the daughter cyst than in the mother cyst, and heterogeneous signal intensity in the posterior lesion; (**b**) T_1WI enhanced scan shows mild enhancement of the cyst wall (the picture was provided by Hui Guo from the First Affiliated Hospital of Xinjiang Medical University, thanks)

4. Ultrasonography.
   (a) Cystic type: It is characterized by cystic masses in muscle tissues, with smooth and complete cyst wall. The endocyst is separated from the external wall. Ultrasonography can clearly show the double-layer wall structure, a very narrow and uniform sonolucent area filled with (anechoic) fluid between the two layer cyst walls, and multiple hyperechoic light banded septa in the cyst. The signals in the cyst in the changed position are heterogeneous, showing a "snowfall sign," which is the basis for distinguishing it from the general simple cyst, and banded hypoechoic inflammatory response can be observed around the lesion.
   (b) Polycystic type: Most cysts are elliptic or oval in shape, with clear boundaries with peripheral tissues, regular edges, and thick cyst walls. There are small daughter cysts of different sizes and numbers inside the mother cyst, which are honeycomb or wheel-like and gather inside the mother cyst, presenting characteristic "cyst in cyst." The diagnostic accuracy rate can reach 100% [98].

Key Points of Diagnosis

1. The patients are those who have a clear epidemiological contact history, and contact with animals such as dogs, cattle, sheep, and foxes and their fur before the onset of the disease, residents living in pastoral areas, people with a history of tourism and hunting in pastoral areas, and occupational groups.
2. Soft tissue echinococcosis is mostly secondary, with no subjective symptoms in the early stage, slow development, and is characterized by painless swelling. Most of the patients present with soft tissue masses, hard toughness of local masses to touch, elasticity to press, and tremor to percussion, often accompanied by hepatic and pulmonary echinococcosis.
3. Laboratory test: Echinococcus ELISA is positive, and the etiological examination mainly finds hydatid cyst wall, daughter cysts, protoscolices, or hooks mainly in the lesions or excretions.
4. CT is the most valuable method for diagnosis of echinococcosis. CT shows single or multiple circular or quasi-circular cysts with a thickness of 2 ~ 5 mm in wall, homogeneously watery low density, and well-defined border. For the polycystic type, a mother cyst contains daughter cysts with lower density presenting "bunch of grapes" appearance, and septa, with cyst walls of arc-shaped or eggshell-like calcification which can be used as the main basis for diagnosis.
5. On MRI, cysts present hypointense on T_1WI and hyperintense on T_2WI. For the polycystic type, daughter cysts are arranged in the mother cyst in the shape of rosette or mulberry, and the daughter cysts show significantly lower signal intensity on T_1WI and more hyperintense on T_2WI compared with the mother cyst. The cyst wall and septa are clearly shown, with hypointense capsule at the periphery, in which hypointense is found on T_1WI and T_2WI. The enhanced scan demonstrates mild enhancement in cyst wall. The cyst rupture as a complication is manifested as internal capsule dissection, showing ribbon sign.
6. The ultrasonography can clearly reveal double-walled structure of simple cysts, and intracystic signals present falling snowflakes sign with the change in the patient position. A polycystic echinococcus cyst is characterized by the change of the mother cyst containing daughter cysts.

Differential Diagnosis

1. **Pyogenic soft tissue abscesses.** Pyogenic soft tissue abscesses are mostly caused by bacterial infection and present acute onset accompanied by high fever, chills, and obvious systemic poisoning symptom. The total leukocyte count significantly increases. Local soft tissue is manifested as redness, swelling, fever, and pain. There is no distinct border between red skin and peripheral normal skin tissue. The abscess is well-demarcated and gives a sense of fluctuation in touching. The enhanced scan demonstrates obvious ring enhancement in the abscess wall but no enhancement in the internal necrotic area. The abscess may be combined with pneumatosis, presenting the change of hypointense or extreme hypodensity. If a patient with a soft tissue abscess does not have a history of epidemiology or develop cystic lesions in other parts of the body, the patient can be diagnosed with a soft-tissue abscess by a microscopic examination and bacterial culture of purulent fluid extracted. Moreover, the abscess can be distinguished from echinococcus cyst.
2. **Tuberculous soft tissue abscess.** Most patients with tuberculous soft tissue abscesses have a history of pulmonary tuberculosis, gastrointestinal tuberculosis, and other relevant diseases. This disease causes obvious tuberculosis poisoning symptoms mostly including fatigue, night sweats, and afternoon low-grade fever. The tuberculin test shows positive. The erythrocyte sedimentation rate (ESR) is elevated. A tuberculous abscess is a cold abscess with clear margin. Most of paravertebral abscesses are psoas abscesses. The lesions often develop to the extent exceeding the length of the affected vertebra, with saltatory osteoclast migration, and may involve the destruction of adjacent vertebral end plate and intervertebral disc. CT shows that a juxta-articular abscess is well-demarcated from peripheral tissues, adjacent articular bones may be destroyed, and sequestrum or calcification can be found in the abscess. In the enhanced scan, the

ring enhancement is presented and deep multiple abscesses are formed. The enhanced scan reveals ring enhancement in the abscess walls. A patient can be diagnosed with a juxta-articular abscess after bacterial culture of purulent fluid extracted from his joints.

3. **Soft tissue lipoma.** Soft tissue lipoma is a benign tumor composed of mature adipocytes. It is often a single, slow-growing, and painless mass. Its clinical manifestations are associated with the location and shape of tumor. The circular or quasi-circular tumor can produce compression symptoms. The mass is smooth in edge and well-demarcated from peripheral tissues, of which shape may change with muscular contraction. The CT value is −120 ~ -80HU. The capsule and septa are found in the mass on CT. The enhanced scan shows no enhancement. The MRI examination presents characteristic fat signals, that is, hyperintense on T_1WI and hyperintense on T_2WI, which are the same as subcutaneous fat signals. Fat signals of the lipoma may be suppressed on the fat-suppressed sequence. The enhanced scan shows no enhancement.
4. **Subcutaneous or soft tissue hematoma.** Patients with subcutaneous or soft tissue hematoma often have a history of trauma of different degrees. Most hematomas are located in subcutaneous or intramuscular tissue and can result in tenderness. They can be resolved automatically. A diagnosis can be made based on relevant medical history. On CT, the hematoma in the acute stage is manifested as hyperdensity, and the hematoma in the subacute stage and chronic stage shows changes of isodensity or slightly high density. Moreover, fluid–fluid levels can be seen in some hematomas. Hematoma further progresses to present liquid low density. The enhanced scan shows no enhancement. Hematoma may also be associated with peripheral tissue infection. MRI signal changes of a hematoma in different stages are different. The acute hematoma is often accompanied by peripheral soft tissue edema, with poorly defined border, and shows slightly hypointense on T_1WI and hyperintense on T_2WI. The subacute hematoma presents slightly hyperintense in T_1WI and T_2WI sequences, in which a few of patchy hypointense shadows can be seen. The chronic hematoma shows a hypointense hemosiderin ring at the periphery. Typical clinical history and imaging changes of hematoma can be used for its differentiation [99]. Biopsy can be performed for differential diagnosis of hematoma when necessary.
5. **Soft tissue and muscle cyst.** Sacral canal cyst, sebaceous cyst, popliteal cyst, ganglion cyst, and other soft tissue and muscle cysts are mostly cystic masses in different size with relatively smooth wall on imaging, and no enhancement in the enhanced scan. These cysts do not contain typical daughter cysts of echinococcus cyst. There is no cystic mass in other parts of its patient. In addition, a patient with aforesaid lesion often has records of onset age, clinical manifestations, and dysplasia of relevant diseases without a history of epidemiology. The lesion can be confirmed by an intracutaneous test showing negative.

Status Quo and Progress of Research

1. **DWI** is the only imaging method that can be used to observe micro-motion of in vivo water molecules. This method can detect early changes in morphology and physiology related to change in water content of tissue. ADC values, as an intrinsic characteristic of tissue, can quantitatively evaluate diffusion changes and reflect the rate and range of diffusion motion of water molecules. Generally, the ADC value increases when diffusion is fast in tissue. A echinococcus cyst is composed of endocyst and ectocyst. Endocyst fluid is secreted from the germinal layer. Ectocyst is a fibrous capsule formed by the host tissue in response to the echinococcus cyst. The difference of motion limitation of water molecules in endocyst and ectocyst results in the difference in ADC values and DWI signals. Especially, when the echinococcus cyst is associated with infection, ADC values are valuable for diagnosis, differential diagnosis, and analysis of pathological components of echinococcus cyst.
2. **MRS** is the only noninvasive method to observe energy metabolism of in vivo muscular tissue and allows the observation for energy metabolism of muscular tissue at the cellular level. MRS can test and analyze the metabolites of phospholipid metabolism and energy metabolism and intracellular pH changes in skeletal muscles. Substances observed on phosphorus magnetic resonance spectroscopy (P-MRS) include PCr, Pi, and PCr as reference for chemical shift in phosphorus metabolism. The chemical shift of Pi relating to phosphocreatine can be used for noninvasive determination of intracellular pH. A muscular echinococcus cyst causes abnormal changes in the metabolic rate of affected muscular tissue, which can be reflected by changes on P-MRS. Specifically, the peak value of PCr decreases, the peak value of Pi increases, the pH value of cytoplasm significantly rises, and free ADP also markedly increases.
3. **DCE-MRI** can reflect morphological and physiological characteristics of a lesion at the microcirculation level and quantitatively analyze affected tissue based on the microvascular changes. DCE-MRI can reflect the enhancement characteristics of the lesion in a more objective manner compared with conventional enhanced MRI. Echinococcus cyst without typical features can be differentiated from tumorous lesions to some extent by microvascular changes reflecting the characteristics of infiltration zone around the lesion.

8.5 Other Rare Pathogen Infections

Junyan Yang and Peng Zhang

8.5.1 Non-tuberculous Mycobacterial Infection

Overview

Mycobacteria is a group of bacteria with acid-fast staining property, including Mycobacterium tuberculosis, Mycobacterium leprae, and non-tuberculous mycobacteria. Non-tuberculous mycobacteria (NTM) were previously known as atypical mycobacteria. Up to now, more than 200 species of NTM have been identified, most of which are opportunistic pathogens. NTM is mainly found in sewage, soil, aerosols, unpasteurized milk, animals, and plants. Cases of relevant diseases caused by over 50 species of NTM have been reported in China [100]. Non-tuberculous mycobacteriosis is a chronic disease attributable to NTM infection. NTM infection was mostly reported in developed countries. NTM infection may occur in all tissues and organs of human, most common in lungs, followed by lymph nodes, skin soft tissues, and bones. Pathogens that can infect skin and soft tissue include Mycobacterium marinum, Mycobacterium abscessus, Mycobacterium chelonae, Mycobacterium fortuitum, and Mycobacterium ulcerans [101]. In recent years, with the increase in the application of hormones and immunosuppressive agents, severe burns and wounds, organ transplantation, tumor patients and AIDS patients, the incidence of NTM infection has been increasing year by year [102].

Most of NTM infections are single and a few may involve several systems. Disseminated NTM infection may occur in immunocompromised patients, affecting liver, lymph node, and gastrointestinal tract, and be complicated by osteomyelitis, with various clinical manifestations. Patients with pulmonary infection often have such tuberculosis poisoning symptoms as cough, expectoration, low fever, night sweats, and fatigue which are less severe than those of tuberculosis. NTM often invades lymph nodes to cause lymphnoditis, which is common in preschool children, involving cervical and submandibular lymph nodes. Quick malacia may occur in lymph nodes, and the sinus is formed after ulcer rupture. NTM also invades synovial membrane, tendinous sheath, and bursa mucosa in skeletal system, resulting in joint deformity and dysfunction in the advanced stage. NTM is easy to cause skin and soft tissue infection, which is common in dermal and subcutaneous adipose tissue, and skins of extremities including hand, feet, elbows, knees, and other parts, as well as possible in deep muscle tissue. Clinical manifestations vary with different pathogens or different stages of the disease. Affected skin and soft tissue present with redness, swelling, fever, and pain, with commonly local abscesses. The ulceration caused by skin infections may result in the formation of necrotic ulcers (Buruli ulcers).

Laboratory tests include acid-fast staining (smear staining microscopy), bacterial culture and histopathology, immunological diagnosis, among which bacterial culture and histopathology are main criteria for diagnosis of NTM infection. In recent years, the introduction of molecular biological techniques has facilitated and accelerated the identification of related mycobacteria and sources of transmission.

Pathophysiology

Pathological changes caused by NTM infection are similar to those of tuberculosis. These changes are milder and the body tissue response is weaker due to the weak virulence of NTM and rare caseous necrosis. For most NTM infections, the primary focus in the respiratory tract spreads to all organs and tissues through lymph and hematogenous dissemination. Immunodeficient or immunocompromised individuals are susceptible to NTM infection. In the early stage, acute inflammatory reactions occur, mainly with inflammatory exudation and edema. The lesion further develops into form soft tissue nodules, abscesses, and sinuses. The main pathogens of NTM infection in skin and soft tissue are Mycobacterium abscessus and Mycobacterium fortuitum. Its main pathological manifestations include granulomatous lesion and non-specific chronic pyogenic inflammation. The granulomatous lesion is tuberculous granuloma dominated by epithelioid cells and lymphocytes. In addition to epithelioid cells and lymphocytes, infiltration of such inflammatory cells as neutrophils, plasma cells, and multinucleated giant cells may occur, presenting infectious granuloma structure of mixed cell infiltration [103, 104]. Mycobacterium abscessus may cause chronic pyogenic inflammation, mainly purulent tuberculous granuloma, with small abscesses in the lesion center.

Imaging Findings

1. **X-ray.** X-ray mainly demonstrates soft tissue swelling in the lesion area, accompanied by ulceration, with unclear soft tissue stratification and blurred intermuscular space and fat space. Multiple spotted and nodular calcifications can be seen in the focus. The lesion may progress to involve surrounding bones and result in bone destruction.
2. **CT.** In the early stage, CT mainly shows inflammatory hyperemia and edema of soft tissue, swelling of local soft tissue, increased density in fat space, local cord-like shadows and grid-like shadows presenting honeycomb changes, ill-defined border of the focus with peripheral tissues, and liquid density shadows representing effusion.

The lesion further develops into soft tissue nodules, and the enhanced scan shows mild enhancement. Soft tissue abscesses are formed, with well-defined borders; the enhanced scan demonstrates ring enhancement in abscess wall and no enhancement in internal necrotic area. There may be multiple spotted calcifications. The lesion involves adjacent osteoarticular region, which is manifested as worm-eaten bone destruction, and accompanied by hyperostosis and sclerosis at the periphery.

3. **MRI.** It mainly reveals diffuse swelling and edema in soft tissue of the lesion area, which may be combined with effusion and exudative changes, and ill-defined borders with peripheral tissues, as well as mild enhancement in the enhanced scan. Combined soft tissue nodules show changes in hypointense on T_1WI and hyperintense on T_2WI, and mild enhancement on the enhanced MRI. Some foci may further develop into abscesses mostly in quasi-circular shape which are localized and well-demarcated from peripheral tissues. T_1WI shows heterogeneous hypointense. The signal in abscess wall is higher than that in pus. T_2WI sequences show isointense or slightly hypointense in abscess wall and hyperintense in pus, homogeneously or heterogeneously. DWI sequences demonstrate hyperintense in vomica. The enhanced scan reveals enhancement in abscesses and no enhancement in internal necrotic area. Sinus formation is shown as a tubular or strip-shaped hypointense shadow on T_1WI and an isointense or hypointense shadow on T_2WI. Pus in sinus presents hyperintense on T_2WI. Abnormally irregular signals in bone marrow indicate invaded adjacent bones.
4. **Ultrasonography.** It mainly shows skin discontinuity, unclear soft tissue stratification, diffuse swelling, enhanced echo, ill-defined borders with peripheral tissues, blood flow signals observed locally, exudative inflammatory changes in the focus. Sinus formation may be found in some cases. The ultrasonography can guide surgery and efficacy evaluation.

Key Points of Diagnosis

1. **Epidemiological contact history.** Patients have a history of skin wounds and have been in contact with fishes or suspected water sources, or medical equipment without standard disinfection.
2. **Susceptible population.** NTM infection usually occurs in immunodeficient or immunocompromised population, such as patients with autoimmune diseases, organ transplantation, tumor, long-term use of antibiotics and glucocorticoid (GC), AIDS, and severe underlying diseases.
3. **Laboratory test.** Direct microscopy, bacterial culture, and biochemical test are used. Acid-fast bacilli are found by acid-fast staining [105], and mycobacteria are isolated or their DNA is detected through bacterial culture. Other tests are used for auxiliary diagnosis. For instance, a tuberculin test shows strong positive. A mycobacterium antibody test shows positive.
4. **Histopathology.** In addition to tuberculous granuloma dominated by epithelioid cells and lymphocytes, the infiltration of such inflammatory cells as neutrophils, plasma cells, and multinucleated giant cells occurs [106].
5. **Skin lesion.** Skin soft tissue infection is often found in dermal and subcutaneous adipose tissue and possibly in deep muscle tissue. Infection in extremities, especially hands, is common, which is manifested as papules, nodules, plaques, and local abscesses developing slowly. For nosocomially rapidly growing mycobacterium infection, skin lesions often occur in injection sites or surgical incision sites with swelling, pain, or ulceration.
6. **Imaging findings.** There is soft tissue swelling and blurred subcutaneous fat layer in lesion area. Effusion and exudative changes may be combined. The lesion area is not clearly demarcated from peripheral tissues. Soft tissue nodules can be seen locally and further develop into abscesses which are localized and shown as circular or quasi-circular shape and heterogeneous density (signal). The abscess walls show isointense or slightly hypointense on T_1WI and T_2WI and vomica shows hyperintense on T_2WI. The enhanced scan demonstrates enhancement in abscess wall and no enhancement in internal necrotic area. Sinus formation is shown as tubular or strip-shaped hypointense on T_1WI and isodensity or hypointense on T_2WI. Pus in sinus presents hyperintense on T_2WI. There may be multiple punctate calcifications.

Differential Diagnosis

1. **Ganglion cysts.** Ganglion cysts are mostly unilocular quasi-circular cystic lesions and often occur in dorsal wrist and dorsum of foot, common in young women. The lesion has a clear margin and watery density (signal) inside. T_1WI sequences show hypointense and T_2WI sequences show more hyperintense. The enhanced scan shows no enhancement.
2. **Gouty arthritis.** With acute attack, the disease presents with obvious soft tissue swelling in the early stage. The first MTP joint is mainly invaded, followed by such joints as ankles, hands, and knees. Nodular calcification (tophus) occurs in peripheral soft tissues. Its signal characteristics depend on the calcium salt content. The disease presents various signals. T_1WI shows hypointense and T_2WI shows hyperintense or homogeneous isointense. The focus shows homogeneous enhancement on the enhanced scan. Hyperuricemia is a typical characteristic in a laboratory test. Irregular or lobulated erosion and destruction is often found in bone cortex of lesion area.

3. **Tuberculous soft tissue inflammation.** The imaging findings are similar to those of NTM soft tissue infection. Tuberculous soft tissue abscesses are more common than abscesses combined with NTM. In the early stage of NTM infection, there also may be thickening of soft tissues, tuberculation, and combination of multiple calcification. The lesion may be differentiated with tuberculous soft tissue infection.

Status Quo and Progress of Research
NTM, as an environmental mycobacterium, is mostly found in immunodeficient or immunocompromised population. Its imaging findings are similar to those of tuberculosis and other diseases, lacking specificity, which easily leads to misdiagnosis and missed diagnosis. Therefore, it is very important to improve the knowledge of the disease and know well its clinical features and imaging findings. When the acid-fast bacilli are positive and normal anti-tuberculosis treatment is poorly effective, as well as imaging findings are mainly chronic inflammatory lesions, NTM infection should be highly suspected in clinical diagnosis. Subsequently, bacterial culture, biochemical identification, and molecular biological test are required for final confirmation.

8.5.2 Actinomycotic Infection

Overview
Actinomycetes are a genus of filamentous or catenulate, and branching prokaryotic microorganism including mycelium and spore. Actinomycetes are bacteria with branching mycelium between bacteria and fungi. Actinomycetes are widely spread in nature, mainly in soil, air, and water as a mycelium or spore. There are a wide range of actinomycetes. Pathogenic actinomycetes are mainly flora in actinomyces and nocardia. Actinomyces is normal flora in human and lives in oral cavity, upper respiratory tract, stomach, intestinal tract, and urogenital tract in human and animal. Actinomyces may cause endogenous infection in immunodeficient or immunocompromised individuals. Actinomyces israelii has high pathogenicity to human. Nocardia is saprophyte and widely exists in soil, causing exogenous infection.

Actinomycosis is a zoonotic infectious disease caused by actinomycetes with slow progress, subacute to chronic course, and no significant specificity. Actinomycosis often occurs in faciocervical region as well as thoracic and abdominal regions, so its clinical classification includes faciocervical, thoracic, abdominal, pelvic actinomycosis, and actinomycosis of central nervous system based on the route of infection and difference in organs involved. Faciocervical infection is the most common, manifested as faciocervical swelling, continuously new nodules, multiple abscesses and sinus formation. Symptoms of pulmonary actinomycosis are cough, hemoptysis, fever, chest pain, and other symptoms similar to tuberculosis. Abdominal infection usually results in palpable abdominal mass, abdominal wall adhesion, hematochezia, and difficult defecation. Spinal actinomycotic infection has mild early symptoms presenting neck and back pain, and the vertebral canal is invaded to compress spinal cord or nerve roots in the advanced stage. Primary dermoactinomycosis is often caused by trauma or insect bites, which causes subcutaneous nodules, nodule softening, ulceration, and sinus formation.

Actinomycetes are gram-positive bacteria, non-acid-fast filamentous bacteria without spore, capsule, and flagellum, with the best culture temperature of 37 °C. Small yellow granules visible to the naked eyes can be found in pus from the focus tissue and sinus in a patient, which are called sulfur granules. In addition, metabolites of actinomycetes have important biological functions and are closely related to human production and life [107]. In a laboratory test, the diagnosis can be confirmed by finding sulfur granules in pus, sputum, and tissue sections and characteristic chrysanthemum mycelium in radial arrangement under a microscope. Moreover, hematoxylin-eosin staining and microscopic examination of tissue sections may be performed to observe pathological features of sulfur granules for confirmed diagnosis. When necessary, actinomycetes may be isolated and cultured, and actinomyces and nocardia are further distinguished by acid-fast staining. In recent years, the heavy use of antibiotics, corticoid, and immunosuppressive agents has led to dysbacteriosis in body and sharp increase in incidence of superinfection caused by actinomycetes. It should be specially noted that a variety of specific antibodies can be detected in serum of patients with actinomycetes, but these antibodies do not have immunoprotective effect and the immunity of patients to actinomycetes mainly depends on cellular immunity [108].

Pathophysiology
Actinomycosis causes purulent inflammation of soft tissue. If there is no secondary infection, chronic granuloma changes are mostly presented, often accompanied by multiple sinus and fistula formation, as well as characteristic sulfur granules can be found in pus. Basic pathological changes of actinomycosis are multiple abscesses, sinus formation, granulation tissue hyperplasia, and fibrous changes. In the early focus, multiple neutrophils can be seen around the actinomycetes. The lesion is localized. Multiple abscesses in different size are formed, and some of the abscesses fuse together to form a purulent mass. Abscesses connect with each other and form intricate sinuses from which pus may be discharged. Small yellow or yellowish white granules with diameters of several millimeters can be found in the pus, namely sulfur granules. Filamentous bacilli masses are seen microscopically in radial arrangement and the mycelium end

is expanded in rod-like appearance, resembling chrysanthemum. Neutrophils and monocytes can be observed around the masses. The infection may spread to deep muscle tissue. Abscesses are surrounded by granulation tissue and fibrous tissue and fibrosis of some tissues may form scars. A large number of foamy macrophages and epithelioid cells can be observed to accumulate in some tissues, resembling tuberculous granuloma [111].

Imaging Findings

1. **X-ray** Main findings include swelling and increased density in local soft tissue, blurred fat space and intermuscular space, and clear margin; peripheral muscles are compressed and displaced when an abscess forms; the irregularly slightly low-density shadow is seen in the increased density zone; swelling gives a sense of fluctuation in local touching; the slightly low-density tubular shadow connecting with the body surface can be seen in sinus formation; pus and yellow granules flowed out inside.
2. **CT** mainly shows swelling of soft tissue in the lesion area, thickened and blurred subcutaneous fat space, increased density and disordered structure, which are manifested as grid-like shadows and cord-like shadows, subcutaneous tissue in honeycomb changes, ill-defined borders with peripheral tissues, and mild enhancement on the enhanced scan. The focus may further develop into soft tissue nodules and small multiple abscesses that can fuse with each other, with well-defined borders. A low-density necrotic area can be seen in the lesion center, with uniform thickness of abscess walls. The enhanced scan shows obvious ring enhancement in abscess walls and no enhancement in central necrotic area. Abscesses may spread to deep intermuscular space to form deep multiple abscesses. Soft tissue nodules may be ruptured to form sinuses, shown as low-density pipe-like structure connecting with the body surface, from which pus and yellow granules flow out. Affected tissues indicate heterogeneous enhancement on the enhanced scan.
3. **MRI.** Main findings include diffuse thickening of soft tissue in the lesion area presenting inflammatory exudation and edema changes, and unclear soft tissue stratification. The soft tissue is ill-defined from peripheral tissues. The lesion shows localized strip-shaped hypointense on T_1WI and hyperintense on T_2WI in adipose tissue with hyperintense, presenting grid-like and cellular changes. The enhanced scan shows mild enhancement. The hypointense on T_1WI and hyperintense on T_2WI are present between subcutaneous tissue and muscle when effusion is combined with the lesion. The inflammation is localized or further progresses to form soft tissue nodules or abscesses. The lesions are well-demarcated from peripheral tissues. T_1WI sequences show heterogeneous hypointense. The signal in abscess wall is higher than that in pus. T_2WI sequences show isointense or slightly hypointense in abscess wall and hyperintense in pus. The enhanced scan presents ring enhancement in abscess wall and no enhancement in central necrotic area. Pus shows significant hyperintense on DWI. Abscesses may form deep multiple abscesses along joint space, intermuscular space or intervertebral space. Abscesses protrude into the vertebral canal to form intraspinal epidural abscesses, shown as fusiform or strip-like abnormal signals. The dural sac and adjacent nerve roots may be compressed at different degrees. The infection is protracted and sinus is formed locally, manifested as strip-like and tubular soft tissue signal foci. Signals in lumen are heterogeneous due to purulent secretion inside. MRI can clearly demonstrate the formation direction and scope of deep multiple abscesses.
4. **Ultrasonography** Main findings include diffuse swelling, enhanced echo, and ill-defined borders with peripheral tissues in soft tissue, and blood flow signals and exudative inflammatory changes observed locally. The hyperplasia of blood vessels is a non-specific manifestation of local inflammation. The echo of infectious exudate is stronger than that of normal exudate. The combination with effusion and empyema is presented with blurred borders or circumscribed sonolucent area with (anechoic) fluid. Ultrasound can guide puncture and treatment.

Key Points of Diagnosis

1. **Susceptible population.** Actinomyces is a normal flora in human and belongs to opportunistic pathogens, which usually occurs in immunodeficient or immunocompromised population with dysbacteriosis, such as patients with long-term use of antibiotics, autoimmune diseases, organ transplantation, tumor, AIDS, and severe underlying diseases.
2. **Actinomycetes.** Actinomycetes are gram-positive. Finding sulfur granules in pus, sputum, and tissue sections is used as specific diagnosis. Characteristic chrysanthemum mycelium in radial arrangement is seen under microscopy. The main diagnosis basis is to find actinomycetes masses in bacterial isolation and culture or pathological sections.
3. **Clinical manifestation** Actinomycosis is a purulent inflammation of soft tissue which often occurs in faciocervical region. Most patients with actinomycosis have a history of stomatitis, tooth extraction, or mandible fracture. Primary dermoactinomycosis is manifested as subcutaneous nodules, abscesses, sinus or fistula formation, sulfur granules found in pus.

4. **Imaging findings.** Findings include swelling of soft tissue observed, ill-defined borders in the lesion area, thickened subcutaneous fat and heterogeneous density (signal) presenting honeycomb and reticular changes. Soft tissue nodules and abscesses are formed in the lesion area, often accompanied by sinuses connecting with the body surface which are presented as strip or tubular soft-tissue signal shadows. Signals are heterogeneous in lumen. Pus shows hyperintense on T_2WI sequences, and DWI also shows obvious hyperintense. The enhanced scan reveals marked enhancement in abscess wall and lumen wall, and no enhancement in central necrotic area. MRI shows the formation direction of deep multiple abscesses and sinus course and range.

Differential Diagnosis

1. **Pyogenic soft tissue inflammation.** Pathogens are mostly caused by Staphylococcus aureus and hemolytic streptococcus. Its manifestations are acute onset, accompanied by chill, fever, headache, and other symptoms, as well as increased neutrophils. The lesion is extensive, and rapidly progresses and expands to the periphery. There is no distinct border between red skin and normal peripheral skin tissue. The early imaging finding is diffuse swelling in local soft tissue with fuzzy border, possibly accompanied by enlargement of local lymph nodes. The lesion presents marked enhancement on the enhanced scan. The swelling may be associated with pneumatosis and effusion and develop into abscesses. Pneumatosis presents hypointense change on T_1WI and T_2WI. Actinomycosis is an opportunistic pathogen, rarely associated with pneumatosis change. The lesion is relatively localized, mostly with the formation of sinus from which typical sulfur granules flow out. The differential diagnosis of the two diseases can be further confirmed through bacteria culture.
2. **Tuberculous soft tissue inflammation** Most of the patients have a relevant medical history such as pulmonary tuberculosis and intestinal tuberculosis and present tuberculosis poisoning symptoms including fatigue, night sweats, and afternoon low-grade fever. The tuberculin test shows positive and erythrocyte sedimentation rate is elevated. The disease adjacent to the osteoarticular area should be differentiated with bone tuberculosis with abscess. Bone destruction of tuberculosis of bone and joint presents saltatory osteoclast migration in which sequestrum and calcification focus can be found. The paravertebral abscess is psychrapostema and well-demarcated from peripheral tissues, with thin and smooth wall. Sequestrum and calcification can be seen in such an abscess. Microscopic examination and bacterial culture of purulent fluid can help to clearly differentiate both diseases.

Status Quo and Progress of Research

DWI, as functional imaging, can detect early lesions. DWI is of great value in diagnosis and differentiation of inflammatory mass, abscess, and tumorous lesion based on different ADC values.

Actinomycetes are opportunistic pathogens and a group of prokaryotic microorganisms between bacteria and fungi. Actinomycosis is insidious in onset. Its clinical manifestations have no obvious specificity and mainly include nodules of subcutaneous soft tissue, abscesses, and sinus formation, as well as sulfur granules seen in pus. Therefore, clinicians need to improve their knowledge on the disease to avoid missed diagnosis and misdiagnosis. Imaging cannot be used as the main basis for the diagnosis of actinomycosis, but the typical signs of soft tissue infection can be used as the basis for its direct diagnosis. The confirmed diagnosis of actinomycosis depends on isolation and culture of the pathogen.

References

1. Jaswal A, Jana AK, Sikder B, et al. Simultaneous complete branchial and thyroglossal fistula a rare presentation. Indian J Otolaryngol Head Neck Surg. 2008;60(1):94–6.
2. Lee CS. Congenital dermal sinuses: an clinical analysis of 20 cases. J Korean Neurosurg Soc. 2005;37(1):29–33.
3. Wang Y, Gang K, Huafa Q, et al. Treatment of superficial sinus and fistula by external application of traditional. Chin Med. 2011;20(6):41–3.
4. Ren W, Zhi K, Zhao L, et al. Presentations and management of thyroglossal duct cyst in children versus adults: a review of 106 cases. Oral Surg Oral Med Oral Pathol Oral Radiol Endod. 2011;111(2):51–6.
5. Ranga U, Aiyappan SK, Veeraiyan S. Computed tomography fistulography demonstrating thyroglossal fistula: a case report. Oral Surg Oral Med Oral Pathol Oral Radiol. 2012;114(3):48–50.
6. Limin Z, Xiaoyan L. One case of congenital midline cervical cleft. Chinese Archives of Otolaryngol-Head and Neck Surg. 2012;19(4):224.
7. Thottam PJ, Bathula SS, Poulik JM, et al. Complete second branchial cleft anomaly presenting as a fistula and a tonsillar cyst: an interesting congenital anomaly. Ear Nose Throat J. 2014;93(10/11):466–8.
8. Bajaj Y, Ifeacho S, Tweedie D, et al. Brachial anomalies in children. Int J Pediatr Otorhinolaryngol. 2011;75(9):1020–3.
9. Hu M. Application of high-frequency ultrasonography in the diagnosis of branchial cysts and branchial fistulas in children. China Med Device Information. 2018;24(22):101–3.
10. Bo Z, Xiao Y, Yuxin J, et al. Sonographic characteristics of branchial cysts and branchial fistulas. Medical Journal of Peking Union Medical College Hospital. 2014;5(3):312–7.
11. Thomas B, Shroff M, Forte V, et al. Revisiting imaging features and the embryologic basis of third and fourth branchial anomalies. AJNR Am J Neuroradiol. 2010;31(4):755–60.
12. Chauhan NS, Sharma YP, Bhagra T, et al. Branchial fistula arising from pyriform fossa: CT diagnosis of a case and discussion of radiological features. Clin Imaging. 2012;36(5):591–4.
13. Huanyu X, Hanjun T, Huafa Q, et al. Treatment of 103 cases of complex sinus and fistula by removing erosion and generating muscle. Shanghai J Traditional Chinese Med. 2005;39(4):34–6.

14. Odom RB, James WD, Berger TG. Andrews' diseases of the skin (9th edition). Trans. Xu Shi et al. Beijing: Science Press; 2004.
15. Yuanjun L, Xiaoming L. Clinical research Progress of panniculitis. J Military Surgeonin in Southwest China. 2012;14(1):111–3.
16. Badri T, Kenani N, Benmously R, et al. Isolated genital annular lichen planus. Acta Dermatovenerol Alp Pannonica Adriat. 2011;20(1):31–3.
17. Kuboi T, Kusaka T, Okazaki K, et al. Subcutaneous fat necrosis after selective head cooling in an infant. Pediatr Int. 2013;55(2):23–4.
18. Kralj D, Ceroved M, Anic B. Etiology of erythema nodosum in rheumatology outpatient clinic. Lijec Vjesn. 2011;133(12):370–6.
19. Kisacik B, Onat AM, Pelilivan Y. Multiclinical experiences in erythema nodosum: rheumatology clinics versus dermatology and infection disease clinics. Rheumatol Int. 2013;33(2):315–8.
20. Mert A, Ozaras R, Tabak F, et al. Primary tuberculosis cases presenting with erythema nodosum. J Dermatol. 2004;31(1):66–8.
21. Bian Z. China clinical dermatology (3rd). Nanjing: Jiangsu Science and Technology Press; 2010.
22. Xufeng X, Lixin L. Clinicopathological features of 28 cases of SPTCL. China Med Pharmacy. 2013;3(5):141–2.
23. Risulo M, Rubegni P, Sbano P, et al. Subcutaneous panniculitis lymphoma: erythema nodosum-like. Clin Lymphoma Myeloma. 2006;7(6):239–41.
24. Aldape MJ, Bryant AE, Stevens DL. Clostridium sordellii infection: epidemiology, clinical findings, and current perspectives on diagnosis and treatment. Clin Infect Dis. 2006;43(6):1436–46.
25. Hui Z, Lingyan C, Wang F, et al. Etiological analysis of severe orbital cellulitis in children. J Clin Ophthalmol. 2013;21(3):281–3.
26. Wang Y, Ming Z, Ma S. Application value of MRI in the diagnosis of orbital cellulitis. J Modern Med Imaging. 2015;24(3):313–6.
27. Yulin L. Pathology. 9th ed. Beijing: People's Health Publishing House; 2018.
28. Lope LA, Hutcheson KA, Khademian ZP. Magnetic resonance imaging in the analysis of pediatric orbital tumors: utility of diffusion- weighted imaging. J AAPOS. 2010;14(3):257–62.
29. Norrby-Teglund A, Muller MP, McGeer A, et al. Successful management of severe group a streptococcal soft tissue infections using an aggressive medical regimen including intravenous polyspecific immunoglobulin together with a conservative surgical approach Scand. Infect Dis. 2005;37(8):166–72.
30. Lemke AJ, Kazi I, Felix R, et al. Magnetic resonance imaging of orbital tumors. Eur Radiol. 2006;16(10):2207–19.
31. Fischer M, Bhatnagar J, Guarner J, et al. Fatal toxic shock syndrome associated with Clostridium sordellii after medical abortion. N Engl Med. 2005;35(3):2352–60.
32. Lee MC, Rios AM, Aten MF, et al. Management and outcome of children with skin and soft tissue abscesses caused by community-acquired methicillin-resistant Staphylococcus aureus. Pediatr Infect Dis. 2004;23(5):123–7.
33. Stevens DL, Bisno AL, Chambers HF, et al. Practice guidelines for the diagnosis and management of skin and soft-tissue infections. Clin Infect Dis. 2005;41(6):1373–406.
34. Zhijie H. Research progress in diagnosis and treatment of necrotizing fasciitis. Shijiazhuang: Hebei Medical University; 2018.
35. Karkas A, Chahine K, Schmerber S, et al. Optimal treatment of cervical necrotizing fasciitis associated with descending necrotizing mediastinitis. Br J Surg. 2010;97(4):609–15.
36. Luo N, Lihui Z. Research progress of necrotizing fasciitis with diabetes mellitus. Med Recapitulate. 2017;23(24):4921–5.
37. Uluğ M, Gedik E, Girgin S, et al. The evaluation of microbiology and Fournier's gangrene severity index in 27 patients. Int J Infect Dis. 2009;13(6):424–30.
38. Hua X, Jinqing L. Clinical and imaging findings of necrotizing fasciitis. J Clin Radiol. 2002;21(5):400–2.
39. Kuncir EJ, Tillou A, St Hill CR, et al. Necrotizing soft-tissue infections. Emerg Med Clin North Am. 2003;21(4):1075–87.
40. Yahav D. Monomicrobial necrotizing fasciitis in a single center: the emergence of gram-negative bacteria as a common pathogen. Int J Infect Dis. 2014;28(1):13–6.
41. Lancerotto L, Tocco I, Salmaso R, et al. Necrotizing fasciitis: classification, diagnosis, and management. J Trauma Acute Care Surg. 2012;72(3):560–6.
42. Schulze M, Overkamp D, Joanoviciu S, et al. CT findings of necrotizing fasciitis. Radiological Practice. 2008;23(11):1290–1.
43. Goh T, Goh LG, Ang CH, et al. Early diagnosis of necrotizing fasciitis. Br J Surg. 2013;101(1):119–25.
44. Yang X, Feng D, Xianbao L, et al. 153 cases of neonatal infectious gangrene of subcutaneous tissue. J Clin Pediatric Surg. 2007;6(5):41–2.
45. Xueping Z. Nursing care of one case of neonatal infectious gangrene of subcutaneous tissue. Chinese General Practice Nursing. 2018;16(20):2550–1.
46. Quirke M, Saunders J, O'Sullivan R, et al. A pilot cross sectional study of patients presenting with cellulitis to emergency departments. Ir Med J. 2014;107(10):316–8.
47. Xiaomei S, Hongmao Y, Xiaoshan Q. Practice of neonatology. 4th ed. Beijing: People's Health Publishing House; 2011.
48. Jinzhe Z, Pan S, Chengru H. Practical pediatric surgery. Beijing: People's Health Publishing House; 2005.
49. Chira S, Miller LG. Staphylococcus aureus is the most common identified cause of cellulitis: a systematic review. Epidemiol Infect. 2010;138(3):313–7.
50. Yulan Y. Two cases of neonatal infectious gangrene of subcutaneous tissue. Chinese J Neonatol. 2002;17(4):176–7.
51. Kulshrestha S, Kulshrestha M. Ischaemic gangrene of the scalp in the neonate. BJOG. 2005;112(5):1334–5.
52. Shulin S, Aifang L. Clinical efficacy evaluation of hyperbaric oxygen in the treatment of neonatal infectious gangrene of subcutaneous tissue. Heilongjiang Med Jl. 2005;18(6):460–1.
53. Jianhua S, Xuehong Z, Zhenchao S. Diagnosis and treatment of neonatal infectious gangrene of subcutaneous tissue. Ningxia Med J. 2009;31(1):81–2.
54. Dong M, Xiaojun Z. Neonatal acute necrotizing fasciitis. Chinese Pediatric Emergency Med. 2005;12(2):147–8.
55. Köhler JR, Casadevall A, Perfect J. The spectrum of fungi that infects humans. Cold Spring Harb Perspect Med. 2015;5(1):192–7.
56. Enoch DA, Ludlam HA, Brown NM. Invasive fungal infection: a review of epidemiology and management options. J Med Microbiol. 2006;55(7):809–18.
57. Fan L, Xu Z. Medical Microbiology. 9th ed. Beijing: People's Medical Publishing House; 2018.
58. Tribble DR, Rodriguez CJ. Invasive fungal wound infection associated with combat. Chur Fungal Infect Rep. 2014;8(4):277–86.
59. Benedict K, Park BJ. Invasive fungal infections after natural disasters. Emerg Infect Dis. 2014;20(3):349–55.
60. Park YW, Kim DY, Yoon SY, et al. "Clues" for the histological diagnosis of tinea: how reliable are they? Ann Dermatol. 2014;26(2):286–8.
61. Schram AM, Kim B, Carlos C, et al. Primary cutaneous Candida tropicalis infection in a patient with B-cell lymphoma. Cutis. 2014;93(3):204–6.
62. Buchanan PJ, Mast BA, Lottenberg L, et al. Candida albicans necrotizing soft tissue infection: a case report and literature review of fungal necrotizing soft tissue infections. Ann Plast Surg. 2013;70(6):739–41.
63. Ping C, Yabin Z, Dongming L. Retrospective analysis of deep skin and soft tissue infections caused by candida. Chinese J Mycol. 2018;13(4):217–22.
64. Demiraslan H, Alabay S, Kilic AU, et al. Cutaneous candidiasis caused by Candida glabrata in a HIV/AIDS patient. Int J STD AIDS. 2013;24(9):753–4.
65. Wang D. Medical mycology - a guide to laboratory testing. Beijing: People's Medical Publishing House; 2005.

66. Guo WJ. Imaging diagnostic pathology. Xi'an: Fourth Military Medical University Press; 2007.
67. Gamaletsou MN, Rammaert B, Bueno MA, et al. Aspergillus osteomyelitis: epidemiology, clinical manifestations, management and outcome. J Infect. 2014;68(5):478–93.
68. Gamaletsou MN, Kontoyiannis DP, Sipsas NV, et al. Candida osteomyelitis: anus −207 cases of children and adults (1970-2011). Clin Infect Dis. 2012;55(10):1338–51.
69. Cheng C, Yong Z, Yang C, et al. MRI features and diagnostic value of spinal tuberculosis. Magn Reson Imaging. 2016;7(5):371–5.
70. Bureau of Disease Prevention and Control, Ministry of Health. Brucellosis Control Manual. Beijing: Ministry of Health, 2008.
71. Hongjun L. Radiology of infectious diseases. Beijing: People's Medical Publishing House; 2014.
72. Nielsen K, Yu WL. Serological diagnosis of brucellosis. Prilozi. 2010;31(1):65–89.
73. Christopher S, Umapathy BL, Ravikumar KL. Brucellosis: review on the recent trends in pathogenicity and laboratory diagnosis. Lab Physicians. 2010;2(2):55–60.
74. Oztekin O, Calli C, Adibelli Z, et al. Brucellar spondylodiscitis: magnetic resonance imaging features with conventional sequences and diffusion-weighted imaging. Radiol Med. 2010;115(5):794–803.
75. Pengfei Z, Gao Y, Guangming N. Progress in magnetic resonance imaging of brucellar spondylitis. Magn Reson Imaging. 2016;7(8):625–9.
76. Hadush A, Pal M. Brucellosis-an infectious re-emerging bacterial zoonosis of global importance. IJLR. 2013;3(1):28–34.
77. Bozgeyik Z, Aglamis S, Bozdag PG, et al. Magnetic resonance imaging findings of musculoskeletal brucellosis. Clin Imaging. 2014;38(5):719–23.
78. Hao PF, Gao Y, Niu GM. The research progress of MR diagnosis of spondylitis caused by brulles infection Chin. Magn Reson Imaging. 2016;7(8):625–9.
79. Niu H, Niu GM. Quantitative dynamic contrast-enhanced MRI in spinal tumor. Trans Med. 2015;4(5):302–5.
80. Chelli Bouaziz M, Ladeb MF, Chakroun M, et al. Spinal brucellosis: a review. Skelet Radiol. 2008;37:785–90.
81. Koubaa M, Maaloul I, Marrakchi C, et al. Spinal brucellosis in south of Tunisia: review of 32 cases. Spine J. 2014;14(8):1538–44.
82. Sourbron SP, Buckley DL. Classic models for dynamic contrast enhanced MRI. NMR Biomed. 2013;26(8):1004–27.
83. Ak Ç, Aypak A, Aypak C. Comparative analysis of tuberculous and brucellar spondylodiscitis. Trop Dr. 2011;41(3):172–4.
84. Choi HS, Kim AH, Ahn SS, et al. Glioma grading capability: comparisons among parameters from dynamic contrast-enhanced MRI and ADC value on DWI. Korean Radiol. 2013;14(3):487–92.
85. Pengfei Q, Guangming N. The value of quantitative analysis by dynamic contrast-enhanced magnetic resonance in staging Brucellar spondylitis. Magn Reson Imaging. 2017;8(12):908–11.
86. Ioannou S, Chatziioannou S, Pneumaticos SG, et al. Fluorine-18 fluoro-2-deoxy-D-glucose positron emission tomography, computed tomography scan contributes to the diagnosis and management of brucellar spondylodiskitis. BMC Infect Dis. 2017;7(13):73–6.
87. Arslan F, Karagoz E, Arslan BY, et al. Spinal brucellosis diagnosed with positron emission tomography combined with computed tomography (PET/CT). Spine J. 2016;16(6):381–2.
88. Kern P. Menezes da Silva a, Akhan O, et al. the echinococcoses: diagnosis, clinical management and burden of disease. Adv Parasitol. 2017;96(20):259–61.
89. Pedrosa I, Saíz A, Arrazola J, et al. Hydatid disease: radiologic and pathologic features and complications. Radiographics. 2000;20(3):795–817.
90. Changchun Q, Guoqiang H. Cystic hydatid disease in left femoral muscles: report of one case. Chinese J Practical Surg. 2011;31(11):1063–4.
91. Dapeng L, Xie Z, Rui Z, et al. Diagnosis and treatment of bone hydatid disease. Chinese J Orthopaedics. 2004;24(7):403–7.
92. Christopher P, Cannon MD, Scott D, et al. Soft tissue echinococcosis. CORR. 2001;11(4):186–91.
93. Dazhong S. New progress in treatment of hydatid disease. Parasitic Dis Foreign Med Sci. 2001;28(5):230–2.
94. Junhua L. CT findings of hydatid disease in rare locations of human. J Med Imaging. 2011;21(1):69–71.
95. Abulizi A, Haliya B. Imaging of bone hydatid disease. Chinese Computed Med Imaging. 2009;15(4).354–7.
96. Karaoglanoglu N, Gorguner M, Eroglu A. Hydatid disease of rib. Rev Mal Respir. 2001;71(1):372–3.
97. Liping F. Ultrasonographic features of hepatic hydatid disease and their diagnostic values. Chinese J Med Imaging. 2009;17(1):69–71.
98. Kayaalp C, Dirican A, Aydin C. Primary subcutaneous hydatid cyst: review of 22 cases. Int J Surg. 2011;21(9):117–9.
99. Saiman L. The mycobacteriology of non-tuberculous mycobacteria. Paediatr Respir Rev. 2004;56(5):221–3.
100. Smith MB, Schnadig VJ, Boyars mc, et al. clinical and pathologic features of mycobacterium fortuitum infections. An emerging pathogen in patients with AIDS. Am J Clin Pathol. 2001;116(3):225–32.
101. Wentworth AB, Drage LA, Wengenack NL, et al. Increased incidence of cutaneous nontuberculous mycobacterial infection, 1980 to 2009: a population-based study. Mayo Clin Proc. 2013;88(1):38–45.
102. Zi'an G. Bases and clinics of atypical mycobacteria. Tianjin: Tianjin Science and Technology Press; 1998.
103. Yuanyuan X, Libing F, Lei X, et al. One case of nontuberculous mycobacterial infection in children's skin. The Chinese J Dermatovenereol. 2012;26(9):833–4.
104. Zautner AE, Schmitz S, Aepinus C, et al. Nontuberculous mycobacterial lung disease prevalence at four integrated health care delivery systems. Am J Respir Crit Care Med. 2010;182(7):970–6.
105. Xun Z, He X, Hui L. Chronic skin ulcer caused by nontuberculous mycobacterial infection. J Clin Dermatol. 2007;36(8):508–10.
106. Zautner AE, Schmitz S, Aepinus C, et al. Subcutaneous fistulae in a patient with femoral hypoplasia due to actinomyces europaeus and actinomyces turicensis. Infection. 2009;37(3):289–91.
107. Zhu L, Guozhi Z. Lumbar soft tissue actinomycosis: one case and literature review. Chinese General Practice. 2014;17(7):844–5.
108. Xinqi F, Changlong B, Song L, et al. Actinomycetic epidural abscess: one case and literature review. J Int Neurol Neurosurg. 2018;45(5):492–4.
109. Georgakopoulos CD, Eliopoulou MI, Stasinos S, et al. Periorbital and orbital cellulitis: a 10 year review of hospitalized children. Eur J Ophthalmol. 2010;20(6):1066–72.

9 Lesions of Bones and Joints Associated with Rheumatism

Jun Zhou, Fengzhe Wang, Yuan Qu, He Sun, and Zhen Liu

9.1 Rheumatoid Arthritis

Jun Zhou and Fengzhe Wang

Overview

Rheumatoid arthritis (RA) is a common systemic immune disease mainly characterized by symmetrical and chronic inflammation of peripheral polyarticular synovium. The lesion first involves joint synovium followed by articular cartilage, subchondral bone, tendon and ligament, mostly affecting small joints of hands and feet. The involvement distribution is often symmetrical. The lesion gradually invades multiple joints throughout the body, eventually leading to joint deformity and dysfunction. As RA is a systemic disease, it can also have many extra-articular manifestations, such as fever, fatigue, rheumatoid nodules, lung involvement, pericarditis, peripheral neuropathy, vasculitis, and blood system involvement. RA was originally described as a type of gout. In 1776, Scheele, a Swedish chemist, isolated uric acid from the renal calculus of a gouty patient, clearly distinguishing RA from gout. In 1858, Gaarod first proposed the name of RA. In the early twentieth century, scientists discovered the rheumatoid factor (RF) in basic research. In 1966, American College of Rheumatology (ACR) officially announced the names of rheumatoid arthritis (RA) and ankylosing spondylitis (AS). In 1987, ACR put forward recognized RA classification criteria. In 2010, ACR and European League Against Rheumatism (EULAR) jointly revised the RA classification criteria into new ones. Over the past 20 years, a number of basic and clinical studies have changed the diagnosis and treatment models for RA in modern medicine. Serum anti-cyclic citrullinated peptide (anti-CCP) antibodies are deemed as biomarkers with diagnostic and prognostic value. The development of magnetic resonance imaging techniques allows the early detection of degree and number of joint destruction caused by RA. The application of highly targeted biological agents can benefit patients in the early stage and verify the effect of relevant genes and molecular pathways on pathogenesis [1].

RA can occur at all ages, more common at 25 ~ 55 years of age, with an increasing incidence. The incidence is in the platform stage at 55 ~ 75 years of age and then decreases with the age. The overall prevalence of RA is 0.3% ~ 1%. The prevalence varies by territory and race. The prevalence of RA in mainland China is somewhat lower (0.42%) while it is higher in Europe and America. As with many autoimmune diseases, women are more likely to develop RA than men, with a men-to-women ratio of 1 to (2 ~ 4) while the ratio of women with RA to men with RA is even up to 8 to 1 in some African and Latin American countries.

RA is an autoimmune disease with abnormal cellular immunity. At present, the etiology and pathogenesis are not completely clear. Many studies suggest that pathogen infection, genetic factors, environmental factors, and endocrine dyscrasia are related to its onset to certain degree, and any of these factors alone is insufficient to cause the disease. It is currently considered that the following factors are associated with RA: (1) Genes play an important role in susceptibility to RA and severity of disease, and especially, genes encoding 5 amino acid sequences in the hypervariable region (HVR) of human leukocyte antigen (HLA)-DR4 are the most important genetic factors related to RA. Genome-wide association study (GWAS) demonstrates that genes encoding protein tyrosine phosphatase-22 (PTPN22), peptidyl arginine deiminase type IV (PADI4) and many cytokines are associated with the onset

J. Zhou (✉)
Department of Radiology, The Fourth People's Hospital of Shenyang, Shenyang, Liaoning, China
e-mail: zjzj99991000@163.com

F. Wang · Y. Qu
Department of Radiology, The Fourth People's Hospital of Shenyang, Shenyang, Liaoning, China

H. Sun
Department of Radiology, The Fourth Affiliated Hospital of China Medical University, Shenyang, Liaoning, China

Z. Liu
Department of Radiology, Shengjing Hospital of China Medical University, Shenyang, Liaoning, China

H. Li et al. (eds.), *Radiology of Infectious and Inflammatory Diseases - Volume 5*,
https://doi.org/10.1007/978-981-16-5003-1_9

of RA. The polymorphism of such genes suggests genetic factors relating to RA are very complex. (2) Hormone milieu has an important effect on cells involved with the onset of RA. Due to high prevalence in women, numerous theories have attempted to explain the role of estrogens in onset of RA that estrogens can stimulate the secretion of a cytokine (TNF-α), very important in pathogenesis of RA. But the mechanism for women's susceptibility to RA is still not defined. In addition, tobacco environment is considered as an influential factor in the incidence of RA and may be related to the natural immune system activating the respiratory tract and PADI. The production of anti-CCP antibodies in the bronchi leads to repeated activation of natural immune system, further possibly causing autoimmune response and occurrence of RA. (3) Various pathogens are associated with the onset of RA, including viruses, retroviruses, and mycoplasma. For example, Epstein-Barr virus (EBV) has been detected in synovial fluid and synovial cells in patients with RA. Serological evidence of prodromic infection with mycoplasma and parvovirus B19 can also be found. However, these associations are mostly used as direct evidence. The evidence for the presence of a specific pathogen causing RA has not been discovered. (4) A close relationship between autoantibodies like rheumatoid factors (RFs) and anti-CCP antibodies and RA confirms the involvement of autoimmune responses in the onset of disease. These autoantibodies contribute to synovial inflammation through several mechanisms including activation of complement system [2].

The condition and natural course of RA are complex and see significant individual differences. They are affected by the age of onset, sex, genotype, disease phenotype, comorbidity, and other factors. These factors enable RA to become a truly heterogeneous disease. The vast majority of patients (55% ~ 65%) show chronic insidious onset and persistent and progressive course. The disease activity goes up and down with time. A minority of patients present with intermittent and fulminant arthritis, accompanied by remission. Very few patients with RA present with inexorably acute, progressive, and destructive arthritis. Clinical manifestations of RA include prodromata, such as fatigue, anorexia, weight loss, musculoskeletal pain, and other non-specific manifestations. Joint lesions are the early manifestations of the disease. The more frequently affected joints are metacarpophalangeal (MCP), proximal interphalangeal (PIP), and wrist joints. Monoarticular pain or stiffness lasts for weeks or months, and then involves more joints of the body. Overall, small joints present with symptoms followed by large joints, and symptoms are more significant in small joints than in large joints. RA is mostly symmetrical and non-wandering and characterized by swelling, pain, stiffness, and limitation of motion during movement and morning stiffness. Morning stiffness (stiffness and tightness occur at the joints after waking up in the morning, and improve after activity) lasts for at least 30 ~ 45 min. Its advanced manifestations are joint deformity, stiffness, subluxation, atrophy and spasm of periarticular muscles, and dysfunction. For instance, PIP joint hyperextension with distal interphalangeal (DIP) joint flexion (swan-neck deformity), PIP joint flexion with DIP joint hyperextension (boutonniere deformity), and subluxation of first MCP joint with thumb interphalangeal (IP) joint hyperextension (Z-deformity) are caused by destruction of periarticular tendon, ligament, and soft tissue. Unlike spondyloarthropathy, RA rarely involves thoracic vertebra and lumbar vertebra, but importance should be attached to the involvement in atlanto-axial joints. Progressive instability or subluxation of atlanto-axial joints may lead to compressive myelopathy and nerve injury. In addition to joint symptoms, RA can also cause rheumatoid nodules and other extra-articular lesions in heart, lungs, kidneys, peripheral nerves, and eyes. Subcutaneous nodules can be found in 30% ~ 40% of RA patients, which are most common in the area around the elbow joint and hard in texture without tenderness. Pleural disease is the most common pulmonary manifestation of RA and may cause chest pain, dyspnea, pleural friction rub, and pleural effusion. Heart involvement is most common in pericarditis and cardiomyopathy. RA also presents with various inflammatory and non-inflammatory vasculopathy and sensory and motor neuropathy.

Laboratory abnormalities in RA are not specific, but they can provide important evidence for diagnosis of RA. RA patients in the active stage have moderate positive pigment or hypopigmented positive cell anemia, and normal or increased leukocyte count. The level of serum immunoglobulin including IgG, IgM, and IgA may rise at different degrees, and the serum complement level in most patients is normal or increased. A high level of RF is found in 60% ~ 80% of RA patients. Positive RF can be also found in patients with other connective tissue diseases, chronic infection (hepatitis, tuberculosis, etc.), and sicca syndrome, and 1% ~ 5% of healthy population. Anti-CCP antibody has nearly 98% of specificity and about 70% of sensitivity in diagnosis of RA. Anti-CCP antibody is a relatively specific indicator for diagnosis of early RA and of certain prognostic significance. Patients with positive anti-CCP antibodies are often predicted to have a poor prognosis. The erythrocyte sedimentation rate and C-reactive protein are considered as non-specific indicators of RA and can be used to determine RA activities and degree of remission. In the active stage, the erythrocyte sedimentation rate and C-reactive protein (CRP) are increased.

Pathophysiology

RA mainly affects synovial tissues, articular cartilage, and subchondral bone. Normally, synovial membrane is a thin layer of connective tissue. Most articular surfaces are covered by synovial membranes, so are surfaces of tendinous sheath and bursa. A synovial membrane in a joint is attached on the surface of bone and cartilage, adjacent to the bone and at the edge of articular cartilage. A synovial membrane mainly consists of two types of cells: type A synovial cell (from macrophages) and type B synovial cell (from fibroblasts). The latter is more and an important component in the synthesis of collagen, fibronectin, laminin, and synovial matrix. The synovial membrane has many blood vessels and can secrete synovial fluid, of which main components include hyaluronic acid and lubricin, lubricating cartilages on joint surface.

The pathological characteristic of early RA is acute synovitis, manifested as synovial hyperemia, edema, thickening, and increased cell permeability. Vast capillary hyperplasia and increased vascular permeability allow the serous exudate to penetrate through synovial matrix into articular cavity where a large amount of yellowish-green synovial fluid is present. The periarticular soft tissue significantly swells. Fibrin deposition occurs on synovial surface. The synovial membrane is markedly thickened, especially at the margin of articular cartilage. Continuous hyperplasia may lead to the formation of a large, tumor-like synovial structure with many blood vessels.

After acute inflammation, the hypertrophic synovial membrane is resolved and exudate is gradually absorbed. The condition enters a chronic stage. Synovial cells are proliferated actively and vast granulation tissue hyperplasia and pannus occur. New capillaries and hyperplasia and organization of fibrous connective tissues cause irregularly thickened synovial membrane and formation of many villous protuberances into the articular cavity. Hyperplastic granulation tissue and pannus spread to the margin of cartilage, forming stratum lucidum with different thickness on the surface of articular cartilage. It results in enzymatic destruction of cartilage and interferes with normal cartilage metabolism, causing cartilage deformation and destruction.

The articular cartilage destruction first occurs at the margin of cartilage. With the progression of the lesion, pannus gradually covers the surface of articular cartilage and ulcers and erosion begins to form on the surface. Inflammatory pannus can penetrate through the articular cartilage into the subchondral bone and affect other intra-articular tissues, such as meniscus, ligament, and tendon. In the advanced stage, the synovial membrane presents repeated exudation, organization, and scar formation on the surface, the articular capsule is thickened, and fibrous adhesion occurs on the articular surface, further forming fibrous ankylosis. Joint space stenosis, articular capsule fibrosis, loose adjacent ligament, and tendon as well as muscle spasm eventually lead to joint contracture, aggravate poor joint alignment, and cause subluxation and even joint deformity, hypofunction, or loss of function.

Imaging Findings

1. **X-ray** findings of RA are directly related to pathological changes. Major X-ray signs include periarticular soft tissue swelling, osteoporosis, joint space stenosis, and joint bone erosion. Symmetrical arthritis may involve all joints of the whole body, especially hand, wrist, foot, knee, shoulder, elbow, ankle, and hip joints. Among axial bones, cervical vertebra is the most frequently affected site, and thoracic vertebra, lumbar vertebra, and sacroiliac joints are rarely affected. Such cartilaginous joints as intervertebral disc, manubriosternal joint, pubic symphysis, and tendon and ligament attached to bones may be also involved, but the incidence and erosion are much less and less severe than those of seronegative spondyloarthropathy (SPA).

   No positive X-ray findings are shown in early RA. With the progression of the disease, the first sign is periarticular soft tissue swelling with homogeneous density, symmetrical fusiform thickening of swollen soft tissue, and fuzzy subcutaneous fat lines. In the early stage, synovial hyperplasia and exudation and effusion of articular cavity result in widening of joint space, and decreased bone mass and osteoporosis at the epiphysis under the effect of inflammation and edema. However, symmetrically affected joints are difficult to be evaluated in the middle-aged and elderly patients. Then, utricular bone erosion, defect, and irregularity occur at the edge of entheses of the epiphyseal articular capsule with fuzzy bone cortex presenting "dotted line" changes. There are bone erosion of articular cartilage and joint margins, fuzzy articular surface, significant stenosis of joint space, and significant osteoporosis. In the advanced stage, hyperostosis, sclerosis or fusion on the articular surface, severe stenosis or loss of joint space, subluxation or dislocation deformity, and fibrosis and even bony ankylosis of joints occur [3, 4].

   (a) Hand: PIP and MCP joints are the most common affected sites of RA. The earliest changes occur on the radial and ulnar sides of the second and third MCP joints and PIP joints. The change on the radial side is more significant than that on the ulnar side, and the metacarpal radial side is most affected. The bone cortex at the entheses of articular capsule is fuzzy. Subsequently, peripheral soft tissue presents fusiform swelling and peripheral osteoporosis (Fig. 9.1). The joint space starts to narrow. Bone destruction occurs in several and even all PIP and MCP joints. Local marginal erosion may be present in all DIP joints, but its destruction is milder than that in PIP joints. The affected sites may be asymmetrical or unilateral and often accompanied by osteoarthritis.

       With the continuous destruction of articular bones and cartilage, joint space disappears completely, and radioluminescent defects, cystic changes, and pseudocysts are found in the subchondral center of the joint (Fig. 9.2). These cystic changes are connected

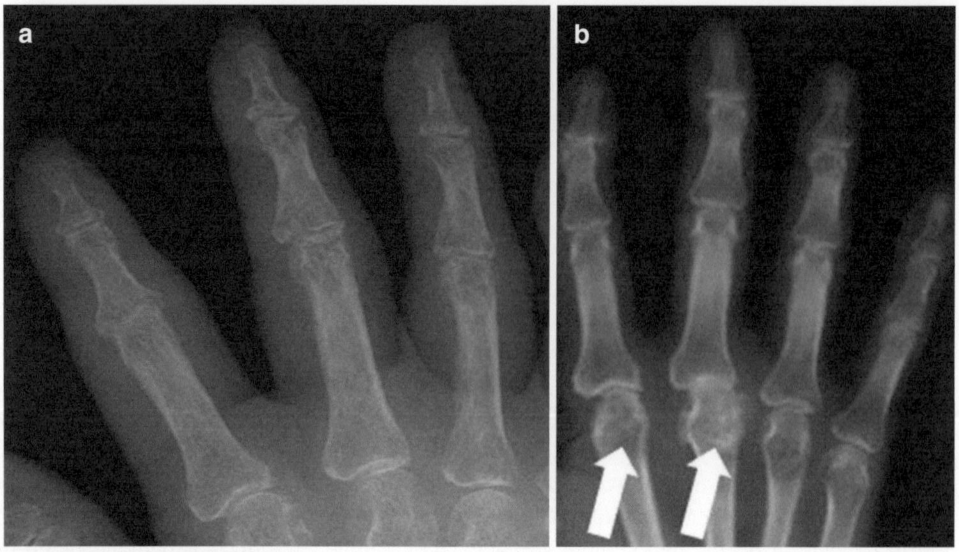

Fig. 9.1 Hand change (1). (**a**) Radiographs show fusiform swelling of soft tissue around the phalanges of fingers of RA patients; (**b**) Bone erosion (white arrows) at the inferior margin of radial and ulnar sides of the second and third MCP joints and osteoporosis at the proximal and middle phalangeal epiphyses

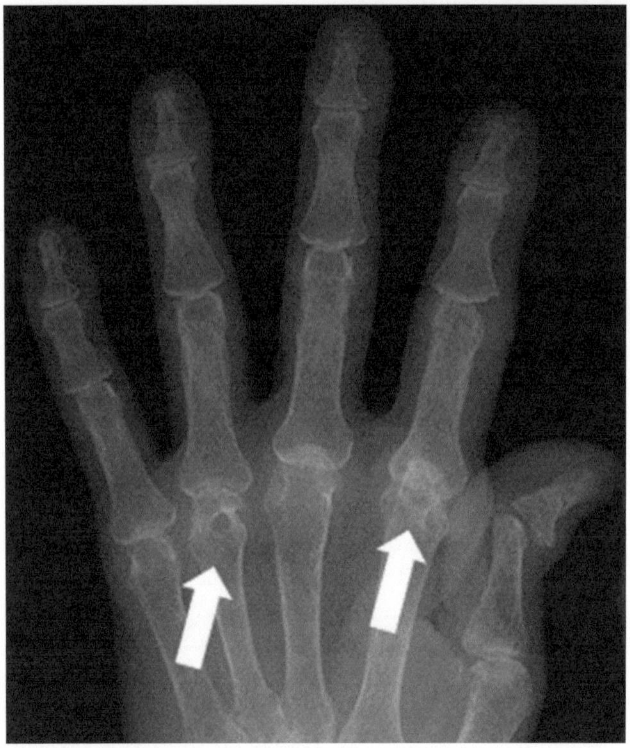

Fig. 9.2 Hand change (2). The radiograph shows diffuse bone erosion of MCP and IP joints of RA patients, joint space stenosis, and locally articular subchondral cystic changes (white arrows)

with the articular cavity as a result of inflammatory pannus throughout cartilage. Severe PIP and MCP arthritis will eventually lead to fibrous ankylosis, rarely bony ankylosis.

A common complication of hands due to RA is abnormal hand axis, causing finger deviation and deformity. (1) Mallet finger: The looseness and disruption of the distal extensor tendon insertion in the distal phalanx can cause a typical mallet finger or drop finger. The looseness of collateral ligament and the further destruction of cartilage and bone may result in DIP joint instability. (2) Boutonniere deformity: It is formed by combining PIP joint flexion and DIP joint hyperextension and caused by RA destroying the tension balance of tendon and ligament of three finger joints (MCP, PIP, and DIP joints). (3) Swan-neck deformity: It is formed by combining PIP joint hyperextension and DIP joint flexion. The main causes include flexor tenosynovitis, hyperextension of long extensor tendon, MCP joint deformity and carpal collapse. (4) MCP joint deformity: RA causes deformity and deviation of multiple MCP joints, including ulnar deviation, extensor tendon subluxation, joint flexion, and palmar subluxation (Fig. 9.3).

(b) Wrist joint: The early findings show soft tissue swelling and bone erosion at the distal ulna and around the styloid process, utricular bone destruction at the styloid process of ulna, and subsequent synovial inflammation causing bone erosion of radial styloid process and adjacent scaphoid bone. Triangular and pisiform bones are the most often affected carpal bones of early RA. Persistent synovial inflammation may lead to extensive narrowing and disappearing of intercarpal, carpometacarpal, and intermetacarpal joint space, and even severe bone erosion and bony ankylosis (Fig. 9.4). The extensive erosion of bones and cartilage, looseness of articular capsules and ligaments, and imbalance of muscles and tendons will cause abnormal alignment and subluxation of multiple radiocarpal, intercarpal, and distal radioulnar joints, which is typically manifested as Z-deformity. This type of deformity is formed by radial deviation of wrist joints and ulnar deviation of MCP joints.

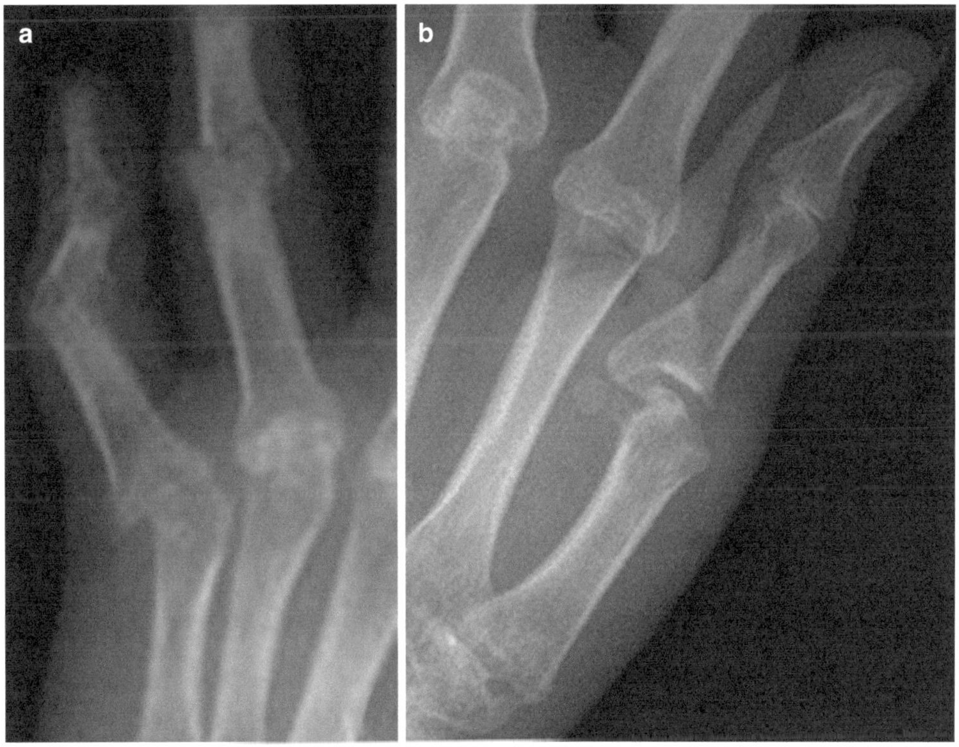

Fig. 9.3 Change in hand deformity. (**a**) Radiographs show hand deformity due to RA, namely boutonniere deformity by PIP joint flexion combined with DIP joint hyperextension; (**b**) Ulnar deviation and subluxation of MCP joint

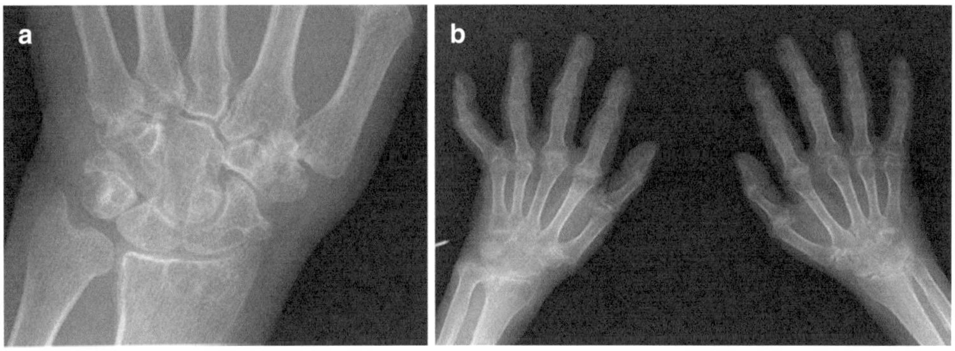

Fig. 9.4 Change in wrist joint. (**a**) Radiographs show multiple bone erosion of carpometacarpal, intercarpal, and radiocarpal joints; (**b**) Peripheral soft tissue swelling, disappearing of joint space presenting bony ankylosis in severe cases

(c) Elbow joint: It is a predilection site of RA. Synovial inflammation destroys bones and cartilage, resulting in typical imaging findings of RA. Joint effusion, soft tissue swelling, and synovial thickening cause the periarticular fat pads to be moved, forming typically positive "fat pad" sign at the distal humerus (Fig. 9.5). There are periarticular osteoporosis, narrowing of joint space, bone erosion in distal humerus, radial head, ulna olecranon, and coronoid process. In severe cases, extensive osteolysis, pathologic fracture, and rare bony ankylosis and subluxation may occur.

(d) Shoulder joint: The early finding is diffuse osteoporosis. Bone erosion occurs at the margin of glenoid cavity and humerus. It is more significant in the latter, presenting as irregularity and cystic changes on the superior lateral surface of the greater tuberosity of humerus (Fig. 9.6). The progressive destruction of articular cartilage leads to joint space stenosis associated with articular surface sclerosis and subchondral cystic changes. Continuous destruction may involve extensive proximal humerus and glenohumeral joint, resulting in upward subluxation of humeral head. Narrow subacromial space and bone changes in the greater tuberosity lead to atrophy or tear of the rotator cuff and eventually pathologic fracture of humerus neck.

(e) Knee joint: The findings in the early soft tissue swelling include bursa suprapatellaris swelling and fuzzy infrapatellar fat pad (Fig. 9.7). Small bone destruction occurs at the lateral margin of femur and tibia, and then inflammatory synovial tissues involve cartilage and the subchondral bone and form multiple subarticular cysts to connect with the articular cavity. The space between the tibiofemoral joint and

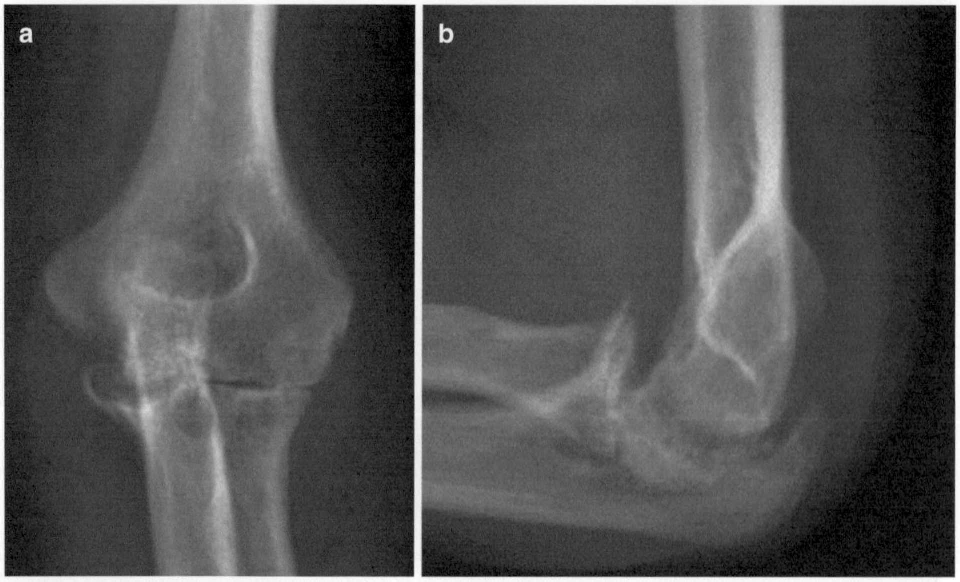

Fig. 9.5 Change in elbow joint. (**a**) Radiographs show osteoporosis of elbow joint, irregular articular surfaces of the coracoid process of ulna and the olecranon, multiple bone destruction, narrowing of joint space, and peripheral soft tissue swelling; (**b**) "Fat pad" sign seen in the distal humerus

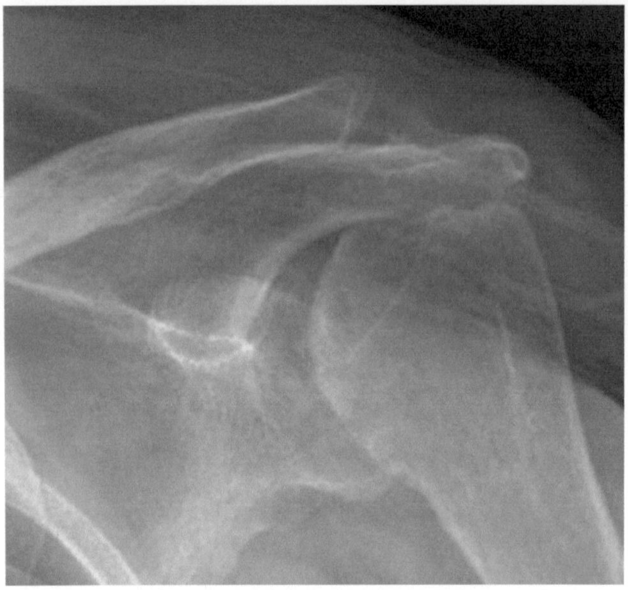

Fig. 9.6 Change in shoulder joint. X-ray shows the osteoporosis change in shoulder joint, narrowing of subacromial joint space, bone erosion and destruction of proximal humerus and glenoid cavity

patellofemoral joint narrows and disappears. The sclerosis of articular surface occurs. Osteophytes and bone fragments are commonly formed (Fig. 9.8). In the advanced stage, knee joints may present knee varus and valgus deformity with or without subluxation, as well as bony ankylosis in rare cases.

(f) Hip joint: Hip joint is often involved bilaterally. The typical early manifestation is centripetal stenosis of joint space, suggesting thinning or defects of articular cartilage on the surface of acetabulum and femur. Bone destruction and cystic changes are common imaging findings of RA in hip joint. The bright area is generally found near the margins of femoral and neck bone cartilage, as well as in femoral head and acetabulum with irregular surface, no sclerosis. For patients with a long course of disease, osteosclerosis and a small number of osteophytes may occur around the hip joint, possibly as a result of bone and cartilage self-repairing. At this time, it is difficult to differentiate osteoarthritis alone from RA with osteoarthritis. In the advanced stage, the hip joint space disappears completely and the femoral head and acetabulum protrude into the pelvic cavity. Arthrokatadysis is a typical characteristic of RA. The prognosis often involves fibrous ankylosis, rare bony ankylosis.

(g) Ankle joint: RA in ankle joint is rare. The early findings include osteoporosis, swelling of the articular capsule and peripheral soft tissues, diffuse stenosis of tibiotalar joint space, and extensive bone destruction and subchondral cystic changes (Fig. 9.9). The late findings include collapsed articular surface of ankle and even ankylosis, possibly with subluxation and stress fracture in ankle joint.

(h) Foot: It is one of the most frequently affected parts of RA. The MTP joints and the hallux PIP joint are mainly involved. The imaging changes occur earliest, even earlier than hand and wrist changes. The early findings include soft tissue swelling, periarticular osteoporosis, joint space stenosis, and bony defects at the edge and center of the joint (Fig. 9.10). RA mainly involves the medial side of the first to fourth metatarsal head and medial and lateral sides of the fifth metatarsal head. With the progression of the disease, hyperostosis, sclerosis, and periostitis may occur. Bony ankylosis is very rare. In addition to the

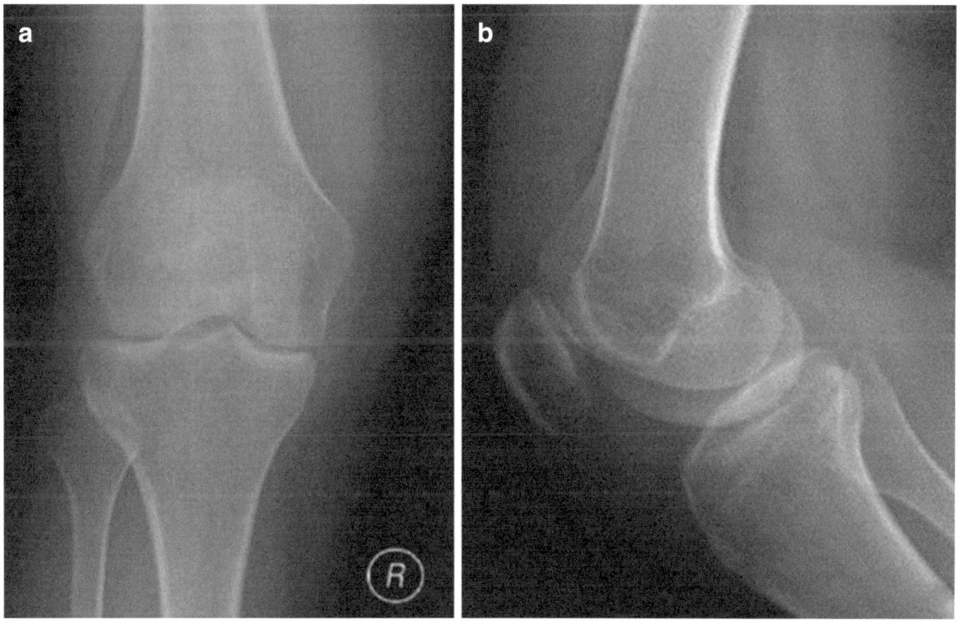

Fig. 9.7 Change in knee joint (1). Radiographs show decreased bone density in knee joint, narrowing of joint space and peripheral soft tissue swelling

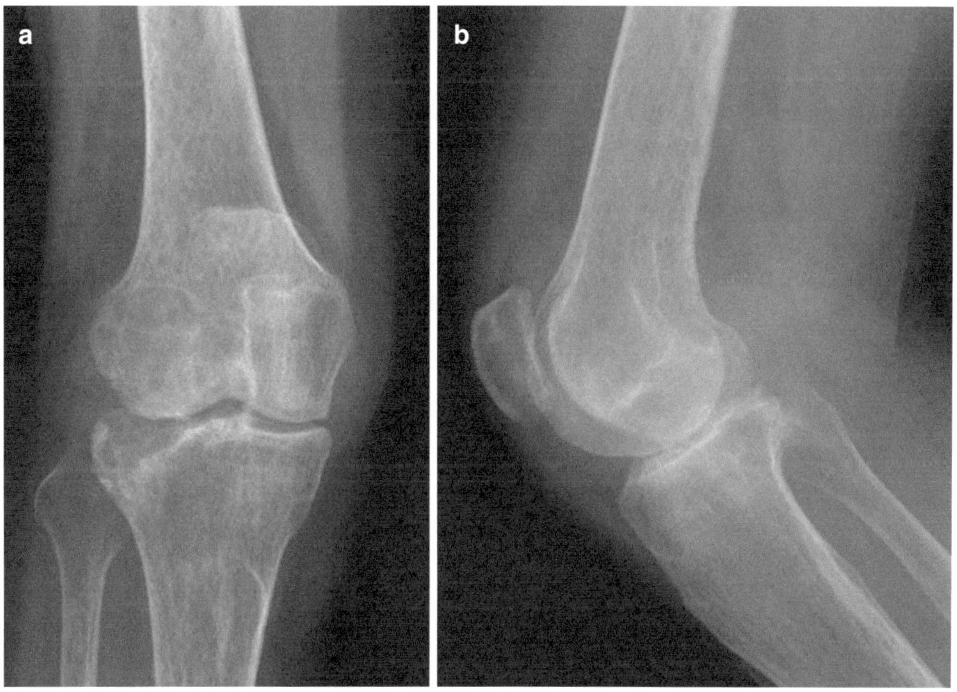

Fig. 9.8 Change in knee joint (2). Radiographs show osteoporosis in knee joint, significant narrowing of joint space and peripheral soft tissue swelling. Multiple bone erosion is found in distal femur, proximal tibia and patella, with local marginal sclerosis and collapsed lateral tibial plateau

above findings, the metatarsal head and PIP joint of hallux also present with osteoporosis and adjacent sesamoid destruction. In the advanced stage, such deformities as metatarsus dislocation, valgus, and pronation may be found. The tarsal joint may also be involved (Fig. 9.11), often in talocalcaneonavicular joints. The findings include diffuse disappearing of joint space, local osteosclerosis, and osteophyte formation. Bone erosion is mild and rare. Bone fusion may be observed occasionally. Achilles tendinitis in calcaneus may have reactive spur-like hyperostosis and bone erosion, and bursitis and swelling of mass-like soft tissue above calcaneus.

(i) Spine: For the spine, RA mainly involves cervical vertebra and is most common in atlanto-axial joints. All synovial joints, uncovertebral joints, and entheses of tendons and ligaments may be affected, which is manifested as osteoporosis, narrowing of intervertebral space, hyperostosis of the vertebral body, and facet joint sclerosis. The involvement of ligaments and tendons leads to cervical curvature instability and subluxation and luxation of atlanto-axial joints.

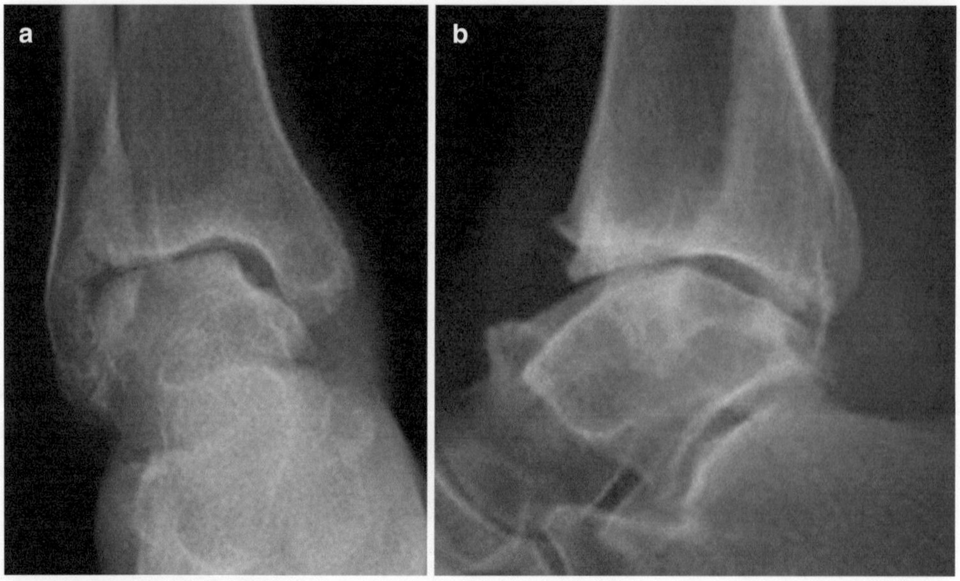

Fig. 9.9 Change in ankle joint. Radiographs show distal tibiofibular and talar hyperostosis, destruction of distal tibiofibular cartilage, multiple bone erosion seen, narrowing of tibiotalar and tibiofibular joint space, and swelling of peripheral soft tissue of the ankle joint

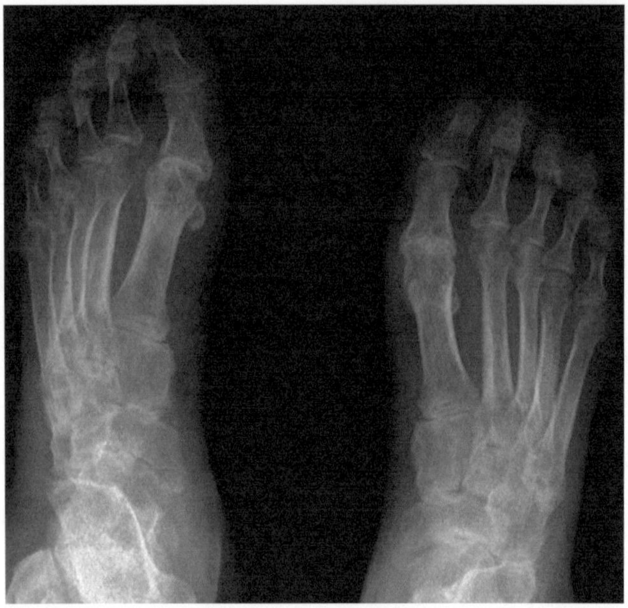

Fig. 9.10 Foot change (1). The radiograph shows osteoporosis in both feet, multiple bone destruction in IP joint and tarsus, sesamoid involved, narrowing of partial joint space, and periarticular soft tissue swelling

2. CT
   (a) CT image is superior to X-ray plain film in periarticular soft tissue swelling and joint effusion.
   (b) The multiplanar reconstruction technique can clearly show the degree of joint space stenosis, intra-articular changes, and minor bone erosion and well assess the synovial cysts and subchondral cystic changes.
   (c) The three-dimensional reconstruction technique can reveal the destruction, dislocation, and deformity of complex joints, such as atlanto-axial joints and acetabulum (Figs. 9.12, 9.13, 9.14, and 9.15).

3. MRI
   (a) Synovitis: In the early stage of RA, acute synovitis leads to joint effusion and synovial thickening. The fluid presents homogeneous changes in hypointense on T_1WI and hyperintense on T_2WI. With the accumulation of effusion for a long time, fibrous tissue components and macromolecular substances are deposited. T_1WI and T_2WI signal intensities are heterogeneous. A normal synovial membrane is not shown on MRI. Imaging of the synovial membrane suggests synovial thickening and/or pannus formation. The thickened synovial membrane is coarse in surface with creep growth along the articular margin and cartilage surface, which shows filamentous slightly hypointense on T_1WI and slightly hyperintense on T_2WI. The thickened synovial membrane shows obvious enhancement on enhanced scan and can be differentiated from joint effusion [5].
   (b) Pannus formation: Pannus is the characteristic change of RA and often in strip, nodule or mass shape (Fig. 9.16). Pannus is classified into inflammatory, fibrous, and mixed pannus according to the type of tissue. Inflammatory pannus shows hypointense on T_1WI and heterogeneous and slightly hyperintense on T_2WI, with marked enhancement on enhanced scan (Fig. 9.17). Fibrous pannus shows hypointense on T_1WI and T_2WI, and weak enhancement on enhanced scan. Mixed pannus is something in between. It shows hypointense on T_1WI and heterogeneous hypointense to hyperintense on T_2WI, and moderate heterogeneous enhancement on enhanced scan. It is generally believed that fibrous pannus suggests RA in the resting stage, while inflammatory and

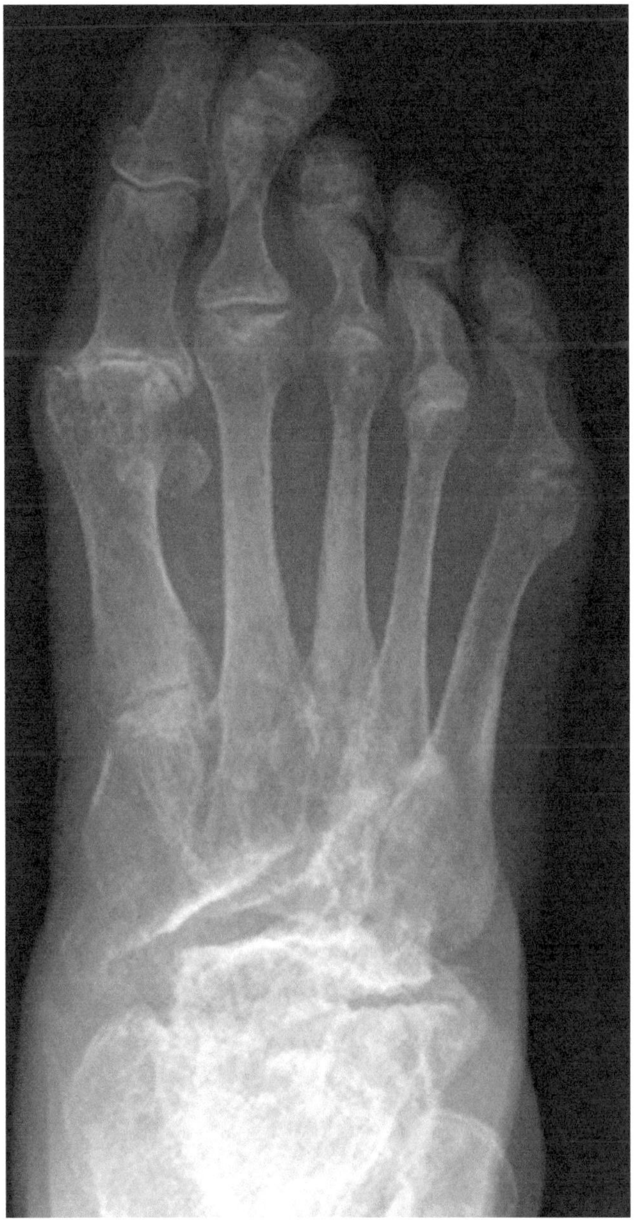

Fig. 9.11 Foot change (2). The radiograph shows osteoporosis in foot, significant bone destruction in tarsus, joint space fusion, and local dislocation and deformity in tarsus

mixed pannus suggests RA in the active stage or semi-active stage [6].

(c) Articular cartilage damage: It first occurs at the margin of cartilage, namely bare area, with small cystic necrosis. As pannus gradually covers the surface of cartilage, the cartilage thins with coarse and uneven surface and utricular defects in local area. The hyperplastic synovial membrane or pannus gradually affects subarticular bone. In the advanced stage, bone erosion is severe with patchy irregular defects.

(d) Bone erosion: Pannus invades the bone. MRI shows the discontinuity of bone cortex signals, bone erosion and destruction, and a subarticular cyst with an irregular hypointense on T_1WI and hyperintense on T_2WI. The bone marrow edema presents as fuzzy patchy hypointense on T_1WI and slightly hypointense or slightly hyperintense on T_2WI, as well as marked hyperintense on STIR sequence (Fig. 9.18).

(e) Periarticular soft tissue changes: MRI may show adhesion and rupture of periarticular tendons and ligaments, peripheral soft tissue edema, involvement of spinal cord, etc.

Key Points of Diagnosis

The clinical diagnosis of RA mainly depends on clinical symptoms and signs of chronic inflammatory arthritis. The laboratory test and imaging changes provide important supplementary information and exclude other diagnoses. The 1987 American College of Rheumatology (ACR) classification criteria (Table 9.1) are widest in clinical application, but the criteria cannot achieve the purpose of early diagnosis of RA. With the application progress of disease-modifying antirheumatic drugs (DMARDs) including methotrexate (MTX) and biological agents, early diagnosis and treatment have become the focus of RA. In 2010, ACR and European League Against Rheumatism (EULAR) jointly revised the RA classification criteria into new ones [7] (Table 9.2), which is regarded as a milestone. Rheumatoid nodules and joint destruction on X-ray image were not included in the new criteria because these manifestations are very rare in the

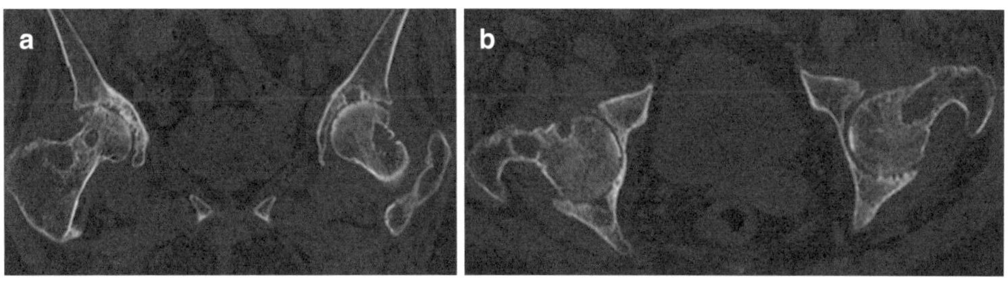

Fig. 9.12 Change in hip joint. CT shows osteoporosis in both hip joints, narrowing of joint space, multiple subarticular bone destruction of bilateral femurs and acetabulum

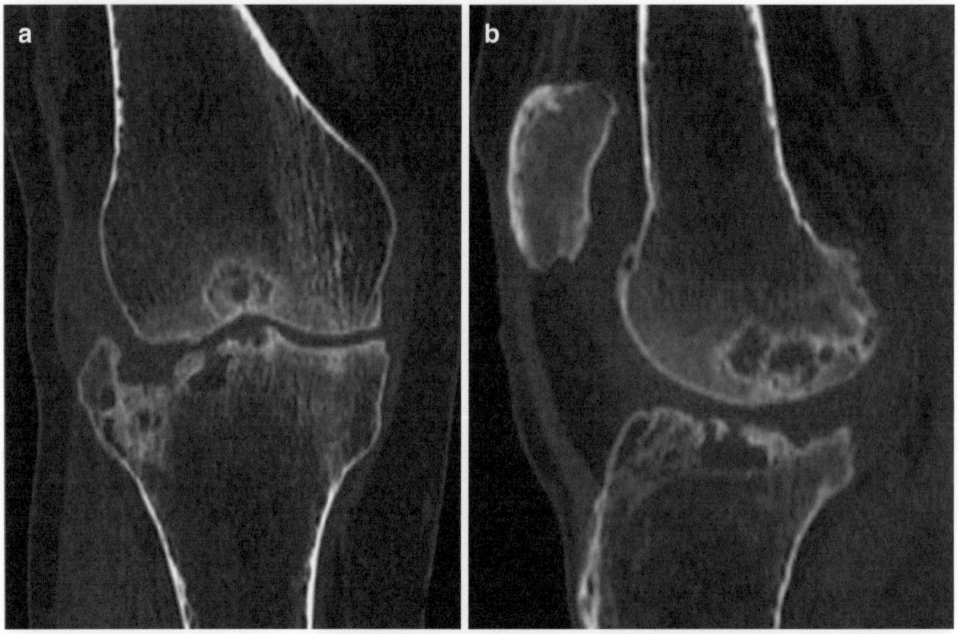

Fig. 9.13 Change in knee joint. CT shows osteoporosis of knee joint, extensive subarticular bone destruction of the distal femur and proximal tibia, local marginal sclerosis, narrowing of joint space and depressed lateral tibial plateau

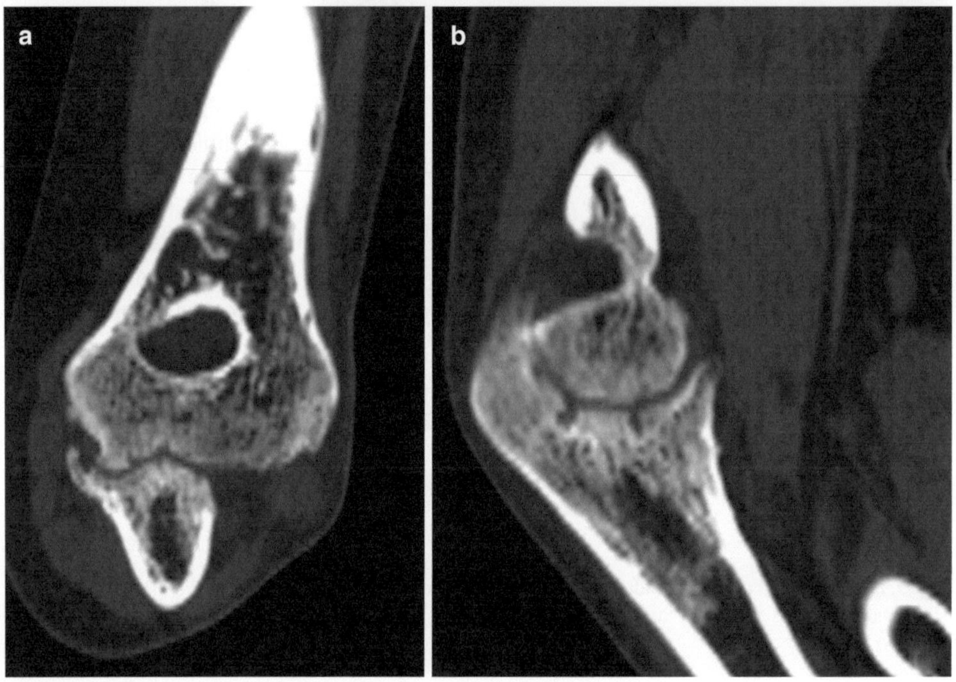

Fig. 9.14 Change in elbow joint. CT reveals narrowing of joint space, irregular articular surface, as well as bone erosion and destruction in humerus, radius, and ulna olecranon

early stage of the disease. The new criteria will aim to identify patients with chronic diseases, who are at high risk of developing persistent synovitis and joint injury at the onset, at an earlier stage, and benefit patients through early use of DMARDs.

Currently, the X-ray plain films of small joints of hands and feet are still preferred in the imaging diagnosis of RA, typically displaying osteoporosis, joint space stenosis, and bone erosion. However, X-ray imaging obviously lacks specificity of diagnosis and ability of early diagnosis. In 95% of RA patients, X-ray changes are not present until 6–12 months after the onset of symptoms. At this time, it is difficult to reverse the progression of the disease with drug treatment. Bone erosion is closely related to diagnosis and treatment improvement. The systematic and complete multi-joint X-ray evaluation is still the evaluation for predilection sites of hands and wrists. The limitations of RA grading system bring challenges to the application of X-ray. CT is rarely used for RA examinations due to its disadvantages in increased radiation dose and inability to display the articular cartilage and synovial membrane, even though CT shows clearer bone erosion changes and improved resolution of soft

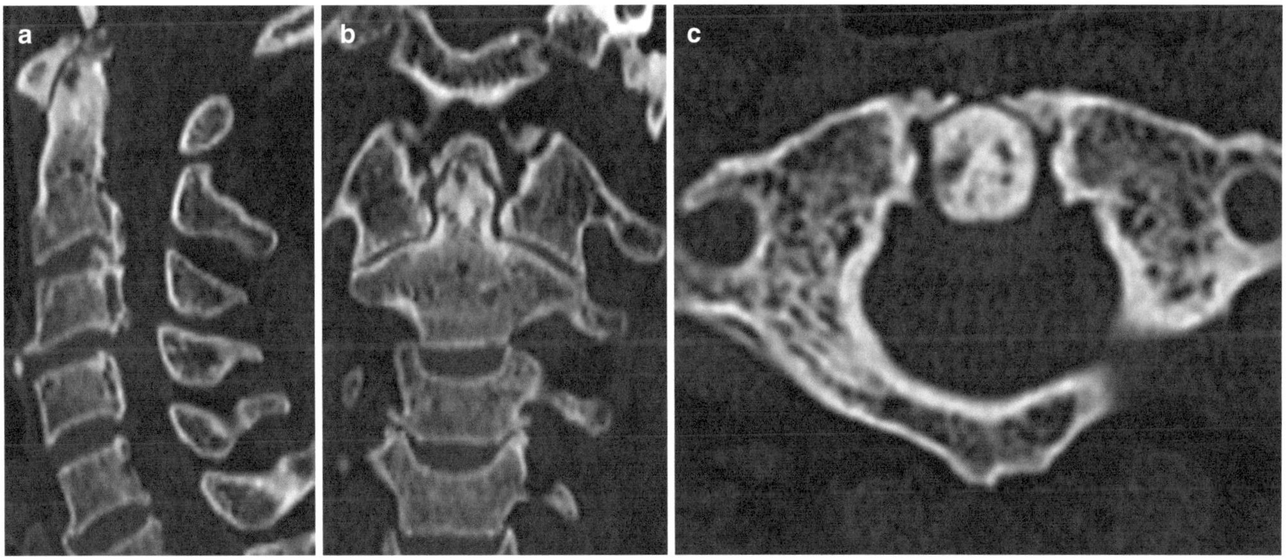

Fig. 9.15 Cervical change. CT demonstrates increased bone density of the axoid odontoid process and atlas, change in low-density bone destruction in the axoid odontoid process, hyperostosis and sclerosis in the vertebral body, and narrowing of atlanto-axial joint space

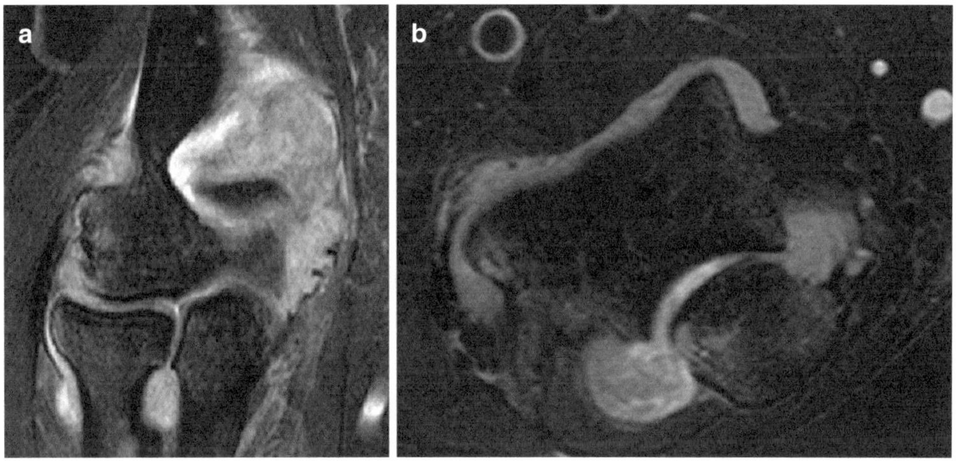

Fig. 9.16 Pannus. MRI STIR shows the development of multiple clumpy synovial pannus around the distal humerus and proximal radius and ulna in elbow joint

tissue compared with X-ray plain films. MRI can show articular cartilage, synovial membranes, bone marrow, ligaments, tendons, and other structures in a noninvasive and clear manner and detect RA-related pathological changes including soft tissue edema, synovial hyperplasia, formation of inflammatory pannus, articular cartilage damage, and bone marrow edema in an early stage. MRI has incomparable advantages over other imaging techniques.

Differential Diagnosis

1. **Osteoarthritis** is more common in middle-aged and elderly people aged over 40 and mainly involves knee, spine, and other weight-bearing joints. Joint pain worsens in movement. There may be joint swelling and effusion, as well as morning stiffness for a short time, less than 30 min. Most of patients with osteoarthritis have a normal erythrocyte sedimentation rate with negative RF. As to its imaging findings, bone destruction mainly occurs in the cartilage coverage area, not bare area. There is lip-like hyperplasia or osteophyte formation at the margin of joints. Joint space is heterogeneous and narrow. Osteoporosis rarely appears. It should be noted that RA mainly affects PIP joints and osteoarthritis involves DIP joints, but both diseases are easily misdiagnosed as the two symptoms often occur together.
2. **Ankylosing spondylitis** is common in young men. The vast majority of patients with AS have positive HLA-B27 and negative RF. AS is also associated with joint lesions in extremities, mainly in axial joints. The sacroiliac joint is first affected. However, the spinal lesions of RA are usually limited to the cervical vertebra, rarely involving the sacroiliac joint. Its main imaging findings are inflammation in tendon and ligament enthesitis with osseous hyperpla-

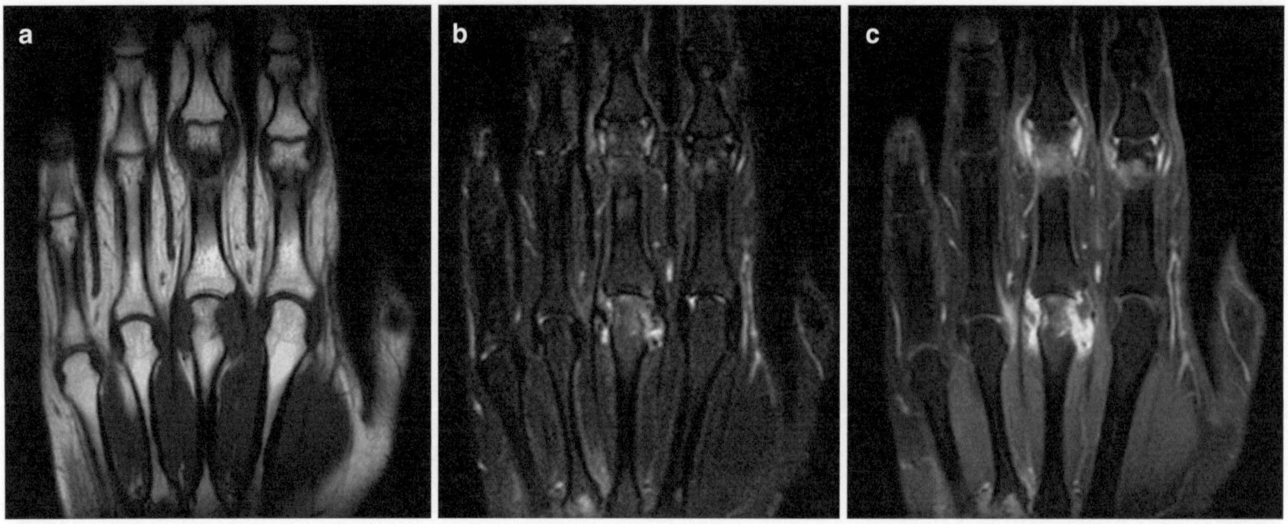

Fig. 9.17 Hand change. (**a**, **b**) MRI reveals synovial thickening around MCP and IP joints, significant for the middle finger, with hypointense on T_1WI. STIR sequences show hyperintense; (**c**) subarticular cartilage damage, bone marrow edema (BME), and marked enhancement of the synovial membrane on enhanced scan

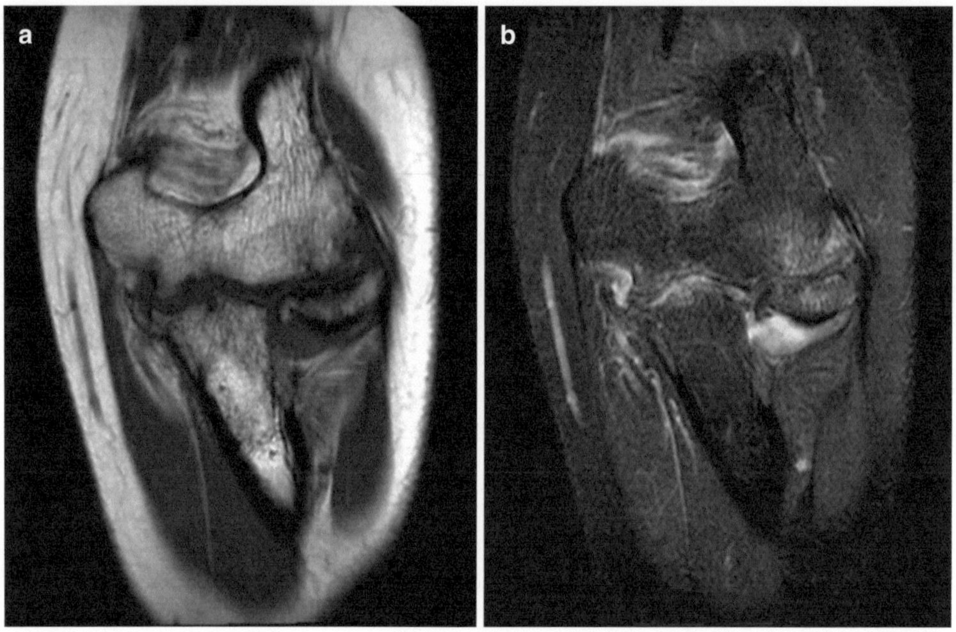

Fig. 9.18 Change in elbow joint. (**a**) MRI shows irregular elbow articular surface with changes in erosive bone destruction, and subarticular multiple hypointense shadows on T_1WI. (**b**) STIR sequences show local subarticular bone marrow edema, obvious destruction of articular cartilage and effusion in the articular cavity

sia and intra-articular bone fusion. AS is manifested as erosion and destruction of the sacroiliac joint, subarticular sclerosis, spine in typical bamboo-like changes, and extensive ossification of collateral ligaments and anterior longitudinal ligaments. AS involves joints of the extremities, with mild joint synovium lesions, rarely severe pannus formation and osteoporosis that do not usually occur.

3. **Gouty arthritis** is common in middle-aged and elderly men. Its predilection sites are the first metatarsophalangeal (MTP) joint or tarsometatarsal joints, and joints including knee, ankle, wrist, and hand may also be affected. The disease often has recurrent attack and juxta-articular tophi can be found. The blood uric acid level is elevated. Gouty arthritis in imaging is an asymmetric joint lesion and characterized by soft tissue swelling, eccentric bone destruction, no joint space stenosis in general or osteoporosis. A specific tophus presents as a juxta-articular irregular soft tissue mass with mild calcification and shows hypointense on T_2WI, which can help distinguish this disease from inflammatory pannus. Some clinical and imaging findings of RA and gouty arthritis are very similar, in particular those on small joints of extremities which should be differentiated through clinical signs and laboratory tests.
4. **Psoriatic arthritis** belongs to seronegative spondyloarthropathy (SPA). Psoriasis is closely related to inflamma-

Table 9.1 American College of Rheumatology (ACR) classification criteria for rheumatoid arthritis (RA) (1987)

Definition	Note
1. Morning stiffness	Stiffness in joints and around the joints lasts for at least 1 h
2. Arthritis in more than 3 areas	A physician observes that soft tissue swelling or effusion (not simple hyperostosis) is present simultaneously in at least 3 areas among 14 following areas (left or right PIP, MCP, wrist, elbow, knee, ankle, and metatarsophalangeal (MTP) joints)
3. Cheirarthritis	At least one area of wrist, MCP, and PIP joints swells
4. Symmetrical arthritis	Joints in the same area on both sides are involved simultaneously (the involvement of bilateral PIP, MCP, or MTP joints may not be symmetrical)
5. Rheumatoid nodules	A physician observes subcutaneous nodules at bony prominences, on extensor surfaces or around joints
6. Positive serum rheumatoid factor	Any detection method shows abnormal content of serum rheumatoid factors, and the positive rate in normal population is less than 5%
7. X-ray changes	PA views of hands and wrists display typical RA changes, including bone erosion or clear bone demineralization of involved joints and their adjacent sites (it is not enough only to include osteoarthritis changes)

Patients who meet 4 or more of above 7 items with other arthritis excluded can be diagnosed with RA. The duration of the symptom in item 1–4 is at least 6 weeks

Table 9.2 American College of Rheumatology and European League Against Rheumatism classification criteria for rheumatoid arthritis (RA) (2010)

Item	Contents	Score
Joint involvement	1 large joint	0
	2–10 large joints	1
	1–3 small joints (with or without involvement of large joints)	2
	4–10 small joints (with or without involvement of large joints)	3
	>10 joints (at least 1 small joint)	5
Serology	Negative	0
(RF or anti-CCP antibody)	Low-level positive result on at least one test (level ≤ 3 times the upper limit of normal)	2
	High-level positive result on at least one test (level > 3 times the upper limit of normal)	3
Duration of synovitis	<6 weeks	0
	>6 weeks	1
Acute-phase reactants	Normal CRP and normal ESR	0
	Increased CRP or ESR	1

Patients with a total score of more than 6 can be diagnosed with RA. Target population: Patients who have at least one joint with definite clinical synovitis (swelling); patients with the synovitis not better explained by another disease

tory arthritis. Patients with psoriatic arthritis have an increased incidence of RA. PsA affects axial bone and bone of the extremities, mainly DIP joints of fingers or toes. It is considered that this disease is characterized by diffuse soft tissue swelling, no osteoporosis in general, bone destruction and absorption occurring in distal phalanges with peripheral hyperostosis, and typical joint fusion forming pencil-in-cup- deformity. In addition, PsA is often accompanied by skin, finger nails, and other extra-articular specific manifestations, which contributes to the differentiation between this disease and RA.

Status Quo and Progress of Research

1. **DCE-MRI.** Enhanced MRI can definitely distinguish enhanced synovial tissues from non-enhanced joint effusion, playing an important role in diagnosis of RA. DCE-MRI is based on the perfusion dynamics of synovial enhancement curves after injection of gadolinium-based contrast agent and can analyze quantitatively parameters of the time-intensity curve. DCE-MRI is closely related to pathological changes of synovial inflammation and bone marrow edema and responses to treatment. DCE-MRI may allow accurate assessment of RA activity based on manual segmentation of synovial tissue in the region of interest [8]. Recently, with the development of machine learning techniques, automated segmentation and texture analysis has made it possible to assess the correlation between RA imaging and pathology, but this method needs further validation and internationally agreed standards.
2. **Whole-body magnetic resonance imaging (WB-MRI).** WB-MRI allows imaging of the entire body in one scanning and has been used in oncology to assess tumor metastases. In rheumatology, WB-MRI is a powerful tool in assessing RA, AS, PsA, and other axial and peripheral polyarticular inflammation [9]. WB-MRI may provide a count of RA involved joints. The number of involved joints detected by imaging mode is one of 2010 ACR/EULAR classification criteria. Improved imaging resolution of small joints of the hands and feet and more assessments in clinical applications are still needed.
3. **DWI.** Except for CE-MRI, conventional MRI sequences are difficult to distinguish synovitis from joint effusion. Both signs show hypointense on T_1WI and hyperintense change on T_2WI and fat-suppressed sequence. However, the detection of synovitis is very important for diagnosis of RA. In addition, conventional MRI sequences are also difficult to differentiate RA-induced bone erosion from osteoarthritic bone cysts, but this differentiation is of

great significance for differential diagnosis. Recent studies have demonstrated that DWI is a new noninvasive imaging method that allows more accurate differentiation between synovitis and joint effusion, as well as bone erosion and bone cysts using ADC values [10]. As the infiltration of inflammatory cells may inhibit the free movement of water molecules, the ADC vale of synovitis is significantly lower than that of joint effusion $(1.63 \pm 0.37) \times 10^{-3}$ mm²/s and $(2.6 \pm 0.36) \times 10^{-3}$ mm²/s, respectively. The sensitivity and specificity reach 91% and 90%, respectively, in differentiation between synovitis and joint effusion using the ADC cut-off value of 2.10×10^{-3} mm²/s. The ADC value of bone erosion is also significantly less than that of a subchondral cyst $(1.61 \pm 0.39) \times 10^{-3}$ mm²/s and $(2.39 \pm 0.34) \times 10^{-3}$ mm²/s, respectively, which proves that they have different pathological processes. The sensitivity and specificity reach 93.5% and 87.5%, respectively, in differentiation between bone erosion and bone cyst using the ADC cut-off value of 2.04 × 10-3 mm²/s. This method still needs to be further improved and validated in improvement of image resolution, selection of the region of interest, and accuracy and repeatability of values.

9.2 Seronegative Spondyloarthropathy

Fengzhe Wang and Yuan Qu

Seronegative spondyloarthropathy (SPA) is a group of joint inflammatory disorders presenting with negative serum rheumatoid factor (RF) and positive human leukocyte antigen B27 (HLA-B27) collectively. SPA often involves the axial bone to cause spondyloarthritis (SpA). SPA includes ankylosing spondylitis (AS), psoriatic arthritis (PsA), reactive arthritis (ReA), and enteropathic arthritis. This group of disorders share many clinical signs, pathological characteristics, and imaging findings. They may involve synovial membrane and cartilaginous joint, bursa mucosa and tendinous sheath, tendon and ligament entheses, tendon, ligament, soft tissue, and bone. But their incidence and distribution vary.

9.2.1 Ankylosing Spondylitis

Overview

Ankylosing spondylitis (AS) is a multi-systematic, progressive, chronic inflammatory spondyloarthropathy and the most common type of SPA. The cause of the disease is unknown. AS mainly involves the sacroiliac joints, axial bones of the spine and peripheral joints. The disease is characterized by sacroiliitis and enthesitis. The term "spondylitis" is derived from spondylos in Greek, meaning vertebra. The term "ankylosis" is derived from ankylos in Greek, meaning stiffness of a joint. Historically, RA has been known by many names, such as spondylitis rhizomelique, pelvospondylitis ossificans, spondylitis ossificans ligamentosa, von Bechterew's syndrome, and rheumatoid spondylitis. In 1963, the American College of Rheumatology adopted the term "ankylosing spondylitis (AS)" which represented differences between AS and rheumatoid arthritis (RA) in clinical and imaging findings. Since then, the term "AS" has been widely used.

AS shows a predilection for young men. The age of onset is usually 15 ~ 30 years, with the male to female ratio of (2 ~ 3):1. The prevalence of AS has a close correlation with the HLA-B27 positive rate. The HLA-B27 positive rate in normal Chinese population is 2% ~ 7%, while the HLA-B27 positive rate in AS patients is up to 90%. However, HLA-B27 is unrelated to the severity of the disease. The prevalence of AS varies by race, population, and territory. For instance, the prevalence is 0.13% ~ 0.22% in the USA, 0.05% ~ 0.2% in Japan, and 0.26% in China. The prevalence of first-degree relatives of AS patients is 11% ~ 25%, and the concordance rate of identical twins is 75%, which indicates that the susceptibility to AS relies on genetic factors to a great extent. HLA-B27 accounts for 50% of genetic factors. The genome-wide single nucleotide polymorphism analysis revealed that other genes relevant to HLA were also associated with the susceptibility to AS, such as genes encoding ERAP1 (chromosome 5q15) and 1 L-23R (chromosome 1p31.3) [11]. Studies have shown that the onset of AS may be associated with bacterial infection. In addition, immune mechanisms, endocrine, metabolic disorders, trauma, and other factors are also considered as possible causes of AS.

AS has insidious onset and slow progression, as well as presentations of benign lesion in the natural course of the disease. Its systemic symptoms are mild, such as weight loss, anorexia, and fever. Inflammatory low back pain is the most common and earliest symptoms of spine. Most patients with the symptom are less than 30 years old with pain of more than 3 months. The pain initially occurs in the low back or hips. It is often insidious dull pain, accompanied by morning stiffness lasting for several hours, and improved with movement. But stiffness occurs again after rest. With the progression of the disease, the low back pain develops from unilaterally to bilaterally, intermittently to persistently, and the pain develops upward to chest and cervical vertebra from lumbar vertebra. After ankylosis occurs at the late stage, these clinical manifestations become mild or are resolved completely. The lesion involves costovertebral joints and sternoclavicular joints, leading to significant chest pain and the pain worsens after coughing or sneezing. Enthesitis may cause bone tenderness at specific sites, such as spinous process, sternocostal joint, ischial tuberosity, tibial tuberosity, and heel. Among peripheral joints, the lesion most commonly involves hip joints and shoulder joints, which is often asymmetrical. The proximal involvement is most significant and may result in severe dysfunction. Typical clinical manifestations include local pain, limitation of motion, muscle contracture and atrophy, and ankylosis. Extra-articular manifestations include uveitis, conjunctivitis, pulmonary fibrosis, pleuritis, ascending aortic inflammation, aortic valve diseases, and nerve and kidney diseases.

There is no specific indicator of laboratory tests for diagnosis and detection of AS. RF is negative. The erythrocyte sedimentation rate is elevated and the C-reactive protein and IgA are increased in the active stage. Approximately 90% of patients are positive for HLA-B27, which has reference value to a certain extent. However, negative HLA-B27 does not mean that patients do not have the disease.

Pathophysiology

Characteristic pathological manifestations of AS are axial arthritis, peripheral large joint inflammation, and enthesitis with subchondral bone marrow edema. Cartilage metaplasia followed by cartilage calcification and ossification formation is also one of the characteristic pathological manifestations of the disease. In the early stage of the lesion, manifestations include the infiltration of synovial membrane and subchondral myelolymphocyte, as well as macrophage and plasma cells, erosion of bone at relevant sites, osteomyelitis, and edema. In the late stage, cartilage calcification and ossification occur at the site of active inflammation and even bone bridges are formed. Pathological changes in synovial joints are similar to those for RA. Synovial thickening, villus hyperplasia, less exudation, and milder pannus can be found. After fibroplasia, cartilage metaplasia, and endochondral ossification may occur, leading to ankylosis and articular capsule ossification [4].

Imaging Findings

X-ray plain film is the preferred method of imaging examination for AS and reveals the involvement degree of bilateral sacroiliac joints, shape of the vertebral body, ligament ossification, and changes in small joints, etc. Internationally recognized diagnostic criteria still use the grading of X-ray results as an important diagnostic basis, but their sensitivity to early diagnosis of AS is not high and their images on early lesions of cartilage, synovial membrane, bone substances, and other structures are not clear. CT is the most sensitive and accurate for the diagnosis of sacroiliitis and superior to X-ray and MRI for the display of bone erosion and sclerosis. CT can also show clearly spinal fracture and spinal stenosis. MRI STIR sequences are very sensitive to detect bone marrow edema and can be used for the diagnosis of AS in the early and active stage. Furthermore, MRI can clearly show inflammatory changes in anterior and posterior borders of vertebral body and intervertebral discs as well as erosion and destruction of articular cartilage.

1. X-ray
   (a) Sacroiliac joint lesion: Sacroiliitis is a characteristic manifestation of AS. The disease is manifested as unilateral or asymmetrical inflammation in the early stage and often bilateral or symmetrical inflammation in the late stage. The symmetrical lesion is an important diagnostic basis for AS and can be used to differentiate AS from other diseases involving sacroiliac joints (such as RA, PsA, and ReA). The sacroiliac joint consists of ear-shaped articular surfaces of the sacrum and the ilium and is divided into synovial and ligament parts. Sacroiliitis mainly involves the ilium. The possible reason is that the cartilage surface of ilium is thinner than that of the sacrum and has degenerative fissures, and inflammatory tissue easily passes through the cartilage surface to the subchondral bone, whereas the cartilage on the surface of the sacrum is thicker and less susceptible to invasion. The early findings are mild periarticular osteoporosis, fuzzy lateral articular surface of the ilium, subsequent erosion and destruction, coarse and uneven articular surfaces, ill-defined subchondral bone plate, low-density bone absorption or destruction area seen, and "pseudo-widening" sign in joint space. With the progression of bone erosion, the articular surface wears significantly and the process of bone destruction is accompanied by reactive osteosclerosis, which eventually causes the sclerosis of entire subchondral bone surface of ilium side with wide and ill-defined sclerosis strap, and irregular stenosis of joint space. In the late stage, when hyperostosis of sacroiliac joints is gradually aggravated, an irregular bone bridge may cross the articular cavity, and joint space narrows and disappears, forming bony ankylosis.

       According to New York diagnostic criteria for AS, X-ray findings of the sacroiliac joint lesion are divided into 5 grades: Grade 0 signifies normal sacroiliac joint. Grade I signifies suspicious sacroiliitis. Grade II signifies mild sacroiliitis, with localized erosion and sclerosis and normal joint space. Grade III signifies moderate sacroiliitis, with significant bone erosion and hyperostosis and osteosclerosis, narrowing and even disappearing of joint space or partial ankylosis. Grade IV signifies complete ankylosis (Fig. 9.19).
   (b) Spinal lesion: The spinal lesion often develops from the sacroiliac joints in a bottom-up approach and gradually involves lumbar vertebra, thoracic vertebra, and even cervical vertebra. Sacroiliac joints do

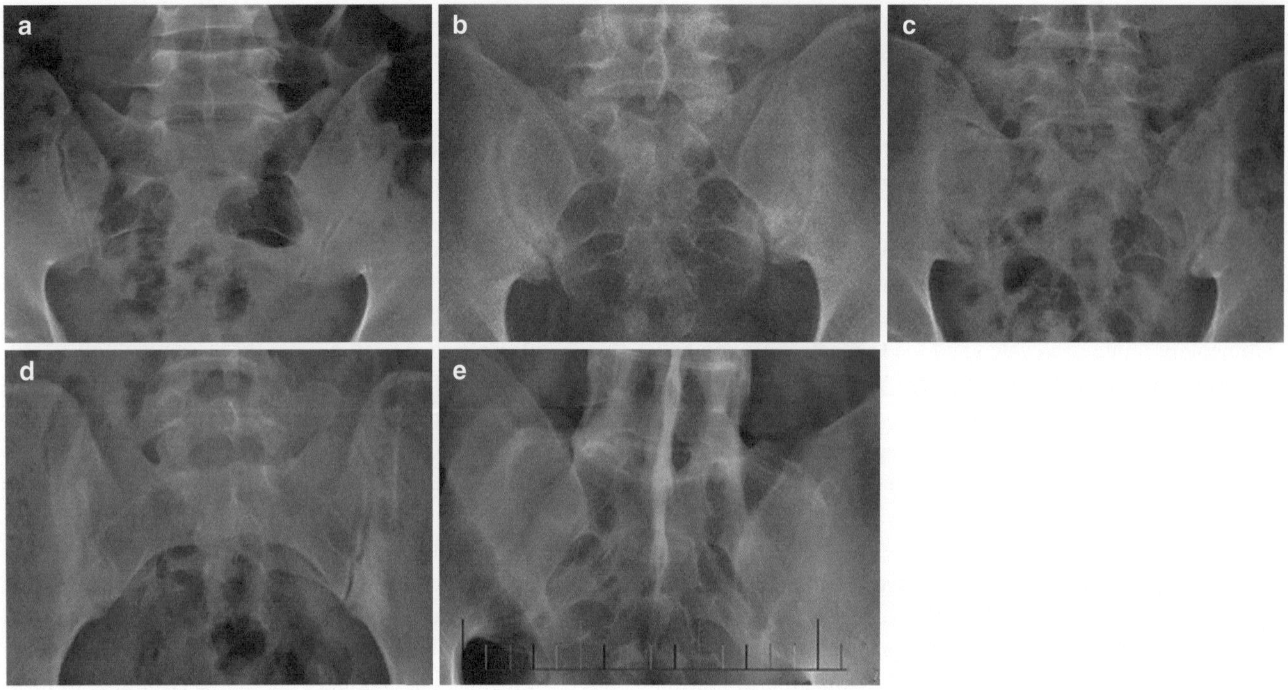

Fig. 9.19 Sacroiliitis (1). (**a**) Radiographs show normal sacroiliac joints, stage 0; (**b**) Fuzzy bilateral sacroiliac joints, suspected sacroiliitis, stage I; (**c**) Fuzzy bilateral sacroiliac joint surfaces, mainly on the right, local bone destruction on the right ilium surface, stage II; (**d**) Narrowing and partial disappearing of bilateral sacroiliac joint space, local bone destruction, sclerosis of articular surfaces, stage III; (**e**) Complete disappearing of bilateral sacroiliac joints, bony ankylosis, stage IV

rarely not have lesions when the spinal lesion occurs. The spinal lesion may involve the discovertebral junction, zygapophyseal joints, costovertebral joints, ligament entheses and atlanto-axial joints. The localized destruction area at the superior and inferior corners of the anterior margin of vertebral body is called Romanus lesion. The lesion is an important early presentation of AS. Bone erosion (osteitis) at superior and inferior corners of the vertebral body combined with bone formation may cause the anterior margin of vertebral body to lose normal concave surface and form "squaring of the vertebral body" sign. After bone erosion has healed, the vertebral body shows the "shiny corner" contour due to reactive osteosclerosis. After fibrous ring of intervertebral disc and anterior longitudinal ligament inflammation, calcification and ossification occur to form syndesmophytes, and ligament calcification grows longitudinally along the long axis of the spine, significant in anterior and lateral spine. Finally, adjoining vertebral bodies are bridged to form the typical bamboo spine (Fig. 9.20). AS leads to erosive destruction at the discovertebral junction to develop spondylodiscitis, which is called Andersson lesion. Cawley et al. classified this lesion into three types. Type I involves the central portion of the discovertebral junction that is covered by cartilage end-plate. Type II involves the peripheral portion of the discovertebral junction not covered by cartilaginous end-plate. Type III involves both the peripheral and central portions of the discovertebral junction. As the lesion progresses, the intervertebral disc may be calcified (Fig. 9.21). The vertebral body has osteoporosis, prone to fracture, which is the most common in the inferior cervical vertebra.

The inflammation of zygapophyseal joints is also a lesion of AS, including bone erosion, sclerosis, and bony ankylosis of articular processes, which may lead to smaller lumbar anterior processes, larger thoracic vertebra posterior processes, and straight or reverse-arch cervical vertebra anterior processes (Fig. 9.22). This lesion may involve the whole spine, but it is rare in PsA and ReA. The costovertebral joints also present as bone erosion, sclerosis, or ankylosis, resulting in less thoracic cage expansion, which is difficult to be displayed on X-ray plain film. As the lesion progresses, calcification and ossification changes may occur in the yellow ligaments, interspinal and supraspinal ligaments of the posterior spine, and extensive ossification causes the completely rigid spine and spinal stenosis. The involvement of atlanto-axial joints may be manifested as odontoid erosion and subluxation.

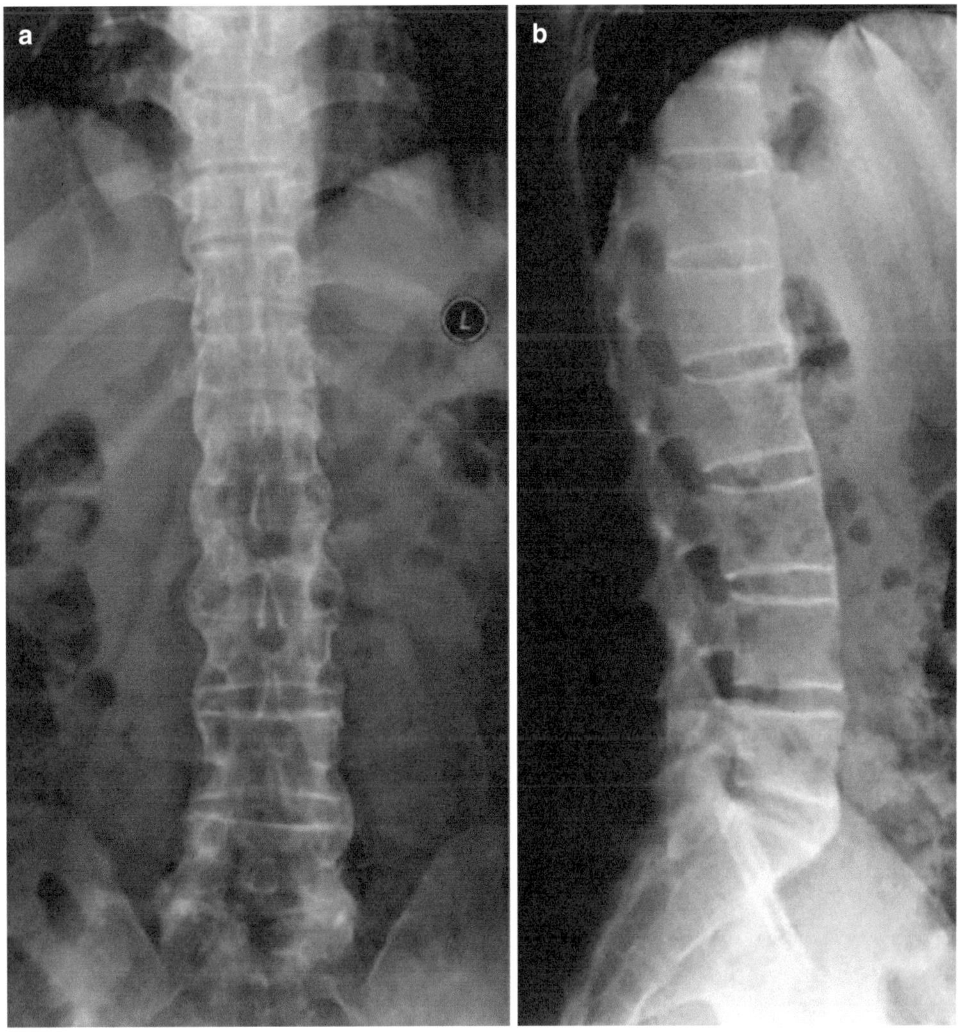

Fig. 9.20 Bamboo spine and ligament ossification. Radiographs show the anterior margin of vertebral body losing normal concave surface, calcification, and ossification of anterior longitudinal ligament to form syndesmophytes, syndesmophytes on the sides of each vertebral body connecting upper and lower vertebral bodies, presenting bamboo-like changes, and normal intervertebral space

(c) Peripheral joint lesion: The hip joints are most commonly involved, manifested as bone erosion and destruction of femoral head and acetabulum, peripheral reactive hyperostosis, secondary osteophyte formation on articular surfaces, and narrowing of joint space, eventually resulting in bony ankylosis. In addition, osteitis changes may occur in bone entheses of tendons and ligaments, such as ischial tuberosity, femur-sized trochanter, pubic symphysis, calcaneal tuberosity and other parts, which present as hyperostosis and osteosclerosis or erosion, and flocculent ossification (Fig. 9.23).

2. **CT** is more sensitive to bone erosion and destruction in sacroiliitis and SpA, allows early imaging of bone changes. CT is the most sensitive and accurate for the diagnosis of sacroiliitis.

Many scholars suggest coronal scanning of sacroiliac joints for more fine diagnosis of inflammatory lesions. Furthermore, the differentiation between normal variation or inflammatory lesions similar to sacroiliitis and sacroiliitis must be considered. According to grading criteria of radiographic AS, the grading of CT results is as follows: Grade 0 means that CT findings are normal or only fuzzy articular surfaces. Stage I means that CT findings are fuzzy articular surfaces, localized osteoporosis and mild erosion in subchondral bone, but normal joint space and ligament joints. Stage II means that CT findings are blurred articular surfaces, localized osteoporosis and sclerosis, bone destruction and tiny cystic changes in subchondral bone, basically normal joint space and locally erosive or normal ligament joints common in the lateral articular surface of the ilium, and bone destruction and cystic changes mostly occurring in lower middle portions of synovial joints. Stage III means that CT findings are significant bone destruction and diffuse sclerosis in subchondral bone, blurred joint margin in brush-like or jagged shape, obviously increased osteoporosis and cystic changes, irregular stenosis of joint space, joint bone destruction and partial ankylosis. Stage IV means that CT findings are complete ankylosis and ligament involvement (Fig. 9.24).

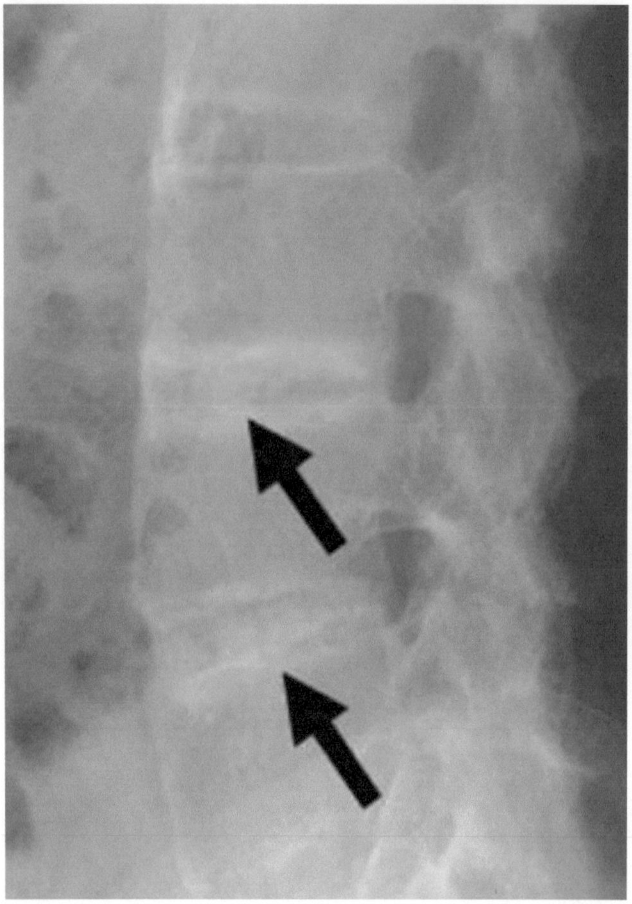

Fig. 9.21 Intervertebral disc calcification. The radiograph shows typical lumbar ligament ossification in patients with long-term AS, intervertebral disc calcification (black arrows), and change in intervertebral disc expansion

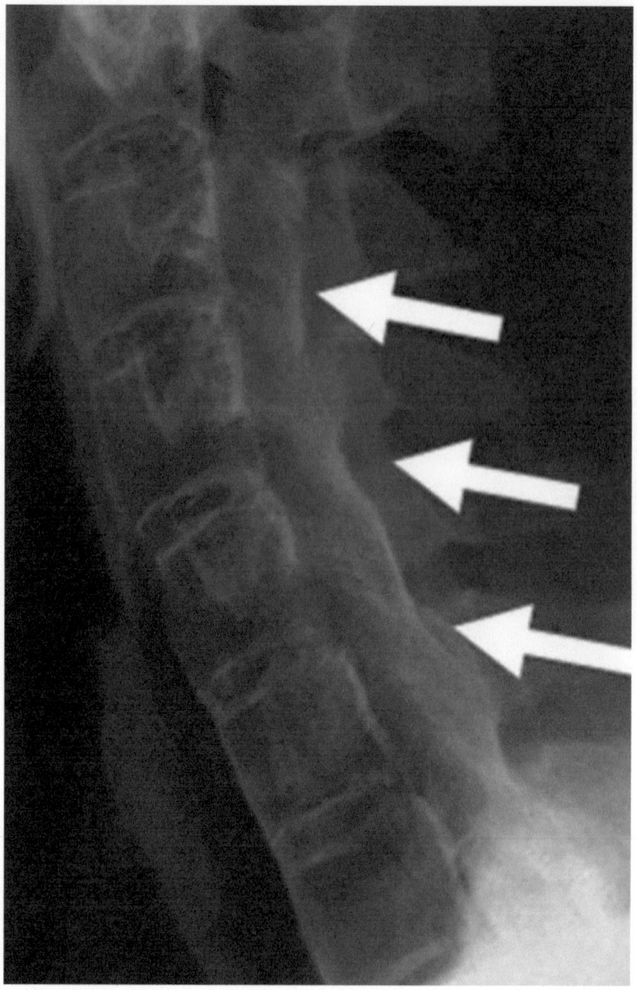

Fig. 9.22 Ankylosis in articular process. The radiograph shows joint narrowing and fusion of articular processes of C2 ~ C6 cervical vertebra segments (white arrows), syndesmophytes, and osteoporosis at the anterior margin of vertebral body

3. **MRI.** MRI is more sensitive to synovial thickening, joint effusion, osteomyelitic edema, and articular cartilage destruction of early AS due to high soft tissue resolution of MRI.
   (a) Cartilage changes: Normal sacroiliac joint cartilage shows strip-shaped isointense on T_1WI and T_2WI. Synovial thickening and inflammatory hyperplasia of pannus cause irregular thickening and distortion of the cartilage surface, showing hypointense on T_1WI and increased signal intensity on T_2WI. With cartilage erosion and destruction, joint space stenosis occurs and hypointense fibrosis or ossification shadows are found on T_1WI and T_2WI.
   (b) Bone changes: There is bone erosion and irregular and uneven subchondral bone surface. Subarticular strip-like or patchy hyperostosis and osteosclerosis occur in the middle and late stages, showing hypointense on T_1WI and T_2WI.

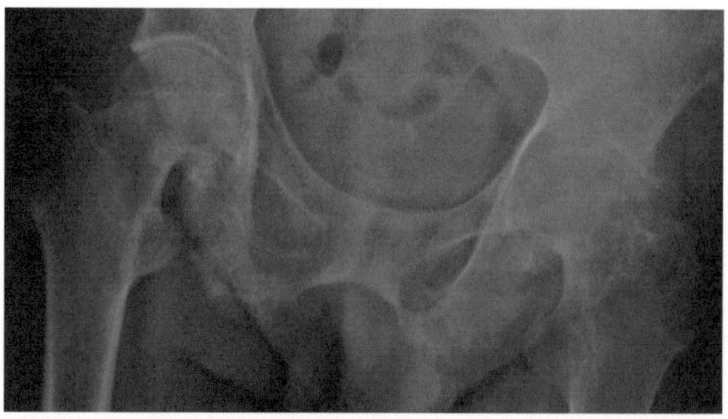

Fig. 9.23 Hip joint lesion. The radiograph shows fuzzy and narrow bilateral hip joint space, mainly on the left, bone erosion seen in femoral head and acetabulum, and multiple hyperostosis and ossification formation in bilateral ischial tuberosity, femoral trochanter and pubic symphysis

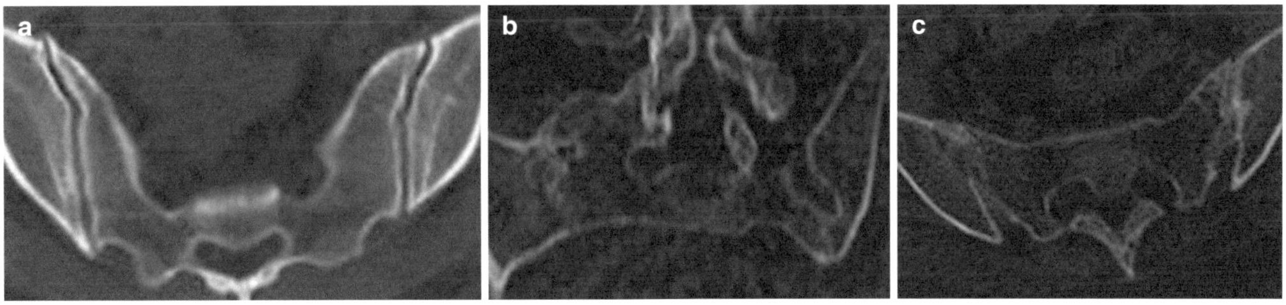

Fig. 9.24 Sacroiliitis (2). (**a**) Radiographs show bilateral sacroiliac joint surface with slightly increased density and irregularity, and normal joint space, in grade II; (**b**, **c**) Narrowed bilateral sacroiliac joint space, with blurred articular surfaces, locally increased change in density and (right sacroiliac joint surface) low-density bone destruction, in grade III

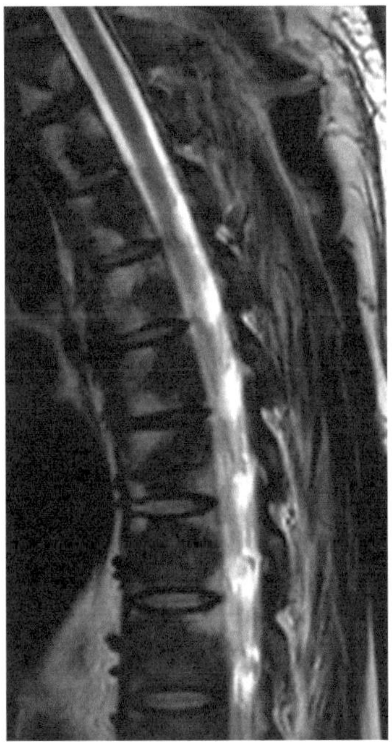

Fig. 9.25 Bone marrow edema. On MRI, T_2WI shows multiple patchy hyperintense at the anterior and posterior corners of the thoracic vertebral body as bone marrow edema, suggesting changes in inflammatory activity

(c) Bone marrow changes: The bone marrow edema presents as spot-like hypointense on T_1WI and fuzzy hyperintense on T_2WI fat-suppressed sequence or STIR sequence, which is considered as the characteristic finding of inflammatory activity (Fig. 9.25).

(d) Bony ankylosis: Joint space narrows and disappears. The signal intensity of hyperplastic bone trabecula on T_2WI decreases (Fig. 9.26).

Key Points of Diagnosis

The diagnosis of AS mainly depends on clinical history, signs, and imaging findings. Young men with chronic low back pain with morning stiffness, family history of AS, positive HLA-B27, and symmetrical sacroiliitis on X-ray plain films should be highly suspicious of the disease. At present, New York criteria in 1966 or revised New York criteria in 1984 are still used for clinical diagnosis of AS. The above criteria are based on definitely radiographic sacroiliitis and have low sensitivity to early patients or patients with mild symptoms. In 2009, the Assessment of Spondyloarthritis international Society (ASAS) proposed new criteria for axial spondyloarthritis (SpA) [12] (Table 9.3). MRI definite diagnosis of active inflammation of sacroiliac joints in these criteria is as important as the definitely radiographic sacroiliitis in New York criteria.

Differential Diagnosis

1. **Condensing osteitis.** Condensing osteitis is common in young and middle-aged women. After natural delivery, women develop mild low back pain and worsened pain with movement. Its onset is generally bilateral and symmetrical. The disease mostly involves the ilium and rarely affects the sacrum. The imaging findings are lamellar or triangular osteosclerosis area below the articular surface of ilium well-demarcated from normal bones without bone destruction, clear articular surfaces, normal joint space, and no changes in cartilage and ligament structures.
2. **Rheumatoid arthritis (RA).** RA is common in women, with positive RF. The spinal lesion is mainly found in the cervical vertebra, rarely involving the thoracic vertebra and lumbar vertebra. The lesions involving sacroiliac joints are distributed bilaterally and asymmetrically. Bone erosion occurs on shallow surfaces with mild sclerosis and no significant bony ankylosis. The main pathological features of RA are synovitis and pannus formation. Enthesitis in tendons or ligaments rarely occurs, with no significant hyperostosis.
3. **Sacroiliac joint tuberculosis and spinal tuberculosis.** The diseases mostly occur in young adults and the elderly, with positive tuberculin. The spinal tuberculosis is mainly

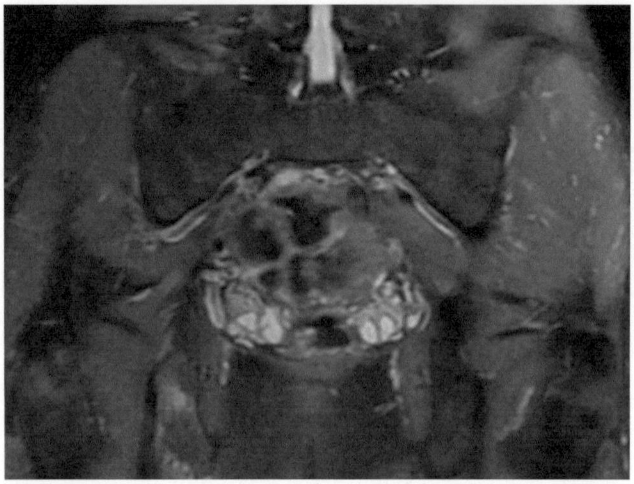

Fig. 9.26 Bony ankylosis. MRI STIR sequence shows disappearing of bilateral sacroiliac joint space and hypointense change in hyperplastic bone trabecula

Table 9.3 Clinical diagnosis criteria for AS

New York criteria (Bennett, Wood, 1966)
1. Limitation of motion of the lumbar vertebra in all 3 planes, including anterior flexion, lateral flexion, and dorsal stretch
2. A history of pain or the presence of pain at the dorsolumbar junction or in the lumbar spine
3. Limitation of thoracic cage expansion less than 2.5 cm
Patients with the following situations may be diagnosed with ankylosing spondylitis (AS)
(a) Radiographs demonstrate stage III ~ IV bilateral sacroiliitis and at least one of the above clinical manifestations is found
(b) Radiographs demonstrate grade III ~ IV unilateral sacroiliitis or grade II bilateral sacroiliitis and at least one or two of the above clinical manifestations are found
Revised New York criteria (Van der Linden, Valkenburg, Cats, 1984)
1. Low back pain for more than 3 months that improves with movement, but is not relieved by rest
2. Limitation of motion of the lumbar vertebra in the anterior and posterior and lateral flexion planes.
3. Limitation of thoracic cage expansion less than normal values for age and gender
4. Bilateral sacroiliitis grade II ~ IV or unilateral sacroiliitis grade III ~ IV
Patients who meet the item 4 and any of items 1 ~ 3 can be diagnosed with ankylosing spondylitis (AS)
ASAS classification criteria for axial spondyloarthritis (Siepr J, Rudwaleit M, Baraliakos X, 2009)
Patients who have back pain for ≥ 3 months and are aged <45 years and meet the following one item can be diagnosed with axial spondyloarthritis
1. Sacroiliitis in radiological findings and at least one characteristic of SpA
MRI reveals active (acute) inflammation in sacroiliac joints, definitely suggesting sacroiliitis related to SpA
Definite radiological changes in sacroiliitis in revised New York criteria
2. Positive HLA-B27 and at least 2 other characteristics of SpA
(1) Inflammatory back pain; (2) Arthritis; (3) Enthesitis (Achilles tendon) (4) Uveitis; (5) Dactylitis; (6) Psoriasis; (7) Crohn's disease or ulcerative colitis (8) Good response to non-steroidal anti-inflammatory drugs (NSAIDs) (9) Family history for SpA; (10) Positive HLA-B27; (11) Increased C-reactive protein

characterized by destruction of the vertebral bodies. The involvement of intervertebral disc causes intervertebral space stenosis. There may be paravertebral abscesses and sand-like sequestrum but no ligament calcification and ossification. The sacroiliac joint tuberculosis is often unilateral and located in the middle and lower portion of sacroiliac joints. Bone destruction, sequestrum formation, blurred and erosive articular surfaces, widened joint space, cold abscess and fistula formation in periarticular soft tissue can be found.

4. **Diffuse idiopathic skeletal hyperostosis (DISH) syndrome.** DISH syndrome is common in men aged over 50. Clinical manifestations and imaging findings are similar to those of AS. But ligament ossification often involves the cervical vertebra and lower thoracic vertebra with thickness and irregularity. There is normal intervertebral space, no erosion in sacroiliac joints and zygapophyseal joints, normal erythrocyte sedimentation rate, and negative HLA-B27.

9.2.2 Psoriatic Arthritis

Overview

Psoriatic arthritis (PsA) is inflammatory arthropathy associated with psoriasis and a type of SPA. The arthritis is typically characterized by dactylitis and enthesitis. Some patients may develop sacroiliitis and spondylitis, with protracted course and easy relapse. Patients with advanced arthritis may be disabled due to ankylosis. Psoriasis is closely related to arthritis. Patients with inflammatory arthritis have an increased incidence of psoriasis, and vice versa. Patients with seronegative arthritis accompanied by psoriasis reach 20%. Before the 1950s, arthritis associated with psoriasis has long been considered as part of RA. With deepening of studies on clinical manifestations, laboratory test, and imaging data, PsA has come to be recognized as an independent and definite disease. In 1964, the American College of Rheumatology first classified PsA as a rheumatic disease. Then PsA is included in spondyloarthropathy as it has similar manifestations with AS and ReA. In 1973, Wright and Moll published five clinical classification criteria including asymmetrical oligoarthritis, symmetrical polyarthritis, (distal interphalangeal) DIP-predominant arthritis, SpA, and arthritis mutilans, which have been widely used and studied up to now. In fact, the above five types have different clinical manifestations and imaging characteristics. So it is difficult to make a definite diagnosis before the occurrence of psoriasis.

PsA may occur at all ages, most likely between 20 and 30 years old. The incidence of PsA in males and females is similar. Due to the lack of unified diagnostic criteria and inclusion criteria for study population, the reported prevalence of PsA varies widely and its exact value is still unknown. A study on large sample reported that the prevalence of PsA was 0.056% ~ 0.28% in the USA, 5% ~ 10% in Russia and Norway, only 0.3% in West Africa, and approximately 1.23‰ in China. The etiology and pathogenesis of PsA are unknown, but they are considered to be related to the interaction of factors, such as heredity, immunity, environment, and infection.

The onset of PsA is insidious. Acute onset is found in 1/3 of patients, with no causes and various joint manifestations. The peripheral joints and the spine may be involved. The arthritis is usually less severe than RA, faster in remission and more common. Sometimes, the arthritis progresses into chronic arthritis and severe disability. Psoriasis occurs before arthritis in 60% ~ 70% of patients; arthritis occurs before psoriasis in 15% ~ 20% of patients; psoriasis and arthritis occur successively within one year in 15% ~ 20% of patients. PsA has a wide spectrum of arthropathy. Its clinical manifestations vary according to clinical classification [13]: (1) Asymmetric oligoarthritis accounts for 70% and mainly involves hands and IP joints in asymmetrical distribution. It is manifested as synovitis and tenosynovitis. Typical cases have sausage-like fingers (toes). (2) Symmetrical arthritis accounts for 15%. It shows similar clinical characteristics to RA. The disease may cause symmetrical involvement, morning stiffness, and fusiform swelling in PIP joints. (3) DIP arthritis, as typical PsA, accounts for 5%. DIP arthritis is related to onychodystrophy, presenting as redness and deformity. (4) SpA accounts for 5%. This disease, similar to AS, presents as syndesmophyte formation, fuzzy sacroiliac joints, and joint space stenosis. Its clinical characteristic is spinal stiffness, which often occurs after rest and in the morning. (5) Arthritis mutilans accounts for 5%. It presents as severe joint destruction and mostly affects multiple joints and sacroiliac joints of hands and feet, which is characterized by progressive paraarticular erosion. However, the above-mentioned joint manifestations are mostly changeable, bringing difficulties to diagnosis. PsA may have characteristic fingernail (toenail) involvement, including pitting, transverse ridging, onycholysis, nail edge yellowing, dystrophic hyperkeratosis, and the above mixed manifestations. Eye involvement may cause conjunctivitis, scleritis, and iritis.

There are no specific diagnosis indicators in laboratory tests. RF negative was regarded as a key to distinguishing PsA from RA. However, 5% ~ 16% of patients may have a low titer of positive RF, antinuclear antibodies in 5% of patients are positive in a low titer, and anti-CCP antibodies in 10% of patients are positive. Furthermore, patients with extensive rashes may have elevated uric acid. In the acute stage, the erythrocyte sedimentation rate and C-reactive protein may be slightly increased.

Pathophysiology

The pathological changes in PsA are similar to those in RA, but have its own characteristics, including synovitis, pannus, enthesitis, hyperostosis, osteolysis, and fibrous and bony ankylosis. The villus hyperplasia and infiltration of lymphocytes and plasma cells can be found in the affected large joint synovium. PsA is characterized prominently by vascular injury and increased number, including endothelial cell swelling, vascular wall thickening, and inflammatory cell infiltration. The early lesion of involved IP joints is synovial thickening and swelling, followed by fibrous hyperplasia, villus formation, and inflammatory cell infiltration. Excessive fibrous tissue hyperplasia may cause joint fusion, especially in PIP joints and wrist joints. The advanced lesions of DIP joints are joint destruction, bone absorption, and hyperostosis at the tendon entheses. Eventually, widened joint space is replaced by fibrous tissue.

Imaging Findings

PsA may involve synovial joints, cartilaginous joints, and entheses of tendons and ligaments of extremities and axial bones. The lesion is usually asymmetrical or unilateral in distribution and may involve joints of both upper and lower extremities. The typical lesion sites are IP joints of hands and feet, MCP joints, MTP joints, calcaneus, sacroiliac joints, and spine. Small joints and larger joints are affected significantly and severely. Imaging findings of PsA lack specificity. Osteoporosis can be observed in the early stage of the lesion, which is only used as a sign to differentiate PsA from RA. Fusiform soft tissue swelling can be found around the affected joints, such as sausage-like swelling of an entire finger (toe). In the facet joints of hands and feet, the destruction of the subchondral bone may widen the joint space. In the large joints including knee, hip, and ankle, the joint space is stenosed extensively. Bone erosion is the main imaging finding of PsA. It often occurs at the joint margin and is accompanied by entheses hyperostosis. With the progression of the lesion, the central area of the joint may also be involved. In the late stage, severe bone erosion may lead to the destruction of phalanges of fingers (toes), intra-articular bone fusion, and even subluxation deformity [3].

1. **Hand.** The arthritis mutilans in DIP joints is the most typical imaging finding of PsA. Bone erosion begins at the joint margin and progresses toward the center, causing the bone surfaces to separate from each other (Fig. 9.27). Fascicular bone absorption can be found in the distal phalanx. Coarse and distorted hyperostosis can be seen at the joint margin, forming a "pencil-in-cup" sign (Fig. 9.28). There may be intra-articular bone fusion.
2. **Foot.** PsA mainly involves IP and MTP joints in bilateral and asymmetrical distribution. PsA presents as bone erosion at the joint margin, hyperostosis, widening or

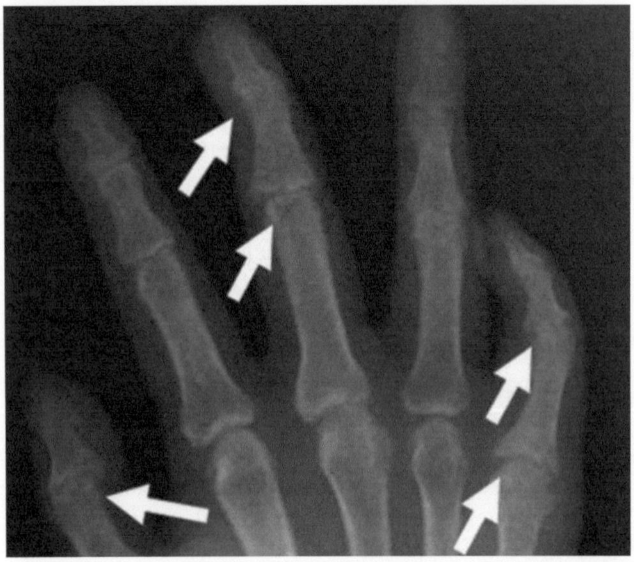

Fig. 9.27 Hand change. The radiograph shows multiple bone erosion of the first, second, and fifth IP joints as well as the fifth MCP joint (white arrows), narrowing and disappearing of joint space and hyperostosis at the joint margin

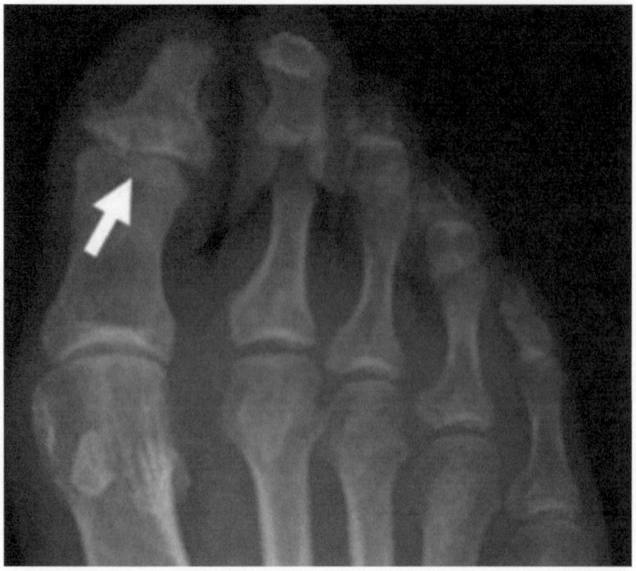

Fig. 9.29 Foot change. The radiograph shows local bone erosion and multiple hyperostosis at the basilar part of distal phalange of the hallux, and slight narrowing of joint space

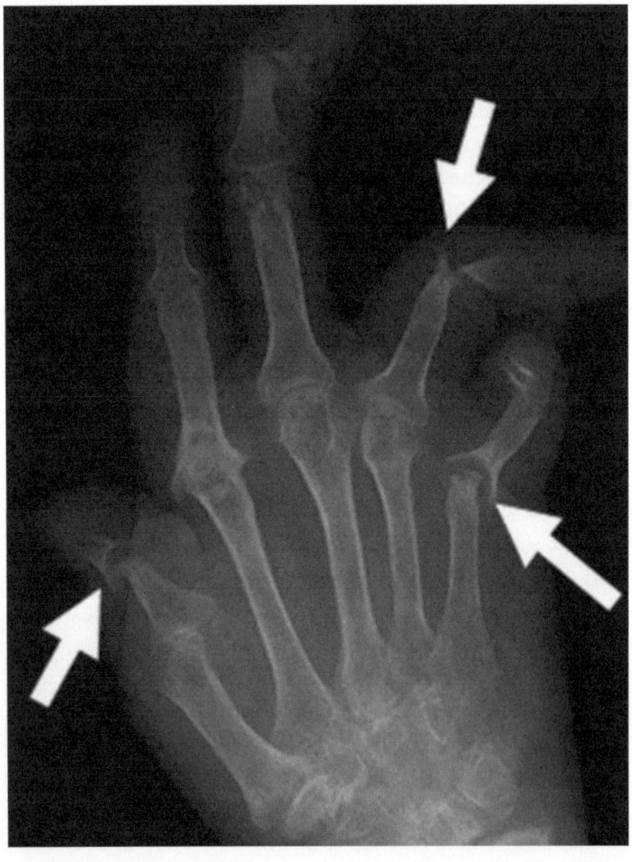

Fig. 9.28 "Pencil-in-cup" sign. The radiograph shows psoriatic arthritis mutilans, with multiple bone erosion in IP and MCP joints, "pencil-in-cup" osteolysis (white arrows) and luxation deformity

stenosis of joint space (Fig. 9.29). Extensive bone destruction in hallux IP joints and increased density in distal phalanges are relatively characteristic.

3. **Calcaneus.** The calcaneal lesions of PsA occur mainly on the posterior and lower surfaces. Retrocalcaneal bursitis may lead to low-density bone erosion on the retrocalcaneal upper surface. Bone erosion on the subcalcaneal plantar surface is often accompanied by hyperostosis at the ligament and tendon entheses, irregular osteophytes and extensive osteosclerosis. Adjacent Achilles tendons may be thickened.
4. **Sacroiliac joint.** The lesion in the sacroiliac joints is generally in bilateral and symmetrical distribution and may not be accompanied by spondylitis. Main imaging findings are erosion and osteosclerosis on the articular surface of the sacrum and widening of joint space. Joint space stenosis and bony ankylosis may also occur, which are less common than those in AS (Fig. 9.30). There may be calcification and ossification in interosseous ligaments and hyperostosis at the tendon entheses including iliac crest and ischial tuberosity.
5. **Spine.** Thoracolumbar paraspinal ossification is the typical imaging finding of PsA. The ossification is distributed unilaterally and asymmetrically and located away from the spine (Fig. 9.31), which is the main characteristic distinguishing PsA from syndesmophyte of AS. The ossification appears unilaterally. There is a wide range of round and arc-shaped high-density shadows in parallel with the vertebral lateral side. The ossification is fused

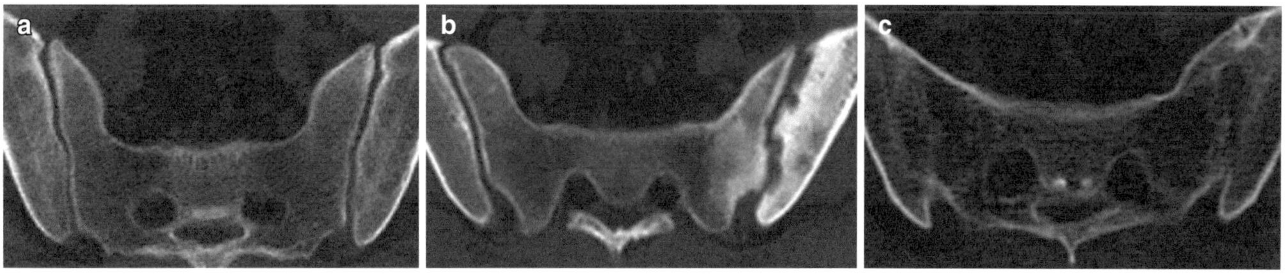

Fig. 9.30 Change in sacroiliac joint. (**a**) CT shows multiple bone erosion on the iliac articular surface of the sacroiliac joint; (**b**) Osteosclerosis and slight widening of joint space; (**c**) Bony ankylosis and joint space stenosis

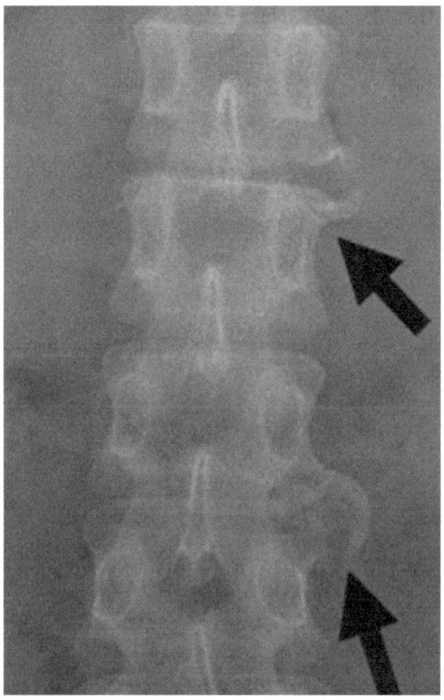

Fig. 9.31 Spinal change. The radiograph shows an asymmetrical distribution of paravertebral ligament osteophytes in the lumbar vertebra (black arrows)

Table 9.4 CASPAR (classification criteria for PsA, 2006)

In order to satisfy CASPAR criteria, patients must have inflammatory arthropathy (arthritis, spondylitis, or dactylitis) and at least three points from the following items:

1. Evidence of psoriasis (any one item of a, b, and c)
   (a) Current psoriasis[a]—Presence of skin or scalp psoriasis judged by a rheumatologist or dermatologist in the visit
   (b) Past history of psoriasis—A history of psoriasis obtained from a patient, family member, dermatologist, rheumatologist, or other qualified health care providers
   (c) Family history of psoriasis—Presence of psoriasis in a first or second degree relative as reported by the patient
2. Psoriatic nail dystrophy—Typical psoriatic nail dystrophy including onycholysis, pitting and hyperkeratosis observed on current physical examination
3. Negative rheumatoid factor (RF)—Preferably using ELISA method or nephelometry for detection
4. Dactylitis (any one item of a and b)
   (a) Swelling of an entire digit observed currently
   (b) Medical history—A history of dactylitis recorded by a rheumatologist
5. Radiographic evidence of periarticular new-bone formation—Ill-defined ossification at the joint margin (excluding osteophyte formation) on X-ray plain film of the hand or foot

[a]Current psoriasis is assigned a score of 2, and other items are assigned a score of 1

with basal tissue of the bony intervertebral disc. The osteitis at the edge of vertebral bodies, change in vertebral body squaring as well as sclerosis and ankylosis of zygapophyseal joints are less common and less severe than those in AS.

Key Points of Diagnosis

As for patients with arthritis occurring before psoriasis, it is difficult to make a diagnosis of PsA. If patients have asymmetrical arthritis combined with dactylitis, enthesitis, or inflammatory low back pain and negative RF, the possibility of PsA needs to be considered, and the diagnosis can be confirmed only after skin and nail lesions occur. At present, CASPAR (classification criteria for the study of psoriatic arthritis study) classification criteria in 2006 [14] (Table 9.4) is commonly used internationally. These criteria include clinical manifestations, signs and imaging findings of psoriasis, and peripheral arthritis or spondyloarthritis in combination with medical history. Such criteria have 99% of specificity and 91% of sensitivity in diagnosis. Imaging examinations can be used as diagnosis clues, contributing to distinguishing PsA from AS, osteoarthritis and gout, etc.

Differential Diagnosis

1. **Rheumatoid arthritis (RA).** In the small joints of hands and feet, typical PsA lesions occur in distal phalangeal joints in asymmetrical and extensive distribution. There are severe erosion and bony ankylosis without osteoporosis at the edge and center of the joint. RA mainly involves PIP joints in bilateral and symmetrical distribution. RA is characterized by osteoporosis, soft tissue swelling, joint space stenosis, and marginal bone erosion. As for spinal lesions, RA primarily affects the cervical vertebra. Thoracolumbar lesions are rare, and paravertebral ossification will not occur. The sacroiliac joint lesion is uncom-

mon in RA, mainly presenting as bone erosion without osteosclerosis.

2. **Other seronegative spondyloarthropathies (SPAs).** The imaging findings of PsA are similar to those of AS and ReA. The above diseases involve synovial joints and cause soft tissue swelling, widening or stenosis of joint space, bone erosion, and hyperostosis without osteoporosis. Moreover, in cartilaginous joints, they are associated with enthesitis changes in tendons and ligaments. However, the three diseases have differences. In terms of lesion distribution, PsA is in asymmetrical multi-joint involvement and often occurs in IP and MTP joints and the spine; AS mainly involves the axial bone, but rarely extremities; ReA is characterized by asymmetrical involvement of lower extremity joints. Bony ankylosis is common In PsA and AS, but rare in ReA. The three diseases may involve the spine and sacroiliac joints, but AS is usually a bilateral and asymmetrical lesion causing filamentous symmetrical syndesmophytes next to the spine, and zygapophyseal joints are affected significantly. PsA and ReA present as asymmetrical broad paravertebral ossification in the axial bone, and osteitis, vertebral body squaring, and zygapophyseal joint lesions are all mild.
3. **Osteoarthritis.** It is common in the elderly. Osteoarthritis mostly involves weight-bearing joints and causes pain. Pain is aggravated with movement and relieved by rest. Inflammatory indicators including erythrocyte sedimentation rate and C-reactive protein are normal. Main imaging findings are hyperostosis, osteosclerosis, and heterogeneous stenosis of joint space. The changes in bone erosion mostly appear under cartilage rather than at the joint margin. Osteolysis rarely occurs in distal fingers (toes). The paraspinal osteophyte is thicker with transverse course parallel to the intervertebral disc. Sacroiliac joint changes rarely appear.

9.2.3 Reactive Arthritis

Overview

Reactive arthritis (ReA) is a sterile arthritis secondary to an infection in another part of the body and mainly refers to SpA occurring after intestinal and urinogenital infections. ReA is characterized by asymmetrical joint involvement in both lower extremities and spinal lesions due to its association with HLA-B27, which is classified as a type of spondyloarthropathy. The correlation between acute arthritis and diarrhea or urethritis was recognized as early as the eighteenth century. In 1916, arthritis, urethritis, and conjunctivitis are collectively known as Reiter syndrome (RS) in numerous cases, often associated with mucous injury. Later, many patients do not present with the complete clinical trial. Meanwhile, ReA has covered RA and both are gradually integrated. At present, RS is only used to describe a reflection of the medical history.

The typical pathogenic bacterium of ReA triggered by a genital tract infection is Chlamydia trachomatis, and 4% of infected individuals will develop ReA. The typical pathogens of ReA triggered by a gastrointestinal infection include Yersinia, Shigella, Salmonella, Campylobacter, and rare Clostridium difficile. ReA occurs most often between ages 18 and 40, but children aged over 5 and the elderly may also develop ReA. ReA triggered by sexually transmitted infections mainly occurs in young men. Women, children, and the elderly usually develop ReA in response to the intestinal bacterial infection. The prevalence due to a triggering infection and genetic susceptibility factors are different among different populations. The flora varies greatly. So it is difficult to obtain the overall prevalence and incidence of ReA. The incidence in Scandinavian Peninsula has been reported to be 10 ~ 30/100,000.

The etiology and pathogenesis of ReA are still unclear, but they are currently believed to be caused by multi-factor interaction of heredity, immunity, and external environment. Among patients treated in hospitals, 60% ~ 80% of patients have positive HLA-B27 and severe arthritis and extra-articular symptoms. The HLA-B27 positive rate in general population only increases slightly or not at all. HLA-B27 appears to promote chronic ReA. One hypothesis holds that there is a cross-reaction between the microbial structure and HLA-B27 or that HLA-B27 may be the target of immune response. ReA-triggered microbes can produce lipopolysaccharides, which have the ability to attack mucosal surface, entering host cells and surviving inside the cells. In studies, DNA and RNA of Chlamydia, Yersinia, Shigella, and Salmonella have been detected in the synovial fluid of ReA patients, but their specificity is unclear. Those can also be found in the synovial fluid of other rheumatoid diseases. Furthermore, other studies have found CD4 + T cells and high-level IL-17 in patients' synovial fluid, which may be associated with weak immune response.

ReA may range from transient monoarthritis to severe multi-system diseases based on clinical manifestations. The typical arthritis appears in 1 ~ 4 weeks after the intestinal or urogenital infections, generally in acute onset. The asymmetric oligoarthritis primarily occurs. Arthritis usually involves large joints of lower extremities, common in knees, ankles, and MTP joints, and wrist and IP joints may also be involved. Diffuse swelling in periarticular soft tissue presenting as sausage fingers (toes), pale skin and increased skin temperature are found. In 30% of patients, their acute low back pain may radiate to the buttocks and worsens at night. Tendinitis and enthesitis have certain characteristics, especially at Achilles tendon, plantar fascia, and spinal entheses. The arthritis may last for 1 ~ 3 months and even half year, then gradually disappears, but it has a tendency to relapse. Urogenital infection lesions may occur throughout the course of disease. Men commonly develop prostatitis and cystitis, and women often have cervicitis or salpingitis with mild symptoms. 50% of patients have skin and mucosal symptoms, presenting as oral ulcer, skin hyperkeratosis, vesicle, erythema, papule, and so on. One-third patients may have conjunctivitis and 5% of patients may have acute iritis, with the risk of blindness if untreated in time. Aortic lesion and cardiac conduction abnormalities are rare.

The only specific laboratory test for ReA is designed to identify pathogens, that is, to isolate pathogenic microorganisms from patient samples. Reactants including leukocyte and C-reactive protein in the acute stage may increase and the erythrocyte sedimentation rate is elevated, without specificity. HLA-B27 testing is often used to support diagnosis.

Pathophysiology

The main pathological change of ReA is synovial inflammation. There is synovial edema, congestion of blood vessels, fibrin exudation, infiltration of neutrophils, lymphocytes and plasma cells, and hyperplasia of synovial cells and fibrocytes in the acute stage. Pannus formation and cartilage erosion may be found in the chronic stage. Lesions including enthesitis and tenosynovitis may occur.

Imaging Findings

ReA may involve synovial joints, cartilaginous joints, and entheses of axial tendons and ligaments. Typical lesions commonly occur in lower extremity joints in asymmetrical distribution. Characteristic affected sites are IP joints, calcaneus, ankle joints, knee joints, sacroiliac joints, and the spine of feet. The imaging findings of ReA are similar to those of AS and PsA, lacking relative specificity, but different from those of RA. Diffuse soft tissue swelling and joint effusion can be found in affected joints, commonly in IP joints of hands and feet, presenting sausage-like change. A large amount of effusion can be seen in knee and ankle joints. Acute inflammation may be accompanied by periarticular osteoporosis, which can be alleviated with the progression of the disease. Joint space stenosis is more common in small joints of hands and feet than in knee and ankle joints. Bone erosion occurs first at the joint margin and then involves gradually the subchondral bone at the joint center, which is often associated with joint space loss. Hyperostosis is the most prominent feature of SPA, which is characterized by linear periosteum hyperostosis, irregular hyperostosis at the tendon and ligament entheses, and intra-articular hyperostosis. The sclerosis of adjacent bones and subchondral bone may occur. Bony ankylosis may appear in small joints of hands and feet, but is uncommon. Tendon calcification and ossification occur more frequently in knee joints and may be related to hyperostosis at entheses.

1. **Foot.** Asymmetrical involvement of MTP and IP joints may occur in 40% ~ 50% of patients. The serious involvement of hallux IP joints often suggests ReA or PsA. Basic imaging findings are osteoporosis, joint space loss, and marginal bone erosion accompanied by adjacent hyperostosis. There may be periostitis in metatarsal and phalangeal diaphysis, as well as erosion and hyperostosis in sesamoid. In severe cases, the subluxation and deformities (known as Launois deformity) of MTP joints may be found.
2. **Calcaneus.** Lesions are the characteristic manifestation of ReA and often associated with clinical symptoms and signs. Both posterior and inferior borders of the calcaneus may be involved, more often bilaterally. Retrocalcaneal bursitis forms radiopaque shadows on the lateral view, resulting in the disappearance of the normal radiolucent area between the top of the calcaneus and the Achilles tendon. Then, bone erosion can be seen on the retrocalcaneal superior border and Achilles tendon is often thickened without osteophyte at its entheses, which is the key to differentiate ReA from AS and PsA. Bone erosion, hyperostosis, and irregular osteophytes at the entheses may be formed on the calcaneal inferior border (Fig. 9.32), which are similar to relevant findings of AS and PsA.
3. **Ankle joint.** Unilateral or bilateral ankle joint lesions may occur in 30–50% of patients, including soft tissue swelling, linear periostitis of distal tibiofibular diaphysis, joint space loss, and marginal bone erosion (Fig. 9.33).
4. **Knee joint.** The most common findings are joint effusion, osteoporosis (Fig. 9.34), periostitis in the distal femur and proximal tibia, and bone erosion.
5. **Sacroiliac joint.** Sacroiliitis is common in ReA, which may be a bilateral symmetrical or asymmetrical lesion,

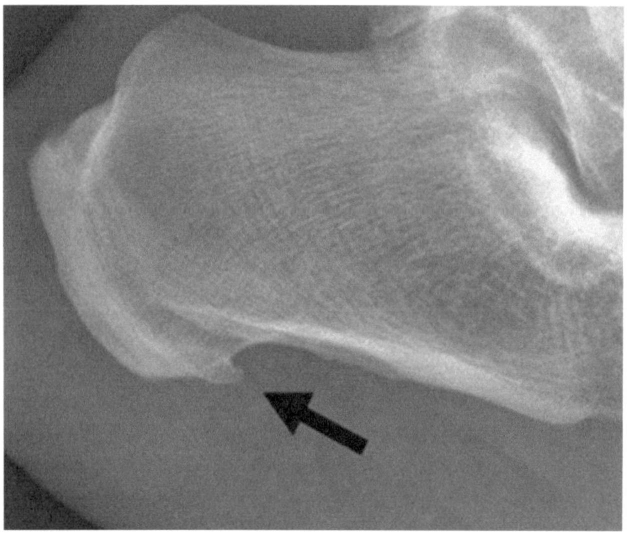

Fig. 9.32 Calcaneal change. The radiograph shows hyperostosis on calcaneal plantar surface (black arrow)

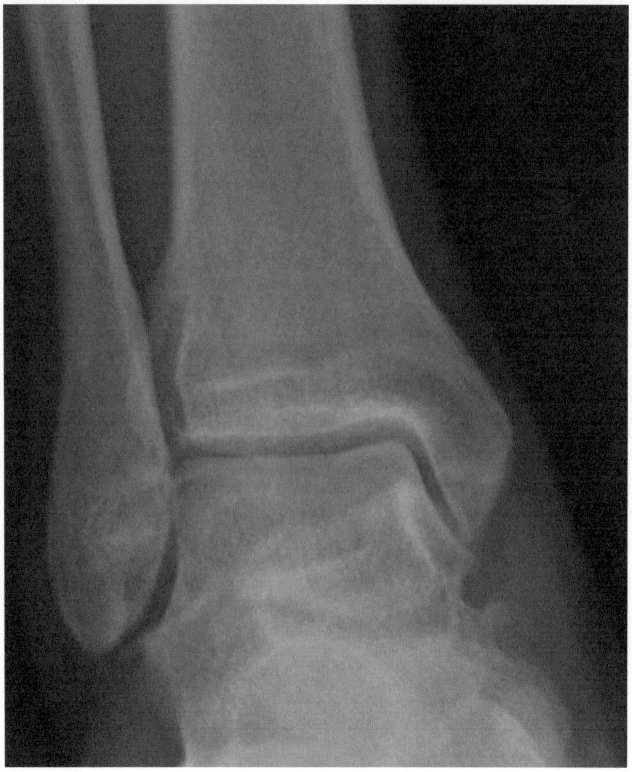

Fig. 9.33 Change in ankle joint. The radiograph shows irregular hyperostosis of medial malleolus and talus, associated with soft tissue swelling

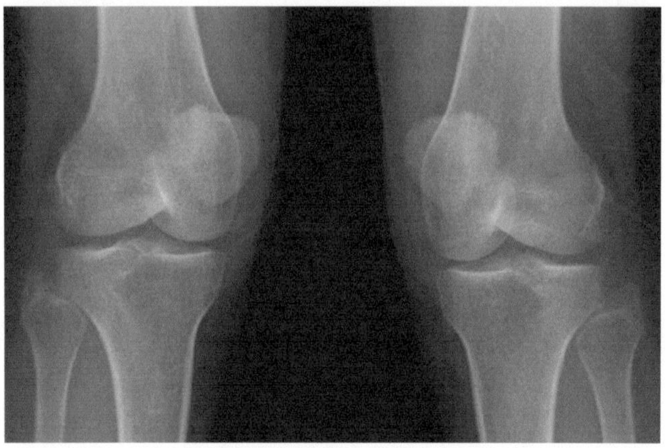

Fig. 9.34 Change in knee joint. The radiograph shows osteoporosis in both knee joints associated with soft tissue swelling

with unilateral onset in some cases. The typical AS is a constant bilateral symmetrical lesion. Bone erosion is more obvious on the ilium surface than on the sacrum surface, and bone sclerosis can be seen (Figs. 9.35 and 9.36). Joint space may be widened in the early stage and narrowed in the late stage, eventually causing bone fusion.

6. **Spine.** The spinal lesion of ReA is similar to that of PsA, but different from that of AS. Thoracolumbar paraspinal ossification is an early finding of ReA. Ossification is in unilateral asymmetrical distribution. The long and narrow longitudinal bone bridge extends across the intervertebral disc and keeps a distinct distance from the intervertebral disc and the external margin of the vertebral body. The ossification has various shapes and eventually fuses with the intervertebral disc and vertebral body below the ossification area to form a large osteophyte. Osteitis at the edge of vertebral bodies and erosion and sclerosis of the zygapophyseal joints are less common.

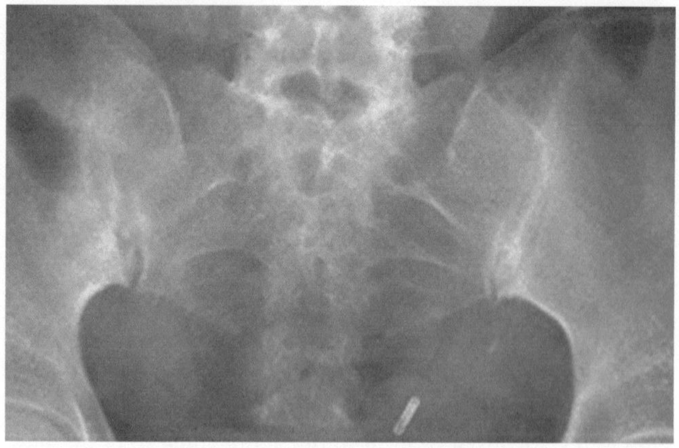

Fig. 9.35 Change in sacroiliac joint (1). The radiograph shows irregular bilateral sacroiliac joint surfaces, and local bone erosion and sclerosis

Key Points of Diagnosis

ReA is a type of SpA associated with intestinal or urogenital infections. ReA is diagnosed clinically without laboratory tests or imaging findings for its definite diagnosis. Thus, when patients have clinical manifestations of spondyloarthropathy, such as asymmetric oligoarthritis of lower extremities, ligament or tendon enthesitis and positive HLA-B27, whether they have a history of diarrhea, dysuria, or other prodromic infections should be asked, if possible. In addition to joint lesions, attention should be paid to the extra-articular involvement including eyes, skin, mucosa, nails, and genitals in physical examination. Serological culture helps confirm the presence of infection.

The classification criteria proposed by Kingsley and Sieper in 1996 are mostly used in the current diagnosis of ReA [15].

1. Asymmetric oligoarthritis, predominantly in lower limbs.
2. Evidence of prodromic infection: (1) Where clear clinical diarrhea or urethritis within preceding four weeks, laboratory evidence is desirable but not essential; (2) Where no clear clinical infection, laboratory evidence of infection is essential.
3. Other causes of oligoarthritis, such as other seronegative spondyloarthropathies, infectious arthritis, Lyme disease, and streptococcal ReA, should be excluded.

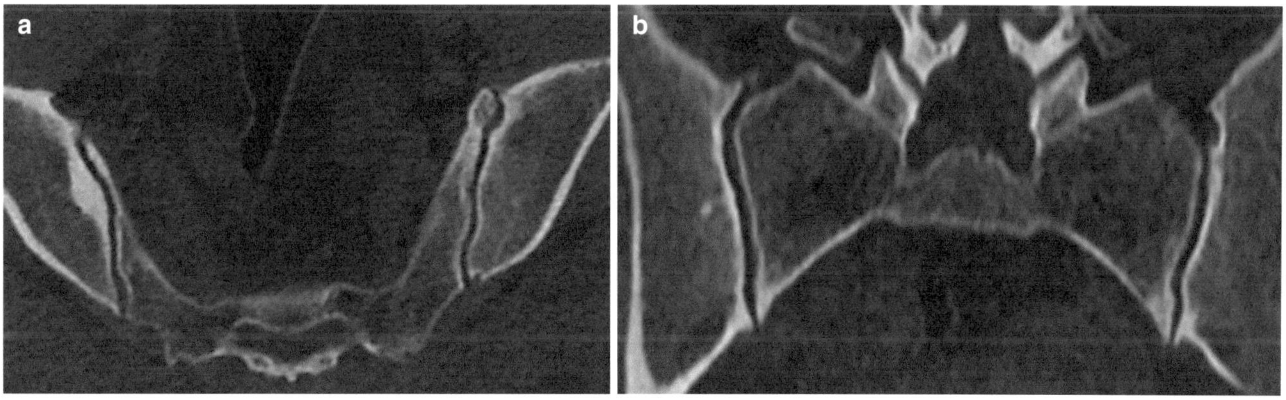

Fig. 9.36 Change in sacroiliac joint (2). CT shows local bone erosion and sclerosis of bilateral ilium surfaces of sacroiliac joint, and no narrowing of joint space

4. The positive HLA-B27 or extra-articular manifestations of ReA (iritis, conjunctivitis, skin, cardiac and nerve system diseases, etc.) or typically clinical features of sacroiliitis (inflammatory low back pain, alternating buttock pain, tendon enthesitis, etc.) are helpful in supporting the diagnosis, but they are not necessary conditions for definite diagnosis.

Differential Diagnosis

1. **Bacterial arthritis.** It is often monoarthritis. The acute-onset arthritis causes high fever, fatigue, and obvious redness, swelling, heat and pain in joints. The pathogens can be found by synovial fluid smear or bacterial culture. Bacterial arthritis may have imaging changes similar to ReA, including soft tissue swelling, osteoporosis, joint effusion, local bone erosion, and periostitis. However, the multiple joint involvement of ReA can achieve the accurate differentiation between ReA and bacterial arthritis.
2. **Other seronegative spondyloarthropathies (SPAs).** The imaging findings of ReA are similar to those of AS and PsA, but ReA has its own characteristics in the lesion distribution. ReA mainly includes symmetrical arthritis of lower extremities, sacroiliitis, and rare spondylitis. AS involves primarily the axial bone; the cervical spondylosis is more common in AS than in ReA, and AS more rarely occurs in peripheral joints than ReA. PsA may involve extremities and axial joints and is more significant in extensive involvement of upper extremities. All the three SPAs may present soft tissue swelling, joint space stenosis, bone erosion, and hyperostosis. Osteoporosis of ReA is more common than that of the other two diseases, and the intra-articular bony ankylosis is less common. The sacroiliac joint and spinal lesions of ReA are essentially identical to those of PsA, but these lesions of PsA have a higher incidence and are more severe. ReA and PsA present with asymmetrical paravertebral osteophytes and symmetrical or asymmetrical sacroiliac joint lesion. AS is apparently different from the two diseases and presents with symmetrical sacroiliac joint lesion and paravertebral osteophytes.
3. **Rheumatoid arthritis (RA).** RA is very different from ReA. RA is common in women, with positive RF and no history of early infection. RA involves small joints of the extremities to present as bilateral symmetrical lesion, and osteoporosis, joint space narrowing, and marginal bone erosion can be seen, with rare hyperostosis. RA involves mainly the cervical vertebra and rarely the thoracolumbar vertebra and the sacroiliac joints.
4. **Gouty arthritis.** Gouty arthritis is common in middle-aged and elderly men. Its predilection site is the first MTP joint. The blood uric acid level is elevated. The disease presents as acute arthritis in recurrent attack, as well as redness and swelling of joints associated with intense pain. Imaging findings show juxta-articular cataclastic calcified tophi, eccentric erosion and destruction of adjacent bone structures, and no joint space stenosis.

9.2.4 Enteropathic Arthritis

Overview

Enteropathic arthritis is an arthritis associated with the inflammatory bowel disease (IBD) and a type of SPA. Enteropathic arthritis is a general term for several different clinical conditions. The association between arthritis and IBD was recognized as early as the 1930s, and then the pathological changes between gastrointestinal and musculoskeletal lesions were further verified. In the 1970s, enteropathic arthritis is incorporated into the concept of spondyloarthropathy. Currently recognized intestinal diseases with rheumatoid manifestations mainly include ulcerative colitis, Crohn's disease, Whipple's disease (intestinal lipodystrophy), and SAPHO syndrome (synovitis, acne, impetigo, hyperostosis, and osteitis). In addition, musculoskeletal disorders may also occur after some intestinal infections and intestinal bypass surgery, which may be complicated with some parenteral diseases, such as biliary cirrhosis, pancreatic diseases, and atrophic portal cirrhosis. The prevalence of ulcerative colitis and Crohn's disease is similar, 0.05% ~ 0.1%. In recent years, the incidences of both diseases have increased. AS and peripheral arthritis are related to IBD. It has been reported that 1% ~ 10% of IBD patients have AS and 10% ~ 50% have peripheral arthritis.

The correlation between IBD and arthritis is unclear, but may be related to multiple theories. First, intestinal pathogens attack joints or infect the intestinal tract and joints. Second, the gastrointestinal tract and joints have same tissue antigens activating immune response, or damage to the normal intestinal mucosal barrier forms immune complexes, then damaging joints. Studies have found that ulcerative colitis, Crohn's disease, and AS all have genetic factors involved and are related to HLA-B27, which increases the susceptibility of human body to infection. GWAS has shown that ulcerative colitis and Crohn's disease have some common susceptibility genes and their own specific genes.

It is difficult to clinically distinguish AS associated with IBD from idiopathic AS. The spinal involvement can be found in 10% ~ 20% of cases, and latent back pain may occur before or after IBD, with no significant difference in gender. Peripheral arthritis may occur in 5% ~ 15% of patients. Patients with Crohn's disease are slightly more than those with ulcerative colitis. The joint lesion may be acute self-limited oligoarthritis or chronic symmetric polyarthritis. Joint erosion and deformity rarely occur. The joint lesion of ulcerative colitis has the same activity as enteropathy, but Crohn's disease is different from ulcerative colitis. Isolated destructive osphyarthrosis is a rare complication of Crohn's disease. The extraintestinal manifestations of IBD include acropachy, uveitis, erythema nodosa, and pyoderma gangrenosum. These manifestations have a high incidence in Crohn's disease.

The laboratory test revealed inflammatory and metabolic manifestations of IBD. Articular synovial fluid is a mildly inflammatory change with synovial cell hyperplasia, fibroblast hyperplasia, and increased vascularization. Positive HLA-B27 may be found in 30% ~ 70% of IBD patients. The erythrocyte sedimentation rate may be elevated and platelets may be increased.

Pathophysiology

IBD-related peripheral arthritis has basically the same pathological features in synovial tissues as other spondyloarthropathies. It has been reported in a study that ulcerative colitis is non-specific synovitis, and Crohn's disease is a granulomatous disease.

Imaging Findings

The imaging findings of IBD-related peripheral arthritis have no specificity. Soft tissue swelling and periarticular osteoporosis are the most common X-ray findings, but can be observed in many diseases related to synovial membranes. Bone erosion, cysts, and joint space stenosis can be rarely seen. IBD-related sacroiliac joint and spinal lesions are indistinguishable from typical AS. The sacroiliac joints are usually involved bilaterally and symmetrically, but occasionally have asymmetrical change, especially in Crohn's disease. The spinal lesion may be characterized by typical squaring of the vertebral body, vertebral erosion and sclerosis, bilateral and symmetrical syndesmophytes, as well as erosion and space stenosis of zygapophyseal joints, which are consistent with relevant findings of typical AS (Fig. 9.37).

Key Points of Diagnosis

Detailed medical history and clinical examinations in combination with imaging examination are considered as important diagnostic tools. Enteropathy and arthritis are common diseases and may co-exist due to multiple causes. When the etiology is related to the pathogenesis, ReA and enteropathic arthritis are the most common causes.

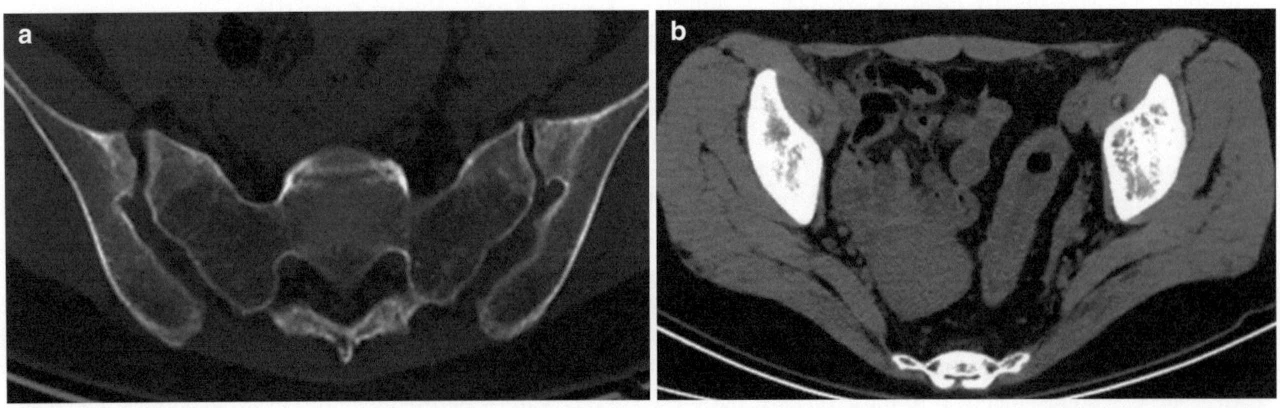

Fig. 9.37 Change in sacroiliac joint (4). (**a**) CT shows no obvious narrowing of the sacroiliac joint space and local irregularity and sclerosis of the articular surface; (**b**) Edema and thickening of the partial sigmoid colon wall; colonoscopic diagnosis as colitis

Differential Diagnosis

1. **Other seronegative spondyloarthropathies (SPAs).** IBD-related spinal and sacroiliac joint lesions are indistinguishable from typical AS, presenting with bilateral symmetrical lesions and paravertebral syndesmophytes, which are different from the manifestations of PsA and ReA. The manifestations of latter two are asymmetrical or unilateral sacroiliac joint lesions and extensive asymmetrical spinal osteophytes.
2. **Rheumatoid arthritis (RA).** IBD-related arthritis of the extremities shows no specific imaging findings. Soft tissue swelling and osteoporosis are the only common findings which may be similar to early findings of RA. The diagnosis of enteropathic arthritis can be basically excluded if joint space stenosis and bone erosion are found.

Status Quo and Progress of Research

Although the above four SPAs vary in lesion distribution, morphology, and degree, overall, their imaging and pathological features are very similar. The current imaging examination still is mainly X-ray plain film. Research on MRI techniques focuses on sacroiliitis, in order to provide more information for early diagnosis, activity predication and response to treatment of diseases.

1. **DCE-MRI.** DCE-MRI is an imaging method that can indirectly reflect the status of blood perfusion and the degree of vascularization in tissue of interest through an intravenous injection of contrast agent. The superior temporal resolution of MRI offers possibilities of contrast agent dynamics modeling with DCE-MRI and the quantitative parameter evaluation. Therefore, DCE-MRI can not only evaluate the changes in capillary permeability, microcirculation, and blood flow in the lesion area but also directly reflect the blood perfusion rate of the lesion area. In the study of sacroiliitis, DCE-MRI is used mainly to evaluate the inflammatory activity and therapeutic effect of sacroiliitis through the degree of vascularization and the blood perfusion in the sacroiliac joint surface bone marrow. The time-intensity curve of the sacroiliac joint is roughly divided into three types: platform, rapid rise and drop, and slow rise and drop. The study of Shi et al. [16] showed that the time-intensity curves of patients with sacroiliitis mainly are rapid rise and drop type (44%) and slow rise and drop type (56%), as well as the enhancement coefficient, enhancement slope, and time to peak (TTP) before and after treatment were different significantly. These results indicate that MRI can be used to evaluate the inflammatory reaction and therapeutic effect of early sacroiliitis to provide reliable imaging evidence for clinical practice.
2. **DWI** is an imaging method to detect the random movement of water molecules in different tissues. The change in the ratio of extracellular water to intracellular water due to inflammatory reaction can result in the relevant change in DWI signal intensity. ADC values are used to quantify the diffusion rate of water molecules. Bozgeyik et al. [17] believed that bone marrow edema can lead to the accelerated movement of water molecules, elevated diffuse rate, and increased ADC value. Therefore, in patients with sacroiliitis, the ADC value of bone marrow edema area increased, and decreased after treatment, which suggested that the infiltration of inflammatory cells and formation of bone marrow edema were reduced after intervention treatment.
3. **IDEAL-IQ sequence.** It is an emerging MR fat quantification imaging method for the assessment of fat fraction (FF) in tissues and organs. This technique corrects factors that affect MR signal intensity, such as T_1 bias, T_2* attenuation, multiple peaks of fat spectrum and noise bias, and can accurately assess fat fraction in tissues, avoid the bias in subjective assessment of fat infiltration. Bone marrow adipogenesis is considered as a possible repair response to inflammation. The study of Ren et al. [18] revealed that fat fraction (65.9% ± 12.1%) of patients with sacroiliitis in the active group was significantly higher than that in the active group (40.2% ± 47.8%) and healthy control group (45.8% ± 8.89%), indicating that fat fraction can be used as an index parameter to evaluate the activity of sacroiliitis.

9.3 Gouty Arthritis

Jun Zhou and He Sun

Overview

Gout is a group of heterogeneous disorders with increased blood uric acid caused by purine metabolism disorder and/or uric acid excretion disorder. Hyperuricemia results in the deposition of urate crystals in articular capsule, bursa, cartilage, bone and other tissues, causing gouty arthritis. There were records on gout in the Babylonian Talmud and the Bible over 2000 years ago. However, it was not until 1683 that gout was first described classically by Thomas Sydenham. In 1798, Antoine Francois de Fourcroy, a French scientist, found an organic acid in normal urine, called uric acid, and then confirmed its close relationship with gout. In 1896, Huber first reported the X-ray findings of gout shortly after the discovery of X-ray. In 1961, McCarty and Hollander's application of a polarizing light microscope to the analysis of synovial fluid is a milestone for gout and other crystal-related diseases. Scientists found that arthritis caused by the deposition of different microcrystals including monosodium urate (MSU), calcium pyrophosphate dihydrate (CPPD), calcium apatite, and calcium oxalate has similar clinical manifestations, but also has significant differences. Gouty arthritis that was believed before the introduction of crystallographic detection techniques into rheumatology is not necessarily a true gout. Therefore, it is greatly important for crystal-induced associated diseases to distinguish different types of crystals through the analysis of synovial fluid.

Kelley and Wortmann classified gout into three types based on its cause [19]: (1) Primary gout is a congenital disease that is neither secondary to an acquired disease nor a secondary manifestation to a birth defect that causes non-gout disease; (2) Secondary gout occurs in the progression process of other diseases or due to drugs. It is usually hyperuricemia caused by excessive uric acid production or inhibition of uric acid excretion arising from drugs, hematopathy, renal failure, and chemoradiotherapy. (3) Idiopathic gout refers to a case that cannot be clearly classified. Gout more often occurs in young and middle-aged men, but also appears in postmenopausal women. The ratio of male to female reaches up to 20 to 1. The peak age of onset is more than 40 years old. The incidence of gout is increasing year by year, and different races and populations have different incidences. The overall prevalence is 1% ~ 15.3%, which is positively correlated with age and the level of blood uric acid.

The natural course of gout may be divided into the following stages [11, 13]: (1) asymptomatic hyperuricemia; (2) acute gouty arthritis; (3) intercritical gout; (4) Chronic tophaceous gouty arthritis. Asymptomatic hyperuricemia is defined as no clinical symptoms or signs with a serum urate concentration of more than 420 μmol/L. The majority of patients with hyperuricemia may remain asymptomatic for life, and only 5% ~ 22% of patients eventually develop gout, as a result of elevated blood uric acid level and accumulation of uric acid. The incidence of gout apparently increases with the age and blood uric acid level. The acute attack of urinary calculi and/or gouty arthritis marks the end of this stage. Typically acute gouty arthritis often breaks out at night for the first time, starting with acute painful arthritis, usually in a single joint. Gout commonly occurs in joints of the lower extremities. The first MTP joint is most frequently involved, and 90% of patients with gout eventually have the lesion in the joint. Other commonly affected joints are IP joint, ankle joint, knee joint, wrist joint, fingers and elbow joint; axial joints are rarely affected. The first episode of acute gouty arthritis usually occurs suddenly in a deep sleep at night. The patient may be awakened by pain and unable to fall asleep. The patient also suffers from redness, swelling, heat and pain in the affected joint, and limitation of motion. The attack lasts for several hours to several weeks and then resolves spontaneously, progressing into intercritical gout. Most patients have the second episode within 6 months to 2 years. As time goes by, untreated patients have increasingly frequent episodes. When the stage of intercritical gout is shortened and affected joints are increased without remission, the disease progresses into chronic tophaceous gouty arthritis. Typical tophi are common in the auricle, first MTP joint, finger and elbow joint. Repeated inflammatory erosion causes joint bone destruction, synovitis, joint effusion and fibrosis, joint swelling, stiffness and deformity, as well as limitation of motion. Urate crystals deposit in the kidney and may form urinary calculi, resulting in decreased renal function and even renal failure.

In a laboratory test, the blood uric acid is often elevated. The uric acid is above 457.5 μmol/L in 95% of patients. In 24-h urine, the uric acid level is not necessarily parallel to the level of blood uric acid. The erythrocyte sedimentation rate and the leukocytes are increased. Urate crystals can be seen in synovial fluid and urine. Birefringent needle-shaped urate crystals can be observed in leukocytes under a polarization microscope, as a specific diagnosis basis for gout.

Pathophysiology

The gross examination shows that urate crystals are deposited in the synovial membrane, articular cartilage, ligament, tendinous sheath and other tissues, there is extensive erosion of articular cartilage, and osseous tissue, and cartilage hyperplasia and osteophyte formation are found at the edge of articular cartilage. Tissue necrosis occurs in the urate deposition area. The necrotic tissue and urate crystals forming a core in the center are combined with peripheral inflammatory tissue to form a topus, as the characteristic lesion of gout. Microscopic findings in the acute stage are synovial hyperemia and edema, as well as hyperplasia of synovial tissues with inflammatory cell infiltration. Microscopic findings in the chronic stage include characteristic gouty granuloma, urate crystals in radial and needle-shaped arrangement, accompanied by calcification or ossification and surrounded by histiocytes and giant cells [4].

Imaging Findings

The diagnosis of gout mainly depends on clinical manifestations and laboratory tests. An imaging examination is primarily used to evaluate the involvement scope and extent of gouty arthritis as well as the presence or absence of tophus formation. Plain radiography is still the preferred imaging examination method for gout. However, the majority of patients do not show joint structure abnormalities on X-ray plain films in many years after clinical symptoms of gout. Periarticular soft tissue swelling appearing in the acute stage is a result of synovial inflammation and soft tissue edema. As the acute stage subsides, the above imaging finding will also disappear. Recurrent arthritis forms chronic tophi, causing permanent imaging abnormalities. CT and MRI play a limited role in gout and are relatively infrequently used. They mainly evaluate sites that cannot be displayed on plain radiographs, such as spine and sacroiliac joints [3].

1. **X-ray**
   (a) Periarticular soft tissue swelling: There is eccentric soft tissue swelling around the affected joint, with the appearance of nodular mass and high density. This sign is common in foot, hand, and ankle, elbow, and knee joints. The eccentric swelling of dorsal soft tissue of the first MTP joint is its typical manifestation (Fig. 9.38).
   (b) Tophus formation: Irregular high-density shadows in intra-articular and periarticular soft tissues denote tophi (Fig. 9.39).
   (c) Soft tissue or intraosseous calcification: Tophus calcification is uncommon and may be found in patients with combined abnormal calcium metabolism. Calcification is deposited around soft tissue masses, presenting as irregular or cloud-like dense shadows, generally with higher X-ray density than tophi (Fig. 9.40). Intraosseous calcification occurs in the intraosseous urate deposition area, spreading from the joint margin, through the articular cartilage surface to spongy bone. Intraosseous calcification of gout is most common in hands and feet. X-ray finding is focal or diffuse calcinoses involving subchondral or subligamentous bony structures. The change is similar to that of enchondroma, bone infarction or infection.
   (d) Changes in joint space: No narrowing of joint space in the early stage is a characteristic of gouty arthritis. In the late stage, homogeneous joint space stenosis is found, similar to RA. Articular cartilage is damaged seriously and may cause ankylosis and deformity, which is rare except for the IP joints.
   (e) Bone erosion: The typical sites are the distal medial and dorsal parts of the first metatarsus. Bone erosion occurs originally at the joint margin, gradually into the joint and away from the articular surface. Destructive foci are single or multiple with different sizes, mostly in round or oval shape, whose long axis is parallel to the long axis of bone structure. Bone

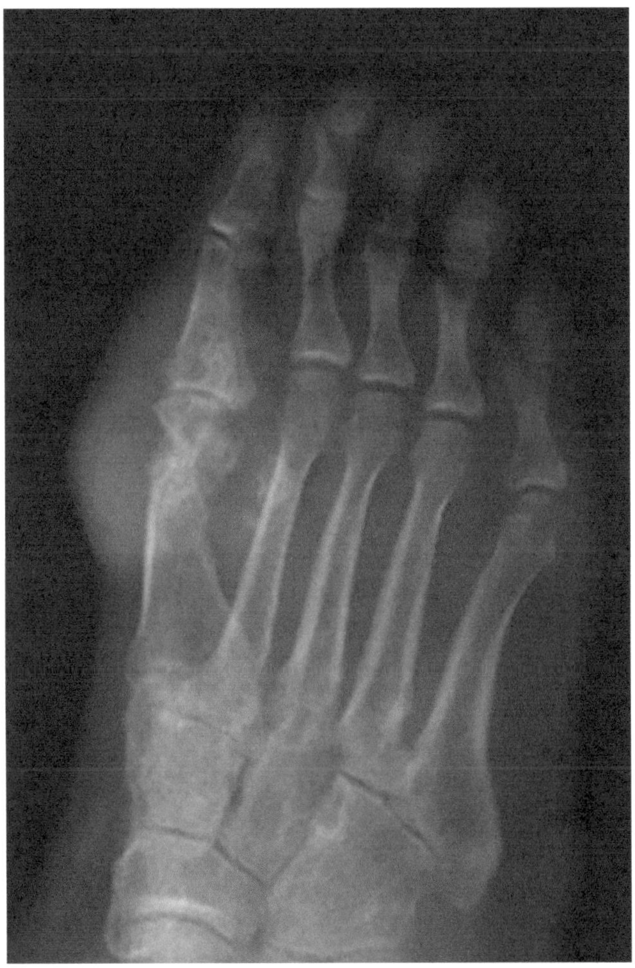

Fig. 9.38 Soft tissue swelling. The plain radiograph shows eccentric swelling of dorsal soft tissue of the first MTP joint, with appearance of mass and high density

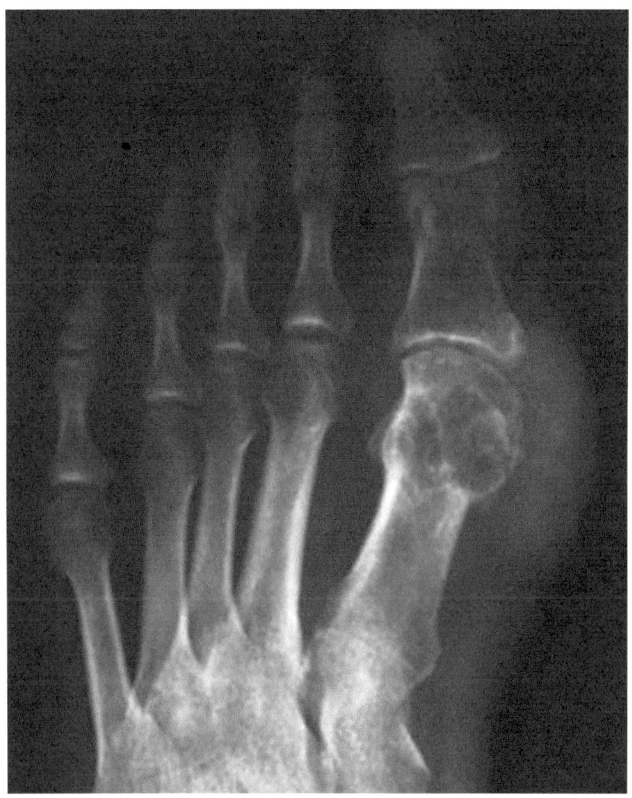

Fig. 9.39 Tophus formation. The X-ray plain film shows formation of slightly high-density fuzzy patchy tophi in medial soft tissue of the first MTP joint

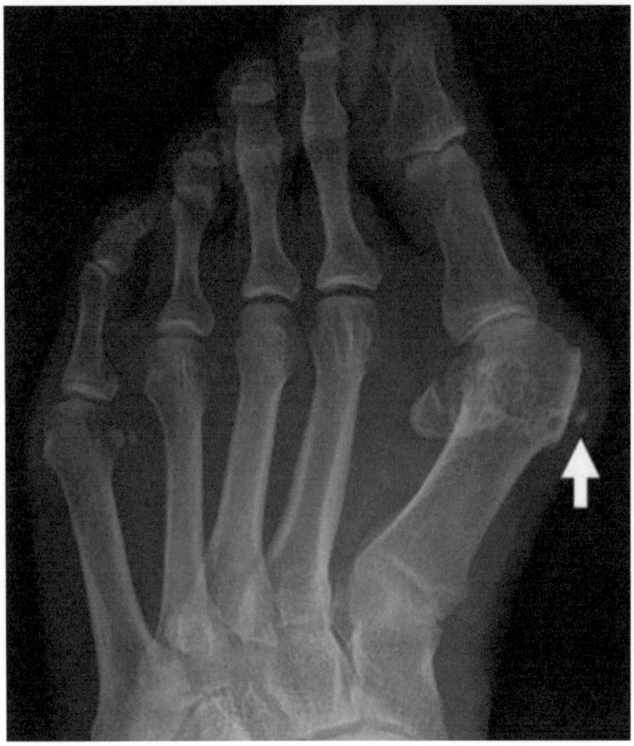

Fig. 9.40 Tophus calcification. The X-ray plain film shows periarticular soft tissue swelling of the first MTP joint and high-density dense calcification in the distal medial soft tissue of the first metatarsus

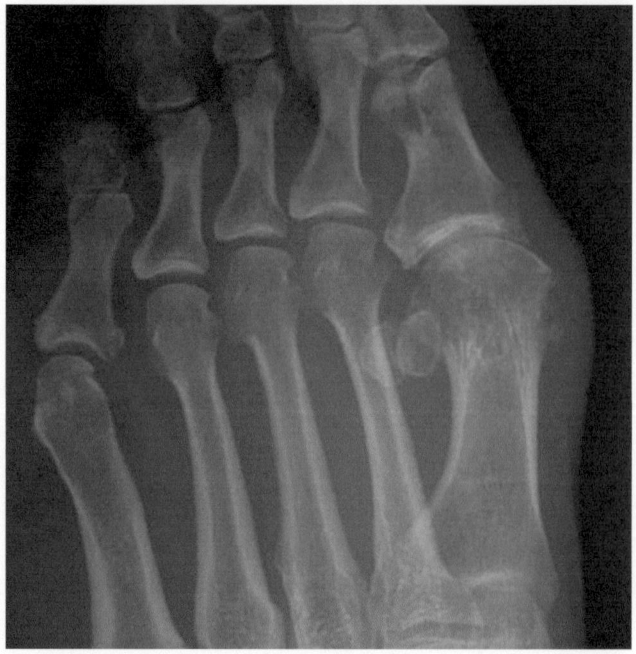

Fig. 9.41 Bone erosion (1). The X-ray plain film shows distal medial subarticular eccentric bone erosion of the first metatarsus, with overhanging edges, protruding in a fish-mouth shape into tophi

destruction has sharp edges with sclerosis straps, presenting "punched out" changes, mostly eccentric. There often are special "overhanging edges" or bone cortex protruding outwards in a fish-mouth shape into intra-articular tophi (Fig. 9.41). In severe cases, multiple bone destruction areas can be fused with each other (Fig. 9.42), presenting honeycomb changes.

(f) Osteoporosis: In the acute stage of gout, due to stimulation of synovial and soft tissue inflammation, localized osteoporosis of the subchondral bone can be seen, manifested as decreased bone mineral density and sparse bone trabecula. These manifestations are not the characteristics of osteoporosis. Osteoporosis is not significant even in the presence of extensive bone erosion. Subchondral osteoporosis can lead to subchondral cysts.

(g) Hyperostosis and bone cortex thickening: Hyperostosis and irregular bone cortex thickening often occur at the edge of bone erosion or bone cortex adjacent to the tophus, which are reactive hyperplasia of bone structure. Irregular spicula or calcification can be found at the tendon and ligament entheses. Gouty arthritis may be secondary to osteoarthritis, presenting as osteophytes and subchondral sclerosis, and common in the first MTP joint, intermetatarsal joint, and knee joint.

2. **CT.** It can determine the scope and extent of gout involvement in joints (Fig. 9.43), but CT examination is rarely performed except for complex anatomical sites. CT can show the deposition of tophi and the CT value is similar to calcification, 160 ~ 170 HU. It is difficult to differentiate between calcified and non-calcified tophi on CT as tophi may be calcified. However, CT scan contributes to distinguishing tophi from other soft tissue masses (xanthomatosis, rheumatoid nodules). The latter has a lower CT value, with soft tissue density.
3. **MRI.** MRI is helpful for comprehensive evaluation of the extent of gout, especially in spine, sacroiliac joint, and other complex anatomical sites. MRI allows the revelation of the involvement of soft tissue, synovial membrane, cartilage, and bone as well as the clear display of bone and cartilage destruction (Fig. 9.44), synovial thickening (Fig. 9.45), and tophi. Typical tophi show mixed signal intensity mainly with hypointense on T_1WI and hypointense on T_2WI (Fig. 9.46), which is related to urate content. The enhanced scan may show homogeneous, heterogeneous, and marginal enhancement and other modes of enhancement.

Key Points of Diagnosis

Gouty arthritis commonly occurs in young and middle-aged men. It often involves feet, hands, wrist, elbow, and knee joints with asymmetrical distribution. The involvement of the first MTP joint is the most common. Typical imaging findings are juxta-articular eccentric lobulated soft tissue mass,

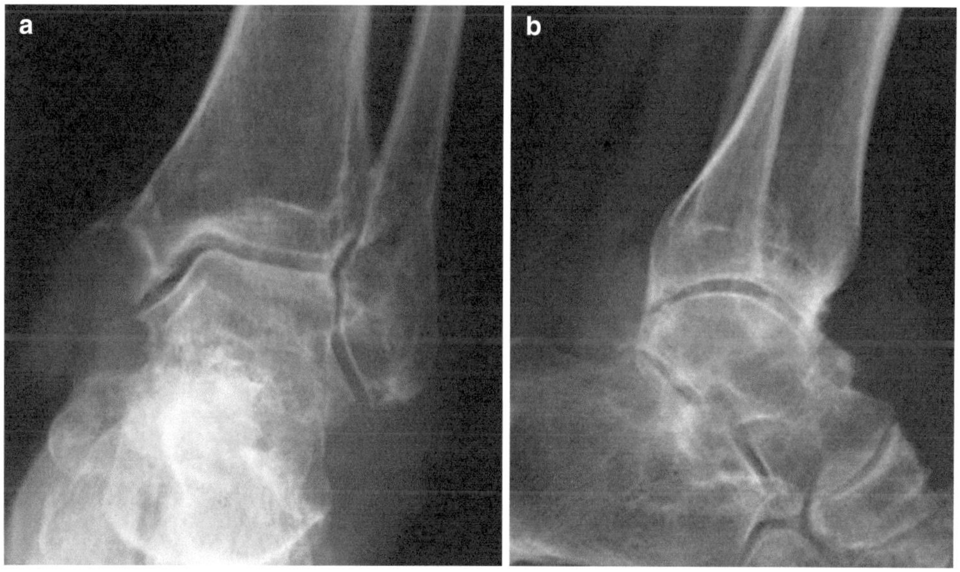

Fig. 9.42 Bone erosion (2). X-ray plain films show decreased bone density in the ankle joints, multiple small cystic low-density shadows with local fusion, eccentric bone erosion and destruction in medial malleoli, periarticular soft tissue swelling with increased density, marked stenosis of ankle joint space, and articular surface sclerosis

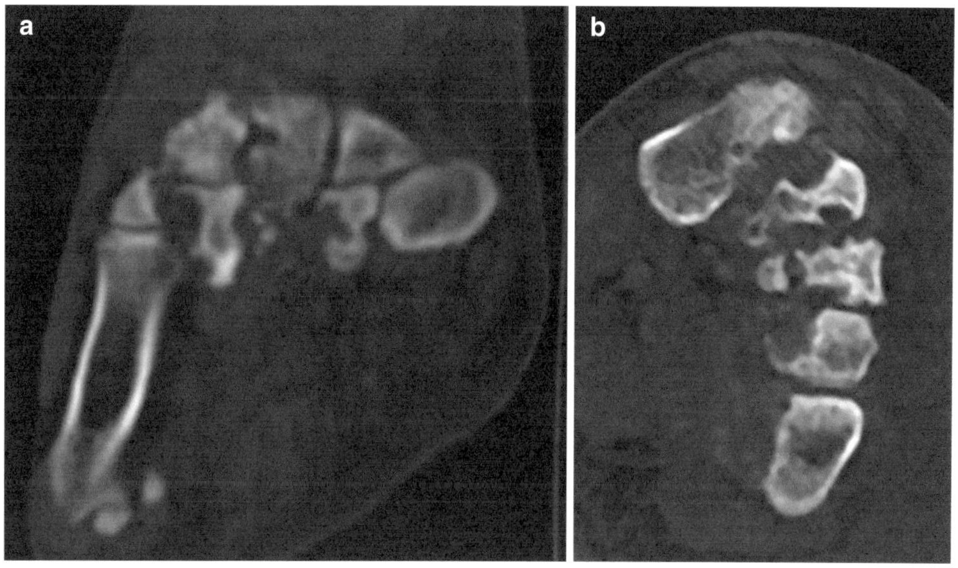

Fig. 9.43 Bone erosion (3). CT shows multiple cystic bone erosion and destruction changes at the edge of metatarsus and tarsus

"punched out" bone destruction at the joint margin, tophi in soft tissue and relatively intact joint space. Such changes mostly occur in the late stage of gouty arthritis. The differentiation of the disease from joint lesion resulting from other causes and pseudogout is required when atypical findings are shown. In 2015, the expert panel of European League Against Rheumatism (EULAR) and American College of Rheumatology (ACR) took the presence of monosodium urate monohydrate (MSU) crystals in bursa or tophus as the gold standard for diagnosis of gout, determined main features of gout through reviewing the literature on imaging findings of gout and using the multi-criteria decision analysis method to reach consensus, and published new classification criteria for gout (Table 9.5). The criteria are more feasible, with the sensitivity of 92% and the specificity of 89% [20].

Differential Diagnosis

1. **Rheumatoid arthritis (RA).** RA often occurs in middle-aged and old women. Its typical imaging findings include symmetrical joint involvement, diffuse soft tissue swelling and local osteoporosis, joint space stenosis in the early stage associated with marginal bone erosion changes. Men have a higher incidence of gout than women. The joint involvement is asymmetrical. On imaging, lobulated eccentric soft tissue masses can be seen and joint space stenosis is rarely found in the early stage, without osteoporosis. Calcification of rheumatoid nodule is occasionally observed, while tophus calcification is more common.
2. **Osteoarthritis.** Osteoarthritis is more common in middle-aged and elderly people of over 40 years old. It

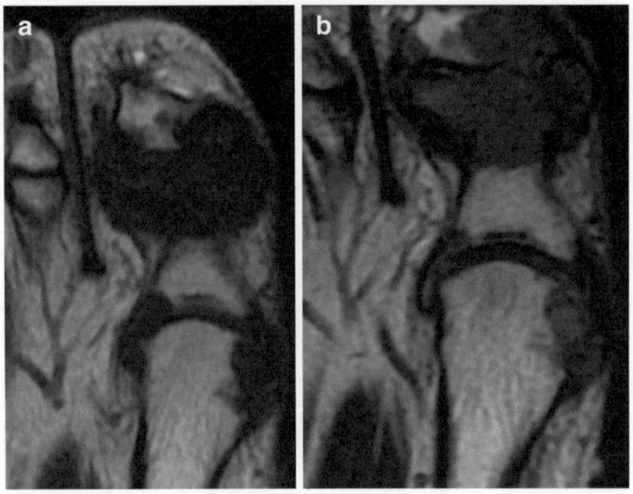

Fig. 9.44 Bone and cartilage destruction. On MRI, T_1WI and T_2WI show isointense multiple masses at the first MTP joint and IP joints, marked erosion and destruction of adjacent bone and articular cartilage

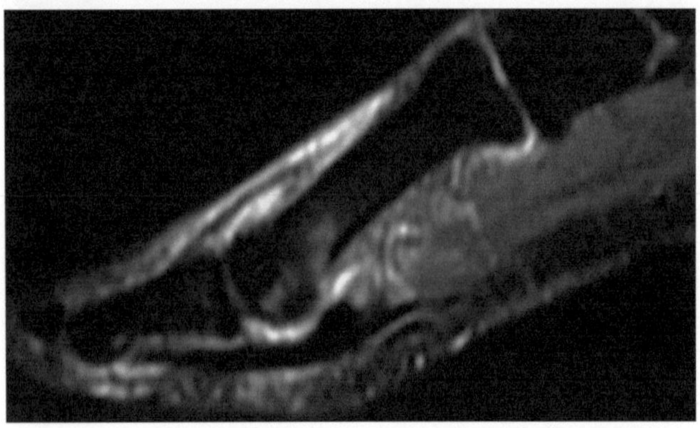

Fig. 9.45 Synovial thickening. On MRI, T_2WI fat-suppressed sequence shows apparent synovial edema and thickening around the first MTP joint, showing diffuse hyperintense changes, and bone marrow edema at the distal end of the first metatarsus

generally involves knee, spine, and other weight-bearing joints, and also small joints of hands and feet. Its imaging findings are heterogeneous stenosis of joint space, and development of labial hyperplasia or osteophyte at the joint margins, occurring in the hands, and possibly developing typical "Heberden" nodule and "Bounchard" nodule. Gouty arthritis may be associated with changes in secondary osteoarthritis, such as osteophyte and subchondral bone sclerosis. These manifestations may cover up characteristics of bone erosion. However, bone erosion in rare sites or atypical abnormalities in imaging characteristics suggest the possibility of gout.

3. **Calcium pyrophosphate dihydrate deposition disease**, also known as pseudogout, is intra-articular deposition of calcium pyrophosphate dihydrate (CPPD). It is common in the elderly. Blood uric acid is also elevated, and its clinical symptoms are the same as gout. Imaging findings are intra-articular and periarticular calcification and degenerative osteoarthrosis, which is extensive and usually symmetrical, as well as involves transparent cartilage and fibrous cartilage. Calcinosis of gout generally is localized and only involves fibrous cartilage. Pseudogout often occurs in wrist, knee, and MCP joints and is associated with osteophyte formation, subchondral bone sclerosis and cystic changes, joint space stenosis and other manifestations of osteoarthritis. If the presence of CPPD crystals is found through synovial fluid puncture, a definite diagnosis of pseudogout can be made. Lobulated soft tissue masses, intact joint space, and bone erosion of typical gout can be used for clear differentiation.
4. Xanthomatosis is a hereditary disorder of lipid metabolism. It is commonly found on extensor tendon surfaces of hands and feet and patellar tendons and Achilles tendons. Its imaging findings are eccentric nodular soft tissue masses, and flabellate bone erosion similar to tophus, which is less common than gout. In addition, hypercholesterolemia is an important laboratory anomaly in xanthomatosis.

Status Quo and Progress of Research

1. **Dual-energy computed tomography (DECT).** DECT is an imaging method based on the principle of different X-ray absorption characteristics of a material's atomic number at different energy levels. High atomic number materials (such as calcium) have a greater difference in attenuation than low atomic number materials (such as urate) when exposed to X-rays of two different energy levels. By scanning tissue with X-ray beams at 80 kV and 140 kV, a post-processing algorithm can be applied to directly convert attenuation differences into different CT values and thus differentiate urate from calcium salts. Therefore, urate (green) and calcium salts (red) can be identified accurately and specifically on DECT images. DECT can accurately analyze the size, quantity, distribution, and shape of urate crystal through the post-processing software. The results of a recent meta-study [21] showed that the sensitivity and specificity of DECT for the diagnosis of gout were 84%. Meanwhile, DECT is also included in 2015 ACR/EULAR classification criteria for gout. When artifacts are removed and green urate crystals are formed, the score increases by 4 points. It can be seen that DECT gets more and more attention in the diagnosis of gout. However, DECT has a low sensitivity to the diagnosis of early gout. The cause for false-positive results may be that urate deposition takes time to accumulate. The detection rate of tiny urate crystals (<2 mm) is limited due to the partial volume effect of CT [22].

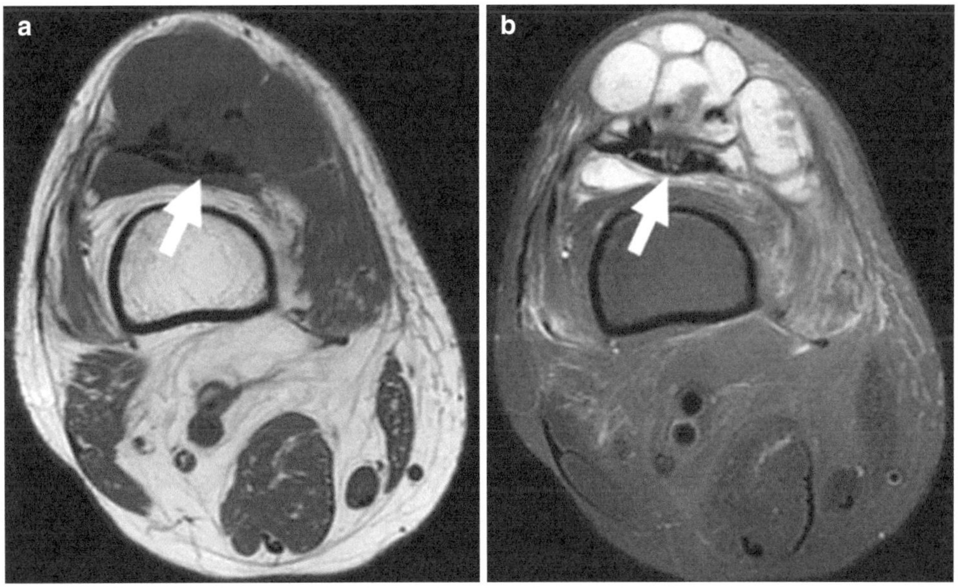

Fig. 9.46 Tophus. MRI shows soft tissue swelling at the anterior femur and isointense diffuse mass on T_1WI inside which hypointense multiple clumpy tophus formation can be seen (white arrows)

2. **MRI** has superior soft tissue resolution and can noninvasively display synovial inflammation, cartilage injury, bone erosion, bone marrow edema, etc. MRI plays an irreplaceable role in rheumatic diseases. A tophus has variable signal intensities and morphological characteristics on MRI images, demonstrating heterogeneity of its components and changes in calcium deposits. Compared with DECT, MRI has a sensitivity of 63% and a specificity of 98% for detecting tophi [23]. The diagnostic efficacy of MRI for gout remains uncertain for lack of data and specific findings, so MRI results were not included in ACR/EULAR classification criteria for gout. Nevertheless, MRI has a great potential in the monitoring of disease activity and progression due to its sensitivity to the diagnosis of non specific inflammation and bone erosion and ability to evaluate affected joints [24].
3. **Radionuclide imaging.** Functional imaging and radionuclide studies have little application data on gout. On PET/CT, uptake of fluorodeoxyglucose (FDG) in tophi and adjacent joints and soft tissue increases [25]. Bone scanning shows increased osteoblastic activity at the site of bone erosion. But these results are non-specific. In a few cases, PET/CT may provide significant diagnostic images when tophi develop to a rare site such as spine.

9.4 Idiopathic Inflammatory Myopathy

Yuan Qu and He Sun

Overview

Idiopathic inflammatory myopathy (IIM) is a heterogeneous group of systemic autoimmune rheumatic diseases characterized by diffuse and non-purulent inflammation of the striated muscles. It is characterized by proximal symmetrical myasthenia and often involves other organs at the same time. Clinical categories mainly include dermatomyositis (DM), polymyositis (PM), and inclusion body myositis (IBM). PM and DM are the commonest ones, where PM usually involves skeletal muscle and skin, while DM involves skeletal muscle only. In the nineteenth century, it has been recognized that such category mainly involves extensive muscular diseases in the trunk and proximal parts of the limbs, with or without inflammatory change of skin. In 1903, Steiner classified inflammatory myopathy as idiopathic polymyositis and myositis arising from bacteria or parasite. Since then, some scholars gradually reported cases of DM in adults and children. Since the 1940s, it has been recognized that the occurrence of PM might be not accompanied by skin lesions and systemic symptoms. Since then, many scholars were devoted to the classification of such disease. But the results have always been controversial due to non-specificity and great variation of clinical symptoms and laboratory tests. In 1975, classification schemes and diagnosis criteria [26] for myositis were first proposed by Bohan and Peter and are still used today, including (1) proximal symmetric myasthenia that persists for weeks to months; (2) increase of serum enzyme or urinary creatinine secretion; (3) abnormal electromyogram (EMG); (4) muscle biopsy conforming to myositis characteristics; (5) characteristic inflammatory change of skin.

The incidence of IIM varies depending on race, age, and gender and is lack of data from large-scale epidemiological studies. As reported by some study data, the annual incidence is (5 ~ 10)/million. PM is common in adults, with the highest incidence between 20 ~ 50 years old; DM shows 2 peaks, 5 ~ 15 years old and 45 ~ 65 years old; while IBM is

Table 9.5 ACR/EULAR classification criteria for gout (2015)

Entry criterion (only apply criteria below to those meeting this entry criterion): At least 1 episode of swelling, pain, or tenderness in a peripheral joint or bursa Sufficient criterion (gold standard, no diagnostic classification required): The polarization microscopy confirms the presence of MSU crystals in a (ever) symptomatic joint or bursa or tophus Classification criterion (to be used if entry criterion met but sufficient criterion not met): A cumulative score of ≥8 can lead to a definite diagnosis of gout	
Clinical characteristic	**Scores**
Pattern of joint involvement: Joint(s) or bursa(e) that had an acute episode (monoarthritis/oligoarthritis)[a]	
Involvement of ankle joints or feet (rather than the first MTP joint)	1
Involvement of the first MTP joint	2
Symptoms of an affected joint in an acute episode: (1) skin redness (patient-reported or physician-observed); (2) tenderness; (3) movement disorder	
One characteristic met	1
Two characteristics met	2
Three characteristics met	3
Typically acute episode: (1) Time to maximal pain <24 h; (2) Resolution of symptoms in ≤14 days; (3) Complete resolution between symptomatic episodes Presence of ≥2 of the above, irrespective of anti-inflammatory treatment	
First episode	1
Recurrent episodes	2
Evidence of tophus: Grayish-white subcutaneous nodule, thin surface skin, sufficient blood supply; Typical sites: joints, auricle, olecranon bursae, fingers, tendons (Achilles tendon)	
Presence of tophus	0
Absence of tophus	4
Laboratory test	
Blood uric acid level: Test when the patient was not receiving UA-lowering treatment and it was >4 weeks from the start of an episode; retest if practicable. Score is calculated based on the highest value	
<4 mg/dl (<240 μmol/L)	−4
4 ~ <6 mg/dl (240 ~ <360 μmol/L)	0
6 ~ <8 mg/dl (360 ~ <480 μmol/L)	2
8 ~ <10 mg/dl (480 ~ <600 μmol/L)	3
≥10 mg/dl (≥600 μmol/L)	4
Synovial fluid analysis: Puncture and polarization microscopy of the symptomatic joint or bursa by an experienced physician	
Not done	0
MSU crystal negative	−2
Imaging characteristic	
Imaging evidence of MSU crystals in a symptomatic (ever) joint or bursa: Joint ultrasonography showing "double-contour sign"[b] or dual energy CT demonstrating MSU crystal deposition[c]	
None (two modalities) or not done	0
Present (either modality)	4
Imaging evidence of gout-related joint destruction: Radiography of the hands and/or feet demonstrates bone erosion in at least one location (cortex destruction, edge sclerosis or edge protrusion)[d]	
None or not done	0
Present	4

[a]Acute episode: Swelling, pain, and/or tenderness occur in a peripheral joint or bursa

[b]Double-contour sign: Irregular hyperechoes occur on transparent cartilage surface, unrelated to the angle of the ultrasonic probe. The double-contour sign that disappears with a change in the angle of the ultrasonic probe is false-positive double-contour sign

[c]MSU crystal deposition with dual energy CT: Scan is performed at 80 kV and 140 kV and specific software is used for material decomposition algorithm, and articular or periarticular MSU crystals are marked with green pseudo color. Nail bed, submillimeter, skin, motion, beam hardening, and vascular artifacts should be differentiated from MSU deposition

[d]The distal IP joints and "gull-wing" sign should be excluded from bone erosion

common in people with an age over 50, it is rare in young people. Women suffering from PM and DM are more common than men, with a female-male ratio greater than 2:1. However, for IBM, the male-female ratio, by contrast, is greater than 2:1. IIM may be combined with other autoimmune connective tissue diseases, such as scleroderma, systemic lupus erythematosus (SLE), rheumatoid arthritis (RA), sicca syndrome, and nodule disease. Studies have confirmed that malignant tumor is associated with IIM, with the highest incidence in DM-combined malignant tumor [27].

The causes and pathogenesis of IIM are not yet clear and may be related to immunoreaction mediated by several factors including heredity, immunity, infection, tumor, and environment. Data from genome-wide association studies (GWAS) about IIM show that IIM is associated with several genes and is genetically heterogeneous. The human leukocyte antigen (HLA) (HLA) allele is the primary genetic risk factor, which is dominated by HLA-DRB1*0301 and its linkage allele DQAl*0501 [28]. Numerous studies have shown that cell-mediated immune mechanisms can cause muscle damage by affecting muscles and adjacent blood vessels. Among patients with DM and PM, 23% of them have been detected antinuclear antibodies (anti-Jo-1) in the blood, accompanied by multiple human leukocyte antigens. Infection may also be the cause of the disease, and multiple viruses are indirectly related to myositis. Although the presence of these viruses has not been confirmed in the muscle biopsy by the polymerase chain reaction (PCR) technology, viroid inclusion bodies have been detected in the skin cells of the patients and relevant evidence has been provided by retroviruses. Correlation between DM and tumor has confirmed that a tumor may promote the development of inflammatory myopathy. The mechanism may be that the tumor activates cross-sensitization of the muscle components, or the combination with muscle components forms a compound allergen.

These three subtypes, DM, PM, and IBM, can all occur independently or exist with other rheumatic diseases and connective tissue diseases, forming an overlap syndrome. DM and PM are characterized by symmetric proximal myasthenia on both sides, especially the muscles of the neck, pelvis, and proximal limbs, mostly difficulties in repetitive actions, such as looking, going upstairs, sitting up, and rising arms. While IBM is characterized by distal limb asymmetric myasthenia and amyotrophy. 20–60% of patients may suffer from joint pain and arthritis, and symmetric arthritis in facet joints of hands and feet is the most common, mostly non-erosive arthritis, but sometimes, they can be aggressive and destructive. 40–60% of patients may suffer from typical or atypical rash. Typical skin symptoms in DM include Gottron sign (reddish scaly rash on joints and extensor surfaces) and purplish rash around the orbit and at the inner canthus, often accompanied by edema around the orbit and upper eyelid capillarectasia (heliotrope rash), generally occurring before muscle symptoms. A purplish rash may also appear in the anterior upper chest (V zone) and posterior upper shoulder back (shawl sign). Some patients show characteristic rash only, without muscle damage, which is called amyopathic dermatomyositis (ADM). Visceral organ damage includes heart disease (arrhythmia and pericarditis), lung disease (pneumonia and interstitial fibrosis), gastrointestinal tract disease (dysphagia, stomachache and constipation), nephropathy, and nervous system disease. It is known that there is a correlation between DM and tumor, especially for elderly patients. The most common tumors include ovarian cancer, breast cancer, melanoma, and rectal cancer.

The most sensitive indicator for a laboratory test is serum creatine kinase (CK). It is significantly increased during the active period and, with the highest value existing in PM patients, and showing normal or slightly increased in DM/IBM patients. CK is a sensitive indicator to evaluate the degree of muscle cell damage, generally indicating the active stage of inflammation. Anti-Jo-1 antibody in the immunologic test is characterized by high specificity and low sensitivity. The antinuclear antibodies are positive for 60–70% of patients. The electromyogram (EMG) test shows myopathic damage. Muscle biopsy shows damaged and necrotic muscle cells and inflammatory cell infiltration.

Pathophysiology

In visual examination, the affected muscle of IIM is often in light red or light yellow, soft and fragile in palpation, or hard and elastic. Percutaneous muscle biopsy may show microscopic changes of affected muscles under the microscope, mainly including extensive or local muscle fiber degeneration, muscle necrosis and chronic inflammatory cell infiltration, muscle cell regeneration, late fibrosis and atrophy. Inflammatory cell infiltration is a characteristic change, which is dominated by lymphocyte and plasma cell (PC), and macrophage, eosinophilic granulocyte, basophilic granulocyte, and neutrophil granulocyte may also exist [4]. PM infiltrating cells are clustered in the endomysium area around the muscle fibers, while DM infiltrating cells are clustered in the epimysium area around the infiltrating fascicle and small vessels. Atrophy is common around the fascicle, while necrotizing vasculitis is rare. Eosinophilic inclusion bodies are visible in IBM myonuclei and sarcoplasm.

Imaging Findings

The imaging findings of DM and PM are mainly abnormal soft tissue and abnormal joints. The former is more common, mainly involving edema and calcification of muscle, fascia, fat, and subcutaneous tissue. Joint damage is less common. Joint deformity is generally caused by soft tissue contracture and muscle imbalance.

1. **Calcification of soft tissue.** This is the characteristic imaging finding of DM and PM, which is highly common in children, commonly found in subcutaneous tissue, intermuscular fascia, aponeurosis, and adipose tissue, featuring wide distribution, various calcification size, and clear boundary. It may appear as strip, mass, or line (Figs. 9.47 and 9.48). Subcutaneous calcification is the most common. Its morphology and distribution are similar to scleroderma, mainly manifested as linear calcium deposits around knee joints, elbow joints and fingers, intramuscular calcification predispositional to proximal limb muscles, varying sizes of calcification intramuscular fascia, and relatively rare calcification in aponeurosis and fat. The soft tissue, especially calcification in muscular system is proportional to the severity of the disease and may progress over the prolonged duration of disease, or spontaneously fade away and absorb with illness improvement [3].

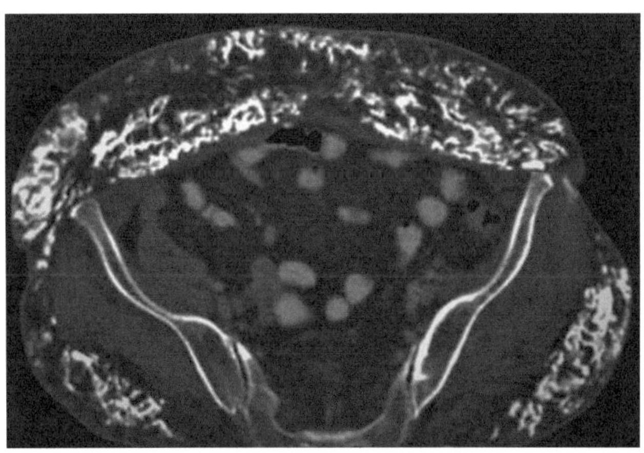

Fig. 9.47 Calcification of soft tissue (1). CT shows a wide distribution of plaque and linear calcification shadows in the subcutaneous soft tissue of hypogastrium, dominated by subcutaneous fat space, which is also visible in anterior abdominal wall muscle

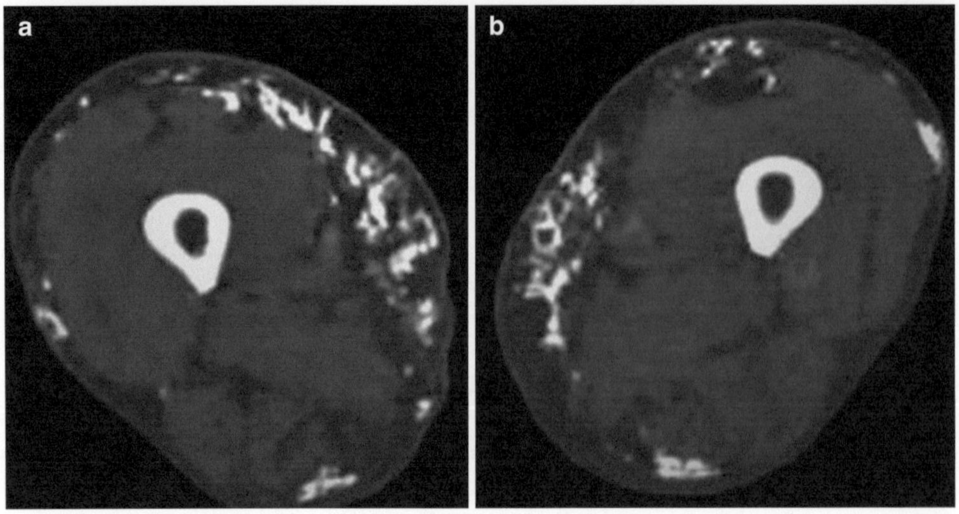

Fig. 9.48 Calcification of soft tissue (2). CT shows scattered speckled calcification shadows in the subcutaneous soft tissue of the thigh

2. **Myositis.** It is manifested as edema of the subcutaneous soft tissue and muscle in the early stage, mainly involving the proximal muscular system, the axilla, the chest wall, the forearm, and the fibular side of the lower extremity X-ray plain film is manifested by increased density of soft tissue, thickening of subcutaneous space, and blurred boundary between subcutaneous tissue and muscle. In the later period, there is obvious fibrosis and amyotrophy, decreased volume of soft tissue and muscle, increased transmittance of soft tissue, and relevant osteoporosis. MRI-based high soft tissue resolution and water sensitivity to water can perform earlier and more precise diagnosis of DM and PM before the affected muscles have not yet shown clinical symptoms. Manifested as diffuse hyperintense on T_1WI and hyperintense on T_2WI, changes in typical hyperintense on T_2WI fat-suppressed sequence and STIR sequence, and significantly higher signal intensity of patients in the active stage than that in the resting stage (Figs. 9.49 and 9.50), the degree of involvement varies with different muscle groups.
3. **Arthrosis changes**. Arthrosis involvement is rare, manifested as osteoporosis around the arthrosis, swelling and calcification of soft tissue, and dominated by metacarpal and interphalangeal joints. Bone erosion is common at the lower ulna, radius, metacarpal and interphalangeal joints, and styloid process of ulna (Fig. 9.51). Joint dislocation is characterized by radial subluxation or dislocation of interphalangeal joints, i.e. "thumb slack sign." In the later period, joint contracture and deformity result from fibrosis of soft tissue.

Key Points of Diagnosis

It is difficult to develop diagnostic criteria and classify to unclear etiology and pathogenesis of IIM, lack of specific diagnosis indicators, and significant variation in clinical symptoms and laboratory test results. In 1975, Bohan and Peter proposed the IIM classification criteria for the first time (B/P criteria). Such criteria are clinically recognized based on five aspects: clinical manifestations, tissue biopsy, serology, electromyogram (EMG), and skin manifestations and are still in use today.

In the following decades, more than 10 IIM classification criteria have been proposed internationally and not been recognized by the academic community. The diagnostic sensitivity fluctuates greatly (49% ~ 100%) since most cases lack muscle biopsy results. However, clear definition of the criteria and differential diagnosis remain ambiguous. In 2017, the European League Against Rheumatism (EULAR) and American College of Rheumatology (ACR) proposed the classification criteria of adult and child IIM and its main subtypes [29] (Table 9.6). With the methods of scoring and weighting, such criteria improved the sensitivity and specificity of disease diagnosis and the accuracy of classification. In the absence of muscle biopsy, the diagnostic sensitivity and specificity of the new criteria are 87% and 82%, respectively. In the presence of muscle biopsy, the sensitivity and specificity reach 93% and 88%, respectively, and the sensitivity and specificity of correct classification are 86% and 91%, respectively. Imaging is not a routine test for diagnosing IIM and is not incorporated in the new criteria but can provide more information or guide muscle biopsy for clinics. With the rapid development of MR function and quantitative imaging, it should play an important role in evaluating disease activity and monitoring therapeutic effect and differential diagnosis.

Differential Diagnosis

1. **Calcification of soft tissue.** It is the common feature of several collagen vascular diseases, especially DM, PM, and scleroderma. In addition, similar imaging findings can also be found in systemic lupus erythematosus (SLE)

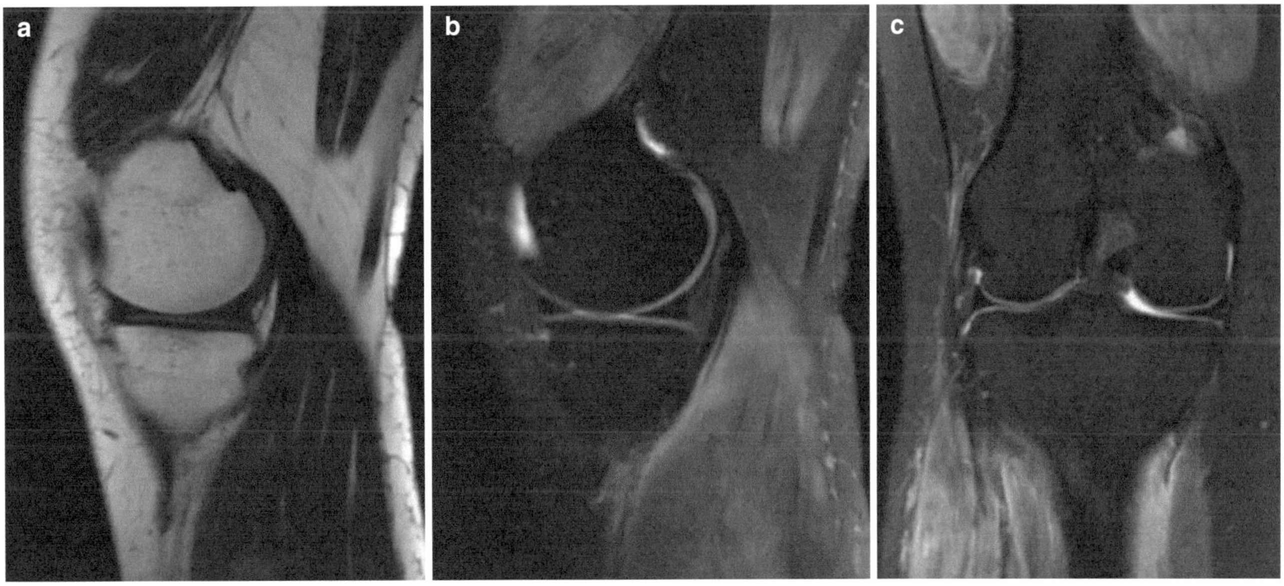

Fig. 9.49 Myositis (1). (**a**) MRI shows slightly hyperintense on T_1WI of muscle around the knee joint; (**b**, **c**) T_2WI fat-suppressed sequence shows significantly increased signal intensity of all muscles

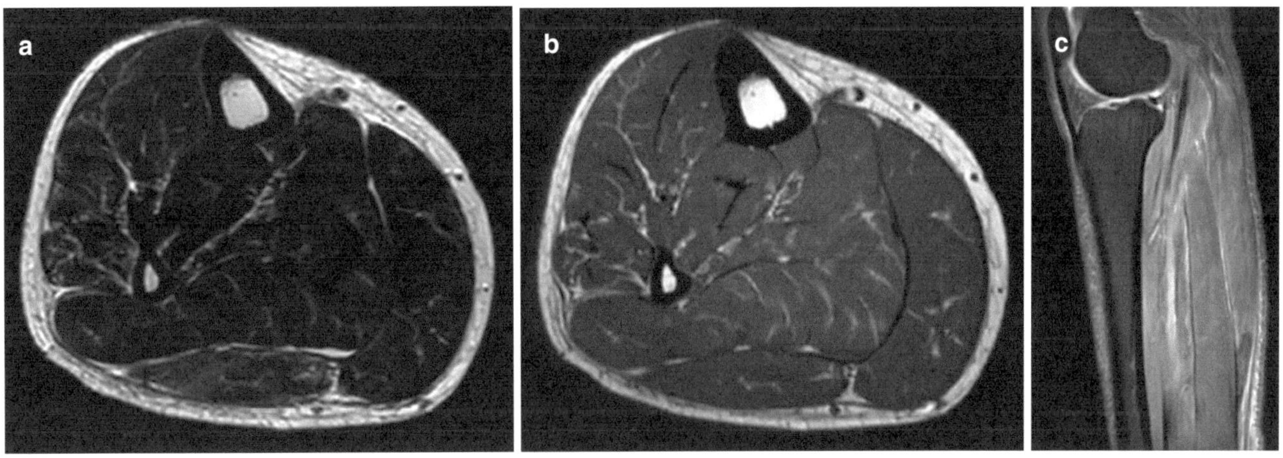

Fig. 9.50 Myositis (2). (**a**, **b**) MRI shows changes in slightly hyperintense on T_1WI and slightly hyperintense on T_2WI of deep layer and shallow layer muscle of leg; (**c**) Fat-suppressed sequence shows increased signal diffusion of the above muscles and increased adjacent subcutaneous fat space signal

and overlap syndrome. In DM and PM, calcification may occur in the intermuscular fascia and is more common and characteristic than other collagen vascular diseases. If calcification of soft tissue is gathered in lines or beams, it is helpful for the diagnosis of inflammatory diseases. Point or line-like calcification around joints can be distinguished from calcification of tumors associated with hyperparathyroidism and hypervitaminosis D.

2. **Myositis.** The imaging findings of inflammatory myopathies on MRI lack specificity. Similar extensive or local muscle abnormalities may occur to many diseases, but in most myositis, there is no local mass and it usually can be distinguished from tumors and infections. Therefore, although MRI can evaluate the degree, scope, and activity of IIM myopathies, it is still necessary to distinguish clinical history and symptoms from myopathies resulting from factors including trauma, infarction, infection, rhabdomyolysis, and denervation.
3. **Arthrosis change.** Articular bone erosion and deformity arthritis caused by DM and PM are not specific and need to be distinguished from abnormal joints associated with other diseases, such as systemic lupus erythematosus (SLE), scleroderma, rheumatoid arthritis (RA), gout, and psoriatic arthritis (PsA).

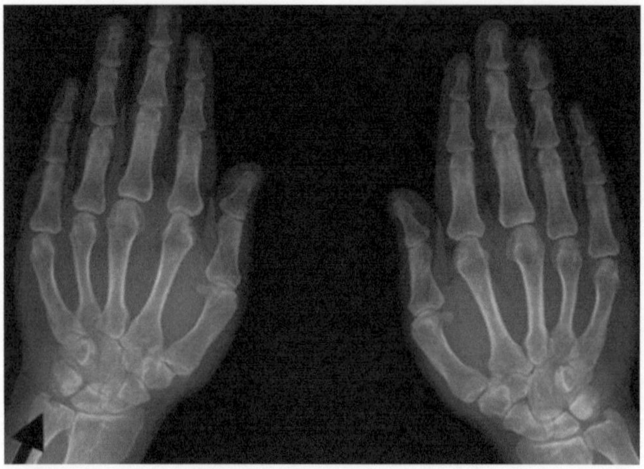

Fig. 9.51 Arthrosis change. X-ray plain film shows osteoporosis of both hands and wrists, swelling of soft tissue, and visible bone erosion (black arrow) in the styloid process of ulna

Status Quo and Progress of Research

1. **MRS.** Phosphorus magnetic resonance spectroscopy (^{31}P-MRS) is a technique to quantify muscle energy metabolism by measuring pH and high-energy phosphate metabolite [such as phosphocreatine (PCr), triphosadenine (ATP) and inorganic phosphate (Pi)]. To measure the phosphate metabolite before, during, and after exercise, metabolic information on oxidative phosphorylation in mitochondria can be provided and has been used to evaluate mitochondrial dysfunction and pathophysiology changes in IIM. The study of Cea et al. [30] has shown that, after exercise, both DM and PM patients have impaired oxidative metabolism indicators, the recovery time of PCr and adenosine diphosphate is 2 times that of the normal control group, the maximum production rate of mitochondria ATP is half of that of the control group, and the proton discharge rate of muscle fiber is significantly lowered. All these changes may be contributed to microangiopathy and perfusion disorder of the affected muscles. Since studies evaluating IBM using MRS are limited, some studies have shown that [31] IBM patients have abnormal resting metabolic rate and normal recovery parameters, indicating that the mitochondrial oxidation capacity of IBM patients is not impaired. In conclusion, MRS is a functional imaging technique for noninvasive evaluation of muscle energy metabolism, providing valuable information for studying the pathogenic mechanism of IIM and the therapeutic responses of different subtypes.
2. **DWI.** ADC values are calculated to reflect the Brownian motion of water molecule in the tissue. The pathologic changes of inflammatory myopathy include degradation and regeneration of muscle fiber, muscle necrosis, inflammatory cell infiltration, and fibroplasia, which may affect the diffusion of water molecule in the muscle. The increased diffusion of water molecule in the edema muscle reflects the activity of disease. By modeling, ADC values can be further divided into diffusion in muscle and perfusion (false diffusion) in capillary bed, separate muscle from vascular structure, and perform function evaluation, which is of great significance to study IIM. The study of Qi et al. [32] has shown increased muscle and capillary perfusion in normal people after exercise, reflecting an increase in water content. However, for the DM and PM patients in resting state, the affected edema muscle is manifested as increased diffusion performance and increased capillary perfusion, but significantly decreased perfusion volume, contributing to the histopathological discovery of capillary beds decreased in the affected muscle of IIM. In addition, lower ADC values shown by fatty infiltrated muscle may be caused by the decreased water content. Therefore, DWI can improve the sensitivity to the detection of affected muscle of inflammatory myopathy and can be used to guide a muscle biopsy, especially to superimpose the whole MRI technology. It will play an important role in the examination of IIM muscle edema.
3. **Magnetic resonance elastography (MRE).** This is a noninvasive imaging technique and capable of evaluating the mechanical properties of human tissues through the propagation of shear waves. At present, MRE has been applied in the musculoskeletal system to evaluate the shear modulus (hardness) of muscle. McCullough et al. [33] used MRE to study PM and DM patients and found, compared with healthy control groups, the hardness of the affected muscle in the patient group is significantly decreased, which may be associated with the destruction of structural proteins by myositis. The above changes may result in decreased transmission of force in the muscles and difficulties in maintaining contraction state, further causing the patients' affected muscles to lack endurance. Considering the complexity of muscle structure and function, the study of MRE in muscle disease remains a challenge. It is expected that the future study can improve the evaluation of IIM therapeutic strategy and contribute to distinguishing the myositis types in the early stage.

9.5 Systemic Lupus Erythematosus (SLE)

Jun Zhou and He Sun

Overview

Systemic lupus erythematosus (SLE) is a chronic connective tissue disease and autoimmune disease mediated by multiple

Table 9.6 Classification criteria of idiopathic inflammatory myopathy of ACR/EULAR (2017)

Variable	Score (muscle biopsy or not) No	Yes	Definition
Age of onset			
≥18 years old, but <40 years old	1.3	1.5	Age ≥ 18 years old but <40 years old when first symptoms associated with this disease appear
≥40 years old	2.1	2.2	Age ≥ 40 years old when first symptoms associated with this disease appear
Myasthenia			
Objective existence of symmetric and progressive proximal myasthenia of upper limb	0.7	0.7	Manual muscle testing or other objective examination, proximal myasthenia of both upper limbs, progressing over time
Neck flexor is weaker than neck extensor	1.9	1.6	Manual muscle testing or other objective examination; neck flexor is weaker than neck extensor
The proximal muscles of lower limb are weaker than distal muscles	0.9	1.2	Manual muscle testing or other objective examination; proximal muscles of lower limb are relative weaker than distal muscles
Rash			
Heliotrope rash	3.1	3.2	Purple, mauve, or red macula distributed around the upper eyelid or orbit, often accompanied by edema around the orbit
Gottron rash	2.1	2.7	Red to fuchsia papules on the extensor articular surface, sometimes accompanied by desquamation, distributed in finger, elbow, knee, ankle, and toe joints
Gottron rash	3.3	3.7	Red to fuchsia macula (not papula) on extensor articular surface
Other clinical manifestations			
Dysphagia or dyskinesia of esophagus	0.7	0.6	Objective evidence of dysphagia or abnormal esophageal motility
Laboratory test			
Anti-Jo-1 (anti-histidyl-tRNA synthetase), positive	3.9	3.8	Serological antibody positive detected by standard test and verification test
Increased level of serum creatine kinase (CK) or lactic dehydrogenase (LD) or aspartate aminotransferase (ASAT/AST/SGOT) or alanine aminotransferase (ALAT/ALT/SGPT)	1.3	1.4	The most abnormal detection value (the highest absolute value of enzyme) in the course of the disease is higher than the upper limit of normal value
The following lesions are found in the muscle biopsy			
Endomysial infiltration of mononuclear cells surrounding, but not invading, myofibres, which are distributed around the muscle fibers not do not invade muscle fibers		1.7	The muscle biopsy shows infiltration of mononuclear cells of perimysium, adjacent to other healthy muscle fiber membrane without muscle fiber necrosis, but no obvious muscle fiber involvement
Infiltration of mononuclear cells around the perimysium and/or blood vessel		1.2	Mononuclear cells are located around the perimysium and/or blood vessel (perimysium or endomysium vessel)
Muscular perifascicular atrophy		1.9	Muscle biopsy shows decreased muscle fiber in the muscular perifascicular compared with the muscle fiber near the center
Rimmed vacuoles		3.1	Rimmed vacuoles of HE staining are in blue, while improved Gomori trichrome staining is in red

(1) IIM is confirmed with a diagnostic possibility of 90% if the total score ≥7.5 (no muscle biopsy) or ≥8.7 (muscle biopsy); (2) IIM is suspected with a diagnostic possibility ≥55% and <90% (recommended diagnostic threshold) if the total score ≥5.5 (no muscle biopsy) or ≥6.7 (muscle biopsy); (3) IIM is doubtful with a diagnostic possibility ≥50% and <55% if the total score ≥5.3 (no muscle biopsy) or ≥6.5 (muscle biopsy); (4) The possibility of diagnosis of IIM is <50% if the total score <5.3 (no muscle biopsy) or <6.5 (muscle biopsy); (5) After IIM is diagnosed, classify subtypes according to the age and clinical features

autoantibodies and immune complex and involving multiple organs and viscera throughout the body. It can involve the skin and mucous membrane, musculoskeletal, kidney, heart, blood system, gastrointestinal system, eyes, central nervous system, and other organ systems. Arthrosis involvement is common, and the course of disease is alternating between recurrent attacks and relief. The word lupus dates from the Middle Ages and describes erosive skin lesions similar to the symptoms after being bitten by wolves. In 1864, a Viennese physician, VonHebra, described a rash on the cheeks as a butterfly and proposed the world lupus erythematosus. In 1872, Kaposi first proposed that this disease is a systemic disease. In the following decades, several scientists confirmed this point and further described the clinical and pathological features of SLE. In 1948, Hargraves from Mayo Clinic and his colleagues discovered the lupus erythematosus cell. This is a major breakthrough in the serological diagnosis of SLE, enabling the characteristic immunological changes of the disease emphasized. Since then, people discovered many antinuclear antibodies, established the animal model of lupus, and discovered that major histocompatibility complex, cytokine, genetic factor, autoimmune and acquired immune systems, and cell apoptosis are associated with this disease, making the understanding of SLE increasingly clear, realizing early diagnosis and providing new therapeutic targets.

SLE is predispositional to the women of reproductive age. The onset age of 65 patients is 16 ~ 65 years old; 20% of patients have an onset of illness before 16 years old; 15% of patients have an onset of illness after 55 years old. The female-male ratio is up to 9:1. The prevalence of SLE varies depending on different regions, races, genders, and ages. The incidence is 51/100,000 people in the USA, 70/100,000 people in China, and up to 115/100,000 people for women. With improved diagnostic levels, the incidence of SLE has tripled in the last 40 years.

The etiology of SLE is unclear, usually attributed to a combination of genetic, hormonal, infectious, immunological, and environmental factors [13]. SLE appears in family aggregation. It is a multigenic disease. Human leukocyte antigen (HLA) presented by some susceptible antigens is the most common susceptibility gene. Due to polymorphism, such susceptibility gene leads to decreased immune complex and apoptotic cell clearance, increased reactivity of B lymphocyte and T lymphocyte, imbalance of cytokine secretion, and promotion of immune and inflammatory reaction, further resulting in abnormal autoimmune and acquired immune responses. The effect of hormones and genetic differences on X chromosome and gender epigenetic differences suggests that women are more susceptible to this disease. Stimulation from various environmental factors may influence the onset or severity of SLE. Ultraviolet irradiation may cause a recurrence of the disease, which may be due to the increased apoptosis of skin cells or its antigenicity by changing DNA and intracellular proteins. In addition, many drugs (such as procaine, hydrazine, quinidine, isoniazid, penicillin, sulfanilamide, and cephalosporin) and infections (such as gonococcus and EB virus) can induce or aggravate this disease.

The clinical symptoms and signs of SLE are variable, depending on the distribution and degree of the affected system lesions. Different degrees of musculoskeletal manifestations may occur in 75% ~ 90% of SLE patients. The clinical manifestations are mainly intermittent and symmetrical polyarthritis, usually involving metacarpophalangeal joints, wrist joints, metatarsophalangeal joints, and knee joints, in symmetrical distribution. Its distribution is similar to that of rheumatoid arthritis (RA), characterized by soft tissue swelling, tenderness, morning stiffness around joints. Joint deformity (hands and feet) occurs to 10% of patients only. There are many extra-articular symptoms of SLE, involving organs and systems including the whole-body skin, respiration, nerves, digestion, lymph, urinary, and eyes. Systematic symptoms mainly include weakness, fever, anorexia, and weight loss. The skin symptoms are diverse, including typical butterfly speckles on face, erythema rash on forehead and neck, erythema below fingernail (toenail), and urticaria. The nervous system symptoms include headache, cognitive disorder, epilepsy, hemiplegia, and peripheral neuropathy, involving possible eye bleeding. Lupus nephritis can lead to hypertension, proteinuria, and nephrotic syndrome. The affected respiratory system may suffer from pneumonia, pleurisy, pulmonary fibrosis, and atelectasis. Cardiovascular anomalies may involve pericarditis, cardiomyopathy, and coronary vasculitis [11].

Value of laboratory test for SLE: (1) confirm or exclude diagnosis; (2) track disease changes, especially indicate a recurrence of the disease or the occurrence of related organ involvement; (3) find adverse reactions to treatment. The laboratory test mainly includes the detection of various autoantibodies. Antinuclear antibody (ANA) is the most important autoantibody, and over 95% of SLE patients are ANA positive. High-titer IgG anti-double-stranded-DNA (ds-DNA) antibody is SLE specific, and its level can vary over time. An increase in anti-ds-DNA antibody accompanied by a decrease in complement C3 or C4 level often indicates recurrence of a disease, especially the recurrence of lupus nephritis or vasculitis. Anti-Sm antibody is also a specific antibody for diagnosing SLE, but generally not associated with disease activity and clinical manifestations. Antiphospholipid antibody (aPL) is not the specific antibody of SLE, but one of the classification criteria of SLE and associated with the formation of arteriovenous thrombosis and thrombocytopenia. Anti-Ro antibody is predictive, not diagnostic. It may indicate the increased risk of occurrence of SLE and sicca syndrome. Other laboratory tests such as complete blood count, blood platelet count, and urine analysis can be used as screening checks to discover abnormalities associated with diagnosis or treatment.

Pathophysiology

The main pathological manifestations of the SLE affected joints are necrotizing angiitis, myxoid edema of the stroma in the early stage, followed by fibrin degeneration of connective tissue of medium and small vessel walls, and formation of necrosis and thrombosis in the later stage, resulting in changes in bleeding and local anemia and development of necrotizing vasculitis, thus causing looseness of supporting structures around joints, atrophy of soft tissue, joint contracture and deformity, and ischemic osteonecrosis [4]. Therefore, lesions around SLE joints are more serious than those in the joints. The synovial fluid analysis of joints shows less inflammatory reaction than RA, and lupus cells can be detected in the synovial fluid. The synovial membrane biopsy shows focal fibrinoid necrosis, accompanied by proliferation of synovial cells and infiltration of mononuclear cells around vessels, generally not so serious as RA patients. Pannus and erosion of bone and cartilage are rare.

Imaging Findings

Typical skeletal muscle abnormalities are common in SLE patients, with complex and varied manifestations, including myositis, symmetrical polyarthritis, deformed non-erosive arthritis, subchondral cyst, ischemic osteonecrosis, spontaneous tendon rupture, calcification of soft tissue, sacroiliitis, osteomyelitis, pyogenic arthritis, and other abnormalities [3].

1. **Myositis.** Muscle involvement may occur in 30% ~ 50% of SLE patients, which may be caused by myositis induced by the pulling of adjacent muscles by the affected joints or corticosteroid. About 4% of SLE patients may show imaging myositis, which mostly occurs in the proximal muscles. MRI fat-suppressed sequence shows obvious hyperintense.
2. **Symmetrical polyarthritis.** Joint manifestations may occur in 75% ~ 90% of SLE patients. The most common manifestation is bilateral symmetrical onset, mainly involving facet joints of hands and large joints of knees, wrists, and shoulders. Most of them are non-corrosive arthritis. X-ray abnormalities are manifested as soft tissue swelling around non-specific joints and limited osteoporosis (Fig. 9.52), similar to rheumatoid arthritis (RA). If no concurrent osteonecrosis is found, damage to cartilage and bone is rare and there is usually no narrowing of joint space. Osteolytic changes or cyst are occasionally seen around joints, but it is different from marginal bone erosion of rheumatoid arthritis (RA).
3. **Deformed non-erosive arthritis.** Its incidence is 5% ~ 40% in SLE patients and it may occur in the early stage. Jaccoud arthropathy may have various manifestations. The typical manifestation is symmetrical interphalangeal joint deformity of hand, including PIP joint hyperextension accompanied by "swan-neck" deformity of distal interphalangeal joint flexion, PIP joint flexion accompanied by "boutonniere" deformity of distal interphalangeal joint hyperextension, interphalangeal joint hyperextension of thumb, and ulnar deflection and subluxation of metacarpophalangeal joint. Deformity of feet includes hallux valgus and subluxation of metatarsophalangeal joints. It is not common to see instability of shoulder joints or knee joints and subluxation of atlanto-axial joints. The joint deformity caused by SLE is often not accompanied by joint space stenosis and bone erosion. Different from joint deformity caused by rheumatoid arthritis (RA), it may be associated with looseness of ligament and tendon and muscle imbalance around joints caused by long-term low inflammatory reaction and fibrosis of joints [34]. Occasionally, there are bone defects (hooked erosion) at the radial side of metacarpal bones, which are associated with the changes in joint pressure, rather than non-pannus bone erosion.
4. **Subchondral cyst.** Mainly involve hands, wrists, and feet, especially carpal bones, metacarpal bones, and metatarsal head. Most cystic lesions are subchondral with relatively normal joint structure (Fig. 9.53), in irregular morphology, single or multiple, and may be accompanied by deformed non-erosive arthritis.
5. **Ischemic osteonecrosis.** SLE and osteonecrosis are highly related. The pathogenesis may be related to the use of corticosteroid. The SLE-related osteonecrosis is symmetrically distributed, predispositional to femur, humerus,

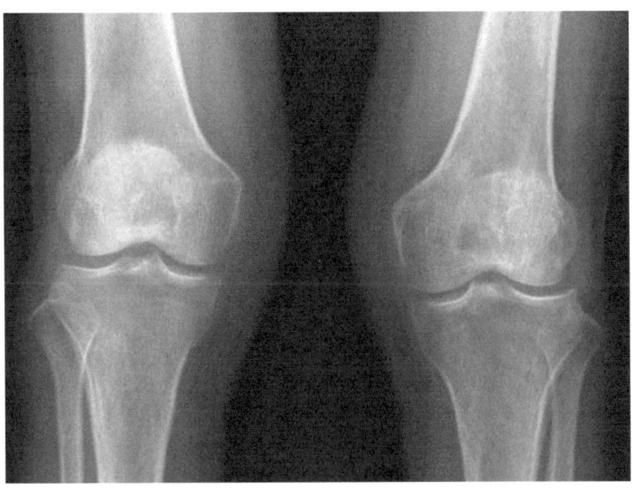

Fig. 9.52 Changes in symmetrical arthritis. X-ray plain film shows osteoporosis around both knee joints, accompanied by obvious swelling of soft tissue around joints

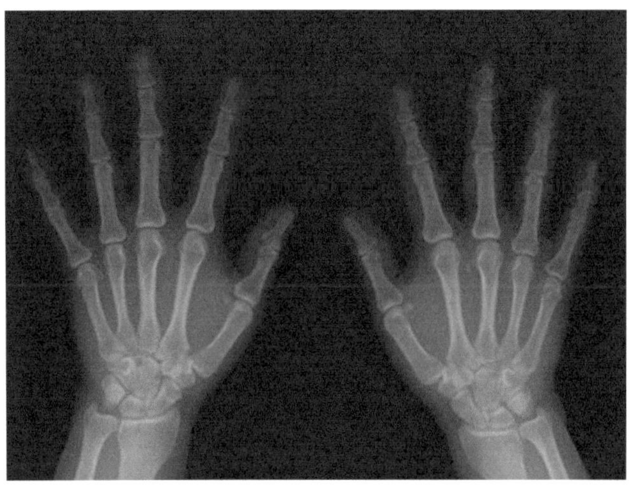

Fig. 9.53 Subchondral cyst. X-ray plain film shows multiple quasi-circular capsule change at the lunate bone and capitate bone of wrist joint and normal joint structure

tibial plateau, huckle-bone, and even hands, wrists, and feet. Its imaging findings are basically consistent with the osteonecrosis not caused by SLE and are difficult to identify. The imaging findings include subchondral cystic change and crescent sign and possible articular surface collapse (Fig. 9.54), narrowing of joint space and bone deformation in the later period, extensive lesion involvement, formation of large patchy patterned bone infarction (Fig. 9.55), and highly sensitive MRI.

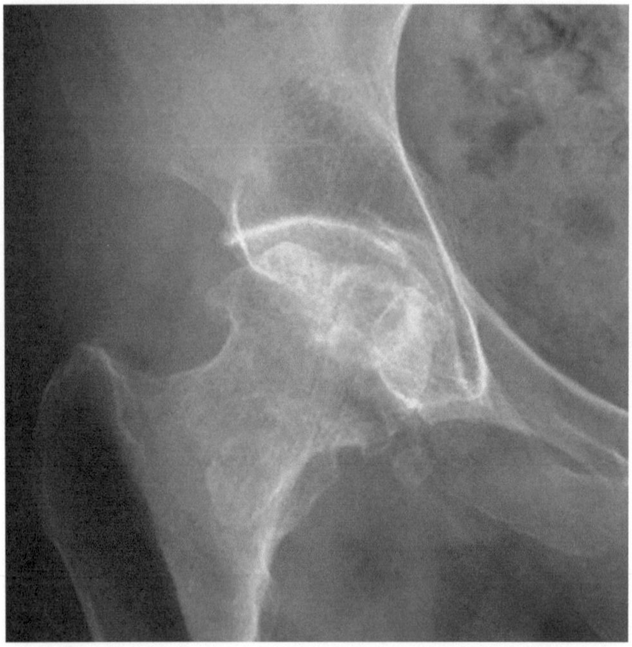

Fig. 9.54 Ischemic osteonecrosis. X-ray plain film shows local collapse of articular surface of right femur, with uneven internal density, cystic ischemic necrosis, and hyperostosis and calcification at the joint edges

6. **Spontaneous tendon rupture.** Almost all spontaneous tendon ruptures in SLE patients are associated with the use of steroid, with possible rupture of one or more tendons, involving many weight-bearing parts, such as Achilles tendon, quadriceps tendon, and patellar tendon. It is also common in biceps tendon and extensor tendon of hand, with various imaging findings.
7. **Calcification of soft tissue.** It occasionally occurs in SLE patients, usually in hips, thighs, and forearms, located under the skin or deep soft tissue, manifested as diffuse linear, striated or nodular calcification, plaque calcification, calcification around joints and arterial calcification (Figs. 9.56 and 9.57).
8. **Sacroiliitis.** It is rare and its X-ray plain film is manifested as joint space stenosis, subarticular bone destruction, and unilaterally or bilaterally distributed reactive osteosclerosis (Fig. 9.58). These changes are similar to osteoarthritis and need to be noted.
9. **Osteomyelitis and pyogenic arthritis.** Bacteria and fungal infection are very common in SLE patients, mainly caused by use of steroid and secondary nephropathy. However, the bone joint infection has a low incidence and may involve several joints, with single joint infection of knee, hip, and ankle joint being the most typical. The main pathogens include Neisseria gonorrhoeae, Neisseria meningitidis, Staphylococcus aureus, Gram-negative bacillus, Mycobacterium tuberculosis, Bacillus typhosus, and Salmonella enteritis.

Fig. 9.55 Bone infarction. (**a**) MRI shows multiple abnormal garland or map signals in distal right femur and proximal tibia, and T_1WI shows slightly hypointense; (**b**) Fat-suppressed sequence shows typical hyperintense changes

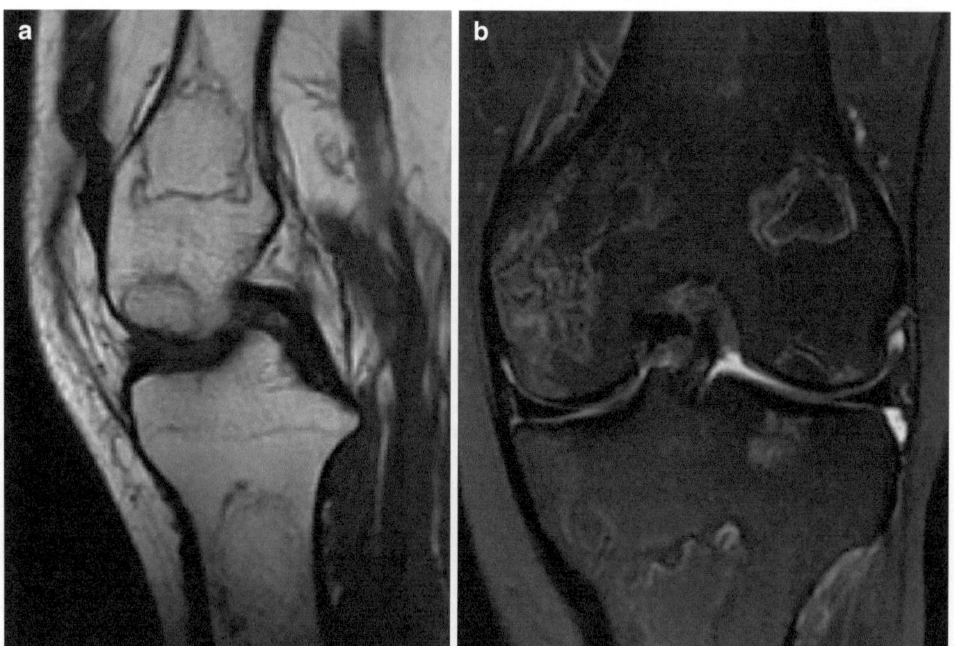

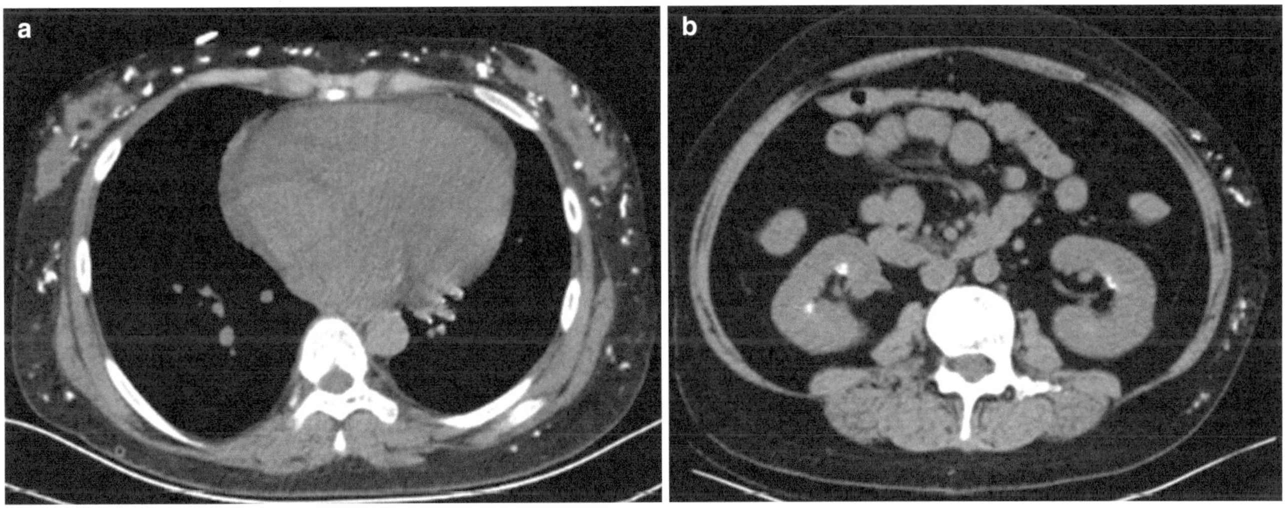

Fig. 9.56 Calcification of soft tissue (1). CT shows scattered high-density calcification shadow in the subcutaneous soft tissue of both chest walls and abdominal wall

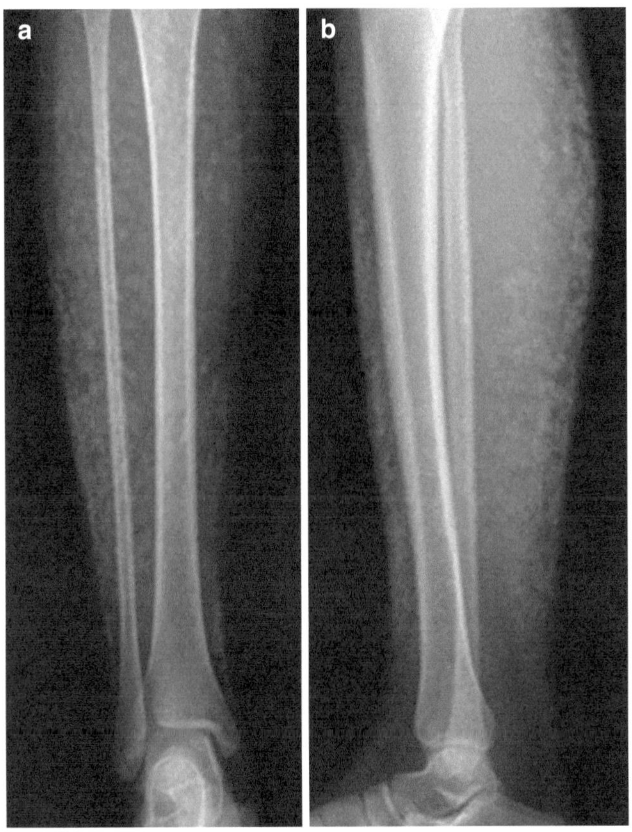

Fig. 9.57 Calcification of soft tissue (2). X-ray plain film shows swelling of subcutaneous soft tissue of right tibia and fibula, blurred subcutaneous fat line, and diffusion high-density nodular calcification shadow in the soft tissue

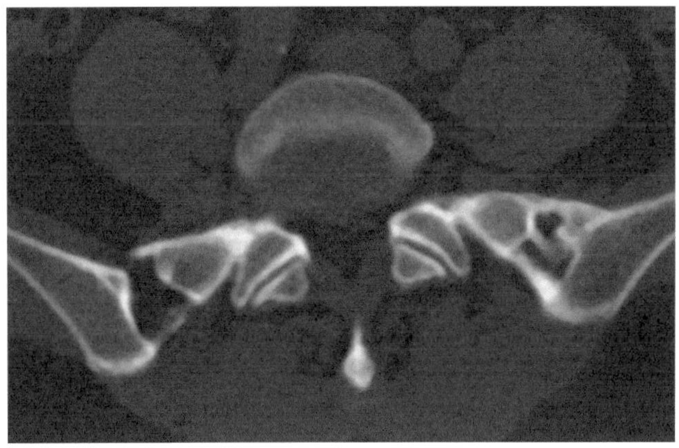

Fig. 9.58 Change in sacroiliac joint. CT shows the development of ossification of sacroiliac ligament on both sides

Key Points of Diagnosis

The diagnosis of SLE is the same as that of other systemic rheumatic diseases, based on the patient's characteristic clinical symptoms, signs, laboratory tests, and imaging and other comprehensive judgment. In 2019, the European League Against Rheumatism (EULAR) and the American College of Rheumatology (ACR) jointly published the latest diagnostic classification criteria for SLE [35] (Table 9.7), which have a higher diagnostic sensitivity (98%) and specificity (96%), providing a new tool that raises ANA positivity to a high diagnostic status and facilitates early clinical diagnosis of SLE. Bone and joint involvement is more generalized, including swelling, effusion, or pressure pain in more than two joints, and morning stiffness, but the weighting score is high. Imaging manifestations of myositis, symmetric polyarthritis, spontaneous tendon rupture, soft tissue calcification, and osteonecrosis are similar or overlapped with rheumatoid arthritis (RA) and other collagen vascular diseases, which need to be further identified.

Differential Diagnosis

1. **Rheumatoid arthritis (RA).** The manifestations of symmetrical polyarthritis of SLE include swelling of soft tis-

Table 9.7 The 2019 EULAR/ACR classification criteria for systemic lupus erythematosus (SLE) (reproduced with permission from [35])

Entry criterion
Antinuclear antibodies (ANA) at a atiter of ≥ 1:80 on HEP-2 cells or an equivalent positive test (ever)
↓
If absent, do not classify as SLE If absent, apply additive criteria
↓
Additive criteria
Do not count a criterion if there is a more likely explanation than SLE. **Occurrence of a criterion on at least one occasion is sufficient.** **SLE classification requires at least one clinical criterion and ≥ 10 points.** **Criteria need not occur simultanceously.** **Within each domain, only the highest weighted criterion is counted toward the total score§.**

Clinical domains and criteria	Weight	Immunology domains and criteria	Weight
Constitutional		***Antiphospholipid antibodies***	
Fever	2	Anti-cardiolipin antibodies OR	
Hematologic		Anti-ß2GP1 antibodies OR	
Leukopenia	3	Lupus anticoagulant	2
Thrombocytopenia	4	***Complement proteins***	
Autoimmune hemolysis	4	Low C3 OR low C4	3
Neuropsychiatric		Low C3 AND low C4	4
Delirium	2	***SLE-specific antibodies***	
Psychosis	3	Anti-dsDNA antibody* OR	
Seizure	5	Anti-Smith antibody	6
Mucocutaneous			
Non-scarring alopecia	2		
Oral ulcers	2		
Subacute cutaneous OR discoid lupus	4		
Acute cutaneous lupus	6		
Serosal			
Pleural or pericardial effusion	5		
Acute pericarditis	6		
Musculoskeletal			
Joint involvement	6		
Renal			
Proteinuria >0.5g/24h	4		
Renal biopsy Class II or V lupus nephritis	8		
Renal biopsy Class III or IV lupus nephritis	10		

Total score:
↓
Classify as Systemic Lupus Erythematosus with a score of 10 or more if entry criterion fulfilled.

sue and osteoporosis. Its X-ray shows no specificity, similar to other diseases dominated by synovitis, such as rheumatoid arthritis (RA). Typical rheumatoid arthritis (RA) often occurs in middle-aged and old women, involving erosive joint diseases in hands and wrists, characterized by joint space stenosis and bone erosion, synovial thickening and development of inflammatory pannus. SLE is a deformed noninvasive arthropathy, featuring ulnar deviation, subluxation, "swan-neck" deformity and "boutonniere" deformity similar to rheumatoid arthritis (RA), but generally not accompanied by obvious joint space stenosis and bone erosion. In few patients, when rheumatoid arthritis (RA) may involve finger deformity without cartilage and bone erosion, and SLE involves development of joint space stenosis, hooked erosion and cyst, their differential diagnosis is more complicated.

2. **Osteoarthritis.** Osteoarthritis is more common in middle-aged and elderly people over 40 years old and generally involves knee, spine and other weight-bearing joints, and even fingers. Joint pain worsens in movement.

There may be joint swelling and effusion, as well as morning stiffness for a short time, less than 30 min. Most of patients with osteoarthritis have a normal erythrocyte sedimentation rate with negative rheumatoid factor (RF). The imaging findings show rare osteoporosis, heterogeneous stenosis of joint space, and development of labial hyperplasia or osteophyte at joint margins, occurring in the hands, and possibly developing typical Heberden nodule and Bounchard nodule. Hyperostosis and osteophyte rarely occur in SLE polyarthritis, without obvious joint space stenosis and bone erosion, but more joint deformities.

3. **Ischemic osteonecrosis.** SLE-related osteonecrosis is basically consistent with the imaging findings of osteonecrosis caused by other diseases. They are hard to identify. But if it occurs in metacarpal bones, metatarsal head, carpal bones, tarsus and other non-osteonecrosis predilection sites, the diagnosis can be confirmed by combining the possibility of SLE suggested with the extra-articular manifestations and damage to multiple organs and viscera.

Status Quo and Progress of Research

1. **DCE-MRI.** Enhanced scan of MRI can definitely distinguish enhanced synovial tissues and non-enhanced joint effusion, with a high sensitivity for diagnosing synovitis. Up to 90% of SLE patients feature the symptoms of bone and muscle involvement, especially inflammatory arthralgia and deformed non-erosive arthritis. CE-MRI can be used to accurately evaluate the affected joint range of SLE patients and determine the degree of bone erosion and bone marrow edema and tendon injury. Early accurate diagnosis is an important treatment strategy to improve the adverse outcome of multiple joint involvement in SLE. It can fully control the inflammatory activity and strictly monitor, relieve, and prevent the progression of tendon and bone injuries [36].
2. **Whole-body magnetic resonance imaging** (WB-MRI). The whole body can be imaged during one scan. The whole-body short time inversion recovery (WB-STIR) is highly sensitive to pathologic changes in soft tissue and bone, and can screen the whole body in an appropriate period, reducing the time and cost for diagnosis and treatment. Ischemic osteonecrosis is a common clinical manifestation in SLE patients, with an incidence of up to 5% ~ 40%, involving femoral head, head of humerus, condyles of femur, tibial plateau, huckle-bone, and even hands, wrists, and feet. WB-STIR can evaluate the involvement range and degree of ischemic osteonecrosis in SLE patients in an early, fast and accurate manner, which is of great clinical significance for screening and prognosis evaluation of high-risk patients [37].
3. **MRS.** It is a quantitative analysis method for specific atomic nuclei and other compounds using magnetic resonance and chemical shift. It is also the only noninvasive technique to observe metabolic and biochemical changes in vivo tissues at present. In the skeletal muscle study, ^{31}P spectrum is the most widely used method. 31P-MRS mainly reflects the energy metabolism level of human tissue cells and confirms the energy state of cell by determining the concentration and distribution of phosphorus metabolite, which is of great significance on studying the energy metabolism changes of skeletal muscle under resting and moving states [38]. Exhaustion syndrome is one of the most common and disabling outcomes for SLE patients. Its pathogenesis is complicated and may be associated with mixing of perimeter and central mechanism. Studies have shown that skeletal muscle dysfunction is related to SLE associated failure. Cheung et al. [39] compared and analyzed the metabolic and structural properties of skeletal muscle of both SLE patients with idiopathic failure and healthy volunteers using multimodal magnetic resonance technology. The results have shown that the half-life recovery time of phosphocreatine (PCr) of skeletal muscle of SLE patients is significantly longer than that of healthy volunteers. PCr half-life recovery time reflects the oxidizing capacity of muscle and is used as a marker of mitochondrial function of muscle. Therefore, the skeletal muscle of SLE patients may suffer from mitochondrial dysfunction, which is associated with exhaustion syndrome.

References

1. Tian X, Zeng X. Harrison's rheumatology. 3rd ed. Beijing: Science Press; 2018.
2. Li Z, Tang F. Kelley's textbook of rheumatology. 8th ed. Beijing: Peking University Medical Press; 2011.
3. Wang X, Chen Z, Ma X, et al. Diagnosis of bone and joint disorders. 4th ed. Tianjin: Tianjin Science & Technology Translation & Publishing Co., Ltd; 2009.
4. Xu J. Rheumatologic imaging. Shanghai: Shanghai Scientific & Technical Publishers; 2007.
5. Baker JF, Conaghan PG, Gandjbakhch F. Update on magnetic resonance imaging and ultrasound in rheumatoid arthritis. Clin Exp Rheumatol. 2018;114(5):16–23.
6. Barile A, Arrigoni F, Bruno F, et al. Computed tomography and MR imaging in rheumatoid arthritis. Radiol Clin N Am. 2017;55(5):997–1007.
7. Aletaha D, Neogi T, Silman AJ, et al. 2010 Rheumatoid arthritis classification criteria: an American College of Rheumatology/European League Against Rheumatism collaborative initiative. Arthritis Rheum. 2010;62(9):2569–81.
8. Øtergaard M, Boesen M. Imaging in rheumatoid arthritis: the role of magnetic resonance imaging and computed tomography. Radiol Med. 2019;124(11):1128–41.
9. Reijnierse M, Helm-Mil AV, Eshed I, et al. Magnetic resonance imaging of rheumatoid arthritis: peripheral joints and spine. Semin Musculoskelet Radiol. 2018;22(2):127–46.

10. Qu J, Lei X, Zhan Y, et al. Assessing synovitis and bone erosion with apparent diffusion coefficient in early stage of rheumatoid arthritis. J Comput Assist Tomogr. 2017;41(5):833–8.
11. Fauci AS. Harrison's rheumatology. 3rd ed. Translated by Tian Xinping et al. Beijing: Science Press; 2018.
12. Siepr J, Rudwaleit M, Baraliakos X, et al. The Assessment of spondyloarthritis international society (ASAS) handbook: a guide to assess spondyloarthritis. Ann Rheum Dis. 2009;68(suppl 2):ii1–44.
13. Firestein GS. Kelley's textbook of rheumatology. 8th ed. Translated by Li Zhanguo et al. Beijing: Peking University Medical Press; 2011.
14. Taylor W, Gladman D, Helliwell P, et al. Classification criteria for psoriatic arthritis development of new criteria from a large international study. Arthritis Rheum. 2006;54(8):2665–73.
15. Kingsley G, Sieper J. Third international workshop on reactive arthritis. 23–26 September 1995, Berlin, Germany. Report and abstracts. Ann Rheum Dis. 1996;55(8):564–84.
16. Shi Z, Han J, Qin J, et al. Clinical application of diffusion-weighted imaging and dynamic contrast-enhanced MRI in assessing the clinical curative effect of early ankylosing spondylitis. Medicine. 2019;98(20):e15227.
17. Bozgeyik Z, Ozgocmen S, Kocakoc E. Role of diffusion- weighted MRI in the detection of early active sacroiliitis. AJR Am J Roentgenol. 2008;191(4):980–6.
18. Ren C, Zhu Q, Yuan H. Mono-exponential and bi-exponential model-based diffusion-weighted MR imaging and IDEAL-IQ sequence for quantitative evaluation of sacroiliitis in patients with ankylosing spondylitis. Clin Rheumatol. 2018;37(11):3069–76.
19. Kelley WN, Wortmann RL. Gout and hyperuricemia. Textbook of rheumatology. 5th ed. Philadelphia: WB Saunders; 1997.
20. Neogi T, Jansen TL, Dalbeth N, et al. 2015 Gout classification criteria: an American College of Rheumatology/European League Against Rheumatism collaborative initiative. Ann Rheum Dis. 2015;74(10):1789–98.
21. Buckens CF, Terra MP, Maas M. Computed tomography and MR imaging in crystalline-induced arthropathies. Radiol Clin N Am. 2017;55(5):1023–34.
22. Teh J, McQueen F, Eshed I, et al. Advanced imaging in the diagnosis of gout and other crystal arthropathies. Semin Musculoskelet Radiol. 2018;22(2):225–36.
23. McQueen FM, Doyle A, Reeves Q, et al. Bone erosions in patients with chronic gouty arthropathy are associated with tophi but not bone oedema or synovitis: new insights from a 3T MRI study. Rheumatology. 2014;53(1):95–103.
24. Davies J, Riede P, van Langevelde K, et al. Recent developments in advanced imaging in gout. Ther Adv Musculoskel Dis. 2019;11:1–12.
25. Wimmer G, Stoecklegger S, Stojakovic T, et al. Evaluation of tophaceous gout by FDG-PET/CT and bone scan. Curr Mol Imaging. 2013;2(2):117–9.
26. Bohan A, Peter JB. Polymyositis and dermatomyositis (first of two parts). N Engl J Med. 1975;292(7):344–7.
27. Fanci AS. Kelley's textbook of rheumatology. 8th ed. Translated by Li Zhanguo et al. Beijing: Peking University Medical Press; 2011.
28. Firestein GS. Harrison's rheumatology. 3rd ed. Translated by Tian Xinping et al. Beijing: Science Press; 2018.
29. Lundberg IE, Tjärnlund A, Bottai M, et al. 2017 European League Against Rheumatism/American College of Rheumatology classification criteria for adult and juvenile idiopathic inflammatory myopathies and their major subgroups. Ann Rheum Dis. 2017;76(12):1955–64.
30. Cea G, Bendahan D, Manners D, et al. Reduced oxidative phosphorylation and proton efflux suggest reduced capillary blood supply in skeletal muscle of patients with dermatomyositis and polymyositis: a quantitative ^{31}P-magnetic resonance spectroscopy and MRI study. Brain. 2002;125(Pt 7):1635–45.
31. Day J, Patel S, Limaye V. The role of magnetic resonance imaging techniques in evaluation and management of the idiopathic inflammatory myopathies. Semin Arthritis Rheum. 2017;46(5):642–9.
32. Qi J, Olsen NJ, Price RR, et al. Diffusion-weighted imaging of inflammatory myopathies: polymyositis and dermatomyositis. J Magn Reson Imaging. 2008;27(1):212–7.
33. McCullough MB, Domire ZJ, Reed AM, et al. Evaluation of muscles affected by myositis using magnetic resonance elastography. Muscle Nerve. 2011;43(4):585–90.
34. Tani C, D'Aniello D, Possemato N, et al. MRI pattern of arthritis in systemic lupus erythematosus: a comparative study with rheumatoid arthritis and healthy subjects. Skelet Radiol. 2015;44(2):261–6.
35. Aringer M, Costenbader K, Daikh D, et al. 2019 European League Against Rheumatism/American College of Rheumatology classification criteria for systemic lupus erythematosus. Arthritis Rheumatol. 2019;71(9):1400–12.
36. Tani C, Carli L, Stagnaro C, et al. Imaging of joints in systemic lupus erythematosus. Clin Exp Rheumatol. 2018;114(5):68–73.
37. Castro TC, Lederman H, Terreri MT, et al. The use of joint-specific and whole-body MRI in osteonecrosis: a study in patients with juvenile systemic lupus erythematosus. Br J Radiol. 2011;84(1003):621–8.
38. Jones DEJ, Hollingsworth KG, Taylor R, et al. Abnormalities in pH handling by peripheral muscle and potential regulation by the autonomic nervous system in chronic fatigue syndrome. J Intern Med. 2010;267(4):394–401.
39. Cheung SM, Keenan K, Senn N, et al. Metabolic and structural skeletal muscle health in systemic lupus erythematosus related fatigue: a multi-modal magnetic resonance imaging study. Arthritis Care Res (Hoboken). 2019. doi:https://doi.org/10.1002/acr.23833.

Correction to: Radiology of Infectious and Inflammatory Diseases - Volume 5

Correction to:
H. Li et al., Radiology of Infectious and Inflammatory Diseases - Volume 5 - Musculoskeletal system, https://doi.org/10.1007/978-981-16-5003-1.

The original version of this chapter was revised by modifying the affiliation of editors in the copy right page and by modifying the affiliation of associate editors and contributors under the section 'Editors and contributors' in the front matter. Their affiliation is also modified accordingly in the chapters they have contributed.

The updated original version for this book can be found at https://doi.org/10.1007/978-981-16-5003-1

H. Li et al. (eds.), *Radiology of Infectious and Inflammatory Diseases - Volume 5*,
https://doi.org/10.1007/978-981-16-5003-1_10